Role of Medical Imaging in Cancers

Role of Medical Imaging in Cancers

Volume 1

Editors

Stefano Fanti
Laura Evangelista

MDPI • Basel • Beijing • Wuhan • Barcelona • Belgrade • Manchester • Tokyo • Cluj • Tianjin

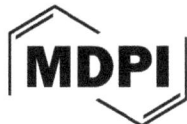

Editors
Stefano Fanti
University of Bologna
Italy

Laura Evangelista
Veneto Institute of Oncology IOV—IRCCS
Italy

Editorial Office
MDPI
St. Alban-Anlage 66
4052 Basel, Switzerland

This is a reprint of articles from the Special Issue published online in the open access journal *Cancers* (ISSN 2072-6694) (available at: https://www.mdpi.com/journal/cancers/special_issues/imaging_cancer).

For citation purposes, cite each article independently as indicated on the article page online and as indicated below:

LastName, A.A.; LastName, B.B.; LastName, C.C. Article Title. *Journal Name* **Year**, *Volume Number*, Page Range.

Volume 1
ISBN 978-3-0365-0180-2 (Hbk)
ISBN 978-3-0365-0181-9 (PDF)

Volume 1-2
ISBN 978-3-0365-0208-3 (Hbk)
ISBN 978-3-0365-0209-0 (PDF)

© 2021 by the authors. Articles in this book are Open Access and distributed under the Creative Commons Attribution (CC BY) license, which allows users to download, copy and build upon published articles, as long as the author and publisher are properly credited, which ensures maximum dissemination and a wider impact of our publications.

The book as a whole is distributed by MDPI under the terms and conditions of the Creative Commons license CC BY-NC-ND.

Contents

About the Editors ix

Preface to "Role of Medical Imaging in Cancers" xi

Laura Evangelista and Stefano Fanti
What Is the Role of Imaging in Cancers?
Reprinted from: *Cancers* **2020**, *12*, 1494, doi:10.3390/cancers12061494 1

Melanie A. Kimm, Maxim Shevtsov, Caroline Werner, Wolfgang Sievert, Wu Zhiyuan, Oliver Schoppe, Bjoern H. Menze, Ernst J. Rummeny, Roland Proksa, Olga Bystrova, Marina Martynova, Gabriele Multhoff and Stefan Stangl
Gold Nanoparticle Mediated Multi-Modal CT Imaging of Hsp70 Membrane-Positive Tumors
Reprinted from: *Cancers* **2020**, *12*, 1331, doi:10.3390/cancers12051331 5

Giulia Polverari, Francesco Ceci, Valentina Bertaglia, Maria Lucia Reale, Osvaldo Rampado, Elena Gallio, Roberto Passera, Virginia Liberini, Paola Scapoli, Vincenzo Arena, Manuela Racca, Andrea Veltri, Silvia Novello and Désirée Deandreis
^{18}F-FDG Pet Parameters and Radiomics Features Analysis in Advanced Nsclc Treated with Immunotherapy as Predictors of Therapy Response and Survival
Reprinted from: *Cancers* **2020**, *12*, 1163, doi:10.3390/cancers1205 23

Anna Myriam Perrone, Giulia Dondi, Manuela Coe, Martina Ferioli, Silvi Telo, Andrea Galuppi, Eugenia De Crescenzo, Marco Tesei, Paolo Castellucci, Cristina Nanni, Stefano Fanti, Alessio G. Morganti and Pierandrea De Iaco
Predictive Role of MRI and ^{18}F FDG PET Response to Concurrent Chemoradiation in T2b Cervical Cancer on Clinical Outcome: A Retrospective Single Center Study
Reprinted from: *Cancers* **2020**, *12*, 659, doi:10.3390/cancers12030659 39

Yan Jin, James W. Randall, Hesham Elhalawani, Karine A. Al Feghali, Andrew M. Elliott, Brian M. Anderson, Lara Lacerda, Benjamin L. Tran, Abdallah S. Mohamed, Kristy K. Brock, Clifton D. Fuller and Caroline Chung
Detection of Glioblastoma Subclinical Recurrence Using Serial Diffusion Tensor Imaging
Reprinted from: *Cancers* **2020**, *12*, 568, doi:10.3390/cancers12030568 53

Rossana Castaldo, Katia Pane, Emanuele Nicolai, Marco Salvatore and Monica Franzese
The Impact of Normalization Approaches to Automatically Detect Radiogenomic Phenotypes Characterizing Breast Cancer Receptors Status
Reprinted from: *Cancers* **2020**, *12*, 518, doi:10.3390/cancers12020518 65

Natalia Samolyk-Kogaczewska, Ewa Sierko, Dorota Dziemianczyk-Pakiela, Klaudia Beata Nowaszewska, Malgorzata Lukasik and Joanna Reszec
Usefulness of Hybrid PET/MRI in Clinical Evaluation of Head and Neck Cancer Patients
Reprinted from: *Cancers* **2020**, *12*, 511, doi:10.3390/cancers12020511 91

Angelo Castello, Francesco Giuseppe Carbone, Sabrina Rossi, Simona Monterisi, Davide Federico, Luca Toschi and Egesta Lopci
Circulating Tumor Cells and Metabolic Parameters in NSCLC Patients Treated with Checkpoint Inhibitors
Reprinted from: *Cancers* **2020**, *12*, 487, doi:10.3390/cancers12020487 107

Manuela Andrea Hoffmann, Hans-Georg Buchholz, Helmut J. Wieler, Matthias Miederer, Florian Rosar, Nicolas Fischer, Jonas Müller-Hübenthal, Ludwin Trampert, Stefanie Pektor and Mathias Schreckenberger
PSA and PSA Kinetics Thresholds for the Presence of ^{68}Ga-PSMA-11 PET/CT-Detectable Lesions in Patients with Biochemical Recurrent Prostate Cancer
Reprinted from: *Cancers* **2020**, *12*, 398, doi:10.3390/cancers12020398 123

Serena Monti, Valentina Brancato, Giuseppe Di Costanzo, Luca Basso, Marta Puglia, Alfonso Ragozzino, Marco Salvatore and Carlo Cavaliere
Multiparametric MRI for Prostate Cancer Detection: New Insights into the Combined Use of a Radiomic Approach with Advanced Acquisition Protocol
Reprinted from: *Cancers* **2020**, *12*, 390, doi:10.3390/cancers12020390 145

Matteo Bauckneht, Selene Capitanio, Maria Isabella Donegani, Elisa Zanardi, Alberto Miceli, Roberto Murialdo, Stefano Raffa, Laura Tomasello, Martina Vitti, Alessia Cavo, Fabio Catalano, Manlio Mencoboni, Marcello Ceppi, Cecilia Marini, Giuseppe Fornarini, Francesco Boccardo, Gianmario Sambuceti and Silvia Morbelli
Role of Baseline and Post-Therapy 18F-FDG PET in the Prognostic Stratification of Metastatic Castration-Resistant Prostate Cancer (mCRPC) Patients Treated with Radium-223
Reprinted from: *Cancers* **2020**, *12*, 31, doi:10.3390/cancers12010031 157

Domenico Albano, Riccardo Laudicella, Paola Ferro, Michela Allocca, Elisabetta Abenavoli, Ambra Buschiazzo, Alessia Castellino, Agostino Chiaravalloti, Annarosa Cuccaro, Lea Cuppari, Rexhep Durmo, Laura Evangelista, Viviana Frantellizzi, Sofya Kovalchuk, Flavia Linguanti, Giulia Santo, Matteo Bauckneht and Salvatore Annunziata
The Role of 18F-FDG PET/CT in Staging and Prognostication of Mantle Cell Lymphoma: An Italian Multicentric Study
Reprinted from: *Cancers* **2019**, *11*, 1831, doi:10.3390/cancers11121831 171

Stefano Fanti, Wim Oyen and Elisabetta Lalumera
Consensus Procedures in Oncological Imaging: The Case of Prostate Cancer
Reprinted from: *Cancers* **2019**, *11*, 1788, doi:10.3390/cancers11111788 183

Concetta Schiano, Monica Franzese, Katia Pane, Nunzia Garbino, Andrea Soricelli, Marco Salvatore, Filomena de Nigris and Claudio Napoli
Hybrid ^{18}F-FDG-PET/MRI Measurement of Standardized Uptake Value Coupled with Yin Yang 1 Signature in Metastatic Breast Cancer. A Preliminary Study
Reprinted from: *Cancers* **2019**, *11*, 1444, doi:10.3390/cancers11101444 195

Jeong Won Lee, Sung Yong Kim, Hyun Ju Lee, Sun Wook Han, Jong Eun Lee and Sang Mi Lee
Prognostic Significance of CT-Attenuation of Tumor-Adjacent Breast Adipose Tissue in Breast Cancer Patients with Surgical Resection
Reprinted from: *Cancers* **2019**, *11*, 1135, doi:10.3390/cancers11081135 211

Christopher Montemagno, Laurent Dumas, Pierre Cavaillès, Mitra Ahmadi, Sandrine Bacot, Marlène Debiossat, Audrey Soubies, Loic Djaïleb, Julien Leenhardt, Nicolas De Leiris, Maeva Dufies, Gilles Pagès, Sophie Hernot, Nick Devoogdt, Pascale Perret, Laurent Riou, Daniel Fagret, Catherine Ghezzi and Alexis Broisat
In Vivo Assessment of VCAM-1 Expression by SPECT/CT Imaging in Mice Models of Human Triple Negative Breast Cancer
Reprinted from: *Cancers* **2019**, *11*, 1039, doi:10.3390/cancers11071039 227

Mariarosaria Incoronato, Anna Maria Grimaldi, Peppino Mirabelli, Carlo Cavaliere,
Chiara Anna Parente, Monica Franzese, Stefania Staibano, Gennaro Ilardi, Daniela Russo,
Andrea Soricelli, Onofrio Antonio Catalano and Marco Salvatore
Circulating miRNAs in Untreated Breast Cancer: An Exploratory Multimodality Morpho-Functional Study
Reprinted from: *Cancers* **2019**, *11*, 876, doi:10.3390/cancers11060876 . . . . **241**

Francesco Fiz, Helmut Dittmann, Cristina Campi, Matthias Weissinger, Samine Sahbai,
Matthias Reimold, Arnulf Stenzl, Michele Piana, Gianmario Sambuceti
and Christian la Fougère
Automated Definition of Skeletal Disease Burden in Metastatic Prostate Carcinoma: A 3D Analysis of SPECT/CT Images
Reprinted from: *Cancers* **2019**, *11*, 869, doi:10.3390/cancers11060869 . . . . **263**

Katsuo Usuda, Shun Iwai, Aika Funasaki, Atsushi Sekimura, Nozomu Motono, Munetaka
Matoba, Mariko Doai, Sohsuke Yamada, Yoshimichi Ueda and Hidetaka Uramoto
Diffusion-Weighted Imaging Can Differentiate between Malignant and Benign Pleural Diseases
Reprinted from: *Cancers* **2019**, *11*, 811, doi:10.3390/cancers11060811 . . . . **277**

Noriyuki Fujima, Yukie Shimizu, Daisuke Yoshida, Satoshi Kano, Takatsugu Mizumachi,
Akihiro Homma, Koichi Yasuda, Rikiya Onimaru, Osamu Sakai, Kohsuke Kudo
and Hiroki Shirato
Machine-Learning-Based Prediction of Treatment Outcomes Using MR Imaging-Derived Quantitative Tumor Information in Patients with Sinonasal Squamous Cell Carcinomas:
A Preliminary Study
Reprinted from: *Cancers* **2019**, *11*, 800, doi:10.3390/cancers11060800 . . . . **287**

About the Editors

Stefano Fanti Fanti is born in Bologna (Italy) where completed all his studies and finally graduated at University of Bologna. Started working in conventional nuclear medicine in the '90, then involved in the project of PET Unit at S.Orsola Policlinic Hospital, participating to site planning then appointed as medical director in 2002. Last year the PET Unit carried out more than 14000 exams, resulting one of the most active in Europe; in particular the PET Center in Bologna is known for the nonFDG scans, in both clinical routine and research area. At present he is full time employed in Nuclear Medicine as Full Professor of Diagnostic Imaging as well as Director of Nuclear Medicine Division and of PET Unit at the S.Orsola Policlinic Hospital. Author of more than 1000 papers, including 450 full articles published in peer reviewed international journals (more than 18000 citations and H-index of 73 on Google Scholar, 60 on Scopus), dozen of books and chapters; invited lecturer at more than 200 national and international meetings.

Laura Evangelista is a researcher of Diagnostic Imaging at University of Padova (Italy), Vice-Director of the Nuclear Medicine residency program since 2019. Dr. Evangelista received an undergraduate degree in medicine in 2004 and the Nuclear Medicine degree in 2009, both from University of Napoli (Italy). Author of more than 250 publications, including about 200 original papers in international peer-reviewed journals, more than 300 abstracts, 15 books or chapters; H-index: 18; invited speakers in more than 50 international meetings. Dr. Evangelista's current research is currently focused on PET/MRI imaging in oncology and non-oncology settings. She is currently focused on the evaluation of the additional value of hybrid PET/MRI scanners in the management of oncological patients.

Preface to "Role of Medical Imaging in Cancers"

Medical imaging comprises a huge amount of imaging techniques, from ultrasound and computed tomography (CT) to molecular imaging comprising magnetic resonance imaging (MRI) and positron emission tomography (PET).

Molecular imaging allows for the remote, noninvasive sensing and measurement of cellular and molecular processes in living subjects. It provides a window into the biology of cancer from the sub-cellular level to the patient undergoing a new, experimental therapy. Conventional imaging, and mainly CT, remains critical to the management of patients with cancer, while molecular imaging provides more specific information, such as early detection of changes with therapy, identification of patient-specific cellular and metabolic characteristics, that have a considerable impact on morbidity and mortality.

Molecular imaging has developed rapidly in the last years, particularly in the oncological field. The development of new hybrid scanners, like digital PET/CT, PET/MRI and single photon emission tomography (SPET)/CT, has significantly improved the detection of tumors, in all phase of disease (from the initial staging to the evaluation of response to therapy). Moreover, the introduction of various radiopharmaceutical agents has opened new scenarios for the in-vivo molecular characterization of cancer.

This Special Issue will highlight the role of medical imaging, with particular interest to molecular imaging in cancer management, covering some important aspects by focalizing the attention of new discoveries for the big killers, like prostate cancer, lung cancer, breast cancer and colon cancer.

Stefano Fanti, Laura Evangelista
Editors

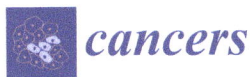

Editorial

What Is the Role of Imaging in Cancers?

Laura Evangelista [1,*] and Stefano Fanti [2]

1. Nuclear Medicine Unit, Department of Medicine (DIMED), University of Padua, 35128 Padua, Italy
2. Department of Nuclear Medicine, Sant'Orsola-Malpighi Hospital, University of Bologna, 40138 Bologna, Italy; stefano.fanti@aosp.bo.it
* Correspondence: laura.evangelista@unipd.it; Tel.: +39-0498211310; Fax: +39-0498213008

Received: 3 June 2020; Accepted: 4 June 2020; Published: 8 June 2020

In the issue entitled "Role of Medical Imaging in Cancers", 33 papers have been collected (23 original articles, 8 reviews, 1 brief report and 1 perspective). All the papers focus on different topics, mainly on the role of positron emission tomography (PET) imaging in the management of oncological patients.

Table 1 shows a summary of the topics and the papers included for each topic [1–33]. The majority of papers are focused on prostate cancer (PCa) and radiomics. The first topic has continuously gained interest in last years, in particular after the introduction of prostate specific membrane antigen (PSMA)-based radiopharmaceuticals, as extensively reported by Hoffmann et al. [18] in a cohort of more than 580 patients with recurrent PCa, showing that, after radical prostatectomy, PSMA PET/computed tomography (CT) was able to detect the presence of recurrent disease in more than 50% of patients with a PSA level < 1.24 ng/mL. Moreover, Treglia et al. [24], in a meta-analysis, clearly demonstrated the high detection rate of 18F-labeled PSMA also in patients with a PSA levels < 0.5 ng/mL. Nevertheless, Fanti et al. [20] underlined that, although there is a large amount of data on PSMA PET in PCa, the diagnostic procedures are still underutilized in clinical practice. The role of imaging in PCa was also analyzed by using different radiopharmaceutical agents and specific software. Laudicella et al. [23] tested the utility of 18F-FACBC (or fluciclovine) in recurrent PCa, showing a high diagnostic performance for the detection of local recurrence, mainly in the prostatic fossa. Bauckneht et al. [19] support the role of 18F-Fluorodeoxyglucose (FDG) PET/CT as a tool for patient selection and response assessment in metastatic castrate resistant PCa patients undergoing 223Ra administration. Furthermore, in this latter setting of patients, a segmentation-based tumor load at 99mTc-dysphonate SPECT/CT was linked with clinical outcome [21]. Finally, a radiomic approach with a specific magnetic resonance imaging (MRI) protocol can be useful to appropriately detect and characterize PCa [31]. Radiomics is an emerging field, defined as the extraction of quantitative data from medical images by using specific software. It can be applied to all medical imaging, such as CT, MRI, PET/CT or PET/MRI. In the last years, a large amount of data has been published, such as in the current issue of *Cancers*, in order to apply this in diverse settings of disease. Castaldo et al. [30] and Schiano et al. [32] evaluated the role of radiomics in breast cancer. The first group of authors concluded the ability of radiomic features by MRI to discriminate major breast cancer molecular subtypes, thus potentially guiding a personalized treatment [30]. The second group by Schiano et al. [32] showed that the combination of radiomic features by FDG PET/MRI and molecular data are able to predict the synchronous metastatic disease more accurately than a single information. Fujima et al. [33] found a correlation between the clinical outcome and machine-learning algorithm using various MRI-derived data in patients with sinonasal squamous cell carcinomas.

Table 1. Summary of articles in the special issue.

Topic (in Alphabetic Order)	Type of Paper	
	Original Articles (ref)	Reviews or Brief Article or Perspectives (ref)
Breast cancer	None	Salvatore et al. [1], Hildebrandt et al. [2]
CT imaging	Kimm et al. [3], Lee et al. [4]	None
Immunotherapy	Castello et al. [5]	Frega et al. [6], Decarez et al. [7]
Lymphoma	Albano et al. [8]	Voltin et al. [9]
Meningioma	None	Laudicella et al. [10]
MRI	Jin et al. [11], Usuda et al. [12]	None
Pancreas	None	Serafini et al. [13], Montemagno et al. [14]
PET/MRI	Samolyk-Kogaczewska et al. [15], Incoronato et al. [16]	None
Preclinical	Montemagno et al. [17]	None
Prostate and genito-urinary	Hoffmann et al. [18], Bauckneht et al. [19], Fanti et al. [20], Fiz et al. [21], Zattoni et al. [22]	Laudicella et al. [23], Treglia et al. [24]
Response to therapy or predictors	Perrone et al. [25], Sachpekidis et al. [26], Perrone et al. [27], Surov et al. [28]	None
Radiomics	Polverari et al. [29], Castaldo et al. [30], Monti et al. [31], Schiano et al. [32], Fujima et al. [33]	None

Indeed, radiomics can be used as a tool for the prediction of outcomes in terms of response to therapy or prognosis in patients undergoing immune check point inhibitors, as stated by Polverari et al. [29]. The use of imaging as a predictive biomarker of response to immunotherapy has been discussed by some authors [5–7], in the present issue. Both in the reviews and in the original articles, nuclear medicine images can be considered as a non-invasive method that is able to predict the response to immunotherapy, mainly in combination with other clinical or biological markers. Moreover, FDG PET/CT can be helpful in predicting the response to therapy in patients with head and neck squamous cell carcinoma, due to the high correlation between micro-vessel density and FDG uptake in terms of SUVmax [28]. This latter semiquantitative parameter is predictive of overall survival in patients with recurrent ovarian cancer [25]. The same author [27] reported that PET/CT can predict more accurately than MRI the response to concurrent chemoradiation treatment in T2 cervical cancer patients. Finally, from a German experience in a small cohort of patients ($n = 16$) affected by high-risk soft tissue sarcoma, the authors of [26] found that FDG kinetic analysis can be considered as a marker of response to pazopanib in soft-tissue sarcoma, and therefore it could guide anti-angiogenetic therapy.

The residual papers focused on different topics by analyzing diverse imaging modalities from preclinical [17], to gold nanoparticles for CT imaging [3,4], to specific pathologies (i.e., breast cancer [1,2] or pancreas [13,14] or meningioma [10]), to multicenter trials [8,22]. The common conclusion of these contributions is the current and future support that medical imaging can add to clinical information. The continuous developments of new radiopharmaceutical agents or the production of new technologies (i.e., scanners or software) will lead to increasingly personalized medicine.

Funding: This research received no external funding.

Conflicts of Interest: The authors declare no conflict of interest.

References

1. Salvatore, B.; Caprio, M.G.; Hill, B.S.; Sarnella, A.; Roviello, G.N.; Zannetti, A. Recent Advances in Nuclear Imaging of Receptor Expression to Guide Targeted Therapies in Breast Cancer. *Cancers* **2019**, *11*, 1614. [CrossRef] [PubMed]
2. Hildebrandt, M.G.; Lauridsen, J.F.; Vogsen, M.; Holm, J.; Vilstrup, M.H.; Braad, P.-E.; Gerke, O.; Thomassen, M.; Ewertz, M.; Høilund-Carlsen, P.F.; et al. FDG-PET/CT for Response Monitoring in Metastatic Breast Cancer: Today, Tomorrow, and Beyond. *Cancers* **2019**, *11*, 1190. [CrossRef] [PubMed]

3. Kimm, M.A.; Shevtsov, M.; Werner, C.; Sievert, W.; Zhiyuan, W.; Schoppe, O.; Menze, B.H.; Rummeny, E.J.; Proksa, R.; Bystrova, O.; et al. Gold Nanoparticle Mediated Multi-Modal CT Imaging of Hsp70 Membrane-Positive Tumors. *Cancers* **2020**, *12*, 1331. [CrossRef]
4. Lee, J.W.; Kim, S.Y.; Lee, H.J.; Han, S.W.; Lee, J.E.; Lee, S.M. Prognostic Significance of CT-Attenuation of Tumor-Adjacent Breast Adipose Tissue in Breast Cancer Patients with Surgical Resection. *Cancers* **2019**, *11*, 1135. [CrossRef] [PubMed]
5. Castello, A.; Carbone, F.G.; Rossi, S.; Monterisi, S.; Federico, D.; Toschi, L.; Lopci, E. Circulating Tumor Cells and Metabolic Parameters in NSCLC Patients Treated with Checkpoint Inhibitors. *Cancers* **2020**, *12*, 487. [CrossRef] [PubMed]
6. Frega, S.; Dal Maso, A.; Pasello, G.; Cuppari, L.; Bonanno, L.; Conte, P.; Evangelista, L. Novel Nuclear Medicine Imaging Applications in Immuno-Oncology. *Cancers* **2020**, *12*, 1303. [CrossRef] [PubMed]
7. Decazes, P.; Bohn, P. Immunotherapy by Immune Checkpoint Inhibitors and Nuclear Medicine Imaging: Current and Future Applications. *Cancers* **2020**, *12*, 371. [CrossRef]
8. Albano, D.; Laudicella, R.; Ferro, P.; Allocca, M.; Abenavoli, E.; Buschiazzo, A.; Castellino, A.; Chiaravalloti, A.; Cuccaro, A.; Cuppari, L.; et al. The Role of 18F-FDG PET/CT in Staging and Prognostication of Mantle Cell Lymphoma: An Italian Multicentric Study. *Cancers* **2019**, *11*, 1831. [CrossRef]
9. Voltin, C.-A.; Mettler, J.; Grosse, J.; Dietlein, M.; Baues, C.; Schmitz, C.; Borchmann, P.; Kobe, C.; Hellwig, D. FDG-PET Imaging for Hodgkin and Diffuse Large B-Cell Lymphoma—An Updated Overview. *Cancers* **2020**, *12*, 601. [CrossRef]
10. Laudicella, R.; Albano, D.; Annunziata, S.; Calabrò, D.; Argiroffi, G.; Abenavoli, E.; Linguanti, F.; Albano, D.; Vento, A.; Bruno, A.; et al. Theragnostic Use of Radiolabelled Dota-Peptides in Meningioma: From Clinical Demand to Future Applications. *Cancers* **2019**, *11*, 1412. [CrossRef]
11. Jin, Y.; Randall, J.W.; Elhalawani, H.; Al Feghali, K.A.; Elliott, A.M.; Anderson, B.M.; Lacerda, L.; Tran, B.L.; Mohamed, A.S.; Brock, K.K.; et al. Detection of Glioblastoma Subclinical Recurrence Using Serial Diffusion Tensor Imaging. *Cancers* **2020**, *12*, 568. [CrossRef] [PubMed]
12. Usuda, K.; Iwai, S.; Funasaki, A.; Sekimura, A.; Motono, N.; Matoba, M.; Doai, M.; Yamada, S.; Ueda, Y.; Uramoto, H. Diffusion-Weighted Imaging Can Differentiate between Malignant and Benign Pleural Diseases. *Cancers* **2019**, *11*, 811. [CrossRef] [PubMed]
13. Serafini, S.; Sperti, C.; Brazzale, A.R.; Cecchin, D.; Zucchetta, P.; Pierobon, E.S.; Ponzoni, A.; Valmasoni, M.; Moletta, L. The Role of Positron Emission Tomography in Clinical Management of Intraductal Papillary Mucinous Neoplasms of the Pancreas. *Cancers* **2020**, *12*, 807. [CrossRef] [PubMed]
14. Montemagno, C.; Cassim, S.; Trichanh, D.; Savary, C.; Pouyssegur, J.; Pagès, G.; Fagret, D.; Broisat, A.; Ghezzi, C. 99mTc-A1 as a Novel Imaging Agent Targeting Mesothelin-Expressing Pancreatic Ductal Adenocarcinoma. *Cancers* **2019**, *11*, 1531. [CrossRef]
15. Samolyk-Kogaczewska, N.; Sierko, E.; Dziemianczyk-Pakiela, D.; Nowaszewska, K.B.; Lukasik, M.; Reszec, J. Usefulness of Hybrid PET/MRI in Clinical Evaluation of Head and Neck Cancer Patients. *Cancers* **2020**, *12*, 511. [CrossRef] [PubMed]
16. Incoronato, M.; Grimaldi, A.M.; Mirabelli, P.; Cavaliere, C.; Parente, C.A.; Franzese, M.; Staibano, S.; Ilardi, G.; Russo, D.; Soricelli, A.; et al. Circulating miRNAs in Untreated Breast Cancer: An Exploratory Multimodality Morpho-Functional Study. *Cancers* **2019**, *11*, 876. [CrossRef]
17. Montemagno, C.; Dumas, L.; Cavaillès, P.; Ahmadi, M.; Bacot, S.; Debiossat, M.; Soubies, A.; Djaïleb, L.; Leenhardt, J.; De Leiris, N.; et al. In Vivo Assessment of VCAM-1 Expression by SPECT/CT Imaging in Mice Models of Human Triple Negative Breast Cancer. *Cancers* **2019**, *11*, 1039. [CrossRef]
18. Hoffmann, M.A.; Buchholz, H.-G.; Wieler, H.J.; Miederer, M.; Rosar, F.; Fischer, N.; Müller-Hübenthal, J.; Trampert, L.; Pektor, S.; Schreckenberger, M. PSA and PSA Kinetics Thresholds for the Presence of 68Ga-PSMA-11 PET/CT-Detectable Lesions in Patients with Biochemical Recurrent Prostate Cancer. *Cancers* **2020**, *12*, 398. [CrossRef]
19. Bauckneht, M.; Capitanio, S.; Donegani, M.I.; Zanardi, E.; Miceli, A.; Murialdo, R.; Raffa, S.; Tomasello, L.; Vitti, M.; Cavo, A.; et al. Role of Baseline and Post-Therapy 18F-FDG PET in the Prognostic Stratification of Metastatic Castration-Resistant Prostate Cancer (mCRPC) Patients Treated with Radium-223. *Cancers* **2020**, *12*, 31. [CrossRef]
20. Fanti, S.; Oyen, W.; Lalumera, E. Consensus Procedures in Oncological Imaging: The Case of Prostate Cancer. *Cancers* **2019**, *11*, 1788. [CrossRef]

21. Fiz, F.; Dittmann, H.; Campi, C.; Weissinger, M.; Sahbai, S.; Reimold, M.; Stenzl, A.; Piana, M.; Sambuceti, G.; la Fougère, C. Automated Definition of Skeletal Disease Burden in Metastatic Prostate Carcinoma: A 3D Analysis of SPECT/CT Images. *Cancers* **2019**, *11*, 869. [CrossRef] [PubMed]
22. Zattoni, F.; Incerti, E.; Dal Moro, F.; Moschini, M.; Castellucci, P.; Panareo, S.; Picchio, M.; Fallanca, F.; Briganti, A.; Gallina, A.; et al. 18F-FDG PET/CT and Urothelial Carcinoma: Impact on Management and Prognosis—A Multicenter Retrospective Study. *Cancers* **2019**, *11*, 700. [CrossRef] [PubMed]
23. Laudicella, R.; Albano, D.; Alongi, P.; Argiroffi, G.; Bauckneht, M.; Baldari, S.; Bertagna, F.; Boero, M.; Vincentis, G.D.; Sole, A.D.; et al. 18F-Facbc in Prostate Cancer: A Systematic Review and Meta-Analysis. *Cancers* **2019**, *11*, 1348. [CrossRef] [PubMed]
24. Treglia, G.; Annunziata, S.; Pizzuto, D.A.; Giovanella, L.; Prior, J.O.; Ceriani, L. Detection Rate of 18F-Labeled PSMA PET/CT in Biochemical Recurrent Prostate Cancer: A Systematic Review and a Meta-Analysis. *Cancers* **2019**, *11*, 710. [CrossRef]
25. Perrone, A.M.; Dondi, G.; Lima, G.M.; Castellucci, P.; Tesei, M.; Coluccelli, S.; Gasparre, G.; Porcelli, A.M.; Nanni, C.; Fanti, S.; et al. Potential Prognostic Role of 18F-FDG PET/CT in Invasive Epithelial Ovarian Cancer Relapse. A Preliminary Study. *Cancers* **2019**, *11*, 713. [CrossRef]
26. Sachpekidis, C.; Karampinis, I.; Jakob, J.; Kasper, B.; Nowak, K.; Pilz, L.; Attenberger, U.; Gaiser, T.; Derigs, H.-G.; Schwarzbach, M.; et al. Neoadjuvant Pazopanib Treatment in High-Risk Soft Tissue Sarcoma: A Quantitative Dynamic 18F-FDG PET/CT Study of the German Interdisciplinary Sarcoma Group. *Cancers* **2019**, *11*, 790. [CrossRef]
27. Perrone, A.M.; Dondi, G.; Coe, M.; Ferioli, M.; Telo, S.; Galuppi, A.; De Crescenzo, E.; Tesei, M.; Castellucci, P.; Nanni, C.; et al. Predictive Role of MRI and 18F FDG PET Response to Concurrent Chemoradiation in T2b Cervical Cancer on Clinical Outcome: A Retrospective Single Center Study. *Cancers* **2020**, *12*, 659. [CrossRef]
28. Surov, A.; Meyer, H.J.; Höhn, A.-K.; Wienke, A.; Sabri, O.; Purz, S. 18F-FDG-PET Can Predict Microvessel Density in Head and Neck Squamous Cell Carcinoma. *Cancers* **2019**, *11*, 543. [CrossRef]
29. Polverari, G.; Ceci, F.; Bertaglia, V.; Reale, M.L.; Rampado, O.; Gallio, E.; Passera, R.; Liberini, V.; Scapoli, P.; Arena, V.; et al. 18F-FDG Pet Parameters and Radiomics Features Analysis in Advanced Nsclc Treated with Immunotherapy as Predictors of Therapy Response and Survival. *Cancers* **2020**, *12*, 1163. [CrossRef]
30. Castaldo, R.; Pane, K.; Nicolai, E.; Salvatore, M.; Franzese, M. The Impact of Normalization Approaches to Automatically Detect Radiogenomic Phenotypes Characterizing Breast Cancer Receptors Status. *Cancers* **2020**, *12*, 518. [CrossRef]
31. Monti, S.; Brancato, V.; Di Costanzo, G.; Basso, L.; Puglia, M.; Ragozzino, A.; Salvatore, M.; Cavaliere, C. Multiparametric MRI for Prostate Cancer Detection: New Insights into the Combined Use of a Radiomic Approach with Advanced Acquisition Protocol. *Cancers* **2020**, *12*, 390. [CrossRef] [PubMed]
32. Schiano, C.; Franzese, M.; Pane, K.; Garbino, N.; Soricelli, A.; Salvatore, M.; de Nigris, F.; Napoli, C. Hybrid 18F-FDG-PET/MRI Measurement of Standardized Uptake Value Coupled with Yin Yang 1 Signature in Metastatic Breast Cancer. A Preliminary Study. *Cancers* **2019**, *11*, 1444. [CrossRef] [PubMed]
33. Fujima, N.; Shimizu, Y.; Yoshida, D.; Kano, S.; Mizumachi, T.; Homma, A.; Yasuda, K.; Onimaru, R.; Sakai, O.; Kudo, K.; et al. Machine-Learning-Based Prediction of Treatment Outcomes Using MR Imaging-Derived Quantitative Tumor Information in Patients with Sinonasal Squamous Cell Carcinomas: A Preliminary Study. *Cancers* **2019**, *11*, 800. [CrossRef] [PubMed]

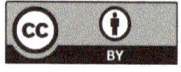

© 2020 by the authors. Licensee MDPI, Basel, Switzerland. This article is an open access article distributed under the terms and conditions of the Creative Commons Attribution (CC BY) license (http://creativecommons.org/licenses/by/4.0/).

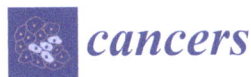

Article

Gold Nanoparticle Mediated Multi-Modal CT Imaging of Hsp70 Membrane-Positive Tumors

Melanie A. Kimm [1], Maxim Shevtsov [2,3,4], Caroline Werner [2], Wolfgang Sievert [2], Wu Zhiyuan [2], Oliver Schoppe [2,5], Bjoern H. Menze [2,5], Ernst J. Rummeny [1], Roland Proksa [6], Olga Bystrova [4], Marina Martynova [4], Gabriele Multhoff [2] and Stefan Stangl [2,*]

[1] Department of Diagnostic and Interventional Radiology, Klinikum rechts der Isar der Technischen Universität München, 81675 Munich, Germany; Melanie.Kimm@tum.de (M.A.K.); Ernst.Rummeny@tum.de (E.J.R.)
[2] Central Institute for Translational Cancer Research (TranslaTUM), Klinikum rechts der Isar der Technischen Universität München, 81675 Munich, Germany; Maxim.Shevtsov@tum.de (M.S.); c.werner@tum.de (C.W.); Wolfgang.Sievert@tum.de (W.S.); zhiyuan2012.wu@tum.de (W.Z.); Oliver.Schoppe@tum.de (O.S.); Bjoern.Menze@tum.de (B.H.M.); Gabriele.Multhoff@tum.de (G.M.)
[3] Pavlov First Saint Petersburg State Medical University, 197022 St. Petersburg, Russia
[4] Institute of Cytology of the Russian Academy of Sciences (RAS), 194064 St. Petersburg, Russia; o3608338@gmail.com (O.B.); mgmart14@mail.ru (M.M.)
[5] Institute for Advanced Studies, Department of Informatics, Technical University of Munich, 85748 Garching, Germany
[6] Philips GmbH Innovative Technologies, Research Laboratories, 22335 Hamburg, Germany; roland.proksa@philips.com
* Correspondence: Stefan.Stangl@tum.de; Tel.: +49-89-4140-6013; Fax: +49-89-4140-4299

Received: 15 April 2020; Accepted: 20 May 2020; Published: 22 May 2020

Abstract: Imaging techniques such as computed tomographies (CT) play a major role in clinical imaging and diagnosis of malignant lesions. In recent years, metal nanoparticle platforms enabled effective payload delivery for several imaging techniques. Due to the possibility of surface modification, metal nanoparticles are predestined to facilitate molecular tumor targeting. In this work, we demonstrate the feasibility of anti-plasma membrane Heat shock protein 70 (Hsp70) antibody functionalized gold nanoparticles (cmHsp70.1-AuNPs) for tumor-specific multimodal imaging. Membrane-associated Hsp70 is exclusively presented on the plasma membrane of malignant cells of multiple tumor entities but not on corresponding normal cells, predestining this target for a tumor-selective in vivo imaging. In vitro microscopic analysis revealed the presence of cmHsp70.1-AuNPs in the cytosol of tumor cell lines after internalization via the endo-lysosomal pathway. In preclinical models, the biodistribution as well as the intratumoral enrichment of AuNPs were examined 24 h after i.v. injection in tumor-bearing mice. In parallel to spectral CT analysis, histological analysis confirmed the presence of AuNPs within tumor cells. In contrast to control AuNPs, a significant enrichment of cmHsp70.1-AuNPs has been detected selectively inside tumor cells in different tumor mouse models. Furthermore, a machine-learning approach was developed to analyze AuNP accumulations in tumor tissues and organs. In summary, utilizing mHsp70 on tumor cells as a target for the guidance of cmHsp70.1-AuNPs facilitates an enrichment and uniform distribution of nanoparticles in mHsp70-expressing tumor cells that enables various microscopic imaging techniques and spectral-CT-based tumor delineation in vivo.

Keywords: gold nanoparticle; heat shock protein 70; molecular imaging; biomarker; spectral-CT

1. Introduction

Detection of all malignant tumor cells in a patients' body is a prerequisite for a successful therapy outcome. In established clinical routine, combined positron emission tomography (PET)/computed tomography (CT) imaging is commonly used for tumors exceeding 0.5–1 cm^3. For standard clinical PET imaging, ^{18}F-glucose is often used as a PET tracer. However, glucose-based PET/CT imaging faces several disadvantages, such as false-positive and/or false-negative signals, e.g., triggered by the fact that only metabolically active but not resting cells can be visualized, the low tumor-to-background contrast, and the relatively low resolution of the technique [1]. With improved settings, a spatial resolution of 2 mm is technically feasible, as demonstrated in patients with prostate cancer [2].

The introduction of gold nanoparticles (AuNP)-based contrast agents added a new value to imaging techniques. Functionalization of novel metal-based nanoparticles with tumor-specific antibodies [3] and their utilization in imaging techniques such as photoacoustic tomography or CT combine the advantages of a molecular, tumor-specific imaging with the unique attributes of AuNP in clinical imaging. For instance, spectral-CT technology employs a photon-counting detector which registers the interactions of individual photons, creating a certain energy spectrum which can subsequently be converted into a color image. At the same time, a nonspectral attenuation image can be acquired. This combination allows a precise spatial information with a high resolution. With the emergence of clinical spectral-CT scanners, the need of tumor-specific contrast agents further increased. In this setting, AuNPs might play a crucial role as the energy-dependent X-ray attenuation properties (K-edge at 80.7 keV) allow an excellent separation from calcium (K-edge at 4 keV) and iodine (K-edge at 33.2 keV) [4].

For in vivo application, it is also essential that the applied nanoparticles are nontoxic, biodegradable or inert, and easily transportable in the blood and/or lymphatic system. Biocompatible camouflage of the NP surface is a prerequisite to avoid immediate uptake by macrophages. Small AuNPs (<100 nm) demonstrated to be beneficial for utilization in clinical applications [5–7]. Apart from the formulation of AuNPs, tumor imaging with nanoparticle-based contrast agents can be further improved and specified by functionalization with antibodies targeting tumor-specific, membrane-bound biomarkers. For an improved signal-to-background ratio and a high tumor specificity, candidate markers should be selectively expressed on tumor cells while being absent on healthy cells. Membrane-bound Heat shock protein 70 (Hsp70, Hsp70-1, HspA1A, #3303) has been found to fulfill these criteria, exhibiting a remarkable tumor-specific targeting capability [8,9]. In addition to the physiological, cytosolic expression in all nucleated cells, Hsp70 is also found on the plasma membrane of malignantly transformed cells. Upon stress, this molecular chaperone has been found to be increased in the cytosol and on the plasma membrane of different murine and human tumor cells. Screening of tumor biopsies of over 1200 patients has shown that the majority of the primarily diagnosed carcinoma samples but none of the tested corresponding normal tissues exhibited a membrane Hsp70-positive phenotype [10–13]. After therapy of tumors with standard regimens, such as radiotherapy or chemotherapy, the membrane expression density of Hsp70 on tumor cells is increased [14], which in turn further improves targeting of membrane Hsp70-positive tumors after standard therapies. Furthermore, an upregulated membrane Hsp70 density could be detected on relapse tumors and metastases compared to primary tumors. In multiple studies, the malignancy of tumors correlates positively with the Hsp70 expression density in the cytoplasm and on the plasma membrane [8,11].

For a specific in vivo tumor targeting which is mediated by membrane-bound Hsp70, we developed the membrane Hsp70-specific antibody cmHsp70.1 [9,15]. To utilize the beneficial features of targeting membrane Hsp70 with the imaging capabilities of gold as a contrast agent, we developed an AuNP formulation, functionalized with cmHsp70.1 monoclonal antibody to target membrane-bound Hsp70 on tumor cells in vitro and in vivo. In previous studies, we could demonstrate a rapid and specific binding, uptake, and internalization of cmHsp70.1-AuNPs into tumor cells in vitro, leading to a high intracellular accumulation. Furthermore, following incubation of viable tumor cells with cmHsp70.1-AuNPs, no severe toxic side effects were observed up to a concentration of 10 µg/mL [16].

2. Results

2.1. Functionalization of AuNPs with cmHsp70.1 Antibody

For the coupling of mouse IgG1 isotype-matched or cmHsp70.1 antibody to AuNPs, we used a standard maleimide coupling reaction (Figure 1A). The size of the mean hydrodynamic diameter of unconjugated AuNPs was determined to be 45 ± 14 nm (Figure 1B, top panel). The sizes of cmHsp70.1 antibody-conjugated cmHsp70-AuNPs were 54 ± 11 nm (Figure 1B, middle panel) and 59 ± 18 nm for IgG1 isotype-matched control antibody-conjugated gold nanoparticles (IgG1-AuNPs) (Figure 1B, bottom panel). No self-aggregation was observed in aliquotes of the conjugated as well as the unconjugated AuNPs in phosphate buffered saline (PBS) at 37 °C during 24 h. After 4 weeks of storage at 4 °C, self-aggregation of the particles was observed. An exemplary size distribution histogram is given in Figure A1. To determine the Hsp70-specific binding capacity of cmHsp70.1-AuNPs, we performed analysis of the interaction of cmHsp70.1-AuNPs as well as IgG-AuNPs with recombinant human Hsp70, using an agglomeration assay, as described by Shevtsov et al. [17]. Following a 4 h incubation period with recombinant Hsp70, the size of the formed clusters, as determined by dynamic light scattering (DLS), was larger after incubation with cmHsp70.1-AuNPs (mean event sizes: 152 nm and 2420 nm) than with IgG1-AuNPs (52.9 nm), indicating the formation of ligand-mediated agglumerates. The hydrodynamic diameter of recombinant Hsp70 was determined to be 9.7 nm (Figure A2).

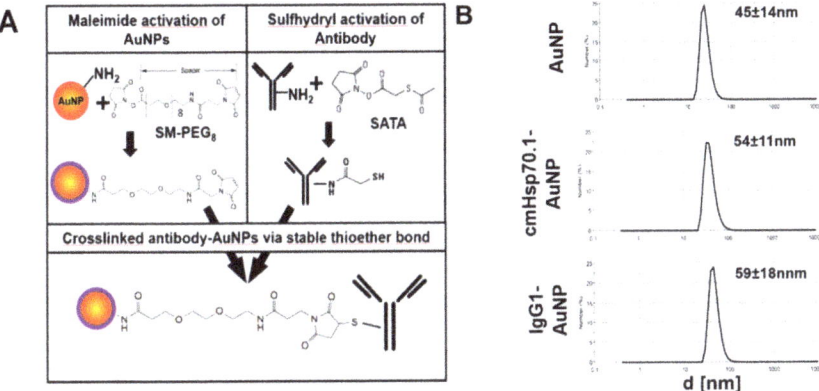

Figure 1. Antibody conjugation of gold nanoparticles (AuNPs) and characterization: (**A**) Coupling reaction of maleimide-activated AuNPs and sulfhydryl-activated monoclonal antibodies. (**B**) Size distribution of the differently functionalized AuNPs, given in size by number histograms.

2.2. Uptake and Internalization of Functionalized AuNPs in Tumor Cells In Vitro

To verify the binding capacities and specific uptake of cmHsp70.1-AuNPs in comparison to control nanoparticles (AuNPs and IgG1-AuNPs) in vitro, we performed binding tests on viable, membrane Hsp70-positive tumor cells. To determine the density of the target antigen, the cell lines 4T1 and CT26 were analyzed for their membrane and cytosolic expression of Hsp70. The Hsp70 high expressing cell line 4T1 showed a membrane Hsp70-positive phenotype on 67% ± 9% of the cells, whereas CT26 cells showed a positive phenotype on 43% ± 6% of the cells (Figure 2A). For determination of the total Hsp70 density in the cell lines, an in-cell ELISA technique was established for cells grown in chamber slides. The Hsp70 mean signal intensity in 4T1 and CT26 cell lines were $150.11 \times 10^3 \pm 24.92 \times 10^3$ a.u. and $89.39 \times 10^3 \pm 17.19 \times 10^3$ a.u., respectively (Figure 2B). These data were verified by a sandwich ELISA of cell lysates derived from 10×10^6 cells of each cell line, resulting in Hsp70 contents of 4.28 ± 1.74 ng/mL and 1.17 ± 0.72 ng/mL for 4T1 and CT26 cells, respectively (Figure 2C). Subsequently, both cell lines were incubated with the three different types of AuNPs for 24 h at 37 °C to mimic the uptake in living cells. In both cell lines, the content of AuNPs was visualized by brightfield and electron microscopy (Figure 3). Compared to blank AuNPs (Figure 3A, left panel) and IgG1-AuNPs (Figure 3A, middle panel), which showed minor cytosolic uptake, cmHsp70.1-AuNPs displayed the strongest accumulation in both 4T1 and CT26 cells (Figure 3A, right panel). In transmission electron microscopy (TEM), the cmHsp70.1-AuNPs have been found to accumulate in intracellular vesicles of both 4T1 and CT26 cells 24 h after incubation. A representative image of cmHsp70.1-AuNPs in 4T1 cells is shown in Figure 3B.

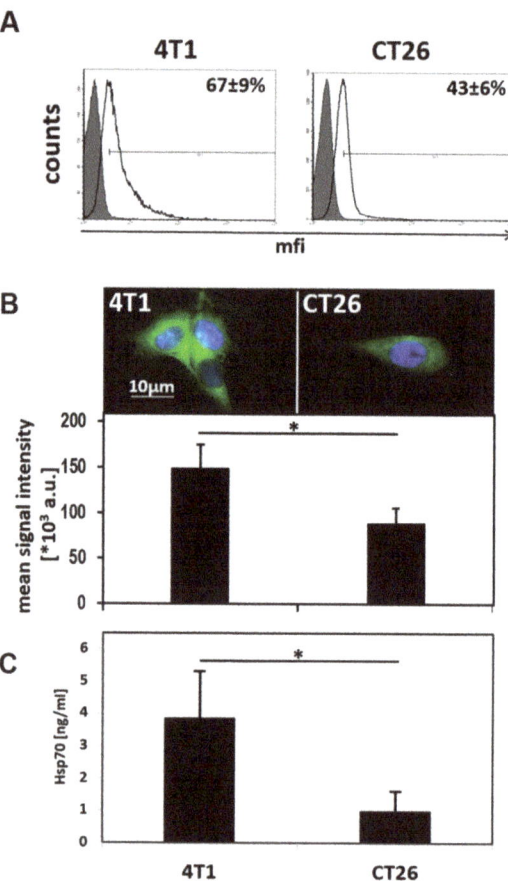

Figure 2. Quantification of Hsp70 in target tumor cell lines: (**A**) Plasma-membrane bound Hsp70 on 4T1 (left) and CT26 (right) cell lines, as determined by flow cytometry. (**B**) Quantitative staining of total Hsp70 in 4T1 and CT26 cells (upper panel) and quantification (lower panel), as determined by an in-cell ELISA technique. (**C**) Quantification of total Hsp70 in whole cell lysates of 4T1 and CT26 cell lines, as determined by an Hsp70 sandwich ELISA. * $p < 0.05$.

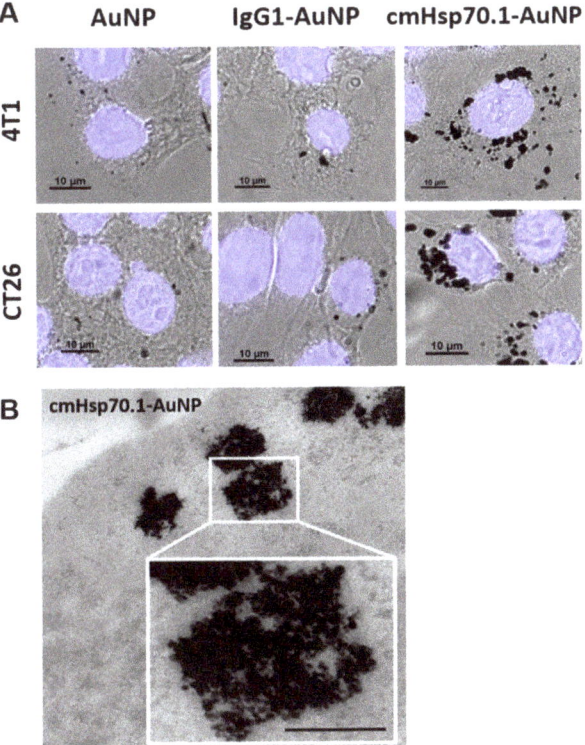

Figure 3. Uptake of AuNPs in tumor cells: (**A**) Intracellular accumulation of blank AuNPs (left), IgG1-AuNPs (middle), and cmHsp70.1-AuNPs (right) in 4T1 (upper panel) and CT26 (lower panel) cells. (**B**) TEM image of intracellular accumulations in 4T1 cells. Magnification is of the indicated area (white box). Scale bar, 1 μm.

2.3. Accumulation of Functionalized AuNPs in Tumors In Vivo

To investigate the specificity and sensitivity of cmHsp70.1-conjugated AuNPs to target tumors in vivo, syngeneic tumor models in Balb/c mice were established. Animals were injected orthotopically (o.t.) with 4T1 and subcutaneously with CT26 tumor cells, respectively. When tumors reached a size of 200 mm³, two times 2.5 mg of AuNPs of each group (AuNP, IgG1-AuNP, and cmHsp70.1-AuNP) were injected i.v. consecutively at an interval of 24 h (Figure 4).

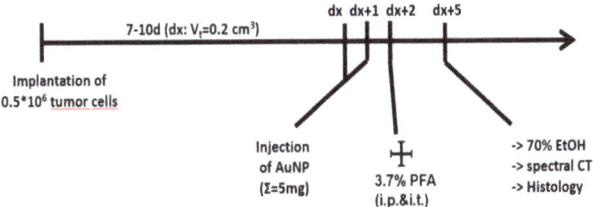

Figure 4. Timeline of the in vivo experiments.

Twenty-four hours after the second injection, mice were euthanized and fixed and subsequently imaged using spectral-CT or tumors and organs were directly applied to histological analysis. In parallel, single cell suspensions of tumors of both models have been analyzed for their plasma membrane Hsp70 status. To characterize the tumor models regarding the main features which determine the accumulation of molecular functionalized contrast agents in vivo, tumors were histologically analyzed for the target antigen content (Hsp70) in the cytosol as well as on the plasma membrane. Their vascularization status (CD31) and the presence of tumor infiltrating macrophages (F4/80) have been investigated as well. Both tumor types, 4T1 (o.t.) and CT26 (s.c.), displayed similar vascularization and infiltration of macrophages, indicating comparable effects on the NP input through these routes. Immunohistological Hsp70 staining revealed a strong expression in both tumor models, featuring cytosolic as well as nuclear Hsp70 expression. However, 4T1 tumors showed a more patterned architecture of the Hsp70 density. To investigate the membrane Hsp70 status of the tumors in vivo, a single cell suspension of freshly dissected tumors was investigated. With 76% ± 7% and 67% ± 13% membrane Hsp70-positive viable tumor cells, 4T1 and CT26 tumors grown in vivo, respectively, showed a slightly higher Hsp70 expression density compared to the in vitro cultured cells. However, the increased width of the cytometric data, as given in histograms, indicates an increased heterogeneity in the membrane Hsp70 expression pattern in in vivo grown tumors (Figure 5).

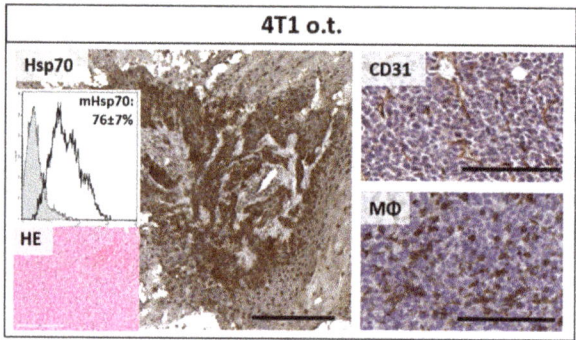

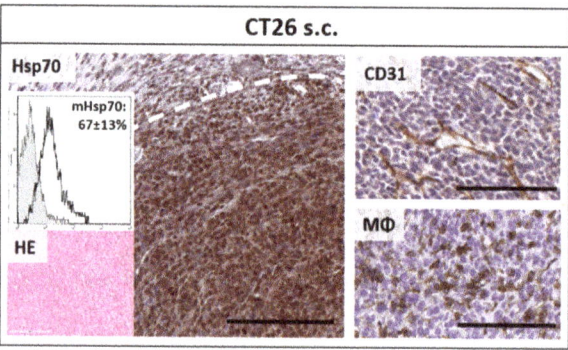

Figure 5. Tumor characterization: Orthotopic (o.t.) 4T1 (upper panel) and subcutaneous (s.c.) CT26 (lower panel) tumors were analyzed with regard to membrane (flow cytometry analysis, upper inlay) and overall (immunohistochemistry, IHC) Hsp70 expression as well as their content of CD31 positive vessels (IHC and CD31) and the infiltration of macrophages (MΦ, IHC, and F4/80). Hematoxylin & Eosin (H&E) was used as an overview stain (lower inlay). Scale bars, 200 μm (Hsp70) and 100 μm (CD31 and MΦ).

In a next step, we investigated the feasibility of cmHsp70.1-AuNPs as a contrast agent in a first cohort of tumor-bearing mice. For this pilot study, three mice with subcutaneous CT26 tumors underwent spectral CT imaging postmortem. Each mouse had received one type of AuNP 24 h before sacrifice. Interestingly, in all animals, we were able to detect AuNPs in the tumors with the highest density of nanoparticles in the tumor periphery. Nevertheless, we also noticed some striking differences. The mouse which was treated with IgG1-AuNPs presented the lowest content of AuNPs inside the tumor (3.3 µg Au/mm^3 tumor) with a very low accumulation of particles within the tumor center (Figure 6C,D). In the mouse which was treated with unconjugated AuNPs, 4.3 µg Au/mm^3 was detected in total but mainly at the periphery of the tumor, with considerably less AuNPs in the tumor center (Figure 6A,B). In case of an injection of cmHsp70.1-AuNPs, 4.4 µg Au/mm^3 was found inside the tumor. Despite similar amounts of different AuNPs in the tumor area, the distribution pattern of the AuNP formulation differed drastically. CmHsp70.1-AuNPs were found to be located in the tumor periphery and highly dispersed in the tumor center (Figure 6E,F).

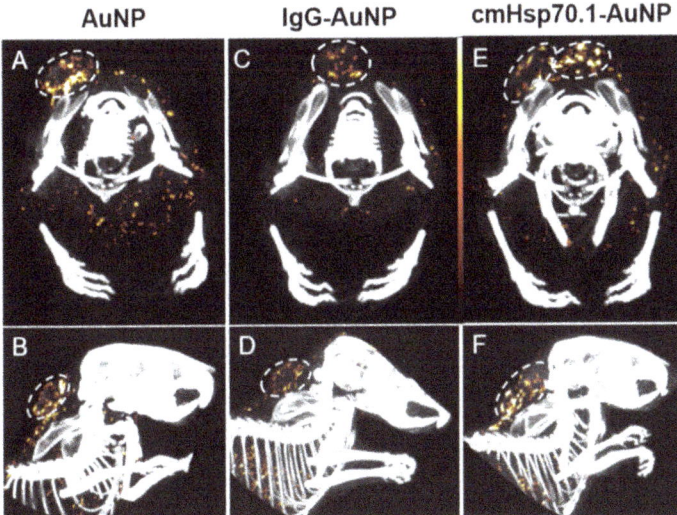

Figure 6. Tumor detection using spectral-CT. Upper Row (**A,C,E**): axial view, bottom row (**B,D,F**): sagital view. AuNP amounts are pseudo-coloured from black (6.5 mg/mL) over red (10 mg/mL) to white (13.5 mg/mL). (**A,B**) spectral CT-views of mice injected with AuNPs; (**C,D**) spectral CT-views of mice injected with IgG-AuNPs; (**E,F**) spectral CT-views of mice injected with cmHsp70.1-AuNPs.

The spectral CT-based biodistribution analysis detected a high accumulation of AuNPs in the spleen, lower amounts in the liver, and very low amounts of AuNPs in the lung. The other organs did not exhibit concentrations which were high enough to generate a signal in the spectral CT measurements. However, to prove data for statistical significance, the number of mice within the study groups have to be increased to relevant numbers in future experiments. The tumors were further analyzed for their gold content by histology (Figure 7).

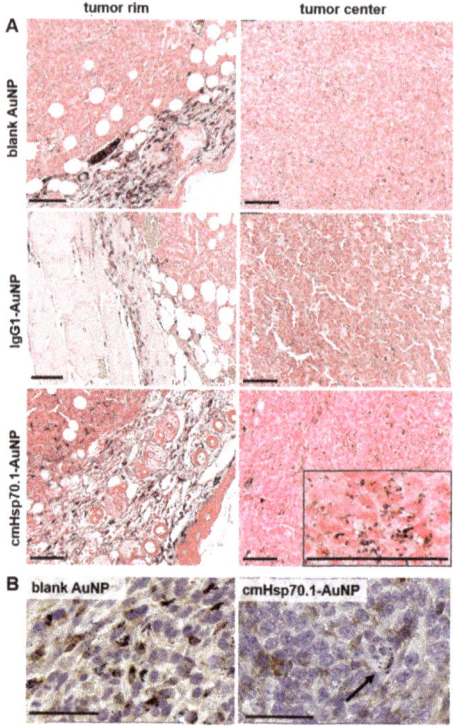

Figure 7. AuNP uptake and distribution in CT26 tumors: (**A**) Silver enhancement of AuNPs. Upper row: blank AuNPs, middle row: IgG1-AuNPs, bottom row: cmHsp70.1-AuNPs. Left: Region of Interest (ROI) at tumor rim area, right: ROI set to tumor center. Scale bars, 100 µm. (**B**) Double staining of Macrophages (F4/80, brown) and silver enhancement of AuNPs (black). Arrow: single-positive cells for AuNPs. Scale bars: 5 µm.

Sections were treated with silver enhancement to visualize AuNPs by light microscopy (Figure 7A). As revealed by spectral-CT, histological analysis confirmed the varying intratumoral distribution of the three groups of AuNPs. In tumors of mice which were treated with cmHsp70.1-AuNPs, a rather homologous distribution of NPs was observed throughout the whole tumor volume compared to the blank AuNPs or IgG1-AuNPs. Notably, the enrichment of AuNPs at the tumor rim following i.v. injection of blank AuNPs was most likely due to F4/80 positive monocyte/macrophage lineages with internalized AuNPs (Figure 7B, left). In contrast, next to the payload introduction via macrophages, cmHsp70.1-AuNPs were also found in large amounts in F4/80-negative tumor cells. Consequently, an extended accumulation of the cmHsp70.1-AuNPs was also detected in the tumor center. In this region, we also identfied less AuNP containing macrophages (Figure 7B, right). IgG1-AuNPs showed the lowest accumulation in all regions of the tumor (Figure 7A, middle). These NPs, besides their lack of targeting ability, exhibited equal biocompatibility to that of cmHsp70.1-AuNPs due to the conjugation of the murine IgG1 antibody. Consequently, these IgG1NPs resulted in the lowest intratumoral accumulation yield.

To obtain the in vivo biodistribution characteristics of cmHsp70.1-AuNPs, 24 h following systemic application, we further analyzed silver enhanced sections of tumors, liver, spleen, kidneys, heart, lungs, and intestines of another group of tumor-bearing Balb/c mice (after subcutaneous and orthotopic injection) (Figure 8).

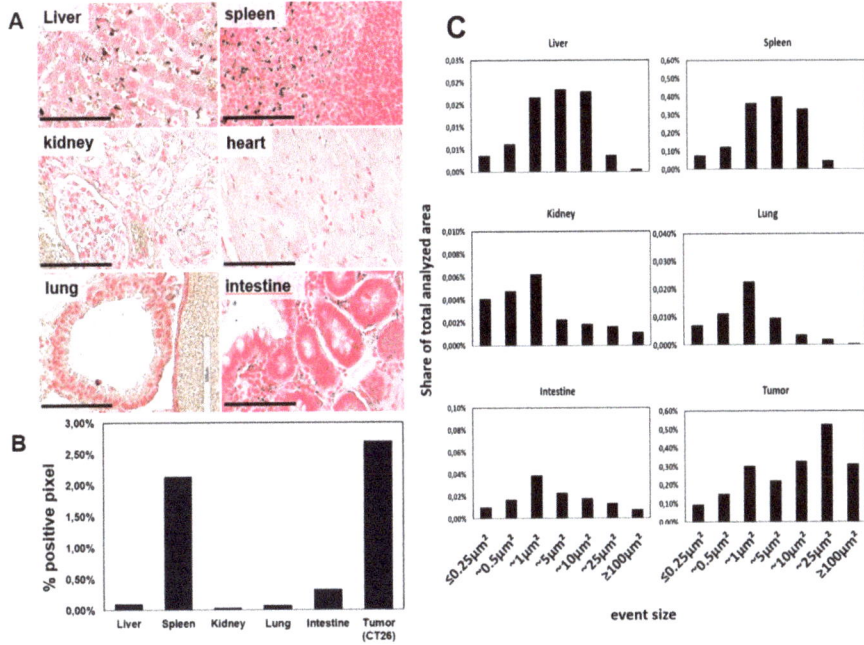

Figure 8. Biodistribution of cmHsp70.1-AuNPs: (**A**) Silver enhancement staining of liver, spleen, kidney, heart, lung, and intestine. Scale bar, 100 μm. (**B**) Pixel analysis of silver enhancement stainings in tumors and organs, given in positive pixel/mm^2 tissue. (**C**) size distribution of silver enhanced cmHsp70.1-AuNP signals in different organs following i.v. injection.

For an improved accuracy of the analysis, we used a machine-learning approach. The algorithm for the analysis of sections was trained on 28 slides in total and was applied for the analysis of 14 slides. In comparison to the organs, the highest accumulation of cmHsp70.1-AuNPs was found in the tumors, with $85.98 \times 10^3 \pm 4.94 \times 10^3$ positive pixel per mm^2, which equals to 2.7% positive pixels per section (Figure 8B). Using the machine-learning approach, we found the majority of the nanoparticles accumulated in spleen ($14.04 \times 10^3 \pm 1.37 \times 10^3$ pixel/mm^2) (2.13% signal/section), liver ($13.34 \times 10^3 \pm 0.7 \times 10^3$ pixel/mm^2) (0.11% signal/section), and intestine ($9.48 \times 10^3 \pm 1.37 \times 10^3$ pixel/mm^2) (0.34% signal/section), followed by lungs ($6.28 \times 10^3 \pm 1.30 \times 10^3$ pixel/mm^2) (0.09% signal/section). In muscle, as represented by heart tissue, the accumulation of AuNPs was below the detection limit. Kidney was rarely affected, indicating an enterohepatic secretion of the AuNPs. In addition to the analysis of the overall entry of AuNPs in the organs and tumors, we utilized the machine-learning approach to analyze the size distribution of the nanoparticle agglumerations within the organs. The majority of positively stained events in liver and spleen resulted in a size range up to 10 μm. Accumulation of events in this size range might be suggested to be due to incorporation of the AuNP by macrophages and Kupffer cells, as indicated also in Figure 7B. The majority of AuNPs in kidney, lung, and intestine yielded in agglumerates of about 1 μm in size. In the tumor, cmHsp70.1-AuNP spots of 25 μm^2 were dominant, followed by spots of 1 μm^2 (Figure 8C). As tumor-associated macrophages exhibit large cytoplasmatic volumes, the accumulation of AuNPs above 10 μm^2 suggest the appearance of this cell type. However, aggregates of 1 μm^2 point to tumor cells with smaller cytoplasmic space as tumor cells. This finding is also supported by microscopical analysis of in vitro grown tumor cells with the majority of NP accumulating in cellular organelles of about 1 μm, following endocytosis (Figure 3).

3. Discussion

The discovery of suitable contrast agents for the visualization of tumors is one of the most important areas in clinical oncology. In tumor imaging, CT imaging is the most commonly used technique featuring fast scanning speed with high spatial resolution of a large portion of the body. Functional molecular imaging can be accomplished with positron-electron-tomography (PET), often used in combination with CT. However, certain limitations affect the quality of tumor visualization. PET imaging using ^{18}F-FDG is highly dependent on a high tumor cell metabolism compared to the surrounding normal tissue. Furthermore, PET tracers need to exert ionizing effects, which in turn increases the patient's risk to accumulate DNA mutations. An approach to overcome the limiting effects of PET/CT led to the development of spectral-CT analyzers [6,18], which use the k-edge discrimination of elements, allowing for their specific identification inside the body [19]. Another advantage of the spectral segmentation is the possibility to utilize multiple contrast agents within one imaging session, which reduces the X-ray expositions of the patient.

One further limitation of PET imaging is the spatial detection limit, leading to a potential miss of small lesions. Therefore, the usage of tumor-specific markers is beneficial.

Herein, the major stress-inducible member of the HSP70 family, Hsp70 (HspA1A), was used as a target for the tumor-specific uptake of functionalized AuNPs in different tumor entities. Hsp70 is expressed on the plasma membrane of a variety of tumor entities, whereas normal cells lack an Hsp70 membrane expression [9]. However, further studies investigate the role of membrane-associated Hsp70 in the context of inflammatory diseases, such as sepsis. It was found that membrane Hsp70 also plays a role in the regulation of inflammatory responses. A study of Hirsch et al. described polymorphonuclear neutrophils (PMNs), expressing mHsp70. These PMNs are recognized and lysed by γδ T-lymphocytes and therefore protect the host cells from inflammation-induced damage [20].

In previous studies, we observed that tumor cell membrane-associated Hsp70 is rapidly internalized and therefore mediates an efficient uptake of Hsp70-binding probes into the cytoplasm, such as fluorescence-labeled cmHsp70.1 antibody [15] and tumor-penetrating peptide (TPP) [21,22]. Since the binding epitope of cmHsp70.1 antibody is identical in mouse and human tumor cells [9], murine CT26 colon and mammary 4T1 tumor cell lines were used in the present study.

The application of AuNPs for imaging in vivo is a promising new approach in the field of in vivo imaging [7,23,24]. The uptake of antibody-conjugated nanoparticles into tumor cells is dependent on several factors: the expression density of receptors, which are expressed on the target cells; the distribution of the target epitopes throughout the cells [25]; the affinity of the tracer to the membrane epitope; and the speed of internalization [21,26].

In order to monitor the efficiency of functionalized AuNPs in vitro and in vivo, we applied different imaging modalities. Dynamic light scattering is a widely used technique to determine the hydrodynamic diameter of AuNPs in the nm–μm range.

Furthermore, the quantification of AuNPs within tumor cells is of relevance to estimate the concentration of nanoparticles that is necessary for noninvasive in vivo imaging of tumors as well as for their use as therapeutic agent. In our in vivo/ex vivo setup, we were able to detect aggregates of AuNPs in tumors and organs in perinuclear areas of around 1–2 μm in diameter as well as larger aggregates of around 25 μm in diameter. The presented machine-learning approach has proven to be beneficial for the analysis of the distribution of AuNPs. Next to calculating the quantity of gold signal within tumors and organs, we were able to separate the signal into groups, which allows for an easy analysis of AuNPs within different cell types. This is important for a more precise prediction of the biodistribution and possible toxic side effects of AuNPs.

Toxic side effects of AuNPs following i.v. application were investigated in previous studies [27,28]. No negative side effects such as loss in body weight or organic dysfunctions were observed in these experiments up to a concentration of 500 μg/mL [29]. Concordantly, in the in vivo experiments of this study, we did not observe any sign of toxicity at the injected concentration of 5 mg AuNPs per mouse. However, additional pharmacological and toxicological studies are needed to prove safety.

On the basis of the specific and quantitative uptake of cmHsp70.1-AuNPs in Hsp70-positive tumor cells and its imaging properties, our approach hints at a possible beneficial use in radiation therapy. Numerous studies have reported on the radiation-enhancing effect of AuNPs within tumor tissue [30,31].

First, promising findings for radiotherapy enhancement of AuNPs were achieved in preclinical mammary carcinoma studies [32]. The results of Hainfeld et al. showed an 86% 1-year survival for a combinatorial therapy of irradiation in presence of NPs compared to 20% for radiotherapy alone. Probable mechanisms involved in radiosensitization are, besides changes in the cell cycle or an elevated reactive oxygen species, the production and the release of secondary Auger electrons by gold in very close proximity to the nucleus [31]. In previous in vitro studies on the intracellular distribution of Hsp70 targeting AuNPs, we observed an increased accumulation of the NPs in close proximity to the nucleus 24 to 48 h after incubation [16], indicating possible beneficial effects of this approach for radiotherapeutical interventions. In summary, we demonstrate that the functionalization of AuNPs with cmHsp70.1 antibody is a highly promising approach for in vivo tumor targeting. Our preclinical studies show that the accumulation of AuNPs within the investigated tumors was sufficient for visualization by spectral-CT which allows 3D reconstructions and quantifications.

4. Materials and Methods

4.1. Antibody Coupling of AuNPs

Coupling of Hsp70-specific antibody (cmHsp70.1, multimmune, Germany) or an isotype-matched control IgG1 antibody (Sigma Aldrich, St. Luis, Mo, USA) to AuNPs (Nanopartz, Loveland, CO, USA) was done as described before [16]. Briefly, polyethylenglycol (PEG)-amine-coated spherical gold nanoparticles of 30 nm diameter were maleimide activated (Pierce, Thermo Fischer Scientific, Rockford, IL, USA) and incubated over night with sulfhydryl-activated antibodies. Antibody-coupled AuNPs or unconjugated AuNPs were analyzed and used for experiments within 24 h. Nanoparticles were analyzed (size, aggregation) by dynamic light scattering (DLS, Zetasizer NanoS, Malvern Instruments, Malvern, UK). Measurements were done in triplets and mean values were calculated.

4.2. Characterization of AuNPs

Antibody-conjugated AuNPs or unconjugated AuNPs were used for experiments directly after coupling. For AuNP characterization and controlling their aggregation, particle size was analyzed by dynamic light scattering (Zetasizer NanoS; Malvern Instruments, Malvern, UK). Only nanoparticles that produced single peaks were used for experiments. For analysis of the specific interaction of differentially functionalized AuNPs with Hsp70, 150 µg/mL nanoparticles dissolved in PBS were incubated with recombinant Hsp70 protein at a concentration of 0.5 µg/mL. Following a 4-h incubation time, the size of the clusters formed by IgG1-AuNP + Hsp70 and cmHsp70.1-AuNP + Hsp70, respectively, was analyzed by DLS.

4.3. Cell Culture

Murine colon carcinoma cell line CT26 (CT26.WT; American type culture collection (ATCC) #CRL-2638) and the mouse mammary carcinoma cell line 4T1 (ATCC #CRL-2539) were cultured in Roswell Park Memorial Institute 1640 medium supplemented with 10% (v/v) heat-inactivated fetal calf serum, 2 mM L-glutamine, 1 mM sodium pyruvate, and antibiotics (100 IU/mL penicillin and 100 µg/mL streptomycin). Cells were incubated at 37 °C in 95% humidity and 5% (v/v) CO_2 and cultivated twice a week.

4.4. Assessment of Hsp70 Content of the Tumor Cells

The Hsp70 membrane phenotype of the cells was assessed by flow cytometry. Single cell suspensions of tumor cell lines were incubated with fluorescein-isothiocyanate (FITC)-conjugated cmHsp70.1 mAb for 30 min on ice. As controls, conjugation of an IgG1 isotype-matched antibody was done. After washing and adding propidium-iodide (PI) for life and dead discrimination, binding of antibodies was measured using a FACSCalibur instrument (BD Biosciences, Heidelberg, Germany). Data were analyzed using CellQuest Pro 6.0 software. Only PI-negative, viable cells were analyzed. To determine the membrane Hsp70 status of tumors grown in vivo, single cell suspension of freshly dissected tumors was generated by combined chopping and trypsin treatment of the tumors. Here, anti-mouse CD45 APC antibody was added to cmHsp70.1-FITC to distinguish tumor cells from mononuclear blood cells and infiltrated macrophages.

In-cell ELISA was performed, as described previously [21]. Briefly, cells grown in chamber slides were fixed with DAKO Fix & Perm kit (DAKO, Jena, Germany) and cellular membranes were permeabilized and incubated with cmHsp70.1-FITC antibody. Following microscopy with comparable settings, quantification of fluorescence signal was determined on the mean signal intensity values by ImageJ 1.52a image analysis software.

Quantification of the Hsp70 content was confirmed by an Hsp70 sandwich ELISA, as described elsewhere [33]. Shortly, after determination of the cell count, cells were lysed by incubation in Tris-HCl-based buffer containing 1% Triton-X100 and SDS. After centrifugation, the Hsp70 concentration in the supernatant was measured by total Hsp70 ELISA kit (R&D systems, Minneapolis, MN, USA) as described by the manufacturer. Each supernatant sample was measured in duplicates.

4.5. Animals

All animal procedures and their care were conducted in conformity with national and international guidelines (EU 2010/63) with approval from the local authorities of the Government of Upper Bavaria and ethical committee of Pavlov First Saint Petersburg State Medical University (St. Petersburg, Russia) (2015/068) and supervised by respective animal care and use committees. Animals were housed in standard animal rooms in individually ventilated cage systems (IVS Techniplast, Buggugiate, Italy) under specific pathogen-free conditions with free access to water and standard laboratory chow ad libitum. In total, 6 female Balb/c mice (aged 10–14 weeks, Charles River Laboratories, Sulzfeld, Germany) were used. Induction of subcutaneous tumors was done under inhalation anesthesia (1.8% isoflurane with medical O_2) by injection of 5×10^5 CT26 cells subcutaneously in the neck area or of 5×10^5 4T1 cells orthotopically in the 4th mammary fat pad. When tumors reached a size of 200 mm^3, AuNPs were intravenously injected using standard procedures. In total, 5 mg unconjugated, IgG1-, or cmHsp70.1-AuNPs, suspended in phosphate buffered saline, were injected in a consecutive pattern of two times 2.5 mg per day within 48 h. Another 24 h after the second application, mice were euthanized under deep anesthesia, fixed in 4% neutral-buffered formalin for 5 days, and stored in 70% ethanol for further analysis.

4.6. Bright Field Microscopy

For light microscopy, cells were grown in 8-well chamber slides (NUNC-Nalgene; Thermo Fisher Scientific, Pittsburgh, PA, USA) at a concentration of 10,000 cells per well. Upon adherence, cells were incubated with AuNPs at a nontoxic concentration of 1 µg/mL. Cellular uptake of AuNPs or quantum dots of the same size were analyzed with a Zeiss Observer Z1 (Zeiss, Germany).

4.7. Transmission Electron Microscopy

Cells were co-incubated with functionalized and non-conjugated AuNPs (at a concentration 100 µg/mL) for 24 h. Following, incubation cells were washed with PBS, fixed for 1 h at 4 °C in 2.5% glutaraldehyde in 0.1 M cacodylate buffer (pH = 7.4), postfixed in 1% aqueous OsO4 (for 1 h), dehydrated, and embedded in Araldite-Epon mixture. Sections were assessed employing Zeiss Libra 120 electron microscope (Carl Zeiss, Germany).

4.8. Histology and Immunohistochemistry

Tumors and organs were either dissected following whole-body fixation of mice or fixed in 3.7% neutral-buffered formaldehyde and embedded in paraffin. Two-μm sections of the organs and tumors were prepared, and the morphology was visualized by standard H&E staining. For immunohistochemistry, the activity of the endogenous peroxidase was blocked with 1% hydrogen peroxide and 0.1% sodium azide. After antigen retrieval in citric acid buffer (pH 6) at 100 °C, sections were incubated with anti-Hsp70 antibody cmHsp70.1, followed by horse radish peroxidas (HRP)-labelled secondary rabbit anti-mouse antibody (Dako, Jena, Germany). Diaminobenzidine (Dako) was used as a chromogen. Sections were counterstained with 1% Mayer's hematoxylin. To visualize the AuNPs by light microscopy, silver-enhancement staining was used according to the manufacturers' protocol (Sigma-Aldrich, Darmstadt, Germany), followed by counterstaining of the nuclei with 0.1% Nuclear Fast Red solution (Morphisto, Frankfurt a.M., Germany). Slides were digitalized with a digital slide scanner (AT2, Leica, Wetzlar, Germany).

4.9. Spectral-CT Imaging and Image Acquisition

Spectral CT images were acquired at a Philips spectral CT scanner, as described before [18]. Briefly, a preclinical spectral photon-counting CT system (Philips Healthcare, Hamburg, Germany) was used to obtain axial scans over 360 ° at a beam voltage of 100 kVp. For optimal discrimination of the signals of AuNPs, a threshold was set at the k-edge energy of gold.

4.10. Spectral CT Image-Based Gold Quantification

Osirix® MD v10.0.5 software (Pixmeo SARL, Bern, Switzerland) was used for analysis. Mean background was measured from several ROIs in the spleen. Gold amounts were calculated over the whole tumor volume (μg gold/mm^3).

4.11. Deep Learning-Based Quantification of AuNP Histology

The biodistribution of silver-stained AuNPs in histological slides was assessed with the help of a deep neural network. Regions of interest in each slide were defined via manual delineation. Slides were subdivided into smaller, slightly overlapping patches of 1000 × 1000 pixels to meet memory constraints. In a first preliminary step, AuNP concentrations were segmented with the help of color-channel-specific dynamic thresholding and morphological operations (opening and closing with fixed kernels). Parameters were manually tuned to optimize results for the majority of slides. In a second step, the best resulting binary masks were manually selected and partially manually corrected. In a third step, a deep neural network was trained to segment AuNP concentrations on this basis. In a final step, the trained network was used to derive segmentations of AuNP concentrations for all slide patches. A k-fold rotation of data splits was applied so that the network yields segmentations on data samples that were not used for training, ensuring that the segmentation represents the result of the learned task rather than replicates the threshold-derived training data. This procedure yielded substantially more accurate and consistent segmentations of AuNP concentrations as compared to the preliminary thresholding procedure. Subsequent re-concatenation of slightly overlapping slide patches ruled out boundary effects and double counting. In a postprocessing step, all individual AuNP concentrations were identified via connected-component analysis, allowing to assess their individual sizes.

The deep neural network follows a U-net like architecture and consists of 4 levels of en- and decoding units. Each layer of encoding units doubles the number of feature channels, starting from 16 and ending at 265 at the deepest [16] level. The network was trained for 10 epochs on a training set of ca. 5000 patches. Details of architecture, implementation, and training procedure follow a previously described protocol [34].

5. Conclusions

Herein, we show that the visualization of tumor cells with AuNPs by addressing membrane Hsp70 is feasible. We present data showing a superior uptake of cmHsp70.1-AuNPs inside Hsp70 membrane-positive tumor cells. Inside the tumor cells, these particles accumulated in the perinuclear region within 24 h. The Hsp70 specificity was shown since unconjugated nanoparticles and nanoparticles conjugated with an irrelevant control antibody were not taken up into Hsp70 membrane-positive tumor cells. Furthermore, Hsp70 knockout tumor cells that do not express Hsp70 in the cytosol and on the plasma membrane showed no uptake of the cmHsp70.1-conjugated nanoparticles [16]. Quantification of the internalized cmHsp70.1-conjugated AuNPs reveals a high sensitivity for the detection of single cells. Experiments are ongoing to study the capability of cmHsp70.1-AuNPs for spectral CT imaging of further Hsp70 membrane-positive and negative tumor models and whether these NPs can be exploited for therapeutic approaches. In the future, these antibody-conjugated AuNPs might be useful for the diagnosis of tumors and for radiotherapeutic interventions.

Author Contributions: Conceptualization, M.A.K. and S.S.; Data curation, M.A.K., M.S., C.W. and S.S.; Formal analysis, M.A.K., C.W., B.H.M., G.M. and S.S.; Funding acquisition, M.A.K., G.M. and S.S.; Investigation, M.S. and S.S.; Methodology, M.A.K., C.W., W.S., W.Z., O.S., R.P., O.B., M.M. and S.S.; Project administration, G.M. and S.S.; Resources, G.M. and S.S.; Supervision, B.H.M., E.J.R., G.M. and S.S.; Validation, M.A.K., C.W., O.S. and S.S.; Visualization, M.A.K., R.P. and S.S.; Writing—original draft, M.A.K. and S.S.; Writing—review and editing, M.A.K., M.S., C.W., W.S., W.Z., O.S., B.H.M., E.J.R., R.P., M.M., G.M. and S.S. All authors were involved in drafting the article or in revising it critically for important intellectual content. All authors have read and agreed to the published version of the manuscript.

Funding: The study was supported by the Russian Foundation for Basic Research (RFBR) according to the research project №20-38-70039 and DFG grant (SFB824/3, STA1520/1-1; ME 3718/5-1), Technische Universität München (TUM) within the DFG funding program Open Access Publishing. Additional financial support was provided by TaGoNaX DFG project №336532926.

Conflicts of Interest: The authors declare no conflict of interest.

Appendix A

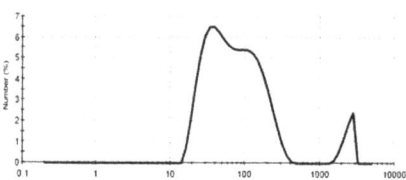

Figure A1. Size distribution of cmHsp70.1-AuNPs after 2 weeks at 4 °C: Size distribution is given in size by number histogram.

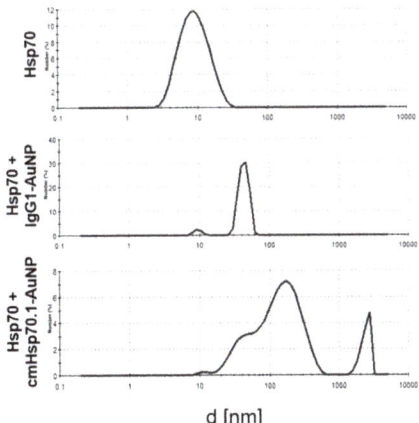

Figure A2. Size distribution of recombinant Hsp70 (upper panel) as well as IgG1-AuNPs (middle panel) and cmHsp70.1-AuNPs (lower panel) following incubation with recombinant Hsp70 for 4 h: Size distribution is given in size by number histograms.

References

1. Vanderstraeten, B.; Duthoy, W.; De Gersem, W.; De Neve, W.; Thierens, H. [18F]fluoro-deoxy-glucose positron emission tomography ([18F]FDG-PET) voxel intensity-based intensity-modulated radiation therapy (IMRT) for head and neck cancer. *Radiother. Oncol.* **2006**, *79*, 249–258. [CrossRef] [PubMed]
2. Bal, H.; Guerin, L.; Casey, M.E.; Conti, M.; Eriksson, L.; Michel, C.; Fanti, S.; Pettinato, C.; Adler, S.; Choyke, P. Improving PET spatial resolution and detectability for prostate cancer imaging. *Phys. Med. Biol.* **2014**, *59*, 4411–4426. [CrossRef]
3. Cormode, D.P.; Naha, P.C.; Fayad, Z.A. Nanoparticle contrast agents for computed tomography: A focus on micelles. *Contrast Media Mol. Imaging* **2014**, *9*, 37–52. [CrossRef]
4. Anjomrouz, M.; Shamshad, M.; Panta, R.K.; Broeke, L.V.; Schleich, N.; Atharifard, A.; Aamir, R.; Bheesette, S.; Walsh, M.F.; Goulter, B.P.; et al. Beam profile assessment in spectral CT scanners. *J. Appl. Clin. Med. Phys.* **2018**, *19*, 287–297. [CrossRef]
5. Chen, W.H.; Chen, J.X.; Cheng, H.; Chen, C.S.; Yang, J.; Xu, X.D.; Wang, Y.; Zhuo, R.X.; Zhang, X.Z. A new anti-cancer strategy of damaging mitochondria by pro-apoptotic peptide functionalized gold nanoparticles. *Chem. Commun.* **2013**, *49*, 6403–6405. [CrossRef]
6. Cormode, D.P.; Roessl, E.; Thran, A.; Skjaaa, T.; Gordon, R.E.; Schlomka, J.P.; Fuster, V.; Fisher, E.A.; Mulder, W.J.; Proksa, R.; et al. Atherosclerotic plaque composition: Analysis with multicolor CT and targeted gold nanoparticles. *Radiology* **2010**, *256*, 774–782. [CrossRef] [PubMed]
7. Shevtsov, M.; Zhou, Y.; Khachatryan, W.; Multhoff, G.; Gao, H. Recent Advances in Gold Nanoformulations for Cancer Therapy. *Curr. Drug Metab.* **2018**, *19*, 768–780. [CrossRef] [PubMed]
8. Sherman, M.; Multhoff, G. Heat shock proteins in cancer. *Ann. N. Y. Acad. Sci.* **2007**, *1113*, 192–201. [CrossRef]
9. Stangl, S.; Gehrmann, M.; Riegger, J.; Kuhs, K.; Riederer, I.; Sievert, W.; Hube, K.; Mocikat, R.; Dressel, R.; Kremmer, E.; et al. Targeting membrane heat-shock protein 70 (Hsp70) on tumors by cmHsp70.1 antibody. *Proc. Natl. Acad. Sci. USA* **2011**, *108*, 733–738. [CrossRef]
10. Hantschel, M.; Pfister, K.; Jordan, A.; Scholz, R.; Andreesen, R.; Schmitz, G.; Schmetzer, H.; Hiddemann, W.; Multhoff, G. Hsp70 plasma membrane expression on primary tumor biopsy material and bone marrow of leukemic patients. *Cell Stress Chaperones* **2000**, *5*, 438–442. [CrossRef]

11. Stangl, S.; Tontcheva, N.; Sievert, W.; Shevtsov, M.; Niu, M.; Schmid, T.E.; Pigorsch, S.; Combs, S.E.; Haller, B.; Balermpas, P.; et al. Heat shock protein 70 and tumor-infiltrating NK cells as prognostic indicators for patients with squamous cell carcinoma of the head and neck after radiochemotherapy: A multicentre retrospective study of the German Cancer Consortium Radiation Oncology Group (DKTK-ROG). *Int. J. Cancer* **2018**, *142*, 1911–1925. [CrossRef] [PubMed]
12. Farkas, B.; Hantschel, M.; Magyarlaki, M.; Becker, B.; Scherer, K.; Landthaler, M.; Pfister, K.; Gehrmann, M.; Gross, C.; Mackensen, A.; et al. Heat shock protein 70 membrane expression and melanoma-associated marker phenotype in primary and metastatic melanoma. *Melanoma Res.* **2003**, *13*, 147–152. [CrossRef] [PubMed]
13. Steiner, K.; Graf, M.; Hecht, K.; Reif, S.; Rossbacher, L.; Pfister, K.; Kolb, H.J.; Schmetzer, H.M.; Multhoff, G. High HSP70-membrane expression on leukemic cells from patients with acute myeloid leukemia is associated with a worse prognosis. *Leukemia* **2006**, *20*, 2076–2079. [CrossRef] [PubMed]
14. Gehrmann, M.; Radons, J.; Molls, M.; Multhoff, G. The therapeutic implications of clinically applied modifiers of heat shock protein 70 (Hsp70) expression by tumor cells. *Cell Stress Chaperones* **2008**, *13*, 1–10. [CrossRef] [PubMed]
15. Stangl, S.; Gehrmann, M.; Dressel, R.; Alves, F.; Dullin, C.; Themelis, G.; Ntziachristos, V.; Staeblein, E.; Walch, A.; Winkelmann, I.; et al. In vivo imaging of CT26 mouse tumours by using cmHsp70.1 monoclonal antibody. *J. Cell. Mol. Med.* **2011**, *15*, 874–887. [CrossRef] [PubMed]
16. Gehrmann, M.K.; Kimm, M.A.; Stangl, S.; Schmid, T.E.; Noel, P.B.; Rummeny, E.J.; Multhoff, G. Imaging of Hsp70-positive tumors with cmHsp70.1 antibody-conjugated gold nanoparticles. *Int. J. Nanomed.* **2015**, *10*, 5687–5700. [CrossRef]
17. Shevtsov, M.; Stangl, S.; Nikolaev, B.; Yakovleva, L.; Marchenko, Y.; Tagaeva, R.; Sievert, W.; Pitkin, E.; Mazur, A.; Tolstoy, P.; et al. Granzyme B Functionalized Nanoparticles Targeting Membrane Hsp70-Positive Tumors for Multimodal Cancer Theranostics. *Small* **2019**, *15*, e1900205. [CrossRef]
18. Schlomka, J.P.; Roessl, E.; Dorscheid, R.; Dill, S.; Martens, G.; Istel, T.; Baumer, C.; Herrmann, C.; Steadman, R.; Zeitler, G.; et al. Experimental feasibility of multi-energy photon-counting K-edge imaging in pre-clinical computed tomography. *Phys. Med. Biol.* **2008**, *53*, 4031–4047. [CrossRef]
19. Ashton, J.R.; Clark, D.P.; Moding, E.J.; Ghaghada, K.; Kirsch, D.G.; West, J.L.; Badea, C.T. Dual-energy micro-CT functional imaging of primary lung cancer in mice using gold and iodine nanoparticle contrast agents: A validation study. *PLoS ONE* **2014**, *9*, e88129. [CrossRef]
20. Hirsh, M.I.; Hashiguchi, N.; Chen, Y.; Yip, L.; Junger, W.G. Surface expression of HSP72 by LPS-stimulated neutrophils facilitates gammadeltaT cell-mediated killing. *Eur. J. Immunol.* **2006**, *36*, 712–721. [CrossRef]
21. Stangl, S.; Tei, L.; De Rose, F.; Reder, S.; Martinelli, J.; Sievert, W.; Shevtsov, M.; Ollinger, R.; Rad, R.; Schwaiger, M.; et al. Preclinical Evaluation of the Hsp70 Peptide Tracer TPP-PEG24-DFO[(89)Zr] for Tumor-Specific PET/CT Imaging. *Cancer Res.* **2018**, *78*, 6268–6281. [CrossRef]
22. Stangl, S.; Varga, J.; Freysoldt, B.; Trajkovic-Arsic, M.; Siveke, J.T.; Greten, F.R.; Ntziachristos, V.; Multhoff, G. Selective in vivo imaging of syngeneic, spontaneous, and xenograft tumors using a novel tumor cell-specific hsp70 peptide-based probe. *Cancer Res.* **2014**, *74*, 6903–6912. [CrossRef] [PubMed]
23. Cormode, D.P.; Si-Mohamed, S.; Bar-Ness, D.; Sigovan, M.; Naha, P.C.; Balegamire, J.; Lavenne, F.; Coulon, P.; Roessl, E.; Bartels, M.; et al. Multicolor spectral photon-counting computed tomography: In vivo dual contrast imaging with a high count rate scanner. *Sci. Rep.* **2017**, *7*, 4784. [CrossRef] [PubMed]
24. Si-Mohamed, S.; Cormode, D.P.; Bar-Ness, D.; Sigovan, M.; Naha, P.C.; Langlois, J.B.; Chalabreysse, L.; Coulon, P.; Blevis, I.; Roessl, E.; et al. Evaluation of spectral photon counting computed tomography K-edge imaging for determination of gold nanoparticle biodistribution in vivo. *Nanoscale* **2017**, *9*, 18246–18257. [CrossRef] [PubMed]
25. Schubertova, V.; Martinez-Veracoechea, F.J.; Vacha, R. Influence of ligand distribution on uptake efficiency. *Soft Matter* **2015**, *11*, 2726–2730. [CrossRef] [PubMed]
26. Lammers, T.; Kiessling, F.; Hennink, W.E.; Storm, G. Drug targeting to tumors: Principles, pitfalls and (pre-) clinical progress. *J. Control. Release* **2012**, *161*, 175–187. [CrossRef] [PubMed]
27. Zhang, X.D.; Wu, D.; Shen, X.; Liu, P.X.; Yang, N.; Zhao, B.; Zhang, H.; Sun, Y.M.; Zhang, L.A.; Fan, F.Y. Size-dependent in vivo toxicity of PEG-coated gold nanoparticles. *Int. J. Nanomed.* **2011**, *6*, 2071–2081. [CrossRef]

28. Alkilany, A.M.; Murphy, C.J. Toxicity and cellular uptake of gold nanoparticles: What we have learned so far? *J. Nanopart. Res.* **2010**, *12*, 2313–2333. [CrossRef]
29. Zhang, X.D.; Wu, H.Y.; Wu, D.; Wang, Y.Y.; Chang, J.H.; Zhai, Z.B.; Meng, A.M.; Liu, P.X.; Zhang, L.A.; Fan, F.Y. Toxicologic effects of gold nanoparticles in vivo by different administration routes. *Int. J. Nanomed.* **2010**, *5*, 771–781. [CrossRef]
30. Dorsey, J.F.; Sun, L.; Joh, D.Y.; Witztum, A.; Kao, G.D.; Alonso-Basanta, M.; Avery, S.; Hahn, S.M.; Al Zaki, A.; Tsourkas, A. Gold nanoparticles in radiation research: Potential applications for imaging and radiosensitization. *Transl. Cancer Res.* **2013**, *2*, 280–291. [CrossRef]
31. Muddineti, O.S.; Ghosh, B.; Biswas, S. Current trends in using polymer coated gold nanoparticles for cancer therapy. *Int. J. Pharm.* **2015**, *484*, 252–267. [CrossRef]
32. Hainfeld, J.F.; Dilmanian, F.A.; Zhong, Z.; Slatkin, D.N.; Kalef-Ezra, J.A.; Smilowitz, H.M. Gold nanoparticles enhance the radiation therapy of a murine squamous cell carcinoma. *Phys. Med. Biol.* **2010**, *55*, 3045–3059. [CrossRef]
33. Rothammer, A.; Sage, E.K.; Werner, C.; Combs, S.E.; Multhoff, G. Increased heat shock protein 70 (Hsp70) serum levels and low NK cell counts after radiotherapy—Potential markers for predicting breast cancer recurrence? *Radiat. Oncol.* **2019**, *14*, 78. [CrossRef]
34. Pan, C.; Schoppe, O.; Parra-Damas, A.; Cai, R.; Todorov, M.I.; Gondi, G.; von Neubeck, B.; Bogurcu-Seidel, N.; Seidel, S.; Sleiman, K.; et al. Deep Learning Reveals Cancer Metastasis and Therapeutic Antibody Targeting in the Entire Body. *Cell* **2019**, *179*, 1661–1676. [CrossRef]

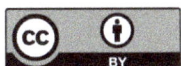

© 2020 by the authors. Licensee MDPI, Basel, Switzerland. This article is an open access article distributed under the terms and conditions of the Creative Commons Attribution (CC BY) license (http://creativecommons.org/licenses/by/4.0/).

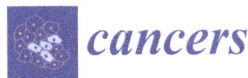

Article

^{18}F-FDG Pet Parameters and Radiomics Features Analysis in Advanced Nsclc Treated with Immunotherapy as Predictors of Therapy Response and Survival

Giulia Polverari [1,2,†], Francesco Ceci [1,*,†], Valentina Bertaglia [3], Maria Lucia Reale [3], Osvaldo Rampado [4], Elena Gallio [4], Roberto Passera [1], Virginia Liberini [1], Paola Scapoli [5], Vincenzo Arena [2], Manuela Racca [5], Andrea Veltri [6], Silvia Novello [3] and Désirée Deandreis [1]

1. Division of Nuclear Medicine, Department of Medical Sciences, University of Turin, AOU Città della Salute e della Scienza, 10126 Turin, Italy; giuliapolverari@yahoo.com (G.P.); passera.roberto@gmail.com (R.P.); v.liberini@gmail.com (V.L.); desiree.deandreis@unito.it (D.D.)
2. PET/CT Center, Affidea IRMET, 10135 Turin, Italy; vincenzo.arena@affidea.it
3. Department of Oncology, University of Turin, San Luigi Gonzaga Hospital, Orbassano, 10043 Torino, Italy; valentina.bertaglia@gmail.com (V.B.); realemarialucia@gmail.com (M.L.R.); silvia.novello@unito.it (S.N.)
4. Medical Physics Unit, S.C. Fisica Sanitaria, A.O.U. Città della Salute e della Scienza, 10135 Turin, Italy; orampado@cittadellasalute.to.it (O.R.); gallio.elena@gmail.com (E.G.)
5. Nuclear Medicine, Istituto per la Ricerca e la Cura del Cancro (IRCC), 10060 Candiolo, Italy; paola.scapoli@ircc.it (P.S.); manuela.racca@ircc.it (M.R.)
6. Radiology Unit, Department of Oncology, University of Turin, San Luigi Gonzaga Hospital, Orbassano, 10043 Torino, Italy; andrea.veltri@unito.it
* Correspondence: francesco.ceci@unito.it
† These authors contributed equally to this work.

Received: 11 March 2020; Accepted: 30 April 2020; Published: 5 May 2020

Abstract: Objectives: (1.1) to evaluate the association between baseline 18F-FDG PET/CT semi-quantitative parameters of the primary lesion with progression free survival (PFS), overall survival (OS) and response to immunotherapy, in advanced non-small cell lung carcinoma (NSCLC) patients eligible for immunotherapy; (1.2) to evaluate the application of radiomics analysis of the primary lesion to identify features predictive of response to immunotherapy; (1.3) to evaluate if tumor burden assessed by 18F-FDG PET/CT (N and M factors) is associated with PFS and OS. Materials and Methods: we retrospectively analyzed clinical records of advanced NCSLC patients (stage IIIb/c or stage IV) candidate to immunotherapy who performed 18F-FDG PET/CT before treatment to stage the disease. Fifty-seven (57) patients were included in the analysis (F:M 17:40; median age = 69 years old). Notably, 38/57 of patients had adenocarcinoma (AC), 10/57 squamous cell carcinoma (SCC) and 9/57 were not otherwise specified (NOS). Overall, 47.4% patients were stage IVA, 42.1% IVB and 8.8% IIIB. Immunotherapy was performed as front-line therapy in 42/57 patients and as second line therapy after chemotherapy platinum-based in 15/57. The median follow up after starting immunotherapy was 10 months (range: 1.5–68.6). Therapy response was assessed by RECIST 1.1 criteria (CT evaluation every 4 cycles of therapy) in 48/57 patients or when not feasible by clinical and laboratory data (fast disease progression or worsening of patient clinical condition in nine patients). Radiomics analysis was performed by applying regions of interest (ROIs) of the primary tumor delineated manually by two operators and semi-automatically applying a threshold at 40% of SUVmax. Results: (1.1) metabolic tumor volume (MTV) ($p = 0.028$) and total lesion glycolysis (TLG) ($p = 0.035$) were significantly associated with progressive vs. non-progressive disease status. Patients with higher values of MTV and TLG had higher probability of disease progression, compared to those patients presenting with lower values. SUVmax did not show correlation with PD status, PFS and OS. MTV ($p = 0.027$) and TLG ($p = 0.022$) also resulted in being significantly different among PR, SD and PD groups, while SUVmax was confirmed to not be associated with response to therapy ($p = 0.427$).

(1.2) We observed the association of several radiomics features with PD status. Namely, patients with high tumor volume, TLG and heterogeneity expressed by "skewness" and "kurtosis" had a higher probability of failing immunotherapy. (1.3) M status at 18F-FDG PET/CT was significantly associated with PFS ($p = 0.002$) and OS ($p = 0.049$). No significant associations were observed for N status. Conclusions: 18F-FDG PET/CT performed before the start of immunotherapy might be an important prognostic tool able to predict the disease progression and response to immunotherapy in patients with advanced NSCLC, since MTV, TLG and radiomics features (volume and heterogeneity) are associated with disease progression.

Keywords: PET/CT; immunotherapy; PD-1; PD-L1; response to therapy; NSCLC

1. Introduction

Lung cancer remains the leading cause of cancer-related death, despite continuous progresses in diagnosis and therapy [1]. Non-small cell lung carcinoma (NSCLC) accounts for 80–85% of all cases of lung cancer [1]. In almost half of the patients, the diagnosis of NSCLC is performed when the disease is already in advanced stages (stage III or stage IV), having an estimated overall 5-year survival rate of 18% [2]. In more than half of patients, the diagnosis of NSCLC is performed when the disease is already in advanced stage with an estimated overall 5-year survival rate of 18% [2,3]. Platinum-based chemotherapy can improve outcome, but the rise of immunotherapy has changed this scenario. Multiple molecules targeting the programmed cell death-1 (PD-1) and the programmed death ligand-1 (PD-L1) axis have been proposed [3]. Different immune checkpoint inhibitors have been approved in the second line setting on the basis of an improving in overall survival (OS) compared to chemotherapy, irrespective to PDL1 expression or with a PD-L1 expression ≥1% for pembrolizumab. Pembrolizumab has also been approved as first-line treatment for advanced NSCLC with PD-L1 higher than 50%, given the significant increase in both progression free survival (PFS) (10.3 versus 6 months) and OS (30 vs. 14.2 months) compared to chemotherapy [3,4]. Moreover, combination strategies of chemo-immunotherapy have recently enriched the upfront therapy approach. However, the benefit with immunotherapy is not seen for the entire population, making the identification of biomarkers and predicting tools a critical step in selecting the ideal candidate population. In NSCLC adenocarcinoma, platinum chemotherapy, plus pemetexered and pembrolizumab, reached a disease control rate of 84.6%, while it was 70.4% for chemotherapy only [5]. However, approximately 15% of positive PD-L1 patients will have disease progression within two months and a median survival of only three months [4]. The inter-patient, inter-tumour and even intra-tumour heterogeneity seem to be the major reasons of such a large prognosis variability, representing a key challenge for the scientific community. In this scenario, the application of new generation image analysis, such as radiomics, might provide further and useful information [6].

Radiomics is an emerging field, defined as the high-throughput extraction of quantitative features from medical images [6,7]. This approach provides high-dimensional data describing the properties of shape and texture of tumors captured in different diagnostic procedures, including PET imaging. The radiomics features are believed to contain information that reflects underlying tumor pathophysiology and allow evaluation of tumor heterogeneity [6,7]. The primary goal of radiomics is to build a clinically relevant predictive, descriptive, or prognostic model using these parameters. Focusing on the relationship between quantitative biological features and cancer prognosis by non-invasive method and aiding clinicians in selecting the appropriate treatments, radiomics is considered a step toward the application of personalized medicine in routine practice. In this respect, NSCLC is a key example to show the advantages of a tailored approach [8,9].

2. Materials and Methods

2.1. Objectives

The objectives of this study were:

(1.1) to evaluate the association between 18F-FDG PET/CT baseline semi-quantitative parameters of the primary lesion in advanced NSCLC patients eligible for immunotherapy with patient's outcome (PFS and OS) and response to immunotherapy,

(1.2) to evaluate the application of radiomics analysis of the primary lesion for texture analysis to extract characteristics (quantitative biomarkers) from PET/CT images to represent tumor pathology or heterogeneity (phenotype),

(1.3) to evaluate if tumor burden assessed by 18F-FDG PET/CT, as nodal (N) and metastatic (M) status, is associated with PFS and OS.

2.2. Study Design and Inclusion Criteria

This is a retrospective, observational study approved by the ethical committee A.O.U. Città della Salute e della Scienza di Torino (IRB number: 0011604; code: IMMUNO PET-19). We analyzed the records and clinical/pathological characteristics of patients referred to Pulmonary Oncology Department, San Luigi Gonzaga Hospital, University of Turin. Eligible patients matched all the following inclusion criteria: (a) biopsy proven advanced NSCLC (stage IIIb/c or stage IV); (b) candidate to immunotherapy targeting the PD-1 or PD-L1; (c) 18F-FDG PET/CT performed at baseline, during the diagnostic work-up, within the start of immunotherapy. Patients with missing data and lost follow-up were excluded from the analysis. Compliance with ethical standards: Ethical approval for all procedures performed in studies involving human participants was in accordance with the ethical standards of the institutional and/or national research committee and with the principles of the 1964 Declaration of Helsinki and its later amendments or comparable ethical standards. Informed consent and local ethical committee approval: informed consent form (ICF) was obtained from all individual participants enrolled in this retrospective analysis. ICF has been provided.

2.3. ^{18}F-FDG PET/CT Image Acquisition and Interpretation

Here, 18F-FDG PET/CT were performed with a standard protocol. Patients were instructed to fast for at least 6 h before the scan, and blood glucose levels were measured before the injection of 18F-FDG. Patients were excluded if their blood glucose levels at the time of the scans exceeded 150 mg/dL. Patient protocol included the intravenous injection of 2.5–3 MBq/kg of 18F-FDG, up to a maximum of 370 MBq (10 mCi), followed by a 60-min uptake period. All patients underwent PET/CT scan in a dedicated tomograph: AOU Città della Salute e della Scienza and IRCSS Istituto di Candiolo (Philips Gemini Dual-slice EXP, Philips Medical Systems, Cleveland, OH, USA)); Affidea-IRMET (Discovery 610, GE Healthcare, Chicago, IL, USA). An attenuation-corrected whole-body scan (base of the skull to mid thighs), 2 to 2.5 min per bed position (with an axial field-of-view of 18 cm per bed position), starting 60 min after tracer injection, was acquired. All patients performed a low-dose CT for attenuation correction and anatomical correlation of PET findings. The tomographs results were validated for a proper quantification and quality of the images recorded. The PET scans were reconstructed by ordered subset expectation maximization (OSEM)-based algorithms. All PET/CT images were analyzed with dedicated workstation (Advantage; GE Healthcare) and were independently interpreted with central reading by two nuclear medicine physicians, aware of clinical data.

2.4. PET Semi-Quantitative Parameters and Radiomics Analysis

Semi-quantitative PET parameters and radiomics features of the primary lesion were extracted using the open-access LIFEx platform v5.1 (IMIV/CEA, Orsay, France) [10]. For each primary lesion were evaluated PET semi-quantitative parameters, including maximum standardized uptake value

(SUVmax), metabolic tumor volume (MTV) and total lesion glycolysis (TLG). The delineation of each primary lung lesion was performed manually, slice-by-slice, independently by two expert operators. Region of interest (ROI) with a threshold at 40% of SUVmax was also applied. MTV represents the volume of the above given ROIs. 3D ROIs based on percentage of SUVmax were applied (3D isocontour at 41% of the maximum pixel value [VOI41]). TLG was calculated as the product of the ROI average SUVmean multiplied by the corresponding MTV. In the longitudinal setting, the quantitative metrics described above were derived using the same approach for all PET/CT examinations in the same patient. Radiomics features were extracted from each of the two ROIs. The following radiomics features were analyzed: size and shape based–features such as volume, maximum diameter along different orthogonal directions, maximum surface, tumor compactness, and sphericity; first-order statistics features reporting the mean, median, maximum, minimum values of the voxel intensities on the image, as well as their skewness (asymmetry), kurtosis (flatness), uniformity, and randomness (entropy) and second-order statistics features include the so-called textural features. Lymph node and systemic metastasis were evaluated and grouped as N and M status.

2.5. Evaluation of the Response to Immunotherapy

Therapy response was routinely assessed by CT evaluation every 4 cycles of therapy and by clinical/laboratory evaluation. The diagnostic assessment of response to immunotherapy was performed with response evaluation criteria in solid tumors (RECIST) 1.1 criteria. Complete response (CR) was the disappearance of the primary tumor, partial response (PR) was a decrease of 30% or more in the longest diameter of the primary tumor, progressive disease (PD) was an increase of 20% or more in the longest diameter of the primary tumor, and stable disease (SD) was noted in patients whose tumors did not show either sufficient shrinkage to qualify for PR or a sufficient increase to qualify for PD [11,12]. When CT evaluation was not feasible for fast disease progression or the worsening of patient clinical condition, the response to immunotherapy was performed by clinical and laboratory evaluation only.

2.6. Outcome Measurements and Statistical Analysis

Demographic and baseline disease characteristics were recorded, censoring the times of observation on July 2019, at a median follow-up of 10 months (IQR 6–14 months). The primary endpoint was PFS, while the secondary one was OS. PFS was defined as the time from the start of immunotherapy to progression/death for any cause. OS was defined as the time from the start of immunotherapy to death as a result of any cause; patients still alive were censored at the date of last contact. The response to immunotherapy was assessed considering both clinical follow-up and RECIST 1.1 criteria.

Patient characteristics were compared using the Fisher's exact test for categorical variables and the Mann–Whitney test for continuous ones. PFS and OS curves were estimated by the Kaplan–Meier method, comparing the two arms by the log-rank test and calculating 95% CIs. All p-values were obtained by 2-sided exact method at the conventional 5% significance level. All statistical analyses were performed in R 3.6.1.

Considering the radiomics analysis, univariate analysis with Kruskal–Wallis test was performed for each variable (histology, PDL-1 expression, disease stage, progression and response to therapy). The intraclass correlation coefficient (ICC) was used to assess intra- (by observer 1) and inter-observer (by observers 1 and 2) differences in texture and evaluate the reproducibility of textural parameters. The ICC was also used to assess differences in texture between manual and semi-automatic segmentation.

3. Results

3.1. Population Characteristics

Fifty-seven patients have been retrospectively enrolled: 17 females and 40 males, with a median age of 69 years old (range 39–84 years old). Three out of 57 patients were non-smokers, 33/57 were former smokers, while 21/57 were current smokers. Sixty-six percent (38/57) of patients had adenocarcinoma (AC), 17.5% (10/57) squamous cell carcinoma (SCC) and 15.7% (9/57) were not otherwise specified (NOS). According to the 8th Edition of TNM in Lung Cancer (8), about half of the patients (47.4%) were stage IVa, 42.1% were IVb and 8.8% of patients were IIIb. The Eastern Cooperative Oncology Group, performance status (ECOG PS) was 0 in 20/57 patients, 1 in 35/57 and two patients had an ECOG PS of 2. All patients were wildtype (no EGFR mutations, no ALK rearrangements detected). The PD-L1 expression on the bioptic specimen was evaluated in 51/57 patients. Notably, 80.4% of patients (41/51) presented a PD-L1 expression higher than 50%, 7.8% (4/51) between 1 and 49% and 11.8% (6/51) patients lower than 1%. All patients' characteristics are listed in Table 1.

Table 1. Overall population ($n = 57$) characteristics.

Characteristics	Value
Age	Median 69 years old (range 39–84)
Sex	
Male	40/57 (70.2%)
Female	17/57 (29.8%)
Smoking Status	
Non-smoker	3/57 (5.3%)
Ex-smoker	33/57 (57.9%)
Current smoker	21/57 (36.8%)
Histological Variant	
Adenocarcinoma	38/57 (66.6%)
Squamous cell carcinoma	10/57 (17.5%)
NOS	9/57 (15.7%)
ECOG PS	
0	20/57 (35.1%)
1	35/57 (61.4%)
2	2/57 (3.5%)
Stage at Diagnosis	
IB	1/57 (1.75%)
IIB	1/57 (1.75%)
IIIA	5/57 (8.8%)
IIIB	7/57 (12.3%)
IIIC	1/57 (1.7%)
IVA	26/57 (45.6%)
IVB	16/57 (28.1%)
Stage before IO	
IIIB	6/57 (8.8%)
IVA	27/57 (47.4%)
IVB	24/57 (42.1%)
PD-L1 expression analysis	
Not Performed	6/57 (10.5%)
<1%	6/57 (10.5%)
1–49%	4/57 (7.0%)
>50%	41/57 (72.0%)
Immunotherapy	
First line IO	42/57 (73.7%)
Second line IO	15/57 (26.3%)

NOS: Not Otherwise Specified; ECOG PS: Eastern Cooperative Oncology Group Performance Status; IO: Immuno-Oncology therapy.

3.2. Immunotherapy Scheme

Treatment was decided by referent physicians considering tumor histology, PD-L1 expression and patients' risk factors. Immunotherapy was performed as a frontline therapy in 42/57 (73.7%) patients and as a second line therapy after chemotherapy in 15/57 (26.3%) patients. The formers were all treated with Pembrolizumab after the assessment of PD-L1 expression higher than 50%. The latter were treated with Pembrolizumab in 5 cases, Nivolumab in 5 cases and Atezolizumab in 5 cases as well. Of these 15 cases treated with immunotherapy as second line, 8 patients received platinum + pemetrexed, 5 patients platinum + gemcitabine and 2 patients platinum + docetaxel. Six out of fifteen patients underwent surgery on the primary lesion before starting immunotherapy. Pembrolizumab, nivolumab and atezolizumab were administered intravenously at the standard dose.

3.3. Follow-Up and Therapy Response to Immunotherapy

The median follow-up was 10 months (range 1.5–68.6; IQR 6–14 months). Forty percent (23/57) of patients died from cancer-related causes, while 59.6% (34/57) were alive with evidence of disease. At the last follow-up, 30 patients were PD, 19 were SD and 8 were PR. No CR was observed. Thirty patients (52.6%) experienced disease progression during therapy. Among patients with progressive disease, 21 had the appearance of new lesions on CT performed as part of monitoring therapy response (RECIST 1.1). In 9 cases, CT evaluation was not feasible (fast disease progression or worsening of patient clinical condition) and disease progression was observed by clinical and laboratory evaluation.

Four patients experienced immunotherapy-induced toxicity (skin reaction, cough and rising liver enzymes) and four patients experienced acute events (transient ischemic attack, pneumonia and acute respiratory failure).

Immunotherapy was suspended in 30/57 patients. The causes of suspension were: progression (clinical and/or radiological) of disease in 27 cases assessed through CT and/or clinical evaluation, severe toxicity in 2 cases and death in 1 case. In 25/57 patients, immunotherapy was ongoing at the time of the last follow-up. The median number of cycles of therapy was 7 (mean = 11; range 1–69).

3.4. ^{18}F-FDG PET/CT Findings

First, 18F-FDG PET/CT was performed as routine diagnostic procedure to stage the disease before the start of immunotherapy. The median time from PET/CT and the start of immunotherapy was 37 days (mean = 45; range 4–133 days). All primary tumors, observed in the 51/57 patients who did not receive surgery and/or radiation therapy with radical intent, exhibited increased FDG uptake.

Twenty-two patients were N0, while 35/57 had positive lymph nodes (N+). In details, 10 were N1 (ipsilateral peribronchial and/or hilar and intrapulmonary), 12 patients were N2 (ipsilateral mediastinal and/or subcarinal nodes), and 13 patients were N3 (contralateral mediastinal or hilar nodes or supraclavicular nodes). Systemic metastases were seen in 34/57 patients, while 23 patients were staged as M0. 18F-FDG PET/CT observed adrenal metastases in 10 cases, contralateral lung nodules in 9, bone metastases in 9, liver lesions in 6, pleural involvement or malignant effusion in 5, extra-pulmonary lymph nodes in 2, soft tissue localization in 2 cases and 1 mesenterial nodule. Eleven patients were classified as M1a (contralateral lung or pleural/pericardial nodule or effusion), six were M1b (single extra-thoracic metastasis) and seventeen were M1c (multiple extra-thoracic metastases).

3.5. PET Semi-Quantitative Parameters Analysis (Objective 1.1)

The values of baseline 18F-FDG PET/CT semi-quantitative parameters of the primary lesion are listed in Table 2. At the Mann–Whitney test, MTV ($p = 0.028$) and TLG ($p = 0.035$) were significantly associated with progressive vs. non-progressive disease status (Table 3). Patients with higher values of MTV and TLG of the primary lesion at the baseline PET/CT had higher probability of disease progression, compared to those patients presenting with lower values. SUVmax values did not show significant association between the two groups (PD vs. non-PD patients) ($p = 0.55$). In the Kaplan–Meier plot analysis, the variables resulted associated with PD vs. non-PD status (MTV and TLG) were compared with PFS and OS (Figure 1). MTV and TLG were stratified according to the median value: upper and lower median value (MTV = 74.1 ml3; TLG = 310.8). Kaplan–Meier curves showed a trend to predict disease progression among patients with MTV and TLG lower or higher the median values. However, the log rank test of the two curves showed them not to be significantly different (Figure 1). In patients with MTV and TLG upper median values, PFS was 5 months, while OS was 15 months. In patients with MTV and TLG lower median values, PFS and OS were not reached (minimum 50% of events at last follow-up not reached).

Table 2. In this table; 18F-FDG PET/CT semi-quantitative parameters: SUVmax, metabolic tumor volume (MTV) and total lesion glycolysis (TLG) values.

PET Parameters	Minimum	Percentile 25	Median	Percentile 75	Maximum
SUVmax (g/mL)	1.4	5.8	9.5	13.5	30.5
MTV (mL^3)	3.1	36.7	74.1	163.3	695.2
TLG	2.8	87.3	310.8	852.9	4639.8

Table 3. SUVmax, MTV and TLG values among patients with progressive (PD) and non-progressive (non-PD) disease.

	Associations Between Baseline PET Parameters and PD vs. non-PD						
PET Parameters	Status	Minimum	Percentile 25	Median	Percentile 75	Maximum	p Value
SUVmax (g/mL)	PD	2.5	5.8	11.5	13.6	30.5	0.55
	non-PD	1.4	5.9	9.3	13.4	28.9	
MTV (mL^3)	PD	3.1	47.0	124.4	203.1	695.2	0.028
	non-PD	3.1	19.7	57.4	86.6	548.5	
TLG	PD	4.5	165.9	536.1	988.1	2820.3	0.035
	non-PD	2.8	55.0	205.8	417.8	4639.8	

In the Kruskal–Wallis test, MTV (p = 0.027) and TLG (p = 0.022) resulted in being significantly different among PR, SD and PD groups (Table 4). SUVmax was confirmed to not be associated with response to therapy criteria (p = 0.427) (Table 4).

Table 4. Association of MTV and TLG with response to immunotherapy, as assessed by response evaluation criteria in solid tumors (RECIST) 1.1 criteria and clinical follow-up.

PET Parameters	Associations Between Baseline PET Parameters and Response to Immunotherapy						
	Status	Minimum	Percentile 25	Median	Percentile 75	Maximum	p Value
SUVmax (g/mL)	PR	1.4	5.8	8.8	13.2	15.3	0.427
	SD	5.7	9.2	11.9	15.0	28.9	
	PD	2.5	6.4	10.7	13.5	30.5	
MTV (mL^3)	PR	3.1	15.3	49.5	79.6	173.9	0.027
	SD	26.9	72.2	75.0	375.9	548.5	
	PD	3.1	44.3	124.3	202.6	695.2	
TLG	PR	2.8	30.4	139.3	251.3	865.6	0.022
	SD	83.4	310.8	417.8	852.9	4639.8	
	PD	4.5	151.3	440.8	979.9	2820.3	

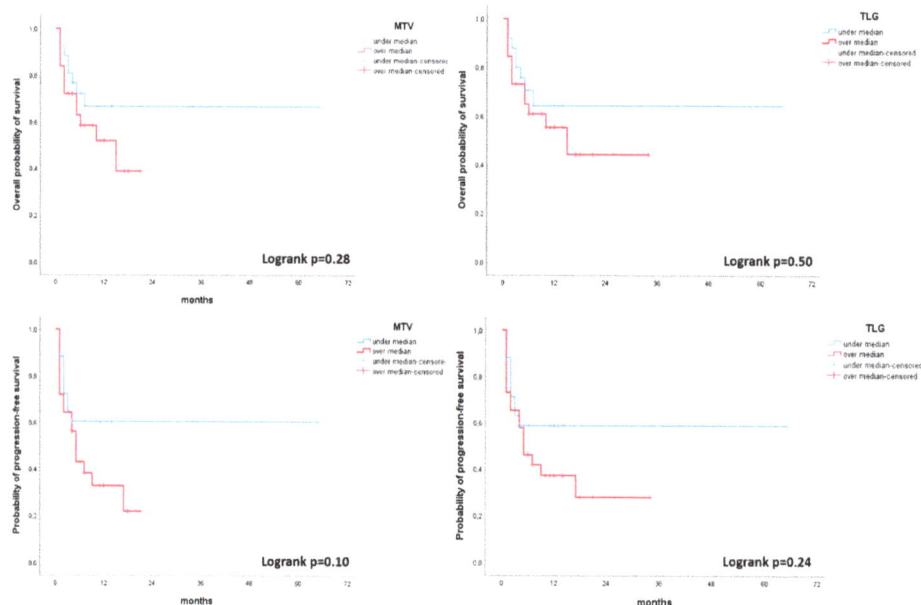

Figure 1. Kaplan–Meier plot analysis for MTV and TLG with both progression free survival (PFS) and overall survival (OS). Population was grouped by the median value of MTV (74.1) and TLG (310.8).

3.6. Radiomics Analysis (Objective 1.2)

The intraclass correlation coefficient (ICC) analysis of the texture parameters of the primary lesion, based on two different delineations generated by two observers, showed that all parameters presented good reproducibility (ICC > 0.95), except for GLZLM_SZLGE (ICC = 0.37). However, when applying a semi-automatic segmentation (threshold = 40% of the SUVmax), only 8 features showed good reproducibility (SUVmax, sphericity, two first-order statistics features and 4 textural features. ICC > 0.95). The univariate analysis with the Kruskal–Wallis test was performed for the following variables: histology, PDL-1 expression, disease stage, progression and response to therapy.

Histological variants: the only feature associated with different histological subtypes was SUVmax (Figure 2). Namely, SCC showed higher SUVmax values than AC and NOS subtype.

PD-L1 expression: several features (including SUVmax, volume, busyness, coarseness, GLZML_ZLNU and GLZML_GLNU) resulted in being significantly different between patients with PD-L1 expression lower than 1%, between 1% and 49% and higher than 50%. Considering the semi-automatic ROIs, only two features (coarseness and GLZLM_ZLNU) maintained the statistical correlation (Figure 3).

Disease stage: radiomics features did not show significant difference between IIIb, IVa and IVb patients at both manual and semi-automatic segmentation.

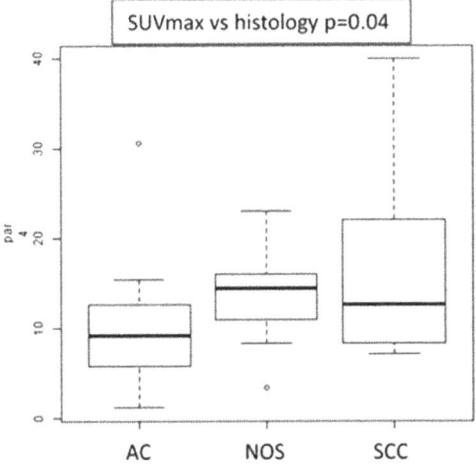

Figure 2. Box plot of SUVmax values showing differences between histological subtypes.

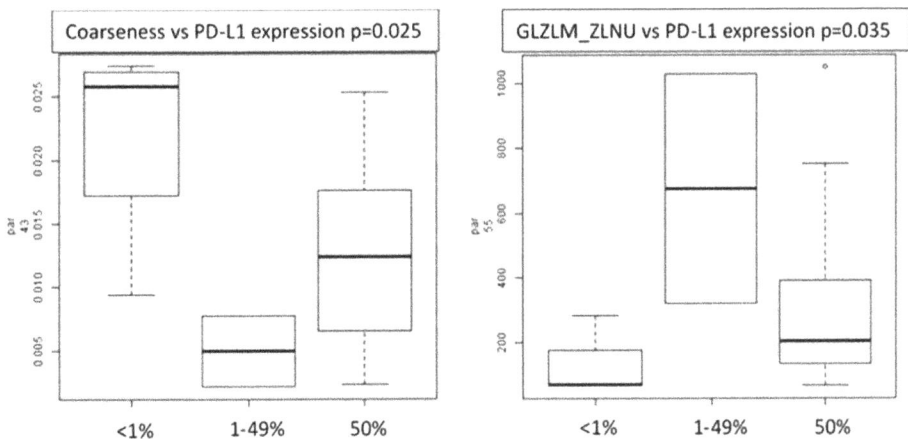

Figure 3. Box plots of radiomics features (coarseness and GLZLM_ZLNU) showing correlation with PD-L1 expression.

Progression status: several features showed differences between PD vs. non-PD patients, such as volume ($p = 0.035$), TLG ($p = 0.037$), three first-order histograms-based features (kurtosis, excess-kurtosis and skewness) and six textural features (GLZLM_LZE, GLRLM_RP, GLRLM_SRE, GLRLM_HGRE, GLRLM_SRHGE and GLCM Homogeneity) (Figure 4). GLZLM represents the grey-level zone length matrix and provides information on the size of homogeneous zones for each grey-level in 3 dimensions. GLZLM_LZE is the distribution of long homogeneous zones in an image. GLRLM represents the size of homogeneous runs for each grey level. "Run" means the presence of elements in the image with the same gray-level on in a row/line. GLCM_homogeneity considers the arrangements of pairs of voxels to calculate textural indices and represents the homogeneity of grey-level voxel pairs.

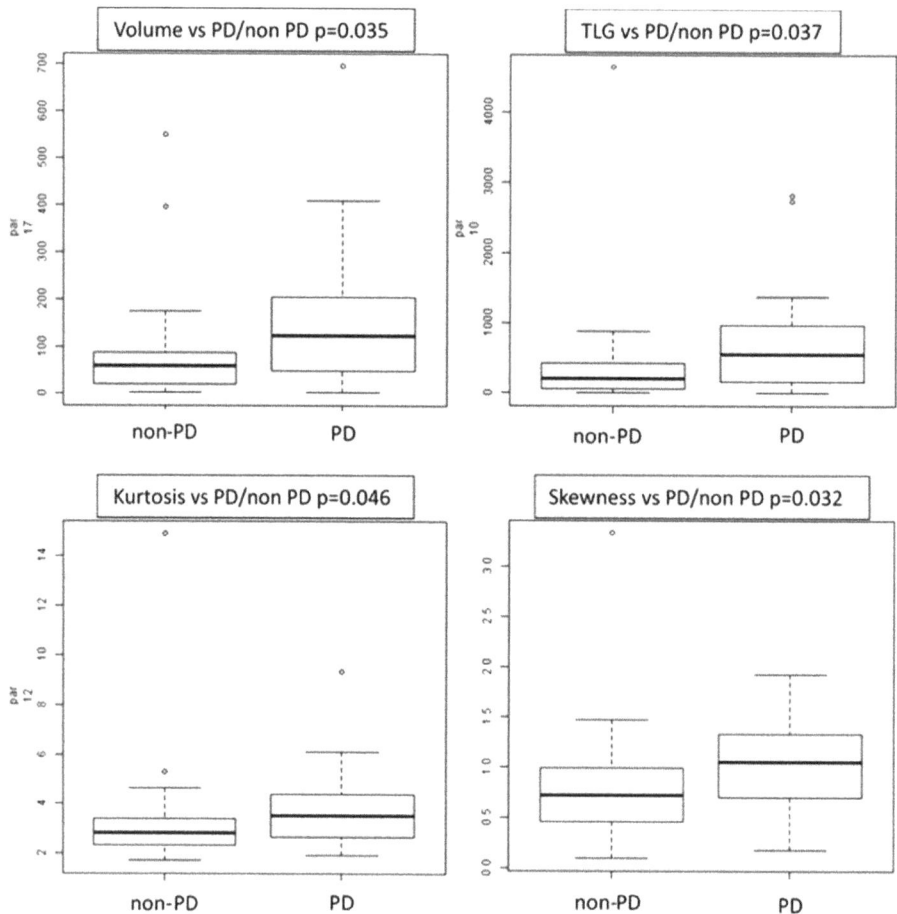

Figure 4. Box plots of radiomics features correlated with progressive (PD) vs. non-progressive disease status (non-PD).

Accordingly, patients with primary lung tumor presenting with higher TLG value, higher volume, higher asymmetry and kurtosis had higher probability to progress.

Response to therapy: TLG, volume and two textural features showed a significant difference between PR, SD and PD patients at both manual and semiautomatic evaluation.

3.7. Tumor Burden Analysis (Objective 1.3)

In the Kaplan–Meier plot analysis, M status (M0, M1a, M1b, M1c) as assessed by 18F-FDG PET/CT was significantly associated with PFS ($p = 0.002$) and OS ($p = 0.049$). Namely, patients with no visible metastases at PET/CT had significantly better outcome compared with those patients presenting with FDG avid metastases. No significant associations were observed for N status (N0, N1, N2, N3) as assessed by 18F-FDG PET/CT and PFS or OS. (Figure 5).

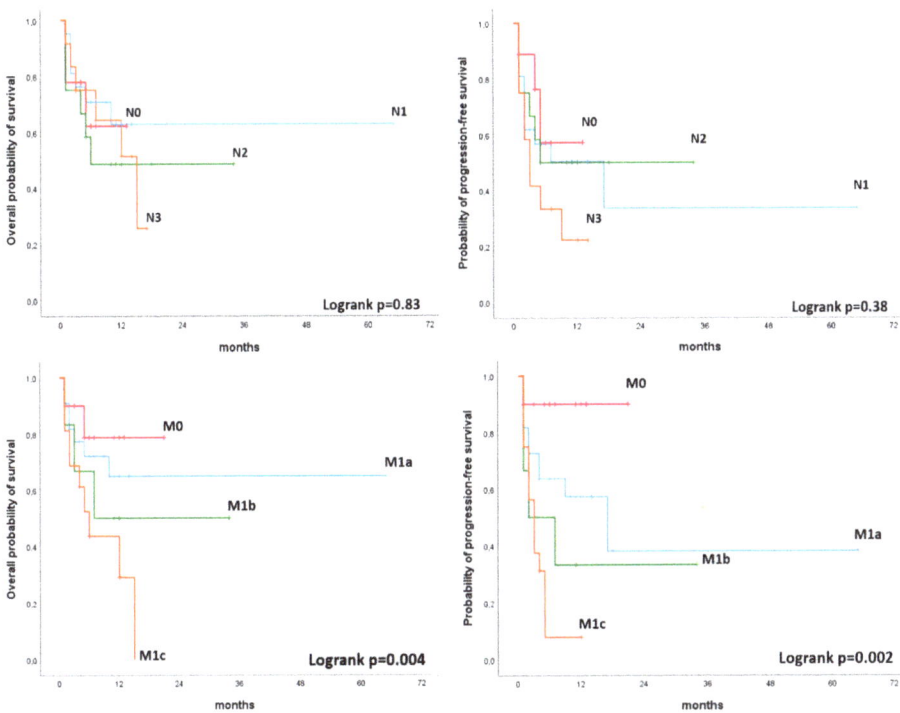

Figure 5. Kaplan–Meier plot analysis for N status (N0, N1, N2, N3) and M status (M0, M1a, M1b, M1c) with PFS and OS.

4. Discussion

Over the past decade 18F-FDG PET/CT demonstrated to be a powerful tool for staging and assessing treatment response in patients suffering from NSCLC [13,14]. Even if PET/CT is widely used in this clinical scenario, limited data are currently available regarding the role of PET/CT semi-quantitative parameters as predictors of patient outcome [15,16]. Findings are generally heterogeneous and this variability might be probably related to the heterogeneity of the population enrolled. Furthermore, the association of semi-quantitative parameters with patients' outcome can be related to the clinical stage of the disease (locally vs. advanced disease) and to the therapy investigated (chemo-radiotherapy vs. biological therapy) [15–18]. At present, SUV values, MTV and TLG are the PET-derived parameters used to assess the tumor metabolic activity in NSCLC [18]. MTV and TLG can easily be calculated in the primary tumor by means of a segmentation technique. The manual or semi-automatic measurement of the pre-treatment MTV has been shown to be better than SUVmax for predicting patients' prognosis in different solid neoplasms such as head and neck cancer, with or without metastases [19,20].

Our study aimed to investigate the relationship between the functional tumor parameters at baseline (SUVmax, MTV, and TLG) and PFS and OS in patients with advanced NSCLC, presenting with stage IIIB, IIIC, IVa and IVb, for whom immunotherapy was shortly planned. A significant association of MTV and TLG of the primary lesions with PD was observed, since lower MTV and TLG values were associated with non-PD status; while, on the contrary, primary lesions presenting with higher values were more likely associated with the progression of the disease during immunotherapy. On the contrary, SUVmax did not show significant association with both PFS and OS. These results are in accordance with recent studies, suggesting a superior correlation of volumetric 18F-FDG PET/CT parameters, rather than SUVmax only [7,9,21,22]. However, despite the fact that in the Kaplan–Meier analysis, MTV and TLG showed a trend in predicting disease progression, the curves associated with PFS and OS were not statistically significant. This is probably due to the relatively small sample size and the limited number of events that occurred.

Grizzi et al., in a preliminary analysis on 27 patients with NSCLC, found an antithetical correlation between 18F-FDG PET/CT pre-treatment parameters and the response to immunotherapy. Authors observed a rapid progression of disease after 8 weeks from the start of immunotherapy in patients with a SUVmax up to 17.1 and a SUVmean up to 8.3, with a sensitivity of 88.9% and 100%, respectively [23]. Similarly, Evangelista et al. investigated the role of semi-quantitative 18F-FDG PET/CT parameters in NSCLC treated with Nivolumab. Authors observed an association between the sum of metabolic parameters of all lesions and PD status, with SUVmax having the strongest association [24]. Their data seem to be in contrast with our analysis. However, authors considered all the lesions together as the cumulative sum of all FDG deposits detected by PET/CT, while we specifically designed our study to analyze semi-quantitative parameters of the primary lesion only, and we analyzed the correlation of the tumor burden (N and M status assessed by 18F-FDG PET/CT) separately, with a dedicated objective (objective 1.3). In our study, MTV and TLG were also significantly associated with immunotherapy response. Patients with SD or PR had lower values of MTV and TLG compared to patients with PD. No correlation was observed again between SUVmax values and response to therapy. Accordingly, since MTV and TLG are parameters that accurately reflect the glycolytic metabolic status of a lesion and thus the disease aggressiveness, 18F-FDG PET/CT might be considered as a prognostic tool to stratify patients presenting with higher metabolic primary tumors that, most likely, will fail immunotherapy. In our study, we also observed a significant association between the M status at 18F-FDG PET/CT and PFS and OS. It is worth noting that 18F-FDG PET/CT offers the possibility of having a single-step whole body examination that can clearly identify distant metastases and select NSCLC patients treated with immunotherapy with a higher probability of experiencing rapid disease progression and poor survival outcomes.

Immunotherapy has completely changed the prognosis and the care of patients with NSCLC. However, the benefit with immunotherapy is not seen for the entire population, making the identification of biomarkers a critical step in selecting the candidate population. Therefore, radiomics aims to identify biomarkers that better predict patient response [25,26]. Radiomics has been investigated in various studies to identify clinical and computational image-based predictors of rapid disease progression phenotypes in NSCLC patients [7,27,28]. However, there are only few studies investigating the application of this new field in patients with NSCLC treated with checkpoint-based immunotherapy and most of them based radiomics analysis on CT images and enrolled heterogeneous population with different primaries (e.g., lung and melanoma) [29,30]. Recently, Mu et al. presented promising data and a novel methodological approach on the application of radiomics analysis in NSCLC treated with immune checkpoint blockades. In their study, authors tested the hypothesis that radiomics features from baseline pretreatment 18F-FDG PET/CT scans can predict the clinical outcomes of NSCLC patients treated with checkpoint blockade immunotherapy. Among other findings, authors reported that when investigating the informative components of multi-parametric radiomics signature (mp-RS) formula, they found that multiple texture features (PET_SRLGE, KLD_SZE) positively correlated, suggesting that the more heterogeneous tumors had a larger probability to have a durable clinical benefit (DCB). These results are slightly in contrast with prior studies, which showed that more heterogeneous tumors with CT textures had worse response to radiation or chemotherapy [31]. Our results were slightly in contrast with Mu et al. [7] as well. In our study, the most interesting difference of features was seen between patients with PD and patients with non-PD. Namely, patients with primary lung tumor presenting with high TLG value, high volume and tumor heterogeneity represented by asymmetry (skewness feature) and kurtosis (how heavily the tails of a distribution differ from the tails of a normal distribution) had a higher probability of progression and were associated with non-response to immunotherapy. However, differences in features extraction methodology and different endpoints (DCB vs. PD) make these findings not completely comparable. Finally, segmentation is currently the rate-limiting step in radiomics analysis. To overcome this issue, in our study, the segmentation of the ROIs was performed manually by two independent operators and semi-automatically, applying a threshold of 40% of the SUVmax.

Limitation

This work is not exempt from limitations. The retrospective design of this analysis might have probably affected population selection. A prospective design would probably offer the chance to recruit a more homogenous population (e.g., same immunotherapy scheme, shorter range for PET scan before immunotherapy, immunotherapy administrated as first-line). Namely, in our cohort, 26.3% of patients received immunotherapy after platinum-based chemotherapy. However, the population enrolled represents the typical cohort of patients generally referred to 18F-FDG PET/CT before immunotherapy in daily clinical practice.

This analysis was performed in a relatively small sample size. A larger cohort would be preferable. In our study, we observed an association of MTV and TLG with PD vs. non-PD status. Nevertheless, this association was not maintained in the Kaplan–Meier analysis and, despite a non-negligible trend, MTV and TLG were not statistically significantly associated with PFS. The limited number of events at the end of follow-up, namely for patients with lower than median values for MTV and TLG, influenced the correlation between these metabolic parameters and PFS and OS. It is probable that our statistical model might rich significance in a larger cohort.

Another limitation is related to the lack of "early intermediate" PET performed while immunotherapy was still on-going, in order to evaluate PET response to therapy. However, since the role of PET imaging during immunotherapy is not yet established, 18F-FDG PET/CT is generally performed in clinical practice at baseline only. Thus, none of the patients enrolled in our study performed a second PET scan.

Considering radiomics analysis, the ideal setting would require a robust validation regarding reconstruction and segmentation on different tomographs. In our analysis, despite similar 18F-FDG PET/CT protocols and using the same reconstruction algorithm, the texture analysis was performed on images derived by three different tomographs. A common issue with radiomics analysis is represented by segmentation process (manual vs. automatic) and a comparison between the two approaches would be preferable. However, to strengthen our analysis, we included two operators who independently perform the segmentation. Furthermore, a threshold of 40% of SUVmax was also applied to both operators' ROI. Finally, in our study, segmentation was performed on PET images only, while low-dose CT images were not segmented, and so not considered in our radiomics analysis.

5. Conclusions

According to our results, baseline 18F-FDG PET/CT performed before the start of immunotherapy might be important, since it offers the chance to evaluate different quantitative parameters potentially associated with different response to therapy in patients with advanced NSCLC. In our study, and considering the limitations exposed above, MTV, TLG and radiomics features (volume and heterogeneity) were associated with disease progression, while metastatic tumor stages assessed with PET/CT were associated with different patients' outcome.

These results, while far from definitive evidence, encouraged us to initiate a prospective trial to investigate the role of radiomics features extracted from 18F-FDG PET/CT in NSCLC eligible to immunotherapy.

Author Contributions: Conceptualization, G.P., F.C., V.B., S.N. and D.D.; methodology, F.C. and R.P.; software, O.R., E.G. and V.L.; validation; F.C., D.D.; formal analysis, R.P., F.C., G.P. and O.R.; investigation, F.C. and G.P.; resources, D.D., S.N. and A.V.; data curation, G.P., V.A., P.S., M.R., V.B., and M.L.R.; writing—original draft preparation, G.P. and F.C.; writing—review and editing, F.C., G.P., D.D., V.B. and S.N.; visualization, F.C., G.P., V.A., M.R. and P.S.; supervision, F.C., A.V., S.N. and D.D.; project administration, G.P. and F.C. All authors have read and agreed to the published version of the manuscript.

Funding: This research received no external funding.

Conflicts of Interest: The authors declare no conflict of interest in relation to the present study.

References

1. Siegel, R.L.; Miller, K.D.; Jemal, A. Cancer statistics, 2018. *CA Cancer J. Clin.* **2018**, *68*, 7–30. [CrossRef] [PubMed]
2. Cancer statistics. *JAMA* **2013**, *310*, 982. [CrossRef] [PubMed]
3. Reck, M.; Rodríguez-Abreu, D.; Robinson, A.G.; Hui, R.; Csőszi, T.; Fülöp, A.; Gottfried, M.; Peled, N.; Tafreshi, A.; Cuffe, S.; et al. Pembrolizumab versus Chemotherapy for PD-L1-Positive Non-Small-Cell Lung Cancer. *N. Engl. J. Med.* **2016**, *375*, 1823–1833. [CrossRef] [PubMed]
4. Mezquita, L.; Auclin, E.; Ferrara, R.; Charrier, M.; Remon, J.; Planchard, D.; Ponce, S.; Ares, L.P.; Leroy, L.; Audigier-Valette, C.; et al. Association of the Lung Immune Prognostic Index with Immune Checkpoint Inhibitor Outcomes in Patients with Advanced Non–Small Cell Lung Cancer. *JAMA Oncol.* **2018**, *4*, 351–357. [CrossRef]
5. Paz-Ares, L.; Luft, A.; Vicente, D.; Tafreshi, A.; Gümüş, M.; Mazières, J.; Hermes, B.; Çay Şenler, F.; Csőszi, T.; Fülöp, A.; et al. Pembrolizumab plus Chemotherapy for Squamous Non-Small-Cell Lung Cancer. *N. Engl. J. Med.* **2018**, *379*, 2040–2051. [CrossRef]
6. Scrivener, M.; de Jong, E.E.; van Timmeren, J.E.; Pieters, T.; Ghaye, B.; Geets, X. Radiomics applied to lung cancer: A review. *Transl. Cancer Res.* **2016**, *5*, 398–409. [CrossRef]
7. Mu, W.; Tunali, I.; Gray, J.E.; Qi, J.; Schabath, M.B.; Gillies, R.J. Radiomics of 18F-FDG PET/CT images predicts clinical benefit of advanced NSCLC patients to checkpoint blockade immunotherapy [published online ahead of print, 2019 Dec 5]. *Eur. J. Nucl. Med. Mol. Imaging* **2019**. [CrossRef]
8. Sollini, M.; Cozzi, L.; Antunovic, L.; Chiti, A.; Kirienko, M. PET Radiomics in NSCLC: State of the art and a proposal for harmonization of methodology. *Sci. Rep.* **2017**, *7*, 358. [CrossRef]
9. Grizzi, F.; Castello, A.; Qehajaj, D.; Toschi, L.; Rossi, S.; Pistillo, D.; Paleari, V.; Veronesi, G.; Novellis, P.; Monterisi, S.; et al. Independent expression of circulating and tissue levels of PD-L1: Correlation of clusters with tumor metabolism and outcome in patients with non-small cell lung cancer. *Cancer Immunol. Immunother.* **2019**, *68*, 1537–1545. [CrossRef]
10. Nioche, C.; Orlhac, F.; Boughdad, S.; Reuzé, S.; Goya-Outi, J.; Robert, C.; Pellot-Barakat, C.; Soussan, M.; Frouin, F.; Buvat, I. LIFEx: A freeware for radiomic feature calculation in multimodality imaging to accelerate advances in the characterization of tumor heterogeneity. *Cancer Res.* **2018**, *78*, 4786–4789. [CrossRef]
11. Eisenhauer, E.A.; Therasse, P.; Bogaerts, J.; Schwartz, L.H.; Sargent, D.; Ford, R.; Dancey, J.; Arbuck, S.; Gwyther, S.; Mooney, M.; et al. New response evaluation criteria in solid tumours: Revised RECIST guideline (version 1.1). *Eur. J. Cancer* **2009**, *45*, 228–247. [CrossRef]
12. Detterbeck, F.C.; Boffa, D.J.; Kim, A.W.; Tanoue, L.T. The Eighth Edition Lung Cancer Stage Classification. *Chest* **2017**, *151*, 193–203. [CrossRef] [PubMed]
13. Huang, W.; Zhou, T.; Ma, L.; Sun, H.; Gong, H.; Wang, J.; Yu, J.; Li, B. Standard uptake value and metabolic tumor volume of 18F-FDG PET/CT predict short-term outcome early in the course of chemoradiotherapy in advanced non-small cell lung cancer. *Eur. J. Nucl. Med. Mol. Imaging* **2011**, *38*, 1628–1635. [CrossRef] [PubMed]
14. Banna, G.L.; Anile, G.; Russo, G.; Vigneri, P.; Castaing, M.; Nicolosi, M.; Strano, S.; Gieri, S.; Spina, R.; Patanè, D.; et al. Predictive and Prognostic Value of Early Disease Progression by PET Evaluation in Advanced Non-Small Cell Lung Cancer. *Oncology* **2017**, *92*, 39–47. [CrossRef] [PubMed]
15. Van de Wiele, C.; Kruse, V.; Smeets, P.; Sathekge, M.; Maes, A. Predictive and prognostic value of metabolic tumour volume and total lesion glycolysis in solid tumours. *Eur. J. Nucl. Med. Mol. Imaging* **2013**, *40*, 290–301. [CrossRef]
16. Visser, E.P.; Philippens, M.E.; Kienhorst, L.; Kaanders, J.H.; Corstens, F.H.; de Geus-Oei, L.F.; Oyen, W.J. Comparison of tumor volumes derived from glucose metabolic rate maps and SUV maps in dynamic 18F-FDG PET. *J. Nucl. Med.* **2008**, *49*, 892–898. [CrossRef]
17. Hofheinz, F.; Van den Hoff, J.; Steffen, I.G.; Lougovski, A.; Ego, K.; Amthauer, H.; Apostolova, I. Comparative evaluation of SUV, tumor-to-blood standard uptake ratio (SUR), and dual time point measurements for assessment of the metabolic uptake rate in FDG PET. *EJNMMI Res.* **2016**, *6*, 53. [CrossRef]

18. Dosani, M.; Yang, R.; McLay, M.; Wilson, D.; Liu, M.; Yong-Hing, C.J.; Hamm, J.; Lund, C.R.; Olson, R.; Schellenberg, D. Metabolic tumour volume is prognostic in patients with non-small-cell lung cancer treated with stereotactic ablative radiotherapy. *Curr. Oncol.* **2019**, *26*, e57–e63. [CrossRef]
19. Sharma, A.; Mohan, A.; Bhalla, A.S.; Sharma, M.C.; Vishnubhatla, S.; Das, C.J.; Pandey, A.K.; Sekhar Bal, C.; Patel, C.D.; Sharma, P.; et al. Role of Various Metabolic Parameters Derived From Baseline 18F-FDG PET/CT as Prognostic Markers in Non-Small Cell Lung Cancer Patients Undergoing Platinum-Based Chemotherapy. *Clin. Nucl. Med.* **2018**, *43*, e8–e17. [CrossRef]
20. Salavati, A.; Duan, F.; Snyder, B.S.; Wei, B.; Houshmand, S.; Khiewvan, B.; Opanowski, A.; Simone, C.B., 2nd; Siegel, B.A.; Machtay, M.; et al. Optimal FDG PET/CT volumetric parameters for risk stratification in patients with locally advanced non-small cell lung cancer: Results from the ACRIN 6668/RTOG 0235 trial. *Eur. J. Nucl. Med. Mol. Imaging* **2017**, *44*, 1969–1983. [CrossRef]
21. Chen, H.H.; Chiu, N.T.; Su, W.C.; Guo, H.R.; Lee, B.F. Prognostic value of whole-body total lesion glycolysis at pretreatment FDG PET/CT in non-small cell lung cancer. *Radiology* **2012**, *264*, 559–566. [CrossRef]
22. Liao, S.; Penney, B.C.; Wroblewski, K.; Zhang, H.; Simon, C.A.; Kampalath, R.; Shih, M.C.; Shimada, N.; Chen, S.; Salgia, R.; et al. Prognostic value of metabolic tumor burden on 18F-FDG PET in nonsurgical patients with non-small cell lung cancer. *Eur. J. Nucl. Med. Mol. Imaging* **2012**, *39*, 27–38. [CrossRef]
23. Grizzi, F.; Castello, A.; Lopci, E. Is it time to change our vision of tumor metabolism prior to immunotherapy? *Eur. J. Nucl. Med. Mol. Imaging* **2018**, *45*, 1072–1075. [CrossRef] [PubMed]
24. Evangelista, L.; Cuppari, L.; Menis, J.; Bonanno, L.; Reccia, P.; Frega, S.; Pasello, G. 18F-FDG PET/CT in non-small-cell lung cancer patients: A potential predictive biomarker of response to immunotherapy. *Nucl. Med. Commun.* **2019**, *40*, 802–807. [CrossRef] [PubMed]
25. Dennie, C.; Thornhill, R.; Sethi-Virmani, V.; Souza, C.A.; Bayanati, H.; Gupta, A.; Maziak, D. Role of quantitative computed tomography texture analysis in the differentiation of primary lung cancer and granulomatous nodules. *Quant Imaging Med. Surg.* **2016**, *6*, 6. [PubMed]
26. Kirienko, M.; Cozzi, L.; Rossi, A.; Voulaz, E.; Antunovic, L.; Fogliata, A.; Chiti, A.; Sollini, M. Ability of FDG PET and CT radiomics features to differentiate between primary and metastatic lung lesions. *Eur. J. Nucl. Med. Mol. Imaging* **2018**, *45*, 1649–1660. [CrossRef]
27. Nappi, A.; Gallicchio, R.; Simeon, V.; Nardelli, A.; Pelagalli, A.; Zupa, A.; Vita, G.; Venetucci, A.; di Cosola, M.; Barbato, F.; et al. FDG-PET/CT parameters as predictors of outcome in inoperable NSCLC patients. *Radiol. Oncol.* **2015**, *49*, 320–326. [CrossRef]
28. Pyka, T.; Bundschuh, R.A.; Andratschke, N.; Mayer, B.; Specht, H.M.; Papp, L.; Zsótér, N.; Essler, M. Textural features in pre-treatment [F18]-FDG-PET/CT are correlated with risk of local recurrence and diseasespecific survival in early stage NSCLC patients receiving primary stereotactic radiation therapy. *Radiat. Oncol.* **2015**, *10*, 100. [CrossRef]
29. Deutsch, E.; Paragios, N. Radiomics to predict response to immunotherapy, bridging the gap from proof of concept to clinical applicability? *Ann. Oncol.* **2019**, *30*, 879–881. [CrossRef]
30. Trebeschi, S.; Drago, S.G.; Birkbak, N.J.; Kurilova, I.; Călin, A.M.; Pizzi, A.D.; Lalezari, F.; Lambregts, D.M.J.; Rohaan, M.W.; Parmar, C.; et al. Predicting Response to Cancer Immunotherapy using Non-invasive Radiomic Biomarkers. *Ann. Oncol.* **2019**, *30*, 998–1004. [CrossRef]
31. Aerts, H.J.; Velazquez, E.R.; Leijenaar, R.T.; Parmar, C.; Grossmann, P.; Carvalho, S.; Bussink, J.; Monshouwer, R.; Haibe-Kains, B.; Rietveld, D.; et al. Decoding tumour phenotype by noninvasive imaging using a quantitative radiomics approach. *Nat. Commun.* **2014**, *5*, 4006. [CrossRef]

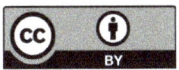

© 2020 by the authors. Licensee MDPI, Basel, Switzerland. This article is an open access article distributed under the terms and conditions of the Creative Commons Attribution (CC BY) license (http://creativecommons.org/licenses/by/4.0/).

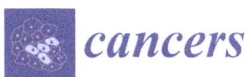

Article

Predictive Role of MRI and ^{18}F FDG PET Response to Concurrent Chemoradiation in T2b Cervical Cancer on Clinical Outcome: A Retrospective Single Center Study

Anna Myriam Perrone [1,2,*], Giulia Dondi [1,2], Manuela Coe [3], Martina Ferioli [4], Silvi Telo [5], Andrea Galuppi [2,4], Eugenia De Crescenzo [1], Marco Tesei [1,2], Paolo Castellucci [5], Cristina Nanni [5], Stefano Fanti [2,5], Alessio G. Morganti [2,4] and Pierandrea De Iaco [1,2]

1. Gynecologic Oncology Unit, Sant'Orsola-Malpighi Hospital, 40138 Bologna, Italy; giulia.dondi@gmail.com (G.D.); eugeniadecrescenzo@gmail.com (E.D.C.); marco.tesei2@gmail.com (M.T.); pierandrea.deiaco@unibo.it (P.D.I.)
2. Centro di Studio e Ricerca delle Neoplasie Ginecologiche (CSR) University of Bologna, 40138 Bologna, Italy; andrea.galuppi@aosp.bo.it (A.G.); stefano.fanti@aosp.bo.it (S.F.); alessio.morganti2@unibo.it (A.G.M.)
3. Department of Specialized, Diagnostic, and Experimental Medicine, Sant'Orsola-Malpighi Hospital, 40138 Bologna, Italy; manuela.coe@aosp.bo.it
4. Radiotherapy Unit, Sant'Orsola-Malpighi Hospital, 40138 Bologna, Italy; m.ferioli88@gmail.com
5. Nuclear Medicine Unit, Sant'Orsola-Malpighi Hospital, 40138 Bologna, Italy; silvi.telo@gmail.com (S.T.); paolo.castellucci@aosp.bo.it (P.C.); cristina.nanni@aosp.bo.it (C.N.)
* Correspondence: myriam.perrone@aosp.bo.it; Tel.: +39-349-8359-048

Received: 22 February 2020; Accepted: 11 March 2020; Published: 12 March 2020

Abstract: Tumor response in locally advanced cervical cancer (LACC) is generally evaluated with MRI and PET, but this strategy is not supported by the literature. Therefore, we compared the diagnostic performance of these two techniques in the response evaluation to concurrent chemoradiotherapy (CCRT) in LACC. Patients with cervical cancer (CC) stage T2b treated with CCRT and submitted to MRI and PET/CT before and after treatment were enrolled in the study. All clinical, pathological, therapeutic, radiologic and follow-up data were collected and examined. The radiological response was analyzed and compared to the follow-up data. Data of 40 patients with LACC were analyzed. Agreement between MRI and PET/CT in the evaluation response to therapy was observed in 31/40 (77.5%) of cases. The agreement between MRI, PET/CT and follow-up data showed a Cohen kappa coefficient of 0.59 (95% CI = 0.267–0.913) and of 0.84 (95% CI = 0.636–1.00), respectively. Considering the evaluation of primary tumor response, PET/CT was correct in 97.5% of cases, and MRI in 92.5% of cases; no false negative cases were observed. These results suggest the use of PET/CT as a unique diagnostic imaging tool after CCRT, to correctly assess residual and progression disease.

Keywords: locally advanced cervical cancer; PET/CT; MRI; concurrent chemoradiotherapy; treatment response; follow up

1. Introduction

Cervical carcinoma (CC) is the third commonest gynecological cancer in women worldwide [1,2]. In the past, CC was routinely staged with the clinical FIGO system but the new ESGO guidelines introduced and recommended a TNM classification with a FIGO staging, too [3–5]. Early CC and locally advanced CC (LACC) represent two different realities with distinct therapeutic approaches and prognosis. Surgery is the preferred approach in the early stage while concurrent chemoradiation (CCRT) is the standard treatment option in LACC [3,6–8]. The target of the external beam radiation therapy

(EBRT) includes the pelvic lymph nodes, but the irradiation field can be extended to the common iliac and para-aortic region in patients with nodal involvement [9,10]. The residual macroscopic tumor is then boosted with brachytherapy (BRT). CCRT allows local control of the disease in 70%–80% of patients, with 66% and 58% 5-year overall survival (OS) and disease-free survival (DFS) rates, respectively [11,12]. Recurrences occur in 22%–41% of patients, mostly within the first two years after the end of treatment. The recurrence site is more frequently loco-regional while distant metastases are rare [13]. Treatment response is evaluated 3-6 months after the end of CCRT, clinically and by imaging techniques [14]. Currently there is no agreement on the gold standard imaging technique to evaluate a tumor's response. Data in the literature are lacking and contradictory. MRI and PET/CT represent the most used imaging techniques [15,16] with different purposes: the assessment of response in the primary tumor (T) performed by MRI and assessment of response of the metastases performed by PET/CT [17,18]. In daily practice, usually MRI represents the first imaging method to evaluate response to therapy and PET/CT is mostly performed only if residual disease is suspected by MRI [3]. However, since clear and reliable data in this field are missing and there is no consensus on which technique should be used, the National Comprehensive Cancer Network (NCCN) [10] recommend both MRI and PET/CT as a post-treatment assessment of tumor response in LACC after CCRT [19].

Considering the uncertainty of current evidence, we retrospectively compared the diagnostic performance of ^{18}F-FDG PET/CT and MRI in the response evaluation after CCRT in LACC stage T2b.

2. Materials and Methods

2.1. Population

The clinical data of all patients with CC referred to our Unit of Gynecologic Oncology of Sant'Orsola Hospital of Bologna (Italy) between June 2007 and January 2017 were retrospectively analyzed. Among these we selected patients with stage T2b treated with CCRT.

Inclusion criteria were (a) histologically proven squamous cell cervical cancer and adenocarcinoma performed by biopsy or cone according to the WHO criteria [20]; (b) clinical stage T2b; c) treatment with CCRT; d) a pre-treatment pelvic MRI and total body ^{18}F-FDG PET/CT and post-treatment pelvic MRI and total body ^{18}F-FDG PET/CT performed in the radiologic service of our institution; and e) adequate follow-up over 24 months.

Exclusion criteria were (a) patients younger than 18 years old; (b) rare (other than squamous or adenocarcinoma) histological type; (c) a previous history of cancer in the last 5 years; (d) other stages different from T2b; (e) previous surgery or chemotherapy; and (f) pre- or post-treatment pelvic MRI and/or total body ^{18}F-FDG PET/CT performed in other centers.

All clinical and pathological data were collected and examined, including age, body mass index (BMI), histological type, TNM staging system [5], radiotherapy and chemotherapy administration.

2.2. Concurrent Chemo-Radiotherapy Scheme

All patients underwent pelvic 3-dimensional conformal EBRT. In patients with para-aortic lymph node metastases, detected by ^{18}F-FDG-PET/CT, the fields were extended up to the level of the renal vessels or even more cranially based on the positive node site. In case of large lymphadenopathy (short axis greater than one centimeter) with high ^{18}F-FDG uptake (SUV$_{max}$ > 3), a highly conformed EBRT boost was prescribed.

Cisplatin (40 mg/m^2) was administered intravenously once a week concurrently with EBRT. After radio-chemotherapy, all patients underwent a BRT boost, using the high dose rate (HDR) or pulsed dose rate (PDR) technique. The EBRT and BRT doses were prescribed according to the International Commission on Radiation Units and Measurements Reports 62 and 38, respectively [21].

2.3. Pelvic MRI Image Analysis

A baseline pelvic MRI was performed before the beginning of the treatment. An area with a high signal intensity in the cervix compared to the cervical stroma on the T2-weighted image with enhancement was considered neoplastic tissue in the pelvic MRI. Images were obtained with a high field magnet 1.5 T MRI system (GE, SIGNA LX HD-xt) using phase arrayed body coils. T2-weighted FSE images were obtained in sagittal, axial and oblique, perpendicular to the axis of the uterine cervix, and coronal with a 3–4 mm thickness and interslice gaps of 0.3/0.4 mm (matrix 320 × 224, FOV 28–32, 4NEX, TE 100, TR 3400) planes. LAVA 3D T1-weighted sequences were obtained before and after the intravenous (i.v.) injection of gadolinium contrast medium. Vaginal distension with aqueous gel (60 cc) was used in order to improve evaluation of the vaginal walls. Patients fasted for 4–6 h before the examination in order to reduce bowel motion artefacts and the bladder must be half full.

2.4. Total Body ^{18}F-FDG PET/CT Image Analysis

Whole body PET and low-dose CT scans were obtained one hour after the i.v. injection of 3.5 MBq/Kg of ^{18}F-FDG (PET scanner Discovery PET-CT 710, GE, Boston, Massachusetts, United States). A low dose Computed Tomography (CT) scan was performed both for attenuation correction and to provide an anatomical map. The CT parameters were 120KV, 80mA and 0.8 s for rotation, and a thickness of 3.75 mm. An iterative 3-D ordered subsets expectation maximization method with two iterations and 20 subsets, followed by smoothing (with a 6-mm 3-D gaussian kernel) with CT-based attenuation, scatter and random coincidence event correction, was used to reconstruct the PET images.

Patients fasted for 6 h and eventual insulin therapy was interrupted at least 6 h before the examination. All patients were positioned supine on the imaging table, arms above, and acquired from the base of the skull to the mid thighs. All ^{18}F-FDG PET/CT scans were reviewed by two expert nuclear medicine physicians with more than ten years of experience and a specific interest in gynecological malignancies. Discrepancies have been solved by consensus. For each scan, together with a visual assessment, a maximum standardized uptake value (SUV$_{max}$) was measured for every area of the focal uptake higher than the background and suspected to be a metastasis based on qualitative interpretation according to the location, the size and the intensity of the ^{18}F-FDG uptake.

2.5. Evaluation of the Response to CCRT

All patients were studied at baseline with pelvic MRI and total body ^{18}F-FDG PET/CT and treatment response was performed 6 months after the end of CCRT in the same tomographs. All radiological images were reviewed by M.C. for MRI and C.N. and P.C. for PET. Response to treatment was defined as complete response (CR), partial response (PR), progressive disease (PD) and stable disease (SD) according to RECIST criteria for the pelvic MRI and EORTC criteria for the ^{18}F-FDG PET/CT [22,23].

2.6. Follow Up

Patients defined as CR by both imaging techniques (^{18}F-FDG PET/CT and MRI) had a follow-up gynecological examination every 4 months in the first 2 years and every 6 months for 3 years. A chest–abdomen CT scan was performed every 12 months or in case of clinical suspicion of a relapse.

Patients defined not complete responders (PR, SD, PD) by one or both techniques were treated according to the localization of the residual or progressive disease (surgery or chemotherapy) or observed periodically with subsequent clinical or instrumental investigations in case of doubt.

Progression-free survival (PFS) was calculated from the first diagnosis to recurrence and overall survival (OS) was obtained from diagnosis to the last follow up or death.

The study was performed according to Helsinki declaration 2013, and all patients signed an informed consent and the local ethical committee of Sant'Orsola-Malpighi Hospital—Bologna approved this study (CE 322/2019/Oss/AUOBo).

2.7. Statistical Analysis

The software IBM SPSS ® 20.0, 2012 (Statistical Package for Social Science), was used for statistical data analysis and a *p*-value < 0.05 was considered statistically significant. Continuous variables were expressed as mean ± SD and categorical variables as percentages. Survival curves were calculated using the Kaplan–Meier method. Cohen's kappa was used to compare the two imaging techniques.

3. Results

3.1. Population

The flow chart of the recruitment is showed in Figure 1. In total, 40 patients met the inclusion criteria (patients with histologically proven squamous cell cervical cancer and adenocarcinoma stage T2b treated with CCRT with a pre-treatment pelvic MRI and total body ^{18}F-FDG PET/CT and post-treatment pelvic MRI and total body ^{18}F-FDG PET/CT performed in the radiologic service of our institution, and with adequate follow-up over 24 months) and were enrolled in the study. The patients' characteristics are reported in Table 1.

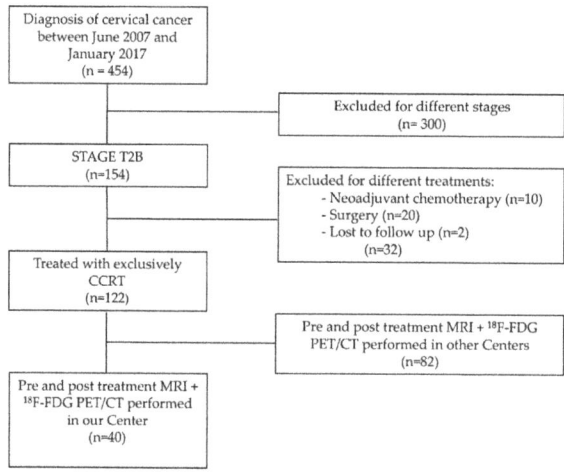

Figure 1. Flow chart of the study. Patient selection from our database of patients with cervical cancer.

Table 1. The population's characteristics.

Characteristics	Values
N	40
Age, years (mean ± SD)	61 ± 16
Mean age at diagnosis (mean ± SD)	55 ± 15
BMI mean (mean ± SD)	24.5 ± 4.2
Histotype	
Squamous *n* (%)	32 (80%)
Adenocarcinoma *n* (%)	8 (20%)
Stage TNM	
T2b	40 (100%)
N0	23 (57%)
N1	17 (43%)
M0	40 (100%)

Note: *n*: number of patients; BMI: body mass index; T: primary tumor; N: nodes; M: metastases.

The mean EBRT total dose was 45 ± 1 Gy, eight patients (20%) needed extended-field pelvic and para-aortic radiotherapy and the mean dose of the boost on the positive nodes was 15.1 ± 6.2 Gy. All patients received weekly Cisplatin at the dose of 40 mg/sm. Eight out of 40 patients (20%) received four cycles, 27/40 (67.5%) patients received five cycles and 5/40 (12.5%) patients received six cycles. All patients received a BRT boost with a mean dose of 28.7 ± 6.3 Gy.

3.2. MRI Parameters

The mean pre-treatment maximum tumor diameter measured by MRI was 45.5 ± 14.4 mm (mean ± SD). In six patients (15%) MRI detected nodal involvement and the mean node short-axis length was 19.5 ± 8.9 mm (mean ± SD). After treatment, a complete response of the primary cervical tumor was recorded in 32 (80%) patients, while residual disease was observed in eight (20%) patients. Only one metastatic lymph node was still present (2.5%) with a short-axis length of 15 mm.

3.3. ^{18}F-FDG PET/CT Parameters

Pathological uptake was present in all primary tumors and lymph node involvement was detected in 17/40 patients (43%). The mean pre-treatment SUV_{max} of the primary tumor was 14.2 ± 5.6 (mean ± SD) and the mean SUV_{max} of pathologic lymph nodes was 6.2 ± 2.6 (mean ± SD). After CCRT in 35 target lesions (87.5%) the uptake of ^{18}F-FDG was normalized and the SUV_{max} of the residual lesions was 9.7 ± 5.6 (mean ± SD). After the CCRT persistence, increased SUV_{max} in the lymph nodes was detected in five patients (12.5%), showing a mean SUV_{max} of 7.5 ± 5.1 (mean ± SD).

3.4. Agreement between MRI and ^{18}F-FDG PET/TC

Agreement between MRI and ^{18}F-FDG PET/CT in the evaluation response to therapy was observed in 31/40 (77.5%) of cases (Table 2 and Figure 2A,B). In these cases, a CR was observed in 28/31 patients (90.3%) and follow-up data showed a strong correlation with the response to therapy. In fact, only five out of 28 patients (18%) with CR experienced a subsequent treatment failure: Two local recurrences after 63 months and 64 months, respectively; one lung metastasis after 15 months; one vertebral metastasis after 24 months; and one patient showed lung and cerebellar metastases after 75 months. A PR was seen in 2/31 (6.5%) of the patients, who underwent rescue therapies. One of them underwent radical surgery and the histological exam confirmed residual disease in the cervix and in pelvic lymph nodes. The second one received palliative treatment because of severe comorbidities. Both patients died due to progressive disease after 12 and 18 months, respectively. One patient showed PD (1/31, 3.2%), and underwent a posterior exenteration (radical hysterectomy, bilateral salpingectomy, total colpectomy, pelvic and para-aortic lymphadenectomy, rectal resection with colorectal termino-terminal anastomosis and ileostomy). The patient died after 18 months.

Table 2. Concordance between MRI and FDG-PET/CT after CCRT.

MRI	^{18}F-FDG PET/CT				
	CR	PR	SD	PD	Total
CR	28	2	0	2	32
PR	3	2	0	2	7
SD	0	0	0	0	0
PD	0	0	0	1	1
Total	31	4	0	5	40

Note: CCRT: concomitant chemo-radiotherapy; CR: complete response; PR: partial response; SD: stable disease; PD: progression disease.

3.5. Disagreement between MRI and ^{18}F-FDG PET/CT

In 9/40 (22.5%) cases, MRI and ^{18}F-FDG PET/CT showed different results in terms of response (Tables 2 and 3). In Cases #1 and #2, MRI showed a CR, while ^{18}F-FDG PET/CT showed a PD due to the detection of distant metastasis in the lung and in a supraclavicular node, respectively. Both patients died after 47 and 33 months.

In Case #3 and #4, MRI showed a PR while ^{18}F-FDG PET/CT showed a PD. In particular, in Case #3 the MRI showed a PR while the ^{18}F-FDG PET/CT showed a CR of the primary lesion but also a vertebral metastasis. The patient underwent chemotherapy and died after 33 months. In Case #4, both imaging techniques showed a PR at the level of the cervical lesion but ^{18}F-FDG PET/CT detected also a common iliac lymph node metastasis. The patient underwent anterior exenteration (radical hysterectomy, bilateral salpingo-oophorectomy, total colpectomy, pelvic and para-aortic lymphadenectomy and total cystectomy with Indiana pouch neobladder reconstruction) followed by chemotherapy. The patient is still alive after 102 months of follow-up with no evidence of disease. The pathological evaluation confirmed the ^{18}F-FDG PET/CT findings.

In Cases #5 (Figure 2C,D), #6 and #7, MRI showed a PR while the ^{18}F-FDG PET/CT showed a CR. Patients #5 and #6 are alive after 48 and 67 months of follow-up, respectively, without evidence of disease and patient #7 died due to unrelated reasons (hearth attack).

In Case #8 both techniques reported CR in the pelvis but a glucose uptake near to the spleen was observed. The patient underwent surgery in order to remove the upper abdominal lesion and the pathological examination showed a desmoids tumor unrelated to CC. The patient is alive after 49 months of follow-up without evidence of disease.

In Case #9, ^{18}F-FDG PET/CT showed a borderline increase uptake in the primary tumor (SUV_{max} was 3.2), interpreted as a suspicious persistence of disease (PR), although MRI showed no sign of disease (CR); the patient is alive after 79 months of follow-up without evidence of disease.

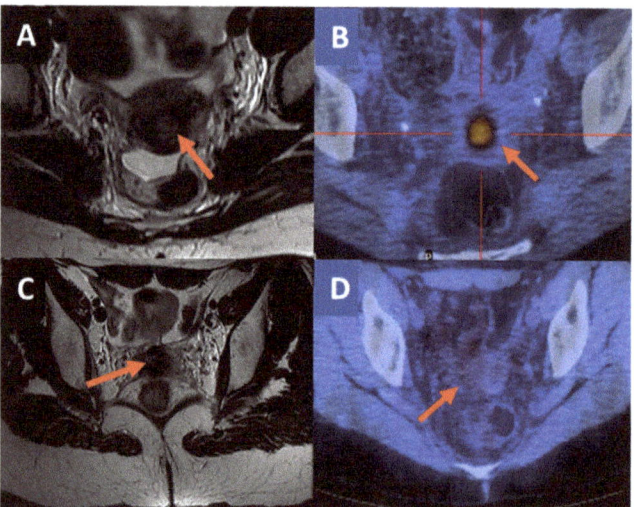

Figure 2. (**A**) and (**B**) show agreement between MRI and ^{18}F-FDG PET/CT after CCRT. The red arrows indicate the residual tumor (partial response). (**C**) and (**D**) show disagreement between MRI and ^{18}F-FDG PET/CT after CCRT. In panel (**C**) the red arrow indicates the residual tumor (partial response) and in (**D**) the red arrow indicates the absence of a tumor (complete response) in MRI and ^{18}F-FDG PET/CT, respectively.

Table 3. Details of discordant cases.

Case	¹⁸F-FDG PET/CT	MRI	FU	Localization of Disease and Treatment	Status to the Last FU
1	PD	CR	PD	Lung metastasis (PET) → chemotherapy	DOD
2	PD	CR	PD	Supraclavicular node metastasis (PET) → chemotherapy	DOD
3	PD	PR	PD	Vertebral metastasis (PET) → chemotherapy	DOD
4	PD	PR	PD	Common iliac lymph node metastasis (PET) → anterior pelvectomy and chemotherapy	NED
5	CR	PR	CR	Follow up → no disease	NED
6	CR	PR	CR	Follow up → no disease	NED
7	CR	PR	CR	Follow up → Died for hearth attack	DOC
8	PR	CR	CR	Uptake near the spleen → Abdominal surgery: desmoid tumor. Follow up → no disease	NED
9	PR	CR	CR	Follow up → no disease	NED

Note: CCRT = concomitant chemo-radiotherapy; CR = complete response; PR = partial response; SD = stable disease; PD = progressive disease; DOD = Died of disease; DOC = Died of other causes; NED = no evidence of disease; FU = follow up.

3.6. Follow-Up Outcomes

According to follow-up data we divided patients in 33 responders (82.5%) and seven non-responders (17.5%) (Table 4). Considering local control and distant metastasis, the number of false positive findings were one for ¹⁸F-FDG PET/CT (Case #9) and three for pelvic MRI (Cases #5, #6 and #7). The number of false negative findings were two (Cases #1 and #2) for pelvic MRI and none for ¹⁸F-FDG PET/CT.

The agreement between pelvic MRI, ¹⁸F-FDG PET/CT and follow-up data showed a Cohen kappa coefficient of 0.59 (95% CI = 0.267–0.913) and of 0.84 (95% CI = 0.636–1.00), respectively.

Considering the evaluation of primary tumor response, ¹⁸F-FDG PET/CT was correct in 97.5% of cases and MRI in 92.5% of cases; no false negative cases were observed with both methods.

The 5-year PFS and OS rates were, respectively, 78% and 88% (Figures 3 and 4).

Table 4. Accuracy in the treatment response evaluation of MRI and FDG-PET/CT compared to the follow-up data.

Response	FU data	¹⁸F-FDG PET/CT	MRI
Responders (CR)	33 (82.5%)	31 (77.5%)	32 (80%)
Non-responders (PR + SD + PD)	7 (17.5%)	9 (22.5%)	8 (20%)
False Positive Findings	-	1	3
False Negative Findings	-	0	2

Note: CCRT: concomitant chemo-radiation therapy; CR: complete response; PR: partial response; SD: stable disease; PD: progressive disease; FU: follow up.

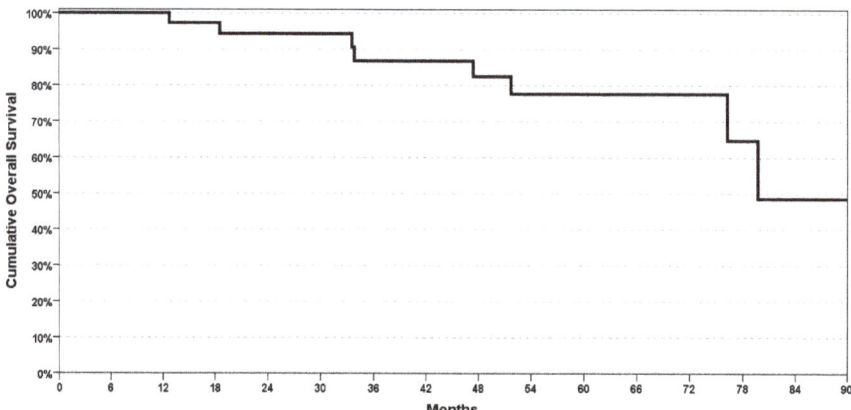

Figure 3. Kaplan–Mayer analysis of overall survival (OS).

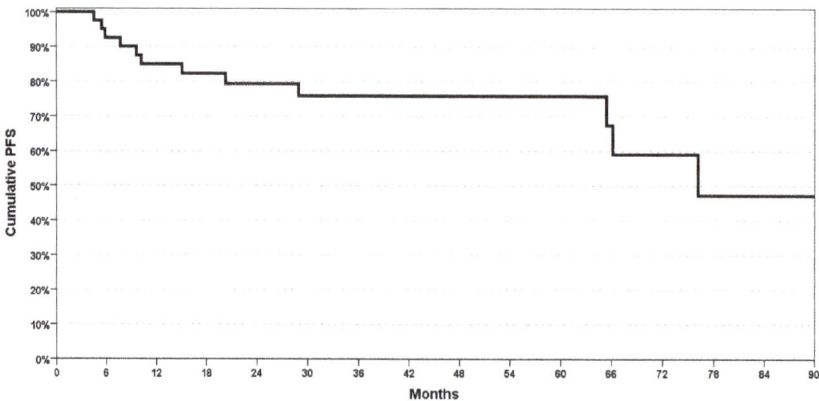

Figure 4. Kaplan–Mayer analysis of progression-free survival (PFS).

4. Discussion

Our retrospective study showed a better correspondence with the follow-up data of ^{18}F-FDG-PET/CT (0.84) with respect to MRI (0.59) in the evaluation of the response to CCR for primary tumor and distant metastasis in T2b CC.

T2b CC represents 38% of CC with the possibility of salvage surgery and complete response to therapy higher than other LACC stages. The persistence of disease in T2b tumors is important to plan salvage surgery. The surgeon's aim is to exclude the diagnosis of disease progression rather than macroscopic parametrial invasion since the therapy is not selective on the parametria but is represented by an exenteration surgery. In the literature, the role of MRI and ^{18}F-FDG-PET/CT before treatment in CC seems well defined. MRI is superior for the assessment of parametrial, vaginal, cervical, bladder and rectum involvement [24,25]. ^{18}F-FDG-PET/CT, instead, is more sensitive in detecting lymph node metastases (pelvic, paraaortic, inguinal and supraclavicular) and peritoneum, mesentery, gastrointestinal tract, pleura and mediastinal involvement [26]. Therefore, both exams are useful in the treatment choice (surgery or CCRT), and in RT planning [27,28]. However, evidence on the evaluation of response to CCRT are weak, although this assessment has a crucial role to decide subsequent treatments [29–32]. To detect residual disease, both clinical and radiological competences are needed. Unfortunately, gynecologic examination after RT is difficult to perform. Indeed, vaginal adhesions and post-RT fibrosis interfere with an accurate visualization of the cervix and with a thorough evaluation of the parametria [33]. Post-RT MRI scans may not optimally evaluate treatment response due to edema/inflammation in T2W hyperintense areas, as well as heterogeneous Gd-contrast enhancement from the main lesion [34]. On the other hand, post radiotherapy necrosis and inflammation may interfere with ^{18}F-FDG-PET/CT evaluation [35]. Therefore, well-defined roles of the two imaging techniques after CCRT are lacking.

In the assessment of primary tumor response, our data found that ^{18}F-FDG-PET/CT is more sensitive (100% versus 80%) and specific (97% versus 89%) than MRI. In fact, three cases correctly diagnosed by PET as CR were false positive using MRI (#5, #6 and #7). When we analyzed the false positive cases found with MRI, we found that probably they were due to the residual fibrosis subsequent to RT as reported in literature [36]. Based on these data, if we had performed only MRI, 20% of our patients would have received an incorrect diagnosis, while with ^{18}F-FDG-PET/CT this percentage would have been of only 3%. False positive results are an important issue: it could require subsequent exams, biopsies and the possibility of over-treatments and complications. These data are supported by a study concluding that MRI accuracy is not enough to select patients who can benefit from completion surgery if residual disease is suspected due to the high false positive rate [37]. In our experience, residual disease with MRI or ^{18}F-FDG-PET/CT after CCRT must be carefully considered before proceeding with further invasive investigations. Instead, in case of negative imaging, no doubt must arise because no false negative cases were observed with both techniques.

The incidence of metastatic progression of disease in LACC is not negligible, particularly in the upper abdomen and chest, even in patients with primary tumor controlled by CCRT. Indeed, in our series, in 10% of cases ^{18}F-FDG PET/CT showed distant metastases (PD) not detectable by pelvic MRI. In our experience, sensitivity and specificity of ^{18}F-FDG PET/CT when we considered distant metastasis was 100% and 97%, respectively; these values were higher than for MRI (71% and 91%, respectively). These values are similar to data from studies reporting 82%–100% and 78%–100% sensitivity and specificity rates for MRI, respectively, and 83%–100% and 50%–100% for ^{18}F-FDG PET/CT, respectively [38,39]. The sensitivity and specificity of PET increases for distant metastases (86% and 100%, respectively). These data highlighted the high diagnostic value of ^{18}F-FDG PET/CT and the importance of a total body evaluation in order to exclude progressive disease even if local control is achieved.

Based on this retrospective analysis we suggest that, after CCRT, ^{18}F-FDG PET/CT is effective in response evaluation and that MRI should only be reserved for special cases. It is not easy to compare the results of our study with those of the literature. To our knowledge there is a lack of studies that focused on the direct comparison between 18F-FDG PET/CT and MRI in in the response evaluation after CCRT in LACC stage T2b.

Waldestrom et al. examined 25 LACC patients (stages IB2–IIIB) with both MRI and ^{18}F-FDG PET/CT before and after CCRT and found that in almost half of the patients the ^{18}F-FDG-PET/CT before treatment provided additional diagnostic information leading to changes in treatment planning compared to information from MRI. MRI, instead, detected pelvic tumor spread not seen on the ^{18}F-FDG-PET/CT in 2/24 patients. [40]. On the contrary, a metanalysis of 15 studies of Maeds et al. evaluated the diagnostic accuracy of additional whole body ^{18}F-FDG PET/CT compared with conventional imaging in women with suspected recurrent/persistent cervical cancer, concluding that the use of ^{18}F-FDG PET/CT in recurrent cervical cancer and its endorsement by national guidelines is not supported by the literature. However, none of the studies included in this metanalysis directly compared additional PET–CT with MRI or CT separately, and the included populations were very heterogeneous and often follow-up periods were short. [41].

The results of other studies are generally based on the analysis of a single imaging technique, ^{18}F-FDG PET/CT [42,43] or CT/MRI [44], or reported that the addition of ^{18}F-FDG PET/CT to other imaging techniques increases the sensitivity and specificity [45]. Finally, no studies compared ^{18}F-FDG PET/CT with MRI and all studies had a short follow-up period. This fact represents an evident problem considering that follow-up accuracy and duration are important to confirm the radiological results, being a pathological response not available in case of CCRT. On the contrary, our study is supported by long-term follow up of 50 ± 26 months (mean ± SD), with overall survival results (Figure 3) consistent with data in the literature.

Some considerations about false positive of ^{18}F-FDG PET/CT are required. Case #8 developed a new and benign tumor, not related to the LACC. We considered this case as FP but probably it should be better considered as a concomitant disease. Case #9 was a borderline glucose case, which was not considered as a positive lesion and therefore the patient received no subsequent treatments.

Limitations of our study were the retrospective nature of the analysis and the small sample size, while strengths of the study could be considered the prolonged follow-up and the well-defined setting of patients. Further studies are needed to confirm our findings in a prospective setting.

5. Conclusions

In conclusion, ^{18}F-FDG PET/CT seems to be superior to pelvic MRI in the evaluation of the treatment response to CCRT in T2b CC. In addition, in some cases ^{18}F-FDG PET/CT detected distant metastasis resulting in a change in the therapeutic strategy. Further studies are needed to confirm that ^{18}F-FDG PET/CT should be the standard option, almost six months after the end of CCRT in LACC, to evaluate the treatment response. These results may suggest that ^{18}F-FDG-PET/CT is a unique diagnostic imaging tool to use after CCRT in order to correctly assess residual and progression disease.

Author Contributions: Conceptualization, A.M.P. and P.D.I.; methodology, S.F. and A.G.M.; software, M.T. and M.F.; validation, A.G. and M.F.; formal analysis, A.M.P and G.D.; investigation, A.M.P and P.D.I.; resources, M.C., P.C. and C.N.; data curation, G.D. and E.D.C.; writing—original draft preparation, A.M.P.; writing—review and editing, G.D. and S.T.; visualization, M.C., C.N. and P.C.; supervision, A.G.M. and S.F.; project administration, P.D.I. All authors have read and agreed to the published version of the manuscript.

Funding: This research received no external funding.

Acknowledgments: The authors are grateful to Stefano Friso for data collection and statistical analysis.

Conflicts of Interest: The authors declare no conflict of interest.

References

1. Jemal, A.; Siegel, R.; Ward, E.; Hao, Y.; Xu, J.; Thun, M.J. Cancer statistics. *CA Cancer J. Clin.* **2009**, *59*, 225–249. [CrossRef] [PubMed]
2. Ries, L.A.G.; Melbert, D.; Krapcho, M.; Stinchcomb, D.G.; Howlader, N.; Horner, M.J.; Mariotto, A.; Miller, B.A.; Feuer, E.J.; Altekruse, S.F.; et al. *SEER Cancer Statistics Review, 1975–2005*; National Cancer Institute: Bethesda, MD, USA, 2008.
3. Cibula, D.; Pötter, R.; Planchamp, F.; Åvall-Lundqvist, E.; Fischerova, D.; Meder, C.H.; Köhler, C.; Landoni, F.; Lax, S.; Lindegaard, J.C.; et al. The European Society of Gynaecological Oncology/European Society for Radiotherapy and Oncology/European Society of Pathology Guidelines for the Management of Patients with Cervical Cancer. *Int. J. Gynecol. Cancer* **2018**, *28*, 641–655. [CrossRef] [PubMed]
4. Bhatla, N.; Berek, J.S.; Fredes, M.C.; Denny, L.A.; Grenman, S.; Karunaratne, K.; Kehoe, S.T.; Konishi, I.; Olawaiye, A.B.; Prat, J.; et al. Revised FIGO staging for carcinoma of the cervix uteri. *Int. J. Gynecol. Obstet.* **2019**, *145*, 129–135. [CrossRef] [PubMed]
5. Brierley, J.; Gospodarowicz, M.K.; Wittekind, C. *TNM Classification of Malignant Tumours*; Wiley: Chichester, UK, 2017.
6. Marth, C.; Landoni, F.; Mahner, S.; McCormack, M.; Gonzalez-Martin, A.; Colombo, N. Cervical cancer: ESMO Clinical Practice Guidelines for diagnosis, treatment and follow-up. *Ann. Oncol.* **2017**, *28*, iv72–iv83. [CrossRef]
7. Fagotti, A.; Anchora, L.P.; Conte, C.; Chiantera, V.; Vizza, E.; Tortorella, L.; Surico, D.; De Iaco, P.; Corrado, G.; Fanfani, F.; et al. Beyond sentinel node algorithm. Toward a more tailored surgery for cervical cancer patients. *Cancer Med.* **2016**, *5*, 1725–1730. [CrossRef]

8. Fanfani, F.; Vizza, E.; Landoni, F.; De Iaco, P.; Ferrandina, G.; Corrado, G.; Gallotta, V.; Gambacorta, M.A.; Fagotti, A.; Monterossi, G.; et al. Radical hysterectomy after chemoradiation in FIGO stage III cervical cancer patients versus chemoradiation and brachytherapy: Complications and 3-years survival. *Eur. J. Surg. Oncol.* **2016**, *42*, 1519–1525. [CrossRef]
9. Ferrandina, G.; Anchora, L.P.; Gallotta, V.; Fagotti, A.; Vizza, E.; Chiantera, V.; De Iaco, P.; Ercoli, A.; Corrado, G.; Bottoni, C.; et al. Can We Define the Risk of Lymph Node Metastasis in Early-Stage Cervical Cancer Patients? A Large-Scale, Retrospective Study. *Ann. Surg. Oncol.* **2017**, *24*, 2311–2318. [CrossRef]
10. Koh, W.-J.; Abu-Rustum, N.R.; Bean, S.; Bradley, K.; Campos, S.M.; Cho, K.R.; Chon, H.S.; Chu, C.; Clark, R.; Cohn, D.; et al. Cervical Cancer, Version 3.2019, NCCN Clinical Practice Guidelines in Oncology. *J. Natl. Compr. Cancer Netw.* **2019**, *17*, 64–84. [CrossRef]
11. Chemoradiotherapy for Cervical Cancer Meta-Analysis Collaboration (CCCMAC) Reducing uncertainties about the effects of chemoradiotherapy for cervical cancer: Individual patient data meta-analysis. *Cochrane Database Syst. Rev.* **2010**, 008285.
12. Onal, C.; Reyhan, M.; Guler, O.C.; Yapar, A.F. Treatment outcomes of patients with cervical cancer with complete metabolic responses after definitive chemoradiotherapy. *Eur. J. Nucl. Med. Mol. Imaging* **2014**, *41*, 1336–1342. [CrossRef]
13. Quinn, M.; Benedet, J.; Odicino, F.; Maisonneuve, P.; Beller, U.; Creasman, W.T.; Heintz, A.; Ngan, H.; Pecorelli, S. Carcinoma of the Cervix Uteri. *Int. J. Gynecol. Obstet.* **2006**, *95*, S43–S103. [CrossRef]
14. Herrera, F.G.; Prior, J.O. The role of PET/CT in cervical cancer. *Front. Oncol.* **2013**, *3*. [CrossRef] [PubMed]
15. Schwarz, J.K.; Siegel, B.A.; Dehdashti, F.; Schwarz, J.K. Association of Posttherapy Positron Emission Tomography with Tumor Response and Survival in Cervical Carcinoma. *JAMA* **2007**, *298*, 2289. [CrossRef] [PubMed]
16. Hricak, H. Cancer of the uterus: The value of mri pre- and post-irradiation. *Int. J. Radiat. Oncol.* **1991**, *21*, 1089–1094. [CrossRef]
17. Saida, T.; Tanaka, Y.O.; Ohara, K.; Oki, A.; Sato, T.; Yoshikawa, H.; Minami, M. Can MRI predict local control rate of uterine cervical cancer immediately after radiation therapy? *Magn. Reson. Med Sci.* **2010**, *9*, 141–148. [CrossRef] [PubMed]
18. Salani, R.; Khanna, N.; Frimer, M.; Bristow, R.E.; Chen, L.-M. An update on post-treatment surveillance and diagnosis of recurrence in women with gynecologic malignancies: Society of Gynecologic Oncology (SGO) recommendations. *Gynecol. Oncol.* **2017**, *146*, 3–10. [CrossRef]
19. Hequet, D.; Marchand, E.; Place, V.; Fourchotte, V.; De La Rochefordière, A.; Dridi, S.; Coutant, C.; Lécuru, F.; Bats, A.-S.; Koskas, M.; et al. Evaluation and impact of residual disease in locally advanced cervical cancer after concurrent chemoradiation therapy: Results of a multicenter study. *Eur. J. Surg. Oncol.* **2013**, *39*, 1428–1434. [CrossRef]
20. Kurman, R.J. World Health Organization Classification of Tumours of Female Reproductive Organs. In *World Health Organization Classification of Tumours*, 4th ed.; International Agency for Research on Cancer: Lyon, France, 2014.
21. International Commission on Radiation Units and Measurements. *Dose and Volume Specification for Reporting Intracavitary Brachytherapy in Gynecology*; (ICRU) Report 38; The Commission: Bethesda, MD, USA, 1985.
22. Eisenhauer, E.A.; Therasse, P.; Bogaerts, J.; Schwartz, L.; Sargent, D.; Ford, R.; Dancey, J.; Arbuck, S.; Gwyther, S.; Mooney, M.; et al. New response evaluation criteria in solid tumours: Revised RECIST guideline (version 1.1). *Eur. J. Cancer* **2009**, *45*, 228–247. [CrossRef]
23. Young, H.; Baum, R.; Cremerius, U.; Herholz, K.; Hoekstra, O.; Lammertsma, A.A.; Pruim, J.; Price, P. Measurement of clinical and subclinical tumour response using [18F]-fluorodeoxyglucose and positron emission tomography: Review and 1999 EORTC recommendations. *Eur. J. Cancer* **1999**, *35*, 1773–1782. [CrossRef]
24. Park, J.J.; Kim, C.K.; Park, B.K. Prediction of disease progression following concurrent chemoradiotherapy for uterine cervical cancer: Value of post-treatment diffusion-weighted imaging. *Eur. Radiol.* **2015**, *26*, 3272–3279. [CrossRef]
25. Freeman, S.; Aly, A.M.; Kataoka, M.Y.; Addley, H.C.; Reinhold, C.; Sala, E. The Revised FIGO Staging System for Uterine Malignancies: Implications for MR Imaging. *Radiographics* **2012**, *32*, 1805–1827. [CrossRef] [PubMed]

26. Yen, T.-C.; Ng, K.-K.; Ma, S.-Y.; Chou, H.-H.; Tsai, C.-S.; Hsueh, S.; Chang, T.-C.; Hong, J.-H.; See, L.-C.; Lin, W.-J.; et al. Value of Dual-Phase 2-Fluoro-2-Deoxy-d-Glucose Positron Emission Tomography in Cervical Cancer. *J. Clin. Oncol.* **2003**, *21*, 3651–3658. [CrossRef] [PubMed]

27. Kusmirek, J.; Robbins, J.; Allen, H.; Barroilhet, L.; Anderson, B.; Sadowski, E. PET/CT and MRI in the imaging assessment of cervical cancer. *Abdom. Imaging* **2015**, *40*, 2486–2511. [CrossRef] [PubMed]

28. Cima, S.; Perrone, A.M.; Castellucci, P.; Macchia, G.; Buwenge, M.; Cammelli, S.; Cilla, S.; Ferioli, M.; Ferrandina, G.; Galuppi, A.; et al. Prognostic Impact of Pretreatment Fluorodeoxyglucose Positron Emission Tomography/Computed Tomography SUVmax in Patients with Locally Advanced Cervical Cancer. *Int. J. Gynecol. Cancer* **2018**, *28*, 575–580. [CrossRef] [PubMed]

29. Lima, G.M.; Matti, A.; Vara, G.; Dondi, G.; Naselli, N.; De Crescenzo, E.M.; Morganti, A.; Perrone, A.M.; De Iaco, P.; Nanni, C.; et al. Prognostic value of posttreatment 18F-FDG PET/CT and predictors of metabolic response to therapy in patients with locally advanced cervical cancer treated with concomitant chemoradiation therapy: An analysis of intensity- and volume-based PET parameters. *Eur. J. Nucl. Med. Mol. Imaging* **2018**, *45*, 2139–2146. [CrossRef]

30. Dessole, M.; Petrillo, M.; Lucidi, A.; Naldini, A.; Rossi, M.; De Iaco, P.; Marnitz, S.; Sehouli, J.; Scambia, G.; Chiantera, V. Quality of Life in Women After Pelvic Exenteration for Gynecological Malignancies. *Int. J. Gynecol. Cancer* **2018**, *28*, 267–273. [CrossRef]

31. Perrone, A.M.; Livi, A.; Fini, M.; Bondioli, E.; Concetti, S.; Morganti, A.; Contedini, F.; De Iaco, P. A surgical multi-layer technique for pelvic reconstruction after total exenteration using a combination of pedicled omental flap, human acellular dermal matrix and autologous adipose derived cells. *Gynecol. Oncol. Rep.* **2016**, *18*, 36–39. [CrossRef]

32. Chiantera, V.; Rossi, M.; De Iaco, P.; Koehler, C.; Marnitz, S.; Ferrandina, G.; Legge, F.; Parazzini, F.; Scambia, G.; Schneider, A.; et al. Survival After Curative Pelvic Exenteration for Primary or Recurrent Cervical Cancer: A Retrospective Multicentric Study of 167 Patients. *Int. J. Gynecol. Cancer* **2014**, *24*, 916–922. [CrossRef]

33. Galuppi, A.; Perrone, A.M.; La Macchia, M.; Santini, N.; Medoro, S.; Maccarini, L.R.; Strada, I.; Pozzati, F.; Rossi, M.; De Iaco, P. Local α-Tocopherol for Acute and Short-Term Vaginal Toxicity Prevention in Patients Treated with Radiotherapy for Gynecologic Tumors. *Int. J. Gynecol. Cancer* **2011**, *21*, 1708–1711. [CrossRef]

34. Jeong, Y.Y.; Kang, H.K.; Chung, T.W.; Seo, J.J.; Park, J.G. Uterine Cervical Carcinoma after Therapy: CT and MR Imaging Findings. *Radiographics* **2003**, *23*, 969–981. [CrossRef]

35. Schwarz, J.K.; Siegel, B.A.; Dehdashti, F.; Rader, J.; Zoberi, I. Posttherapy [18F] Fluorodeoxyglucose Positron Emission Tomography in Carcinoma of the Cervix: Response and Outcome. *J. Clin. Oncol.* **2004**, *22*, 2167–2171.

36. Wang, J.; Boerma, M.; Fu, Q.; Hauer-Jensen, M. Radiation responses in skin and connective tissues: Effect on wound healing and surgical outcome. *Hernia* **2006**, *10*, 502–506. [CrossRef] [PubMed]

37. Vincens, E.; Balleyguier, C.; Rey, A.; Uzan, C.; Zareski, E.; Gouy, S.; Pautier, P.; Duvillard, P.; Haie-Meder, C.; Morice, P. Accuracy of magnetic resonance imaging in predicting residual disease in patients treated for stage IB2/II cervical carcinoma with chemoradiation therapy. *Cancer* **2008**, *113*, 2158–2165. [CrossRef] [PubMed]

38. Viswanathan, C.; Faria, S.; Devine, C.; Patnana, M.; Sagebiel, T.; Iyer, R.B.; Bhosale, P. [18F]-2-Fluoro-2-Deoxy-D-glucose–PET Assessment of Cervical Cancer. *PET Clin.* **2018**, *13*, 165–177. [CrossRef]

39. Otero-García, M.M.; Mesa-Álvarez, A.; Nikolic, O.; Blanco-Lobato, P.; Basta-Nikolic, M.; De Llano-Ortega, R.M.; Paredes-Velázquez, L.; Nikolic, N.; Szewczyk-Bieda, M. Role of MRI in staging and follow-up of endometrial and cervical cancer: Pitfalls and mimickers. *Insights Imaging* **2019**, *10*, 19. [CrossRef]

40. Waldenström, A.-C.; Bergmark, K.; Michanek, A.; Hashimi, F.; Norrlund, R.R.; Olsson, C.E.; Gjertsson, P.; Leonhardt, H. A comparison of two imaging modalities for detecting lymphatic nodal spread in radiochemotherapy of locally advanced cervical cancer. *Phys. Imaging Radiat. Oncol.* **2018**, *8*, 33–37. [CrossRef]

41. Meads, C.; Davenport, C.; Małysiak-Szpond, S.; Kowalska, M.; Zapalska, A.; Guest, P.; Martin-Hirsch, P.; Borowiack, E.; Auguste, P.; Barton, P.; et al. Evaluating PET-CT in the detection and management of recurrent cervical cancer: Systematic reviews of diagnostic accuracy and subjective elicitation. *BJOG: Int. J. Obstet. Gynaecol.* **2013**, *121*, 398–407. [CrossRef]

42. Son, S.H.; Jeong, S.Y.; Chong, G.O.; Lee, Y.H.; Park, S.-H.; Lee, C.-H.; Jeong, J.H.; Lee, S.-W.; Ahn, B.-C.; Lee, J.; et al. Prognostic Value of Pretreatment Metabolic PET Parameters in Cervical Cancer Patients with Metabolic Complete Response After Concurrent Chemoradiotherapy. *Clin. Nucl. Med.* **2018**, *43*, e296–e303. [CrossRef]
43. Ryu, S.-Y.; Kim, M.-H.; Choi, S.-C.; Choi, C.-W.; Lee, K.H. Detection of early recurrence with 18F-FDG PET in patients with cervical cancer. *J. Nucl. Med.* **2003**, *44*.
44. Park, J.J.; Kim, C.K.; Park, S.Y.; Park, B.K. Parametrial Invasion in Cervical Cancer: Fused T2-weighted Imaging and High-b-Value Diffusion-weighted Imaging with Background Body Signal Suppression at 3 T. *Radiology* **2015**, *274*, 734–741. [CrossRef]
45. Grisaru, D.; Almog, B.; Levine, C.; Metser, U.; Fishman, A.; Lerman, H.; Lessing, J.B.; Even-Sapir, E. The diagnostic accuracy of 18F-Fluorodeoxyglucose PET/CT in patients with gynecological malignancies. *Gynecol. Oncol.* **2004**, *94*, 680–684. [CrossRef] [PubMed]

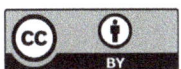

© 2020 by the authors. Licensee MDPI, Basel, Switzerland. This article is an open access article distributed under the terms and conditions of the Creative Commons Attribution (CC BY) license (http://creativecommons.org/licenses/by/4.0/).

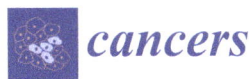

Article

Detection of Glioblastoma Subclinical Recurrence Using Serial Diffusion Tensor Imaging

Yan Jin [1], James W. Randall [1,2], Hesham Elhalawani [1], Karine A. Al Feghali [1], Andrew M. Elliott [1], Brian M. Anderson [3], Lara Lacerda [1], Benjamin L. Tran [1], Abdallah S. Mohamed [1], Kristy K. Brock [3], Clifton D. Fuller [1] and Caroline Chung [1,*]

1. Department of Radiation Oncology, the University of Texas MD Anderson Cancer Center, Houston, TX 77030, USA; yjinz@ucla.edu (Y.J.); jamesran92@gmail.com (J.W.R.); elhalawani.hesham@gmail.com (H.E.); kal1@mdanderson.org (K.A.A.F.); andrew.elliott@mdanderson.org (A.M.E.); lcalvarez@mdanderson.org (L.L.); bltran@mdanderson.org (B.L.T.); asmohamed@mdanderson.org (A.S.M.); cdfuller@mdanderson.org (C.D.F.)
2. The University of Texas Medical Branch, Galveston, TX 77555, USA
3. Department of Imaging Physics, the University of Texas MD Anderson Cancer Center, Houston, TX 77030, USA; bmanderson@mdanderson.org (B.M.A.); kkbrock@mdanderson.org (K.K.B.)
* Correspondence: cchung3@mdanderson.org

Received: 21 December 2019; Accepted: 27 February 2020; Published: 29 February 2020

Abstract: Glioblastoma is an aggressive brain tumor with a propensity for intracranial recurrence. We hypothesized that tumors can be visualized with diffusion tensor imaging (DTI) before they are detected on anatomical magnetic resonance (MR) images. We retrospectively analyzed serial MR images from 30 patients, including the DTI and T1-weighted images at recurrence, at 2 months and 4 months before recurrence, and at 1 month after radiation therapy. The diffusion maps and T1 images were deformably registered longitudinally. The recurrent tumor was manually segmented on the T1-weighted image and then applied to the diffusion maps at each time point to collect mean FA, diffusivities, and neurite density index (NDI) values, respectively. Group analysis of variance showed significant changes in FA ($p = 0.01$) and NDI ($p = 0.0015$) over time. Pairwise t tests also revealed that FA and NDI at 2 months before recurrence were 11.2% and 6.4% lower than those at 1 month after radiation therapy ($p < 0.05$), respectively. Changes in FA and NDI were observed 2 months before recurrence, suggesting that progressive microstructural changes and neurite density loss may be detectable before tumor detection in anatomical MR images. FA and NDI may serve as non-contrast MR-based biomarkers for detecting subclinical tumors.

Keywords: glioblastoma; radiation therapy; recurrence; MRI; diffusion tensor imaging

1. Introduction

Glioblastoma (GBM) is the most common primary malignant brain tumor among adults [1]. Despite treatment with surgical resection, radiation therapy (RT), chemotherapy, and temozolomide, many patients experience intracranial tumor recurrence, and prognosis remains poor, with a median survival time of only 12–15 months [2–4]. In current clinical practice, the onset of recurrence is defined in terms of changes in traditional images, such as contrast-enhanced computed tomography or structural T1-weighted post-contrast magnetic resonance imaging (T1 MRI), followed if possible by histologic verification. However, given the high frequency of recurrence in GBM and the poor survival rate thereafter, early detection of recurrence is key to facilitating timely medical treatment and prolonging survival.

Glioma cells have been shown to migrate into healthy brain tissues along white matter (WM) tracts [5,6]. The molecular mechanism underlying this phenomenon is complex and contains multiple steps, including tumor cell adhesion to components of the extracellular matrix and modification to their compositions, migration by breaking adherence attachments to the matrix, and the degradation of matrix proteins by secreting enzymes [7]. This suggests that examining the integrity of WM tracts within the potential recurrent regions before visible, enhancing tumor recurrence may help further elucidate the mechanism of recurrence.

Diffusion-weighted imaging is a noninvasive MRI technique in which measurements of water diffusion in tissues [8] provide biological and clinically relevant information about the integrity of WM that cannot be provided by other imaging modalities. Diffusion tensor imaging (DTI) applies a mathematical elliptical model to represent the diffusion characteristics at each voxel [9]. A variety of diffusion-derived feature maps, such as fractional anisotropy (FA), mean diffusivity (MD), axial diffusivity (AD), and radial diffusivity (RD), can be extracted from DTI images and have provided complementary information about the integrity of WM in several neurologic diseases, such as multiple sclerosis [10], Parkinson disease [11], and Alzheimer disease [12].

In brain tumors, DTI has previously been used to assess WM disruptions to identify tumor grades [13,14], distinguish tumor tissue from peritumoral tissue [15], and study the patterns of shape (isotropic versus anisotropic) in recurrence [16]. Reduced FA has been linked with decreased fiber density index near tumors in patients with GBM [17]. However, details of how WM tracts are disrupted during the clinical course of recurrence are yet to be elucidated. We hypothesized that tumor cells in the recurrent regions cause microstructural disruptions in WM integrity and these disruptions can be visualized by DTI before tumors can be detected on conventional anatomical MRI. To test this hypothesis, we conducted a retrospective longitudinal study to evaluate whether changes in a series of DTI feature maps precede the clinical onset of recurrence. We also used an advanced diffusion analysis technique, neurite orientation dispersion and density imaging (NODDI) [18], to provide further details on how microstructures in WM are affected at the microscale level.

2. Materials and Methods

2.1. Patients and Image Acquisition

Under an institutional review board-approved protocol (PA18-1113), we extracted MRI data from 30 patients treated for GBM at the University of Texas MD Anderson Cancer Center who had experienced recurrence after RT. All patients had anatomical T1 and DTI brain imaging at four time points: at 1 month after RT (baseline), 4 months before recurrence, 2 months before recurrence, and at recurrence. The average time between baseline and recurrence was 13 months with a standard deviation of 12 months.

All scans were obtained according to a standard protocol developed for GBM follow-up at the University of Texas MD Anderson Cancer Center and were acquired on 1.5 T/3T MRI scanners (GE Medical Systems) with axial orientation. T1 images had a 256 × 256/512 × 512 in-plane acquisition matrix and a voxel resolution of 0.86 × 0.86 × 6.5 mm^3 (TR/TE = 550/8 ms)/0.43 × 0.43 × 5 mm^3 (TR/TE = 967/12 ms). DTI images consisted of 28 volumes with a 256 × 256 in-plane acquisition matrix and a voxel resolution of 0.86 × 0.86 × 6.5 mm^3 (TR/TE = 1000/99 ms)/0.86 × 0.86 × 5 mm^3 (TR/TE = 10,250/94 ms), including one non-diffusion sensitization volume, i.e., T2-weighted b0 volume, and 27 diffusion-weighted volumes (b = 1200 s/mm^2).

2.2. Image Preprocessing

T1 images were first skull-stripped with the open source skull stripping toolkit LABEL [19]. DTI images were also skull-stripped with Brain Extraction Tool in the Functional Magnetic Resonance Imaging of the Brain (FMRIB) Software Library (FSL; https://fsl.fmrib.ox.ac.uk/fsl/fslwiki) [20,21] and then corrected for eddy current-induced distortions and subject movements using EDDY [22] in FSL.

2.3. Microstructural Features with NODDI

We used NODDI, an advanced diffusion analysis technique, to provide additional details about the microstructural features the images represent. Dendrites and axons, known as neural processes or neurites, are the basic units for brain circuits. Using NODDI to investigate variations in branching complexity (i.e., density and orientation) allowed us to characterize changes in microstructural integrity in terms of recurrence. Specifically, NODDI provides three indices to describe such changes: neurite density index (NDI), orientation dispersion index (ODI), and free water fraction (FWF) [23]. NDI and ODI quantify the density and angular variation of neurites, and FWF describes the contamination of tissues by free water at the microstructural level [23].

2.4. Longitudinal Image Processing Pipeline

Our longitudinal image processing pipeline consisted of the following six steps: Step 1. Diffusion Feature Extraction: The following diffusion-derived feature maps were extracted from the DTI images of each patient at each time point by using DTIFIT in FSL: fractional anisotropy (FA), mean diffusivity (MD), axial diffusivity (AD), and radial diffusivity (RD). Next, we calculated the microstructural indices (NDI, ODI, and FWF) at each voxel of the DTI images with the NODDI Matlab Toolbox (http://mig.cs.ucl.ac.uk/index.php?n=Tutorial.NODDImatlab). Step 2. Longitudinal Image Alignment: We applied advanced normalization tools (http://stnava.github.io/ANTs/) [24] to register each patient's T1 images at 1 month after RT, 4 months before recurrence, and 2 months before recurrence to the T1 image obtained at recurrence. Because these T1 images had been acquired at different times, a nonlinear (warping) registration algorithm was used to ensure the best alignment effect. Step 3. Multi-Modality Image Alignment: At each time point, each patient's DTI images were co-registered using linear (rigid) registration with the corresponding T1 images, as both images were acquired during the same imaging session. Step 4. GTV Manual Segmentation: An experienced radiation oncologist manually segmented the tumor recurrence volume on the T1 images at the time of recurrence. Step 5. GTV Transfer: For each patient, the recurrent tumor volume was applied to the T1 images at the previous three time points with the deformation fields generated by nonlinear registrations in step 2. The recurrent tumor volume was then transferred to the corresponding DTI images with the affine matrix generated by linear registrations in step 3. The quality of registration and GTV transfer at steps 2–5 was manually inspected. Step 6. Mean Feature Calculation: The mean values of all diffusion features (FA, MD, AD, and RD) and microstructural features (NDI, ODI, and FFW) within the transferred and original recurrent GTV regions at the four time points were calculated.

2.5. Statistical Analysis

We compared all mean DTI features at the four time points using analysis of variance (ANOVA) to examine potential changes between these time points. Findings are reported as F ratios, i.e., the ratio of the between-group variance to the within-group variance. If any changes were detected, t tests were applied to further investigate changes occurring at each pair of time points.

3. Results

3.1. Diffusion Feature Maps

Mean FA values inside the regions of recurrence over the four time points are shown in box plots in Figure 1a. The ANOVA revealed statistically significant differences between time points (F = 3.4, $p = 0.01$), with a downward trend over time. To further examine which groups were different from one another, we used pairwise t tests to compare the four time points. After Bonferroni correction, the mean FA value at recurrence was significantly lower than those at the three prior time points ($p < 0.05$), with a decrease of 30.8% (95% confidence interval-CI: (18.2%, 43.0%)), 22.9% (95% CI: (11.0%, 38.9%)), and 19.2% (95% CI: (8.7%, 35.4%)) from the farthest to the nearest time point, respectively. Moreover, the mean FA value at 2 months before recurrence was also 11.2% lower than that at 1 month after RT, i.e., the baseline ($p < 0.05$). At the individual level, 14 and 18 out of 30 patients showed a lower mean FA value at 4 months before recurrence and 2 months before recurrence, compared to baseline, respectively.

Findings from the ANOVA of the mean values of the other feature maps (MD, AD, and RD) over time are shown in Figure 1b–d. No statistically significant differences were detected in these feature maps between time points: for MD, $F = 1.38$, $p = 0.25$; for AD, $F = 0.99$, $p = 0.40$; and for RD, $F = 1.57$, $p = 0.20$. Although these values were not statistically different, they demonstrated a trend of increasing values over time, as is evident in those figures. Further pairwise t tests showed that the mean values of MD, AD, and RD at 2 months before recurrence were 9.5% (95% CI: (4.0%, 15.4%)), 7.8% (95% CI: (2.5%, 13.0%)), and 10.9% (95% CI: (4.8%, 17.1%)) higher than those at baseline, respectively ($p < 0.05$ after Bonferroni correction). At the individual level, 18, 16, and 18 patients had a higher mean MD, AD, and RD value at 2 months before recurrence, compared to baseline, respectively.

Changes in these features (FA, MD, AD, and RD) may indicate that WM degeneration occurred at recurrent tumor regions before the tumor became visible on T1.

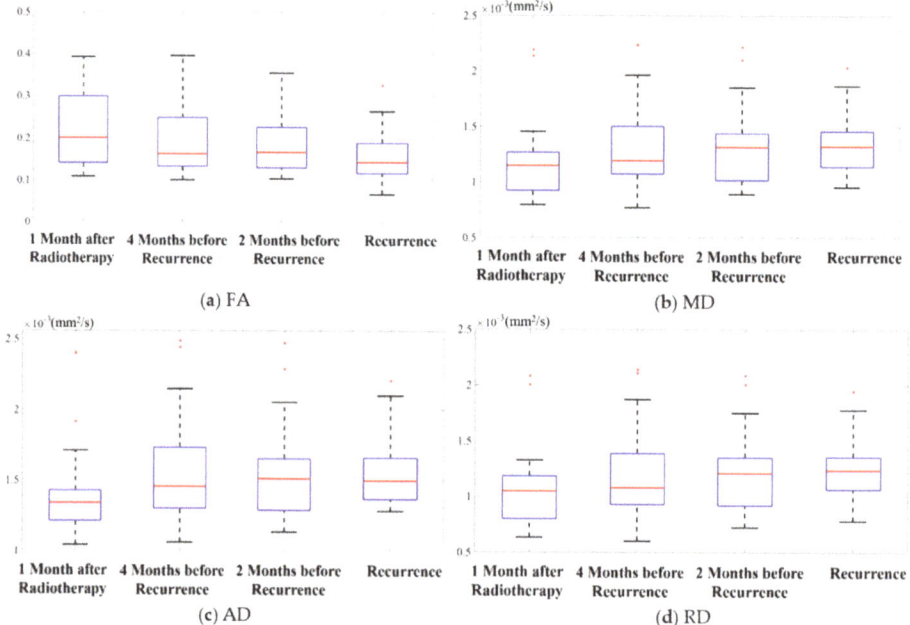

Figure 1. Box plots of the mean values of (**a**) fractional anisotropy (FA), (**b**) mean diffusivity (MD), (**c**) axial diffusivity (AD), and (**d**) radial diffusivity (RD) within recurrent tumor regions over the four time points. The five bars in the box plots indicate, from bottom to top, the minimum, first quartile, median, third quartile, and the maximum. The red dots indicate outliers.

3.2. Microstructural Features

To investigate which WM microstructural components were affected by tumor recurrence, we used the same statistical tests of the mean values of NDI, ODI, and FFW (obtained with the NODDI toolbox) at the regions of recurrence over time. The NDI results were similar to those of the FA findings (Figure 2a). ANOVA revealed differences among the four time points ($F = 5.47$, $p = 0.0015$), with a downward trend over time. Pairwise t tests showed that the mean NDI value at recurrence was significantly lower than baseline and 4 months before recurrence, a relative change of 11.9% (95% CI: (4.3%, 19.5%)), and 7.2% (95% CI: (0.4%, 15.6%)), respectively ($p < 0.05$ after Bonferroni correction).

Furthermore, compared to baseline, the mean NDI values at 4 months before recurrence were 4.2% (95% CI: (1.5%, 6.9%)) lower and the mean NDI values at 2 months before recurrence were 6.4% (95% CI: (3.4%, 9.5%)) lower ($p < 0.05$ after Bonferroni correction). At the individual level, 21 and 20 patients demonstrated a reduced mean NDI value at 4 months before recurrence and 2 months before recurrence, compared to baseline, respectively.

The ANOVA showed no differences in ODI over time (F = 1.16, p = 0.33) (Figure 2b). Similarly, FWF did not change over time according to the ANOVA (F = 0.93, p = 0.43) (Figure 2c).

The observation of a change in NDI but not in ODI before recurrence suggests that microstructural changes in WM due to tumor recurrence may have resulted from a reduction in neurite density rather than a disruption in orientation distribution.

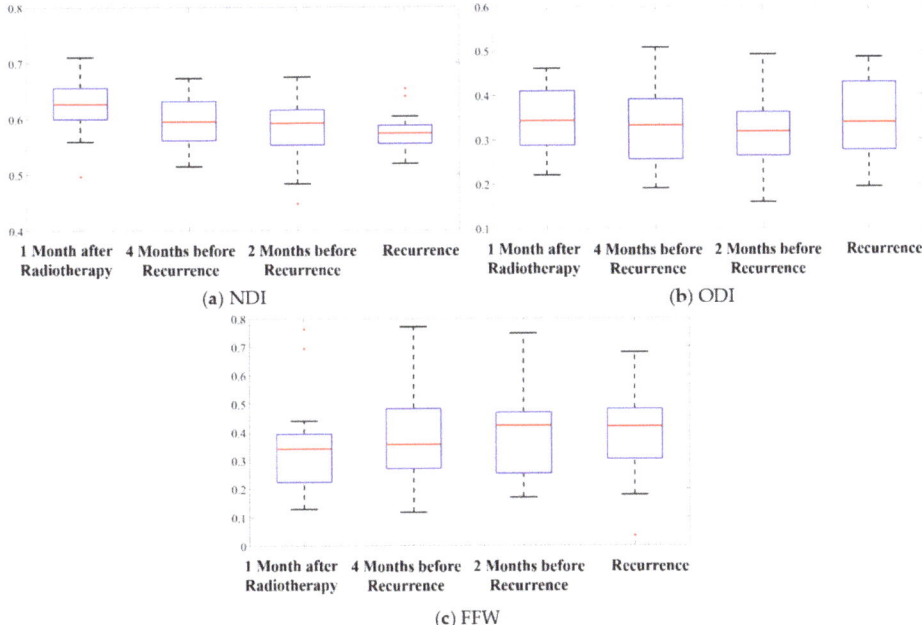

Figure 2. Box plots of the mean values of (**a**) neurite density index (NDI), (**b**) orientation dispersion index (ODI), and (**c**) free water fraction [FWF] within recurrent tumor regions over the four time points. The five bars in the box plots indicate, from bottom to top, the minimum, first quartile, median, third quartile, and the maximum. The red dots indicate outliers.

3.3. Qualitative Comparison

T1 MRI and FA images of a representative patient at each of the four time points are shown in Figure 3. The recurrent tumor (circled in red) was not visible on the three conventional T1 images before the evident time point of recurrence, but WM deterioration at the recurrent region was visibly appreciable on the FA images at 4 months and 2 months before recurrence. Notably, this recurrence appeared at the intersection of the internal capsule and geniculocalcarine tract (optic radiation), which are major WM tracts in the brain. These images corroborate our hypothesis that tumor cells may cause WM disruptions that may be evident on DTI images before the actual tumor is visible in T1 images.

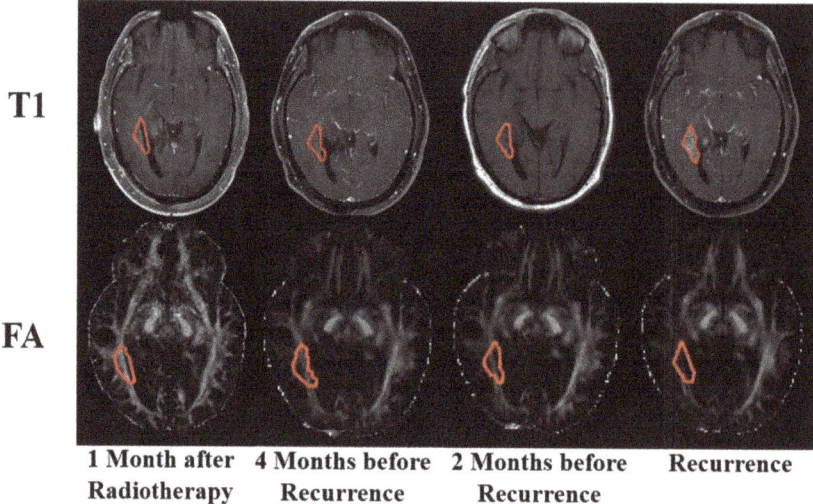

Figure 3. Serial T1 and fractional anisotropy (FA) images of a representative patient. Red outlines indicate the location of the recurrent tumor.

3.4. Radiation Therapy versus Recurrence

It is known that RT would cause dose-dependent white matter damage around treatment areas [25,26]. Therefore, the values of diffusion parameters such as FA would be affected after treatment. In order to distinguish the longitudinal reduction of FA in the study was caused by recurrence or RT, we selected 9 patients from our dataset whose recurrent intervals were longer than 12 months. And we calculated the mean FA values of the recurrence regions at an additional time point—6 months after RT. We performed pairwise t tests at between 6 months after RT and 1 month after RT, 4 months before recurrence, 2 months before recurrence, and recurrence, respectively.

There was no statistically significant change in the mean FA values between 1 month after RT and 6 months after RT ($p = 0.80$, 95% CI: (-12.7%, 12.7%)). However, compared with those at 6 months after RT, the mean FA values were significantly lower at 2 months before recurrence ($p = 0.04$, 95% CI: (0.8%, 28.3%)) and at recurrence ($p = 0.008$, 95% CI: (12.7%, 63.4%)). The mean FA values inside the regions of recurrence over the five time points are shown in box plots in Figure 4. Qualitatively, we showed the FA images at 1 month after RT, 6 months after RT, 2 months before recurrence, and recurrence from two representative patients in Figure 5. The red contours outlined the recurrent tumor regions. White matter inside the contours seemed to be intact at 1 month and 6 months after RT, whereas degeneration could be observed at 2 months before recurrence and at recurrence. Both quantitative and qualitative results indicate that the change in FA in our study may result from tumor recurrence instead of radiation-induced damage.

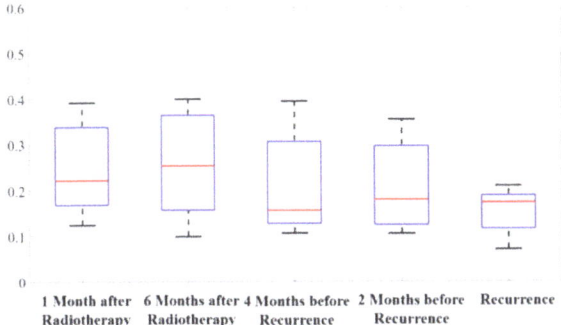

Figure 4. Box plots of the mean values of fractional anisotropy (FA) within recurrent tumor regions over the five time points for selected 9 patients. The five bars in the box plots indicate, from bottom to top, the minimum, first quartile, median, third quartile, and the maximum.

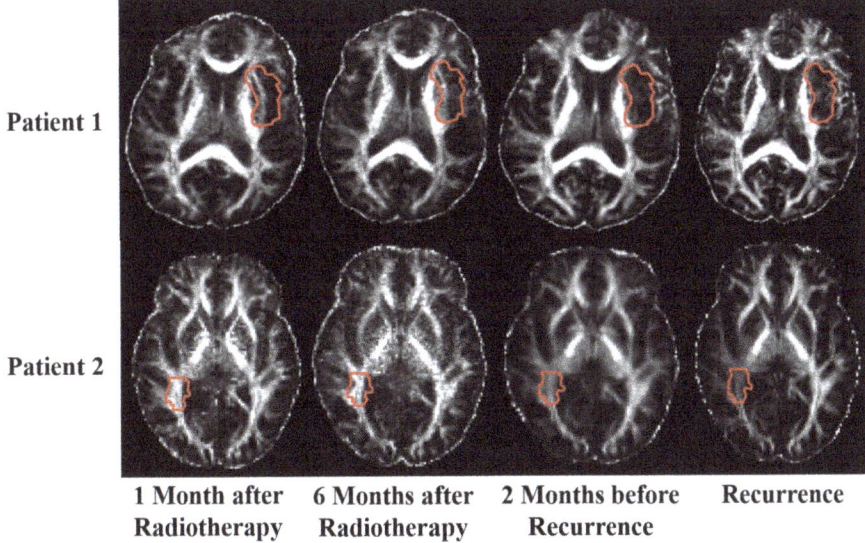

Figure 5. Serial fractional anisotropy (FA) images of two representative patients at four time points, including 6 months after radiation therapy. Red outlines indicate the location of the recurrent tumor.

4. Discussion

Although T1 weighted post contrast MRI remains the gold standard for predicting GBM recurrence, other imaging modalities such as positron emission tomography (PET) and perfusion MRI have been utilized to assist and improve the diagnostic accuracy of tumor recurrence [27,28]. In particular, DTI has the unique capability of displaying information on tissue cellularity, microstructures, and microvasculature by means of noninvasive images [29–31] and thus is increasingly investigated for cancer diagnosis [32] and the prediction of treatment response [33]. Numerous feature maps can be generated from DTI to measure changes in different diffusion properties. For example, FA represents the directionality or the degree of diffusion anisotropy, whereas MD reflects the overall diffusion properties. AD describes the diffusion properties along a particular direction (the principal axis), whereas RD accounts for the diffusion in the other two directions perpendicular to the principal direction [12].

Although DTI has been studied in several types of cancer [34], there are limited studies in GBM. For example, Chang et al. [35] compared the MD values in post-surgical images with those of post-recurrence images in tumor and surrounding tissues to predict tumor recurrence. The current study is one of the first to investigate the utility of DTI for detecting possible changes in WM microstructure before the appearance of a recurrent tumor on conventional MRI.

Our results support our hypothesis that the disruption of WM integrity near the site of recurrence in patients with GBM can precede the appearance of an enhancing tumor on structural MRI. When WM degenerates, the diffusion directionality decreases. When fiber tracts disassociate, water molecules can move freely without obstruction in any direction, and diffusivity usually increases. In general, FA and MD usually move in opposite directions. In our study, we expected that FA values would be lower at recurrence than that at baseline, and that MD would increase as a result of WM degeneration caused by underlying tumor growth. Our findings reflect these expectations, and we found similar trends of increasing values for AD and RD over time. Chang et al. [35] found that MD values were lower inside the tumor than in the surrounding peritumoral region, whereas we found that MD values tended to increase within the tumor region from baseline to recurrence. The pattern of rising MD values, as seen in our study, is consistent with findings in other neurologic diseases, such as Alzheimer disease, where MD values increased in the regions of WM degeneration [12]. Other studies of diffusion MRI brain tumors have speculated that MD is an important marker for tumor response assessment as it is negatively associated with cell density or cellularity, which is a critical measure for tumor progression [34,36,37]. However, our results suggest that the directionality feature (FA) was more sensitive to changes in WM that predicted for GBM recurrence than the other diffusivity features (MD, AD, and RD) suggesting that FA may also be a useful non-contrast imaging biomarker of GBM recurrence.

To further explore changes at the microstructural level and possibly provide more insight into tumor invasion along WM tracts, we used NODDI, a recently developed imaging technique that provides information on specific voxel-wise microstructural substrates via three components, each with values ranging from 0 to 1: NDI describes relative neurite density, ODI quantifies relative angular or morphologic variations, and FWF defines the aggregated free water portion. In the current study, NDI could distinguish recurrence at different stages of development, but the other two components could not. Because changes in FA can result from a combination of NDI and ODI [16], we suspect that the decrease in FA in our study may have been caused by a decrease in NDI rather than in ODI. This in turn suggests that neurite loss (as opposed to neurite morphologic change) may be the main pathologic process for tumor invasion in GBM recurrence, a finding that warrants histologic confirmation in future studies. Not surprisingly, similar patterns of change have also been observed in other neurodegenerative diseases, such as frontotemporal lobar degeneration and amyotrophic lateral sclerosis [23].

In previous studies, diffusion parameters demonstrated significant changes from their baseline values in the areas affected by RT at 6 months after RT [25,26]. In our study, the mean FA values of the region of interest did not show obvious changes between 6 months after RT and baseline (i.e. 1 month after RT) whereas they did show changes between 6 months after RT and 2 months before recurrence in the region of tumor recurrence. Although the small sample size may limit the statistical power, it does imply that the changes we observed from our dataset may be due to white matter deterioration caused by early tumor recurrence rather than radiation.

Despite its promising findings, the current study had several limitations. Our sample size was limited by the difficulty of retrospectively identifying patients treated with concurrent RT and temozolomide with complete sets of serial imaging data at the proposed study time points. With regards to the imaging consistency, the serial DTI images for patients included in this retrospective review were acquired at varying magnet strengths, both 1.5T and 3T without any consistent pattern over time. Although the pattern of image acquisition at varying magnet strengths was random, it may have impacted our results. Additionally, although all the registration results were manually checked after the automated, deformable image registration algorithm, any residual errors in the registration of the GTV to the diffusion images across all four time points have the potential to affect the quantitative measures within these GTV regions before recurrence.

As this is a small retrospective study, the intent of the study was to investigate whether there were suggestive findings that DTI changes may help detect earlier pathological changes prior to traditional anatomical imaging in areas of GBM recurrence based on the hypothesis that an active tumor in a region may lead to the disruption of white matter integrity. For the purpose of this early signal finding study, group analysis enabled statistical analysis. At the individual patient level, we provide several examples of patients with demonstrated changes in DTI at a time point sooner than the clinical onset of recurrence. In our patient cohort, 18 patients of the 30 total group demonstrated changes in FA 2 months prior to confirmed tumor recurrence. Based on these findings, we conclude that DTI changes are promising early biomarkers to help localize areas of GBM recurrence, but further larger prospective studies would need to be done to validate our findings before any clinical implementation could be considered.

5. Conclusions

The results from this retrospective longitudinal study suggest that the disruption of WM integrity near the site of recurrence in patients with GBM can precede the appearance of enhancing tumor on structural MRI. The FA values on images obtained before recurrence were different from those in the baseline images, and the microstructural feature NDI decreased significantly between 2–4 months before recurrence and baseline, suggesting that underlying progressive microstructural changes may precede the appearance of enhancing tumor. We further found that FA was more sensitive than other diffusion-derived features such as MD, AD, and RD for detecting subclinical tumor presence. FA may therefore be useful as an imaging biomarker to predict GBM recurrence, and DTI can provide important complementary information to conventional structural MRI to assist in the clinical diagnosis of recurrence. Our results also suggest that the underlying mechanism for FA reduction may be neurite loss rather than changes in neurite morphology. Future prospective studies of larger cohorts of patients with GBM using a more uniform imaging protocol and more detailed analysis are planned to evaluate the role of DTI in detecting subclinical GBM in a normal-appearing brain and, potentially, to refine the definition of clinical target volume for RT planning and for predicting GBM recurrence.

Author Contributions: Conceived and planned the work, Y.J., J.W.R., H.E., and C.C.; collected the data and performed the analysis, Y.J., J.W.R., and H.E.; took the lead in writing the manuscript, Y.J.; reviewed and edited the manuscript, A.M.E, K.A.A.F., L.L., and C.C.; provided critical feedback during the entire process, A.M.E., B.M.A., B.L.T., A.S.M., K.K.B., C.D.F., and C.C. All authors have read and agreed to the published version of the manuscript.

Funding: The work was supported by the University of Texas MD Anderson Cancer Center Support Grant P30CA01667 and by a ROSI grant from the Division of Radiation Oncology at the University of Texas MD Anderson Cancer Center.

Conflicts of Interest: The authors have no conflicts of interest.

References

1. Thakkar, J.P.; Dolecek, T.A.; Horbinski, C.; Ostrom, Q.T.; Lightner, D.D.; Barnholtz-Sloan, J.S.; Villano, J.L. Epidemiologic and molecular prognostic review of glioblastoma. *Cancer Epidemiol Biomark. Prev.* **2014**, *23*, 1985–1996. [CrossRef] [PubMed]
2. Stupp, R.; Mason, W.P.; van den Bent, M.J.; Weller, M.; Fisher, B.; Taphoorn, M.J.; Belanger, K.; Brandes, A.A.; Marosi, C.; Bogdahn, U.; et al. Radiotherapy plus concomitant and adjuvant temozolomide for glioblastoma. *N. Engl. J. Med.* **2005**, *352*, 987–996. [CrossRef] [PubMed]
3. Ronning, P.A.; Helseth, E.; Meling, T.R.; Johannesen, T.B. A population-based study on the effect of temozolomide in the treatment of glioblastoma multiforme. *Neuro. Oncol.* **2012**, *14*, 1178–1184. [CrossRef] [PubMed]

4. Stupp, R.; Taillibert, S.; Kanner, A.A.; Kesari, S.; Steinberg, D.M.; Toms, S.A.; Taylor, L.P.; Lieberman, F.; Silvani, A.; Fink, K.L.; et al. Maintenance Therapy With Tumor-Treating Fields Plus Temozolomide vs Temozolomide Alone for Glioblastoma: A Randomized Clinical Trial. *JAMA* **2015**, *314*, 2535–2543. [CrossRef] [PubMed]
5. Belien, A.T.; Paganetti, P.A.; Schwab, M.E. Membrane-type 1 matrix metalloprotease (MT1-MMP) enables invasive migration of glioma cells in central nervous system white matter. *J. Cell Biol.* **1999**, *144*, 373–384. [CrossRef]
6. Pedersen, P.H.; Edvardsen, K.; Garcia-Cabrera, I.; Mahesparan, R.; Thorsen, J.; Mathisen, B.; Rosenblum, M.L.; Bjerkvig, R. Migratory patterns of lac-z transfected human glioma cells in the rat brain. *Int. J. Cancer* **1995**, *62*, 767–771. [CrossRef]
7. Lefranc, F.; Brotchi, J.; Kiss, R. Possible future issues in the treatment of glioblastomas: Special emphasis on cell migration and the resistance of migrating glioblastoma cells to apoptosis. *J. Clin. Oncol.* **2005**, *23*, 2411–2422. [CrossRef]
8. Basser, P.J.; Mattiello, J.; LeBihan, D. MR diffusion tensor spectroscopy and imaging. *Biophys. J.* **1994**, *66*, 259–267. [CrossRef]
9. Le Bihan, D.; Mangin, J.F.; Poupon, C.; Clark, C.A.; Pappata, S.; Molko, N.; Chabriat, H. Diffusion tensor imaging: concepts and applications. *J. Magn. Reson. Imaging.* **2001**, *13*, 534–546. [CrossRef]
10. Werring, D.J.; Clark, C.A.; Barker, G.J.; Thompson, A.J.; Miller, D.H. Diffusion tensor imaging of lesions and normal-appearing white matter in multiple sclerosis. *Neurology* **1999**, *52*, 1626–1632. [CrossRef]
11. Atkinson-Clement, C.; Pinto, S.; Eusebio, A.; Coulon, O. Diffusion tensor imaging in Parkinson's disease: Review and meta-analysis. *Neuroimage Clin.* **2017**, *16*, 98–110. [CrossRef] [PubMed]
12. Jin, Y.; Huang, C.; Daianu, M.; Zhan, L.; Dennis, E.L.; Reid, R.I.; Jack, C.R., Jr.; Zhu, H.; Thompson, P.M.; Alzheimer's Disease Neuroimaging, I. 3D tract-specific local and global analysis of white matter integrity in Alzheimer's disease. *Hum. Brain Mapp.* **2017**, *38*, 1191–1207. [CrossRef] [PubMed]
13. Svolos, P.; Kousi, E.; Kapsalaki, E.; Theodorou, K.; Fezoulidis, I.; Kappas, C.; Tsougos, I. The role of diffusion and perfusion weighted imaging in the differential diagnosis of cerebral tumors: a review and future perspectives. *Cancer Imaging* **2014**, *14*, 20. [CrossRef] [PubMed]
14. Darbar, A.; Waqas, M.; Enam, S.F.; Mahmood, S.D. Use of Preoperative Apparent Diffusion Coefficients to Predict Brain Tumor Grade. *Cureus* **2018**, *10*. [CrossRef]
15. Pauleit, D.; Langen, K.J.; Floeth, F.; Hautzel, H.; Riemenschneider, M.J.; Reifenberger, G.; Shah, N.J.; Muller, H.W. Can the apparent diffusion coefficient be used as a noninvasive parameter to distinguish tumor tissue from peritumoral tissue in cerebral gliomas? *J. Magn. Reson. Imaging* **2004**, *20*, 758–764. [CrossRef]
16. Price, S.J.; Jena, R.; Burnet, N.G.; Carpenter, T.A.; Pickard, J.D.; Gillard, J.H. Predicting patterns of glioma recurrence using diffusion tensor imaging. *Eur. Radiol.* **2007**, *17*, 1675–1684. [CrossRef]
17. Roberts, T.P.; Liu, F.; Kassner, A.; Mori, S.; Guha, A. Fiber density index correlates with reduced fractional anisotropy in white matter of patients with glioblastoma. *AJNR Am J. Neuroradiol.* **2005**, *26*, 2183–2186.
18. Zhang, H.; Schneider, T.; Wheeler-Kingshott, C.A.; Alexander, D.C. NODDI: practical in vivo neurite orientation dispersion and density imaging of the human brain. *Neuroimage* **2012**, *61*, 1000–1016. [CrossRef]
19. Shi, F.; Wang, L.; Dai, Y.; Gilmore, J.H.; Lin, W.; Shen, D. LABEL: pediatric brain extraction using learning-based meta-algorithm. *Neuroimage* **2012**, *62*, 1975–1986. [CrossRef]
20. Jenkinson, M.; Pechaud, M.; Smith, S. BET2: MR-based estimation of brain, skull and scalp surfaces. In Proceedings of the Eleventh Annual Meeting of the Organization for Human Brain Mapping, Toronto, ON, Canada, 12–16 June 2005.
21. Jenkinson, M.; Beckmann, C.F.; Behrens, T.E.; Woolrich, M.W.; Smith, S.M. FSL. *Neuroimage* **2012**, *62*, 782–790. [CrossRef]
22. Andersson, J.L.R.; Sotiropoulos, S.N. An integrated approach to correction for off-resonance effects and subject movement in diffusion MR imaging. *Neuroimage* **2016**, *125*, 1063–1078. [CrossRef] [PubMed]
23. Wen, J.H.; Zhang, H.; Alexander, D.C.; Durrleman, S.; Routier, A.; Rinaldi, D.; Houot, M.; Couratier, P.; Hannequin, D.; Pasquier, F.; et al. Neurite density is reduced in the presymptomatic phase of C9orf72 disease. *J. Neurol. Neurosurg. Psychiatry* **2019**, *90*, 387–394. [CrossRef] [PubMed]
24. Avants, B.B.; Tustison, N.J.; Song, G.; Cook, P.A.; Klein, A.; Gee, J.C. A reproducible evaluation of ANTs similarity metric performance in brain image registration. *Neuroimage* **2011**, *54*, 2033–2044. [CrossRef] [PubMed]

25. Connor, M.; Karunamuni, R.; McDonald, C.; White, N.; Pettersson, N.; Moiseenko, V.; Seibert, T.; Marshall, D.; Cervino, L.; Bartsch, H.; et al. Dose-dependent white matter damage after brain radiotherapy. *Radiother. Oncol.* **2016**, *121*, 209–216. [CrossRef] [PubMed]
26. Kassubek, R.; Gorges, M.; Westhoff, M.A.; Ludolph, A.C.; Kassubek, J.; Muller, H.P. Cerebral Microstructural Alterations after Radiation Therapy in High-Grade Glioma: A Diffusion Tensor Imaging-Based Study. *Front. Neurol.* **2017**, *8*. [CrossRef]
27. Lundemann, M.; af Rosenschold, P.M.; Muhic, A.; Larsen, V.A.; Poulsen, H.S.; Engelholm, S.A.; Andersen, F.L.; Kjaer, A.; Larsson, H.B.W.; Law, I.; et al. Feasibility of multi-parametric PET and MRI for prediction of tumour recurrence in patients with glioblastoma. *Eur. J. Nucl. Med. Mol. Imaging* **2019**, *46*, 603–613. [CrossRef]
28. Zhang, J.F.; Liu, H.; Tong, H.P.; Wang, S.M.; Yang, Y.Z.; Liu, G.; Zhang, W.G. Clinical Applications of Contrast-Enhanced Perfusion MRI Techniques in Gliomas: Recent Advances and Current Challenges. *Contrast Media Mol. Imaging* **2017**. [CrossRef]
29. Chen, L.H.; Liu, M.; Bao, J.; Xia, Y.B.; Zhang, J.Q.; Zhang, L.; Huang, X.Q.; Wang, J. The Correlation between Apparent Diffusion Coefficient and Tumor Cellularity in Patients: A Meta-Analysis. *PLOS ONE* **2013**, *8*. [CrossRef]
30. Jiang, R.S.; Ma, Z.J.; Dong, H.X.; Sun, S.H.; Zeng, X.M.; Li, X. Diffusion tensor imaging of breast lesions: evaluation of apparent diffusion coefficient and fractional anisotropy and tissue cellularity. *Brit. J. Radiol.* **2016**, *89*. [CrossRef]
31. Koh, D.M.; Collins, D.J.; Orton, M.R. Intravoxel incoherent motion in body diffusion-weighted MRI: Reality and challenges. *AJR Am. J. Roentgenol.* **2011**, *196*, 1351–1361. [CrossRef]
32. Park, M.J.; Kim, Y.K.; Choi, S.Y.; Rhim, H.; Lee, W.J.; Choi, D. Preoperative detection of small pancreatic carcinoma: value of adding diffusion-weighted imaging to conventional MR imaging for improving confidence level. *Radiology* **2014**, *273*, 433–443. [CrossRef] [PubMed]
33. Tang, L.; Zhang, X.P.; Sun, Y.S.; Shen, L.; Li, J.; Qi, L.P.; Cui, Y. Gastrointestinal stromal tumors treated with imatinib mesylate: apparent diffusion coefficient in the evaluation of therapy response in patients. *Radiology* **2011**, *258*, 729–738. [CrossRef] [PubMed]
34. Tang, L.; Zhou, X.J. Diffusion MRI of cancer: From low to high b-values. *J. Magn. Reson. Imaging* **2019**, *49*, 23–40. [CrossRef] [PubMed]
35. Chang, P.D.; Chow, D.S.; Yang, P.H.; Filippi, C.G.; Lignelli, A. Predicting Glioblastoma Recurrence by Early Changes in the Apparent Diffusion Coefficient Value and Signal Intensity on FLAIR Images. *AJR Am. J. Roentgenol.* **2017**, *208*, 57–65. [CrossRef] [PubMed]
36. Colman, H.; Berkey, B.A.; Maor, M.H.; Groves, M.D.; Schultz, C.J.; Vermeulen, S.; Nelson, D.F.; Mehta, M.P.; Yung, W.K.; Radiation Therapy Oncology, G. Phase II Radiation Therapy Oncology Group trial of conventional radiation therapy followed by treatment with recombinant interferon-beta for supratentorial glioblastoma: results of RTOG 9710. *Int. J. Radiat. Oncol. Biol. Phys.* **2006**, *66*, 818–824. [CrossRef] [PubMed]
37. Pilatus, U.; Shim, H.; Artemov, D.; Davis, D.; van Zijl, P.C.M.; Glickson, J.D. Intracellular volume and apparent diffusion constants of perfused cancer cell cultures, as measured by NMR. *Magn. Reson. Med.* **1997**, *37*, 825–832. [CrossRef]

© 2020 by the authors. Licensee MDPI, Basel, Switzerland. This article is an open access article distributed under the terms and conditions of the Creative Commons Attribution (CC BY) license (http://creativecommons.org/licenses/by/4.0/).

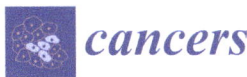

Article

The Impact of Normalization Approaches to Automatically Detect Radiogenomic Phenotypes Characterizing Breast Cancer Receptors Status

Rossana Castaldo, Katia Pane *, Emanuele Nicolai, Marco Salvatore and Monica Franzese

IRCCS SDN, Via E. Gianturco, 113, 80143 Naples, Italy; rcastaldo@sdn-napoli.it (R.C.); enicolai@sdn-napoli.it (E.N.); direzionescientifica@sdn-napoli.it (M.S.); mfranzese@sdn-napoli.it (M.F.)
* Correspondence: kpane@sdn-napoli.it

Received: 2 January 2020; Accepted: 19 February 2020; Published: 24 February 2020

Abstract: In breast cancer studies, combining quantitative radiomic with genomic signatures can help identifying and characterizing radiogenomic phenotypes, in function of molecular receptor status. Biomedical imaging processing lacks standards in radiomic feature normalization methods and neglecting feature normalization can highly bias the overall analysis. This study evaluates the effect of several normalization techniques to predict four clinical phenotypes such as estrogen receptor (ER), progesterone receptor (PR), human epidermal growth factor receptor 2 (HER2), and triple negative (TN) status, by quantitative features. The Cancer Imaging Archive (TCIA) radiomic features from 91 T1-weighted Dynamic Contrast Enhancement MRI of invasive breast cancers were investigated in association with breast invasive carcinoma miRNA expression profiling from the Cancer Genome Atlas (TCGA). Three advanced machine learning techniques (Support Vector Machine, Random Forest, and Naïve Bayesian) were investigated to distinguish between molecular prognostic indicators and achieved an area under the ROC curve (AUC) values of 86%, 93%, 91%, and 91% for the prediction of ER+ versus ER−, PR+ versus PR−, HER2+ versus HER2−, and triple-negative, respectively. In conclusion, radiomic features enable to discriminate major breast cancer molecular subtypes and may yield a potential imaging biomarker for advancing precision medicine.

Keywords: Molecular imaging; breast cancer; miRNA expression; radiogenomics; machine learning; radiomic; diagnosis; biomarker

1. Introduction

Breast cancer is the most frequently diagnosed cancer among women, and it is the second leading cause of death in women [1]. Based on the molecular receptor status, breast cancer can be classified into different subtypes with different response to therapy and prognosis. The three clinically most-useful receptors status to characterize breast cancer cells are the estrogen receptor (ER), progesterone receptor (PR), and human epidermal growth factor receptor 2 (HER2) that can impact therapy and prognosis [2].

Breast cancer is a heterogeneous disease. Indeed, HER2-positive (HER2+) breast cancers are more aggressive and show a poorer prognosis than HER2-negative (HER2−) cancers. Positive hormonal receptor status such as ER-positive (ER+) and PR-positive (PR+) tumor have lower risks of mortality than ER-negative (ER−) and/or PR-negative (PR−) disease [3–7]. Triple negative (TN) tumor (negative for all three receptors) shows a high relapsing rate, and therefore, accounts for a large portion of breast cancer deaths. Therefore, it becomes necessary to identify molecular receptor status and subsequently subtypes to select the appropriate therapy and predict the therapeutic response [8,9].

Radiomics has recently emerged as a promising tool for discovering non-invasive imaging signatures characterizing lesions such as size, shape, descriptors of the image intensity histogram and texture [10,11]. The term 'Radiomics' refers to the high-throughput extraction of quantitative features from medical images, i.e., conversion of images to mineable data, that can potentially capture tumor heterogeneity, aiding precision medicine [12]. A closely related field is 'radiogenomics', which explores the associations between imaging phenotype (radiomic data) and disease genotype (genomic patterns) [13,14]. Two public data resources such as The Cancer Genome Atlas (TCGA) and The Cancer Imaging Archive (TCIA), provide cancer genomic profiling and medical images counterpart, respectively [15,16], to promote cross-disciplinary research including radiogenomic studies [17–19].

In breast cancer, radiomic applications encompass diagnosis and better differentiation of malignant and benign entities as well as identifying ductal carcinoma in situ and invasive ductal carcinoma, for prognosis of metastatic potential, prediction of pathologic stage, lymph node involvement, molecular subtypes, and clinical outcomes [20–30].

Regarding the use of radiomic features for investigating breast cancer molecular receptor status, Agner et al. [28] extracted imaging features to differentiate TN cancers from other molecular subtypes. Yamaguchi et al. [29] investigated the relationship between heterogeneous kinetic curve pattern and molecular subtype. Blaschke et al. [31] showed that HER2-positive tumors have a greater uptake than other molecular subtypes. Li et al. [7] disclosed that the computer-aided tumor imaging phenotypes were able to differentiate between molecular prognostic biomarkers, and statistically significant associations between tumor phenotypes and receptor status were observed. Xie et al. [32] showed that whole-tumor MR multiparametric images offer a non-invasive analytical approach for breast cancer subtype classification and TN cancer cases. Guo et al. [21] demonstrated that the prediction performances by genomics alone, radiomics alone, and combined radiogenomic features showed statistically significant correlations with clinical outcomes (pathological receptors). Yoon et al. [33] used deep neural networks combining both radiomic and genomic features of invasive breast cancer, achieving high classification performance to predict pathological stage and molecular receptor status.

However, an important and often undervalued aspect in radiomic framework of analysis is features normalization relevance. In fact, data normalization methods are essential for radiomic features, due to their basic differences of scale, range, and statistical distributions. Untransformed features may have high levels of skewness, which can result in artificially low p-values in statistical analysis [34]. Moreover, neglecting feature normalization and the use of inappropriate normalization methods may lead to individual features being over or underrepresented and eventually introduce bias into developed models. Recently, normalization transformations are gaining huge interest in the era of machine learning (ML), especially in data preprocessing [35]. In the existing literature, standards to normalize quantitative radiomic features seem to be missing. None of the above-mentioned studies used a normalization method to decrease the overall bias that non-normalized features can generate in the analysis. Only Guo et al. [21] standardized the radiomic and genomic data before applying discriminative models. On the other side, several efforts have been shown to improve normalization procedures for MRI image intensity values as crucial preprocessing step. In fact, image variability and normalization steps are critical correction procedures for imaging-related batch effects before extracting quantitative radiomic features [36–40]. Although image preprocessing normalization steps are decisive to reduce technical variability across images, additional feature normalization steps are still needed and should be not overlooked.

The aim of this study is to evaluate the impact of several normalization methods to study the relationship between radiomic features and breast tumor molecular receptor ER, PR, HER2, and TN status. We integrated data from TCIA-TCGA to analyze 36 MRI radiomic features extracted from 91 biopsy proven invasive breast cancers, T1-weighted Dynamic Contrast Enhancement (DCE) Magnetic Resonance Imaging (MRI), associated with tumor molecular receptor status.

Several feature normalization approaches such as scaling, z-score, robust z-score, log-transformation, quantile, upper quartile, and whitening methods were applied to radiomic features. We compared model predictive power and the impact of radiomic feature normalization using three advanced machine learning methods (Support Vector machine (SVM), Random Forest (RF) and Naïve Bayesian (NB) methods) to differentiate among ER, PR, HER2, and TN cases.

Finally, we included TCGA breast cancer miRNAs expression profiles to explore imaging-miRNA associations.

Our data highlighted that close attention is needed to assess image-based biomarker in radiomic analysis. Thus, the aim of this study is to provide several statistical approaches to generate quantitative MRI-based signature, which may lead to more precise breast cancer prognosis and help clinicians in decision-making towards personalized medicine.

2. Materials and Methods

2.1. Dataset

All patient data used in this study were obtained from The Cancer Genome Atlas (TCGA) (available at: https://tcga-data.nci.nih.gov, accessed October 9, 2019) Breast Cancer initiative. Patients were recruited from five comprehensive cancer centers across the United States. Imaging data processing and feature extraction were conducted by [7,21,27,41]. In order to enforce imaging uniformity, breast MRI studies were acquired by 1.5-Tesla (1.5 T) magnet strength using an MRI system from GE Medical Systems (Milwaukee, Wis). The final dataset included 91 breast MRI cases.

2.1.1. Clinical Data

Table 1 shows breast cancer histological type and molecular receptors status data (ER, PR, and HER2) carried out by Immunohistochemistry (IHC) test. The results of the IHC test can be 0 (negative), 1+ (also negative), 2+ (borderline), or 3+ (positive; the HER2 protein is overexpressed). In addition, TCGA also assessed HER2 receptor protein copies in the cancer cells by Fluorescence in Situ Hybridization (FISH). The ER and PR status for our dataset samples were obtained from the TCGA data portal [21]. The HER2 status of the samples was obtained from [15]. More clinical details are reported in Table S1. Ninety-one invasive breast carcinomas with radiomic imaging profiles were available from TCIA [15,21]. All samples were primary tumors from female patients. We investigated the prediction of ER, PR, and HER2 status and triple negative (TN) of patients using radiomic features alone.

Table 1. Clinical Data.

Variables	Number
Breast Cancer Types	
Ductal carcinoma	79
Lobular carcinoma	10
Mixed	2
Molecular Receptor Status	
Estrogen Receptor (ER)	
Positive	76
Negative	15
Progesterone Receptor (PR)	
Positive	71
Negative	20
Human Epidermal Growth Factor Receptor 2 (HER2)	
Positive	12
Negative	74
Triple Negative (TN)	
Triple negative (ER−, PR−, HER2−)	12
Others	74

2.1.2. Image Data

All MRIs were acquired using a standard double-breast coil on a 1.5T GE whole-body MRI system (GE Medical Systems). In the current study, only T1-weighted, dynamic contrast-enhanced MR images were used. The imaging protocols included 1 pre-contrast image and 3 to 5 post-contrast images obtained using a T1-weighted, 3-dimensional (3D) spoiled gradient echo sequence with a gadolinium-based contrast agent (Omniscan; Nycomed-Amersham, Princeton, NJ). For further information refer to [7,21,27,41].

2.1.3. Radiomic Features

A total of 36 MRI features, computer extracted image phenotypes (CEIPs), were calculated based on the automatically derived 3D tumor segmentations [7,21]. The CEIPs were divided into the following 6 phenotype categories: size (measuring tumor dimensions), shape (quantifying the 3D geometry), morphology (combining shape and margin characteristics), enhancement texture (describing the texture of the contrast uptake in the tumor on the first postcontrast MRIs), kinetic curve assessment (describing the shape of the kinetic curve and assessing the physiologic process of the uptake and washout of the contrast agent in the tumor during the dynamic imaging series), and enhancement-variance kinetics (characterizing the time course of the spatial variance of the enhancement within the tumor) [21]. Data were extracted using version V2010 of the UChicago [27]. The complete dataset was downloaded from the TCGA Breast Phenotype Research Group Data sets (available at: https://wiki.cancerimagingarchive.net/display/DOI/TCGA + Breast + Phenotype + Research + Group + Data + sets, accessed 9 October, 2019). Information about radiomic features, including feature names, label, description, and category is listed in Table S2 and as reported by [21].

2.1.4. miRNA expression data

TCGA breast invasive carcinoma miRNA expression quantification data (raw read count, February 2018) produced on Illumina HiSeq 2000 sequencers (Illumina Ventures, San Diego, CA, USA) were downloaded using the free software R (R version 3.5.2) [42] and TCGAbiolinks R package [43].

TCGA-formatted miRNA-seq data according to the BCGSC miRNA Profiling Pipeline produces miRNA IDs with raw read counts of primary tumor (n = 1096 files for 1078 tumor cases) and normal solid tissue (n = 104 files for 104 normal cases). The miRNA raw counts (n = 1881 miRNAs), were processed as described in [44]. Then, we considered 1625 filtered and normalized miRNAs. We associated the molecular receptor ER, PR, HER2 status from [15], and filtering out NA receptor status.

Samples derived from patients with (n = 504) and without (n = 57) breast cancer were then matched with the 91 patients included in the radiomic analysis. A total of 75 samples along with the respective radiomic and genomic features were included in the radiogenomic framework.

2.2. Statistical Methods

Statistical analyses were carried out for radiomic features and genomic features alone to investigate the statistical significance of the features in detecting molecular receptor status. Associations between radiomics and genomics were also investigated in terms of correlation.

Shapiro–Wilk test was used to determine the normality of radiomic and genomic features [45].

Wilcoxon signed-rank test and Fisher's exact test were adopted to compare continuous and categorical clinical variables, respectively, between molecular receptor status (Table S1). R software (R Core Team. R: A language and environment for statistical computing. R Foundation for Statistical Computing, Vienna, Austria; http://www.R-project.org, 2019) was used to perform statistical analyses.

2.2.1. Radiomic Statistical Analysis

Seven different normalization techniques were used to normalize radiomic features. Features were standardized as the min–max normalization (i.e., scaling method), where each feature was normalized in the range from 0 to 1; z-score normalization, where each feature was normalized as $z = (x - \bar{x})/s$, where $x, \bar{x}$, and s are the feature, the mean, and the standard deviation respectively [46]; robust z-score normalization is calculated from the median absolute deviation and median absolute deviation [47]; log-transformation (base 10), a constant value $a = b - min(x)$ where b is 1 and x is the feature, was added to the data for handling negative values [48]; the upper quartile normalization divides each read count by the 75th percentile of the read counts in its sample [49]; quantile normalization, which transform the original data to remove unwanted technical variation by forcing the observed distributions to be the same and the average distribution, obtained by taking the average of each quantile across samples, is used as the reference [50,51]; lastly, whitening normalization technique from the principle component analysis (PCA), is based on a linear transformation that converts a vector of random variables with a known covariance matrix into a set of new variables whose covariance is the identity matrix, meaning that they are uncorrelated and each have variance equal to one [52].

To investigate the effect of normalization techniques on the radiomic features, Spearman's rank correlation was run between non-normalized radiomic features and normalized radiomic features for each of the seven different normalization methods. A Spearman's ρ value greater than 0.8 and significant p-value (< 0.05) between non-normalized and normalized feature (using scaling, Z-score, robust Z-score, log-transformation, upper quartile, quantile, and whitening methods) was set as threshold to identify the normalized radiomic features that were in agreement with the non-normalized radiomic features. Bland–Altman analysis was also used to investigate the agreement between the features that showed a Spearman's ρ value less than 0.08 and significant p-value. Bland–Altman procedure was used to compute 95% LoA (Limits of Agreement) [53].

For each binary problem, Wilcoxon signed-rank test was performed to investigate radiomic feature variation between two different groups (ER+ vs ER−, PR+ vs PR−, HER2+ vs HER2−, TN vs Others). Median trend or feature trend, using the following convention, was also investigated [54–56]:

- Two arrows, ↓↓ (or ↑↑) were used to report a significant (p-value < 0.05) decrease (or increase) of radiomic feature median in negative receptor status (ER−, PR−, HER2 +, TN);
- One arrow was used for non-significant variations: ↓ (or ↑) indicated a non-significant (p-value > 0.05) decrease (or increase) of a radiomic feature median in negative receptor status (ER−, PR−, HER2+, TN).

The statistical analysis was repeated for each normalization procedure described above. Non-parametric tests such as Wilcoxon signed-rank test and Spearman's rank correlation were used since most of the radiomic features (>90%) were non-normally distributed in the Shapiro–Wilk test. A p-value less than 0.05 was considered significant. Holm's correction was used for multiple hypothesis correction if necessary.

A synthetic scheme of the radiomic analysis carried out in this study is shown in Figure 1.

2.2.2. Genomic Statistical Analysis

Starting from normalized counts we evaluated differentially expressed miRNAs between tumor and normal conditions, applying the Empirical Bayes method for differential expression analysis, edgeR R package [57], combined with the Generalized Linear Model approach (GLM). Differentially Expressed miRNAs (DEmiRNAs) with a |log2 fold-change |> 1.0 (hsa-mir-135b has LogFC 0.93) and with adjusted p-values (FDR) ≤ 0.05, were defined as significant and used for downstream analysis. In addition, differentially expressed miRNAs were analyzed through the use of Ingenuity Knowledge Base, IPA (QIAGEN Inc., https://www.qiagenbioinformatics.com/products/ingenuitypathway-analysis) to assess breast cancer implications.

We investigated DEmiRNAs expression as function of the ER, PR, HER2, and TN molecular receptor status and performed the Wilcoxon signed-rank test for statistical significance.

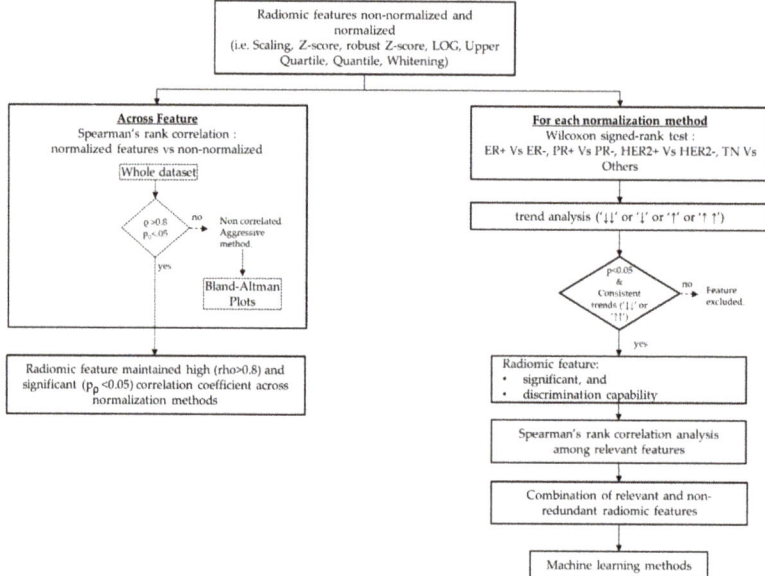

Figure 1. Radiomic analysis framework.

A p-value less than 0.05 was considered significant. Holm's correction was used for multiple hypothesis correction if necessary.

2.2.3. Radiogenomic Statistical Analysis

After identifying the statistically significant radiomic features for each receptor, Spearman's rank correlation was run between DEmiRNAs for each molecular receptor status (ER+ and ER−, PR+ and PR−, HER2+ and HER2−, TN and Others) and radiomic features. In the correlation analysis, two normalization methods were chosen for the radiomic features: upper quartile normalization method as both data types are normalized by upper quartile normalization method, and whitening-transformation method as it is the only normalization method that highlighted a significant change among radiomic features for all receptors' status.

2.3. Machine Learning Classification

The dataset was stratified random split per patient into two folders: Folder 1 (60%) was used to train and validate the classifiers; folder 2 (40%) to test the models. The reason of this split is that a classifier should be tested on an independent set of data to reduce overfitting problems and bias in the overall accuracy of the classifier [55,58].

2.3.1. Feature Selection Methods

Feature selection is a critical step to build a robust model. In fact, the number of features used in the final classifier and its cardinality should be limited by the number of subjects presenting the event to detect in order to minimize the overfitting risk in a machine learning model. Moreover, a significant small set of clinical features powerfully simplifies the clinical interpretation of the results, by pointing the attention only on the most informative and relevant features [58]. Therefore, the feature selection process was based on two main steps: relevance analysis and redundancy analysis [55]. The former was performed using the Wilcoxon signed-rank test to identify the features that changed significantly between two conditions (binary problem). The latter selected only one feature from each cluster of features mutually correlated using Spearman's rank correlation to reduce multicollinearity in the models [55].

2.3.2. Training, Validation, and Testing

Clinical outcomes have unbalanced ratio, which do not meet the assumptions of most machine learning-based models. To tackle this problem, Synthetic Minority Over-sampling Technique (SMOTE) was applied to balance the datasets [59]. It has been shown that SMOTE is a robust technique to overcome unbalanced dataset problems with a variety of classifiers [59,60]. In this study, SMOTE has shown to outperform other sampling methods and thus, it was used to balance the datasets.

Three different machine-learning approaches were considered to develop classifiers aiming to automatically classify receptor status based on MRI phenotypes: Support Vector Machine (SVM), which belongs to a general field of kernel-based machine learning methods and is used to classify both linearly and non-linearly separable data [61]; Random Forest decision trees, an ensemble learning method for classification that operates by constructing a multitude of decision trees during training and outputting the class that is the mode of the classes (classification) [62,63]; Bayesian classifier, a family of simple "probabilistic classifiers" based on applying Bayes' theorem with strong (naïve) independence assumptions between the features [64].

Regarding model parameters, for SVM, polynomial kernel function with the degree from 1 to 5 was used. Random Forest decision trees were developed by changing confidence factor for pruning from 0.05 to 0.5 and minimum number of instances per leaf from 2 to 20. The algorithm parameters were tuned during training on folder 1. Each of those methods was used with all the combinations of relevant and non-redundant radiomic features.

The training of the machine-learning models (including classifier parameter tuning) was performed on folder 1 (around 60% of the total number of patients). Folder 1 was also employed to validate the classifier using a k-fold cross-validation technique. The 3-fold person-independent cross-validation approach was used to validate the models in folder 1 [55]. The model was then tested on folder 2 (around 40% of the total number of patients), in order to assess their ability to automatically detect the receptor status. Binary classification performance measures were adopted according to standard formulae reported in Table 2 [65].

Table 2. Binary performance measures.

Measure	Formula
Total Classification Accuracy (ACC)	$(TP + TN)/(TP + TN + FP + FN)$
Sensitivity (SEN)	$TP/(TP + FN)$
Specificity (SPE)	$TN/(FP + TN)$
Area Under the Curve (AUC)	-

True positive (TP); true negative (TN), false negative (FN); false positive (FP).

2.3.3. Best Model Selection

To evaluate the effect of normalization approaches for radiomic analysis, binary performance was calculated for each ML method across all normalization methods employed in this study. The best normalization technique for each ML model was selected as the one achieving the highest sensitivity, specificity, accuracy and area under the curve (AUC), and the classifier that employed a smaller number of radiomic features (i.e., less computational complexity model). Among the three different ML methods used to train, validate and test the classifiers (SVM, RF, BN), the best-performing model was chosen as the classifier achieving the highest AUC, which is a reliable estimator of both sensitivity and specificity rates; in case of equal AUC, the classifier with less computational complexity was chosen.

3. Results

This study was performed on 91 invasive breast cancers with radiomic imaging profiles from female patients. The patients' average age was 53.6 ± 11.5 years (range of 29–82 years). According to the clinical variables, no statistically significant differences were observed between receptor status (Table S1). For radiogenomic framework, we considered 75 matched samples of 91 invasive breast cancers.

3.1. Radiomics

A correlation analysis was run on the whole dataset to investigate the relationship between non-normalized and normalized radiomic features (i.e., Scaling, Z-Score, Robust Z-Score, Log transformation (LOG), Upper Quartile, Quantile and Whitening (WHT) methods). Spearman's rank correlation was used. Table S3 showed ρ values of the radiomic features with a p-value < 0.05. A graphical representation of the correlation results is presented in Figure 2.

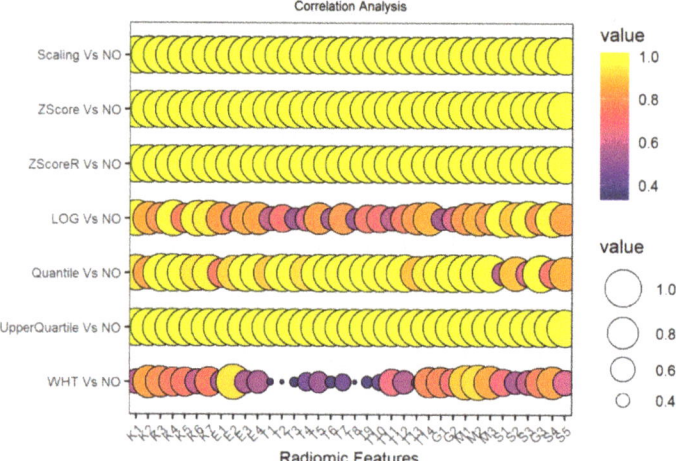

Figure 2. Correlation analysis on the whole dataset between non-normalized and normalized radiomic features. On the x-axis radiomic features are reported; on the y-axis correlation coefficients via Spearman correlation analysis are reported for each comparison between normalization methods and raw features (i.e., non-normalized radiomic features). All correlation p-values resulted less than 0.05. NO: non-normalized features; Scaling normalization method; Z-score normalization method; ZscoreR: Robust Z-score normalization method; LOG transformation; Quantile and Upper Quartile normalization method; WHT: Whitening normalization method.

As shown in Table S3 and Figure 2, non-normalized radiomic features are perfectly correlated with scaling, z-score, robust z-score and upper quartile normalized features. Between LOG transformation method and non-normalized features, only four radiomic features (E1, S1, S3, and S4) showed to be poorly correlated (ρ less than 0.8). Sixteen and thirty out of 36 radiomic features showed a very poor correlation value with the row radiomic features (i.e., non-normalized features) for the quantile and whitening normalization methods respectively.

Bland Altman analysis was also performed to visually investigate the agreement and disruption of normalized methods on the radiomic features that showed a Spearman's rank coefficient less than 0.8 with non-normalized radiomic features. Therefore, the correlation analysis was supported by the visual inspection of the Bland–Altman analysis. An increase in bias and in width of the 95% limits of agreement (LoA) was observed for the radiomic features that showed a Spearman's rank coefficient less than 0.8.

3.1.1. Statistical Analysis per Receptor Status: ER+ vs ER−

Table 3 reports the results of the statistical analysis from Wilcoxon signed-rank test indicating association between MRI phenotype and receptor status ER+ versus ER−, for each normalization method. In Table 3 the radiomic features that showed a significant p-values were reported.

As shown in Table 3 and Figure 3A, 6 out of the 36 radiomic features (T5, T11, S1, S2, S3 and G3) showed significant changes between ER− and ER+ for non-normalized, scaling, z-score, robust z-score, log-transformation and upper quartile radiomic features. Three out of these 6 features (T5, T11, G3) decreased significantly in ER− cases, while the remaining 3 features showed a significant increase trend. For quantile normalization, five features out of 36 radiomic features (T5, T11, S2, S3, and G3) changed significantly between ER− and ER+. As far as whitening normalization method is concerned, only three radiomic features (T11, S2, and G3) showed significant changes between ER− and ER+ and maintained coherent trends with the other normalization methods.

Table 3. Results from the Wilcoxon signed-rank test indicating association between MRI phenotype and molecular classification ER+ versus ER−.

Feature Names	Non-Normalized Pval (Trend)	Scaling Pval (Trend)	Z-Score Pval (Trend)	Robust Z-Score Pval (Trend)	LOG Pval (Trend)	Quantile Pval (Trend)	Upper Quartile Pval (Trend)	WHT Pval (Trend)
T5	0.029 (↓↓)	0.029 (↓↓)	0.029 (↓↓)	0.029 (↓↓)	0.029 (↓↓)	0.029 (↓↓)	0.029 (↓↓)	0.287 (↓)
T11	0.031 (↓↓)	0.031 (↓↓)	0.031 (↓↓)	0.031 (↓↓)	0.031 (↓↓)	0.031 (↓↓)	0.031 (↓↓)	0.002 (↓↓)
S1	0.003 (↑↑)	0.003 (↑↑)	0.003 (↑↑)	0.003 (↑↑)	0.003 (↑↑)	0.003 (↑↑)	0.003 (↑↑)	0.688 (↑)
S2	0.003 (↑↑)	0.003 (↑↑)	0.003 (↑↑)	0.003 (↑↑)	0.003 (↑↑)	0.003 (↑↑)	0.003 (↑↑)	0.004 (↑↑)
S3	0.011 (↑↑)	0.011 (↑↑)	0.011 (↑↑)	0.011 (↑↑)	0.011 (↑↑)	0.011 (↑↑)	0.011 (↑↑)	0.524 (↓)
G3	0.029 (↓↓)	0.029 (↓↓)	0.029 (↓↓)	0.029 (↓↓)	0.029 (↓↓)	0.029 (↓↓)	0.029 (↓↓)	0.029 (↓↓)

↓↓ (or ↑↑): used to report a significant (p-value < 0.05) decrease (or increase) of feature median in negative receptor status (ER−), ↓ (or ↑) indicated a non-significant (p-value > 0.05) decrease (or increase) of a feature median in negative receptor status (ER−).

3.1.2. Statistical Analysis per Receptor Status: PR+ vs PR−

Table 4 reports the results of the statistical analysis from Wilcoxon signed-rank test indicating association between MRI phenotype and receptor status PR+ versus PR−, for each normalization method. In Table 4 the radiomic features that showed a significant p-values were reported.

As shown in Table 4 and Figure 3B, 5 out of the 36 radiomic features (E3, E4, T4, T5, and T6) showed significant changes between PR− and PR+ for non-normalized, scaling, z-score, robust z-score, log-transformation, upper quartile and quantile radiomic features. Three out of these 5 features (E3, E4, T5) showed a significantly decreased value in PR− status, while the remaining 2 features showed a significant increase. As far as whitening normalization method is concerned, only three radiomic features (T2, T5, and S2) showed significant changes between PR− and PR+. T2 and T5 showed a decreased value in PR− status, while S2 showed an increased value in PR− status.

3.1.3. Statistical Analysis per Receptor Status: HER2+ vs HER2−

Table 5 reports the results of the statistical analysis from Wilcoxon signed-rank test indicating association between MRI phenotype and receptor status HER2+ versus HER2−, for each normalization method. In Table 5 the radiomic features that showed a significant p-values were reported.

Table 4. Results from the Wilcoxon signed-rank test indicating association between MRI phenotype and molecular classification PR+ versus PR.

Feature Names	Non-Normalized Pval (Trend)	Scaling Pval (Trend)	Z-Score Pval (Trend)	Robust Z-Score Pval (Trend)	LOG Pval (Trend)	Quantile Pval (Trend)	Upper Quartile Pval (Trend)	WHT Pval (Trend)
E3	0.021 (↓↓)	0.021 (↓↓)	0.021 (↓↓)	0.021 (↓↓)	0.021 (↓↓)	0.021 (↓↓)	0.021 (↓↓)	0.418 (↑)
E4	0.038 (↓↓)	0.038 (↓↓)	0.038 (↓↓)	0.038 (↓↓)	0.038 (↓↓)	0.038 (↓↓)	0.038 (↓↓)	0.867 (↑)
T2	0.071 (↓)	0.071 (↓)	0.071 (↓)	0.071 (↓)	0.071 (↓)	0.071 (↓)	0.071 (↓)	0.046 (↓↓)
T4	0.049 (↑↑)	0.049 (↑↑)	0.049 (↑↑)	0.049 (↑↑)	0.049 (↑↑)	0.049 (↑↑)	0.049 (↑↑)	0.178 (↑)
T5	0.004 (↓↓)	0.004 (↓↓)	0.004 (↓↓)	0.004 (↓↓)	0.004 (↓↓)	0.004 (↓↓)	0.004 (↓↓)	0.02 (↓↓)
T6	0.02 (↑↑)	0.02 (↑↑)	0.02 (↑↑)	0.02 (↑↑)	0.02 (↑↑)	0.02 (↑↑)	0.02 (↑↑)	0.303 (↑)
S2	0.175 (↑)	0.175 (↑)	0.175 (↑)	0.175 (↑)	0.175 (↑)	0.175 (↑)	0.175 (↑)	0.021 (↑↑)

↓↓ (or ↑↑): used to report a significant (p-value < 0.05) decrease (or increase) of feature median in negative receptor status (PR−), ↓ (or ↑) indicated a non-significant (p-value > 0.05) decrease (or increase) of a feature median in negative receptor status (PR−).

Table 5. Results from the Wilcoxon signed-rank test indicating association between MRI phenotype and molecular classification HER2+ versus HER2−.

Feature Names	Non-Normalized Pval (Trend)	Scaling Pval (Trend)	Z-Score Pval (Trend)	Robust Z-Score Pval (Trend)	LOG Pval (Trend)	Quantile Pval (Trend)	Upper Quartile Pval (Trend)	WHT Pval (Trend)
K6	0.054 (↑)	0.054 (↑)	0.054 (↑)	0.054 (↑)	0.054 (↑)	0.054 (↑)	0.054 (↑)	0.008 (↑↑)
T8	0.414 (↑)	0.414 (↑)	0.414 (↑)	0.414 (↑)	0.414 (↑)	0.414 (↑)	0.414 (↓)	0.025 (↑↑)
M3	0.393 (↑)	0.393 (↑)	0.393 (↑)	0.393 (↑)	0.393 (↑)	0.393 (↑)	0.393 (↑)	0.048 (↑↑)

↓↓ (or ↑↑): used to report a significant (p-value<0.05) decrease (or increase) of feature median in negative receptor status (HER2+), ↓ (or ↑) indicated a non-significant (p-value > 0.05) decrease (or increase) of a feature median in negative receptor status (HER2+).

As shown in Table 5 and Figure 3C, none of 36 radiomic features showed significant changes between HER2− and HER2+ for all normalization methods but whitening transformation. As far as whitening normalization method is concerned, three radiomic features (K6, T8, and M3) showed significant changes between HER2− and HER2+. All these features showed an increased value in HER2 positive cases.

3.1.4. Statistical Analysis per Receptor Status: TN vs Others

Table 6 reports the results of the statistical analysis from Wilcoxon Rank test indicating association between MRI phenotype and receptor status TN versus Others, for each normalization method. In Table 6 the radiomic features that showed a significant p-values were reported.

As shown in Table 6 and Figure 3D, 5 out of the 36 radiomic features (E2, G2, S1, S2, and S3) showed significant changes between TN vs Others for non-normalized, scaling, z-score, robust z-score, log-transformation, upper quartile, and quantile radiomic features. All 5 features showed a significantly increased value in TN status. As far as whitening normalization method is concerned, five different radiomic features (E2, T6, T11, G2, and S2) showed significant changes between TN and Others. All features, expect T11, showed an increased value in TN status.

Table 6. Results from the Wilcoxon signed-rank test indicating association between MRI phenotype and molecular classification TN versus Others.

Feature Names	Non-Normalized Pval (Trend)	Scaling Pval (Trend)	Z-Score Pval (Trend)	Robust Z-Score Pval (Trend)	LOG Pval (Trend)	Quantile Pval (Trend)	Upper Quartile Pval (Trend)	WHT Pval (Trend)
E2	0.048 (↑↑)	0.048 (↑↑)	0.048 (↑↑)	0.048 (↑↑)	0.048 (↑↑)	0.048 (↑↑)	0.048 (↑↑)	0.035 (↑↑)
T6	0.107 (↑)	0.107 (↑)	0.107 (↑)	0.107 (↑)	0.107 (↑)	0.107 (↑)	0.107 (↑)	0.024 (↑↑)
T11	0.078 (↓)	0.078 (↓)	0.078 (↓)	0.078 (↓)	0.078 (↓)	0.078 (↓)	0.078 (↓)	0.024 (↓↓)
G2	0.048 (↑↑)	0.048 (↑↑)	0.048 (↑↑)	0.048 (↑↑)	0.048 (↑↑)	0.048 (↑↑)	0.048 (↑↑)	0.019 (↑↑)
S1	0.01 (↑↑)	0.01 (↑↑)	0.01 (↑↑)	0.01 (↑↑)	0.01 (↑↑)	0.01 (↑↑)	0.01 (↑↑)	0.458 (↑)
S2	0.01 (↑↑)	0.01 (↑↑)	0.01 (↑↑)	0.01 (↑↑)	0.01 (↑↑)	0.01 (↑↑)	0.01 (↑↑)	0.021 (↑↑)
S3	0.012 (↑↑)	0.012 (↑↑)	0.012 (↑↑)	0.012 (↑↑)	0.012 (↑↑)	0.012 (↑↑)	0.012 (↑↑)	0.259 (↑)

↓↓ (or ↑↑): used to report a significant (p-value < 0.05) decrease (or increase) of feature median in negative receptor status (TN), ↓ (or ↑) indicated a non-significant (p-value > 0.05) decrease (or increase) of a feature median in negative receptor status (TN).

3.2. Genomics

As previously shown, several MRI radiomic features showed statistically significant variations in ER, PR, HER2, and TN status across different normalization approaches.

Aberrant miRNAs expression is one of the genomic alterations occurring in breast cancer [66], which showed association with some MRI radiomic features [22] Thus, we computed miRNAs differentially expressed among TCGA breast tumor tissues with ER, PR, and HER2 receptor status annotation available. Ten differentially expressed miRNAs (DEmiRNAs, p adjusted ≤0.05), including hsa-mir-4662a, hsa-mir-486.1, hsa-mir-486.2, hsa-mir-526b(mir-515 family), hsa-mir-122, hsa-mir-653, hsa-mir-9.2, hsa-mir-135a.2, hsa-mir-184 and hsa-mir-206 (mir-1 family) were used to investigate relationship between radiomic and genomic features.

Box plots show DEmiRNAs trend as function of ER (Figure S1), PR (Figure S2), HER2 (Figure S3), and triple negative (Figure S4) receptor status, with Wilcoxon test for statistical significance (threshold p-value less than 0.05). Several DEmiRNAs showed to be statistically significant in ER receptor status (hsa-mir-122, hsa-mir-653, hsa-mir-9.2, hsa-mir-135a.2, hsa-mir-184) with a p-value < 0.05 (Figure S1). Three DEmiRNAs expression (hsa-mir-653, hsa-mir-9.2, hsa-mir-184) showed a significant p-values for PR status (Figure S2). Only two DEmiRNAs expression (hsa-mir-653, hsa-mir-135a.2) showed a significant variation in HER2 status (Figure S3). Lastly, four DEmiRNAs expression (hsa-mir-122, hsa-mir-653, hsa-mir-9.2, and hsa-mir-184) had a statistical variation in TN cases (Figure S4).

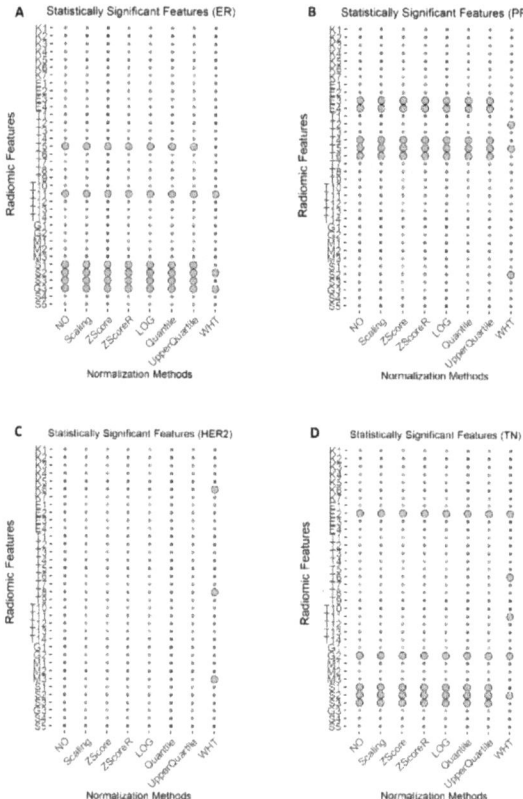

Figure 3. Statistically significant radiomic features. Statistically significant radiomic features across normalization methods are identified with a circle. (**A**) Statistically significant radiomic features for receptor status ER across normalization methods. (**B**) Statistically significant radiomic features for receptor status PR across normalization methods. (**C**) Statistically significant radiomic features for receptor status HER2 across normalization methods. (**D**) Statistically significant radiomic features for receptor status TN across normalization methods. NO: non-normalized features; Scaling normalization method; Z-score normalization method; ZscoreR: Robust Z-score normalization method; LOG transformation; Quantile and Upper Quartile normalization method; WHT: Whitening normalization method.

3.3. Radiogenomics

As shown previously, a set of statistically significant radiomic features emerged from different normalization approaches. In order to assess imaging-genomic associations, considering that the distributions of radiomic and genomic features were not normal, we carried out Spearman's correlation analysis between the statistically significant radiomic features and miRNAs differentially expressed in breast cancer.

Regarding the correlation, we chose radiomic features from two normalization methods: *i)* the upper quartile (UQ) normalized method, since the UQ method was used to normalize miRNA-seq data, and *ii)* the whitening method (WHT), because it provided statistically significant radiomic features for all receptors' status.

The samples were stratified into ER+/ER−, PR+/PR−, and HER+/HER2− and TN status. Greater attention was paid in investigating imaging-genomic associations for ER-negative, PR-negative, HER2-positive, and TN cases, which are more relevant to the clinical practise.

3.3.1. Correlation Analysis per Receptor Status: ER+ vs ER−

Spearman's correlation analysis between UQ normalized radiomic features and miRNAs, for ER negative receptor status, highlighted a statistically significant negative correlation between the shape feature G3 and hsa-mir-526b (p-value adjusted < 0.05, Table S4), representing the ratio surface area to volume based on 3D reconstruction of lesion (Figure 4A). Other correlations included the size feature S3 with hsa-mir-653 and hsa-mir-206, characterizing lesion surface area, and the enhancement texture feature T5, indicating image homogeneity, associated with hsa-mir-9.2 (Figure 4A), although these correlations were not statistically significant (Table S4).

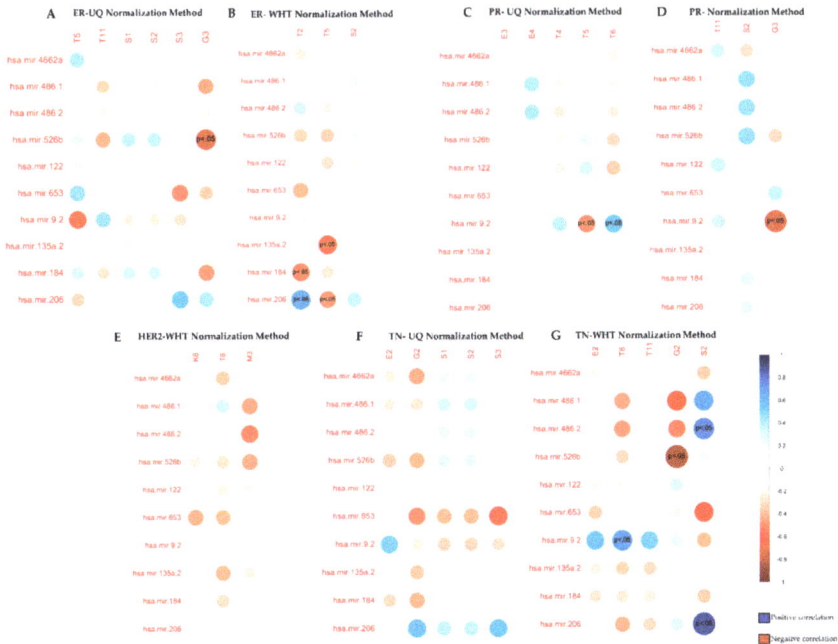

Figure 4. Spearman correlation between miRNAs expression and MRI radiomic features normalized by Upper Quartile and Whitening methods for molecular receptor status. (**A**) Correlation between ER negative breast cancer miRNAs expression and MRI radiomic features normalized by Upper Quartile (UQ) method. (**B**) Correlation between ER negative breast cancer miRNAs expression and MRI radiomic features normalized by Whitening (WHT) method. (**C**) Correlation between PR negative breast cancer miRNAs expression and MRI radiomic features normalized by Upper Quartile (UQ) method. (**D**) Correlation between PR negative breast cancer miRNAs expression and MRI radiomic features normalized by Whitening (WHT) method. (**E**) Correlation between HER2 positive breast cancer miRNAs expression and MRI radiomic features normalized by whitening methods. (**F**) Correlation between TN negative breast cancer miRNAs expression and MRI radiomic features normalized by Upper Quartile (UQ) method. (**G**) Correlation between TN negative breast cancer miRNAs expression and MRI radiomic features normalized by Whitening (WHT) method.

In contrast, when we performed Spearman's correlations for ER negative receptor status, using WHT normalized radiomic features, the shape feature G3 resulted associated with hsa-mir-9.2 (p adjusted < 0.01) in a statistically significant manner (Figure 4B, Table S4).

3.3.2. Correlation Analysis per Receptor Status: PR+ vs PR−

For PR negative receptor status, UQ normalized radiomic features T5 (angular second moment, energy) and T6 (entropy) inversely correlated with hsa-mir-9.2 (p-value adjusted < 0.05) (Figure 4C, Table S4). These enhancement texture features indicate image homogeneity and randomness of the grey levels.

Similarly, for PR negative status, WHT normalized radiomic features (T5 and T2) showed to be correlated (p-value adjusted < 0.05) with different miRNAs (hsa-mir-135a.2, hsa-mir-184, hsa-mir-206) (Figure 4D, Table S4).

3.3.3. Correlation Analysis per Receptor Status: HER2+ vs HER2−

For HER2 positive receptor status, we only performed a correlation analysis using WHT normalized radiomic features, as it was the only normalization method that identified statistically significant radiomic features. In this case, the morphological feature M3 correlated with hsa-mir-486.2, characterizing lesion enhancement structure from the central to a radial pattern, although this association was not statistically significant (Figure 4E, Table S4).

3.3.4. Correlation Analysis per Receptor Status: TN vs Others

We found interesting findings for TN receptor status, comparing UQ and WHT normalized radiomic features.

Correlation analysis of UQ normalized radiomic features highlighted that G2 and S3 were inversely correlated with hsa-mir-653 and hsa-mir-206, respectively (Figure 4F), whereas we found a positive correlation between the enhancement texture feature E2 and hsa-mir-9.2, indicating enhancement variance kinetics. However, none of these correlations were statistically significant (Table S4).

Conversely, when we used WHT normalized radiomic features, we found several statistically significant correlations. Indeed, negative correlations were found between the shape feature G2 measuring irregularity of the lesion with hsa-mir-526b (p adjusted < 0.01), hsa-mir-486-1 and hsa-mir-486-2 (both, p-adjusted n.s.) (Figure 4G, Table S4). We found positive correlations with the size feature S2 indicating effective diameter of a sphere with the same volume of the lesion with hsa-mir-206 (p-value adjusted < 0.01), hsa-mir-486-1 (p-value adjusted n.s.) and hsa-mir-486-2 (p-adjusted < 0.05) and negative correlation with hsa-mir-653 (p-adjusted n.s.) (Figure 4G, Table S4). In addition, we found positive correlations between the enhancement variance kinetics E2, enhancement texture T6 and T11 features with hsa-mir-9.2. Among these associations, only T6 was statically significant (p-value adjusted < 0.05) (Figure 4G, Table S4).

3.4. Machine Learning Per Molecular Classification

Regarding the feature selection process, all possible combinations of relevant and non-redundant radiomic features were investigated for each normalization methods employed in the study. Each machine learning method was trained and validated with all combinations of radiomic features using folder 1. The best feature combination was chosen as the one achieving the best AUC during training. The classifiers were, then, tested on folder 2.

3.4.1. Receptor Status: ER− vs ER+

Figure 5 shows the best performance of the three machine learning classifiers (SVM, RF, and NB) across all normalization methods to automatically detect ER receptor status. For each normalization approach the radiomic features chosen as the one achieving the best performance are reported along with the respective performance in Tables S5–S7.

Figure 6A shows the best classifiers for each of the machine learning methods according to the criteria defined in Section 2.3.3. The classifier achieving the best performances to detect ER− status is Random Forest using only two radiomic features (T11 and S2) normalized via whitening method.

Figure 6B shows the ROC curves for the best classifiers to automatically detect ER receptor status. Box plots of radiomic features chosen by the machine learning methods to automatically detect ER status are shown in Figure S5.

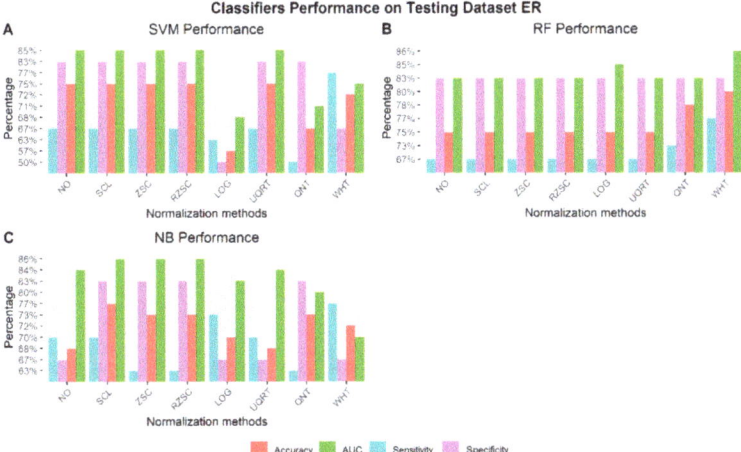

Figure 5. Classifiers performance on testing dataset to identify ER receptor status via radiomic features across normalization methods (NO: non-normalized features; SCL: Scaling normalization method; ZSC: Z-score normalization method; RZSC: Robust Z-score normalization method; LOG transformation; UPQRT: Upper Quartile normalization methods; QNT: Quantile normalization method; WHT: Whitening normalization method). **A**) Support Vector Machine (SVM) Performance on Testing dataset ER+ vs ER−. **B**) Random Forest (RF) Performance on Testing dataset ER+ vs ER−. **C**) Naïve Bayesian (NB) Performance on Testing dataset ER+ vs ER−.

A

Feature Names	Normalization Methods	ML Methods	SEN	SPE	ACC	AUC
T5, T11	NO; Scaling; Z-score; Robust Z-score; Upper Quartile.	SVM	67%	83%	75%	85%
T11, S2	WHT	RF	77%	83%	80%	86%
T5, S2, G3	Scaling	NB	70%	83%	77%	86%

NO: non-normalized features; LOG transformation method; WHT: Whitening normalization method. SVM: Support Vector Machine; RF: Random Forest; NB: Naïve Bayesian; SEN: Sensitivity; SPE: Specificity; ACC: Accuracy; AUC: Area Under the Curve; ML: Machine Learning.

B

a) Support Vector Machine (NO) b) Random Forest (WHT) c) Naïve Bayesian (Scaling)

Figure 6. Classifiers' performance to detect ER receptor status. (**A**) Comparison table among classifiers: ER+ vs ER−. (**B**) ROC curves for the best classifiers to automatically detect ER receptor status. a) Best classifier for Support Vector Machine Method. The normalization methods that achieved the best performance are Scaling, Z-score, Robust Z-score, Upper Quartile normalization methods. They achieved the same performance; therefore, one ROC curve with non-normalized features is reported. b) Best classifier for Random Forest Method. The normalization method that achieved the best performance is the whitening method. c) Best classifier for Naïve Bayesian Method. The normalization method that achieved the best performance is scaling method.

3.4.2. Receptor Status: PR– vs PR+

Figure 7 shows the best performance of the three machine learning classifiers (SVM, RF, and NB) across all normalization methods to automatically detect PR receptor status. For each normalization approach the radiomic features chosen as the one achieving the best performance are reported along with the respective performance in Tables S8–S10.

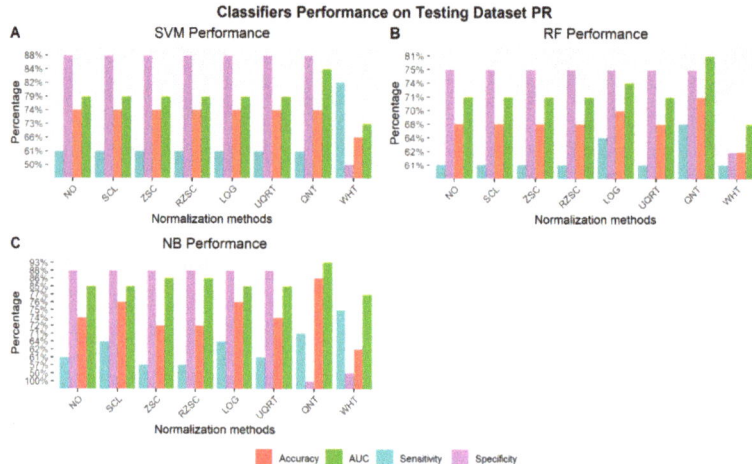

Figure 7. Classifiers performance on testing dataset to identify PR receptor status via radiomic features across normalization methods (NO: non-normalized features; SCL: Scaling normalization method; ZSC: Z-score normalization method; RZSC: Robust Z-score normalization method; LOG transformation; UPQRT: Upper Quartile normalization methods; QNT: Quantile normalization method; WHT: Whitening normalization method). A) Support Vector Machine (SVM) Performance on Testing dataset PR+ vs PR–. B) Random Forest (RF) Performance on Testing dataset PR+ vs PR–. C) Naïve Bayesian (NB) Performance on Testing dataset PR+ vs PR–.

Figure 8A shows the best classifiers for each of the machine learning methods according to the criteria defined in Section 2.3.3. The classifier achieving the best performances to detect PR negative status is Naïve Bayesian model using only two radiomic features (E4 and T5) normalized via quantile method. Figure 8B shows the ROC curves for the best classifiers to automatically detect PR receptor status. Box plots of radiomic features chosen by the machine learning methods to automatically detect PR status are shown in Figure S6.

3.4.3. Receptor Status: HER2– vs HER2+

Figure 9A shows the best classifiers for each of the machine learning methods according to the criteria defined in Section 2.3.3. The classifier achieving the best performances to detect HER2 receptor status is Random Forest model using only two radiomic features (T8 and K6) normalized via whitening normalization method. Figure 9B shows the ROC curves for the best classifiers to automatically detect HER2 receptor status. Box plots of radiomic features chosen by the machine learning methods to automatically detect HER2 status are shown in Figure S7.

3.4.4. Receptor Status: TN vs Others

Figure 10 shows the best performance of the three machine learning classifiers (SVM, RF, and NB) across all normalization methods to automatically detect TN cases. For each normalization approach the radiomic features chosen as the one achieving the best performance are reported along with the respective performance in Tables S11–S13.

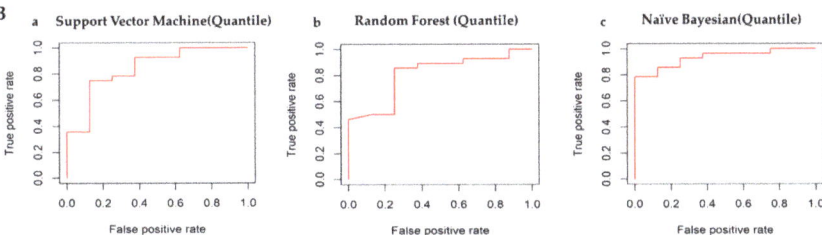

Figure 8. Classifiers' performance to detect PR receptor status. (**A**) Comparison table among classifiers: PR+ vs PR−. (**B**) ROC curves for the best classifiers to automatically detect PR receptor status. a) Best classifier for Support Vector Machine Method. The normalization methods that achieved the best performance is the quantile normalization method. b) Best classifier for Random Forest Method. The normalization method that achieved the best performance is the quantile method. c) Best classifier for Naïve Bayesian Method. The normalization method that achieved the best performance is quantile method.

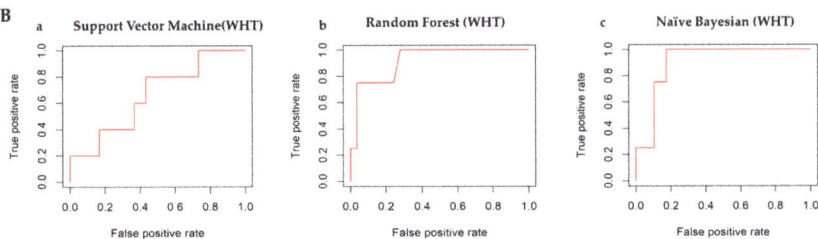

Figure 9. Classifiers' performance to detect HER2 receptor status. (**A**) Comparison table among classifiers: HER2+ vs HER2−. (**B**) ROC curves for the best classifiers to automatically detect HER2 receptor status. Radiomic Feature normalized by whitening methods were considered for the classification task. a) Best classifier for Support Vector Machine Method. b) Best classifier for Random Forest Method. c) Best classifier for Naïve Bayesian method.

Figure 11A shows the best classifiers for each of the machine learning methods according to the criteria defined in Section 2.3.3. The classifier achieving the best performances to detect TN cases is Random Forest model using only two radiomic features (T11 and G2) normalized via whitening method. Figure 11B shows the ROC curves for the best classifiers to automatically detect TN cases. Box plots of radiomic features chosen by the machine learning methods to automatically detect TN cases are shown in Figure S8.

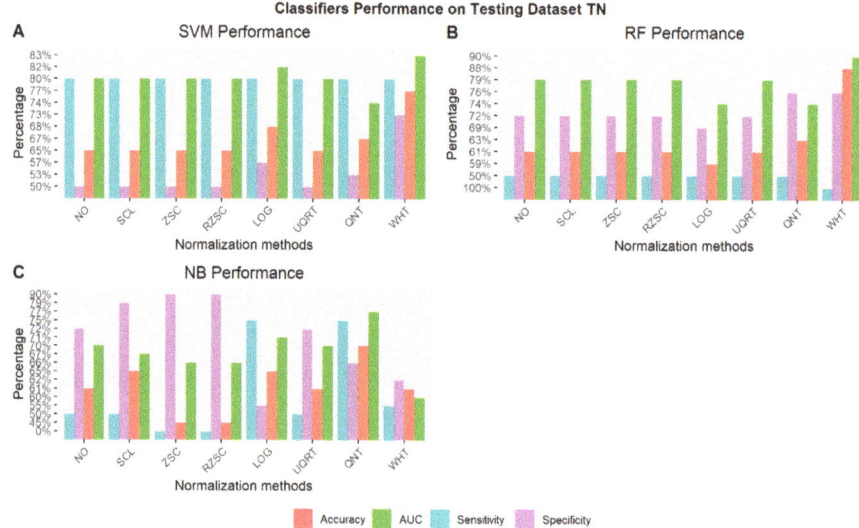

Figure 10. Classifiers performance on testing dataset to identify TN cases via radiomic features across normalization methods (NO: non-normalized features; SCL: Scaling normalization method; ZSC: Z-score normalization method; RZSC: Robust Z-score normalization method; LOG transformation; UPQRT: Upper Quartile normalization methods; QNT: Quantile normalization method; WHT: Whitening normalization method). **A)** Support Vector Machine (SVM) Performance on Testing dataset TN vs Others. **B)** Random Forest (RF) Performance on Testing dataset TN vs Others. **C)** Naïve Bayesian (NB) Performance on Testing dataset TN vs Others.

A

Feature Names	Normalization Methods	ML Methods	SEN	SPE	ACC	AUC
E2, G2	WHT	SVM	80%	73%	77%	83%
T11, G2	WHT	RF	98%	76%	88%	91%
T11, S2	WHT	NB	75%	66%	70%	77%

WHT: Whitening normalization method; SVM: Support Vector Machine; RF: Random Forest; NB: Naïve Bayesian. SEN: Sensitivity; SPE: Specificity; ACC: Accuracy; AUC: Area Under the Curve.

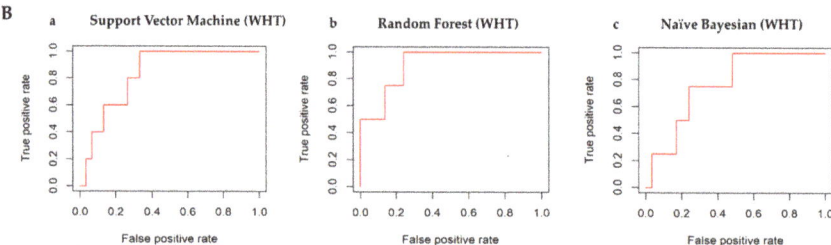

Figure 11. Classifiers' performance to detect TN receptor status. (**A**) Comparison table among classifiers: TN vs Others. (**B**) ROC curves for the best classifiers to automatically detect TN receptor status. a) Best classifier for Support Vector Machine Method. The normalization methods that achieved the best performance is the quantile normalization method. b) Best classifier for Random Forest Method. The normalization method that achieved the best performance is the quantile method. c) Best classifier for Naïve Bayesian Method. The normalization method that achieved the best performance is quantile method.

4. Discussion

The results from this study demonstrate that quantitative radiomic analysis shows potential as a means for high-throughput image-based phenotyping to automatically detect breast cancer receptor status via machine learning methods. Moreover, this study investigates the effect of normalization methods on radiomic features to automatically detect receptor status of breast cancer patients. Altogether our results suggest that quantitative radiomic analysis is influenced by normalization method choice.

The results from the correlation analysis along with visual inspection by Bland–Altman analysis, showed that all radiomic features are perfectly correlated with non-normalized radiomic features using scaling, z-score, robust z-score, and upper quartile normalization methods. Therefore, these methods help reducing bias and do not alter the information carried by the "row" radiomic features. These normalization methods, thus, result less aggressive than log-transformation, quantile, and whitening methods. In fact, four, sixteen and thirty out of 36 radiomic features showed a poorly correlation value with non-normalized radiomic features for log-transformation, quantile, and whitening normalization methods respectively. These results were expected. Log-transformation should be carefully applied to radiomic data as does not always decrease the skewness of the distribution but can make it more skewed than the raw data. Another common use of the log-transformation is to reduce the variability of data, especially in data sets including outliers, but it can often increase the variability of data. Moreover, log-transformation can only be used for positive outcomes, thus, for negative values it is common to add a small positive constant, a, to all observations before applying this transformation. Although this practice can appear quite meaningless, it can have a noticeable effect on the level of statistical significance [67]. Therefore, log-transformation should be carefully used in radiomic studies.

Quantile normalization method transforms original data to remove undesirable technical variation. Technical variation could cause apparent differences between samples. This kind of normalization is achieved by forcing the observed distributions to be the same and the average distribution, obtained by taking the average of each quantile across samples, is used as the reference. This method has worked well in practice, but important information could be wiped out and features that are not statically different across samples can be artificially induced [51]. Therefore, although it could improve the predictive power of the features, it should be used carefully.

Whitening normalization using PCA can make a more substantial normalization of the features to give it zero mean and unit covariance, so that transformed features become decorrelated [68]. One weakness of this transformation is that it can greatly exaggerate the noise in the data, since it stretches all dimensions (including noise) to be of equal size in the input. However, this method is often used as pre-processing step for machine learning models as it improves the overall performance.

Consequently, "aggressive" normalization methods should be carefully assessed based on the nature of the data and the main goal of the analysis.

Regarding the statistical analysis per receptor status, the results are in agreement with the existing literature [69].

Our results indicate that ER-negative cases may have larger volume, diameter and lesion area whereas less homogeneity and brightness than ER-positive cases. Similar observations were also reported by Chen et al. [70] in a correlation study between ER status and breast MRI radiomics and Li et al. [7] that showed an higher effective diameter, irregularity and entropy in ER-negative cases.

Different results were observed using quantile and whitening transformation methods. In fact, less features showed to be significantly different between positive and negative ER cases. One features (S1) and three features (T5, S1, S3) were not statistically significant using whitening and quantile transformation methods compared to the other investigated normalization methods. Moreover, these phenotypes captured on imaging are in agreement with prior literature showing that ER– tumors have higher microvessel density [71], higher levels of vascular endothelial growth factor [72], and higher proliferative activity [72].

Our results indicate that PR-negative cases may have lower enhancement-variance rate and homogeneity while higher entropy. PR-negative cases are also larger, more irregular in shape, more heterogeneous, and have a faster contrast uptake than PR-positive cases as also demonstrated by Li et al. [7]. These observations confirm the existing evidence that PR cancers tend to have high growth factor signaling [73]. Different results were observed using whitening-transformation method. In fact, less features showed to be significantly different between positive and negative PR cases. Three radiomic features showed significant changes between PR cases, while T5 was also captured as significant feature (p-value < 0.05) by other normalization methods, T2 and S2 were not statistically significant using other transformation methods.

As far as HER2 growth factor is concerned, none of 36 radiomic features showed significant changes between positive and negative HER2 cases except for whitening-transformation. Indeed, features normalized by whitening method showed an increased value in enhancement texture, structure and voxel for HER2 positive case.

TN cases showed to be larger, more irregular in shape, heterogeneous, and have a faster contrast uptake rate than all the other cases. Similar results were achieved by Agner et al. [28] showing more lesion heterogeneity in TN breast cancers than non-TN cancers. Li et al. [7] reported that TN cases are larger in size due to the over expression of oncogenes that favor cell proliferation defined by the absence of ER, PR, and HER2 receptors. Youk et al. [74] showed that larger tumor size was significantly associated with TN breast cancer. Using whitening transformation, different radiomic features showed statistical changes between cases but maintained the overall trends.

Overall, imaging phenotypes like enhancement texture, size features convey pathophysiologic characteristics like proliferation and angiogenesis provide clues to more accurate prognosis and optimal treatment. It is interesting to note that enhancement texture (especially heterogeneity) emerged as an important discriminatory indicator. In our study, a decrease in homogeneity was observed in ER–, PR–, and TN cancers relative to ER+, PR+, and non-TN cancers, in agreement with the exiting literature. Enhancement texture homogeneity was also found to be positively associated with tumor stage, suggesting that larger, heterogeneous tumors are potentially linked to more aggressive cancers [7] with higher probability of recurrence [41].

Moreover, we questioned whether radiomic features may be associated with aberrantly expressed breast cancer miRNAs. Thus, we evaluated the correlation degree using two different radiomic features normalization methods. In accordance with the exiting literature, breast miRNAs expression resulted associated especially to MR radiomic features such as shape and enhancement texture features [22]. However, as expected, we showed that various radiomic features normalization approaches capture different imaging-genomic associations. For example, for ER receptor status the upper quartile normalized G3 feature correlated with hsa-mir-526b whereas whitening normalized G3 feature correlated with hsa-mir-9.2. For this reason, once chosen the appropriate radiomic framework of analysis, conspicuous testing of radiomic results on external and independent image datasets are encouraged.

Using machine learning algorithms, enhancement texture features were selected as the most predictive feature for tumor receptor status. Hence, radiomic features have a high predictive power to detect clinical variables related to the genomic status of a tumor, such as ER status and PR status. The machine learning method that better performed to automatically detect ER, HER2, and TN cases is the Random Forest with an AUC of 86%, 91%, and 91% respectively. Naïve Bayesian outperformed the other methods to detect PR cases with 93% AUC.

Compared to the existing literature, the results achieved in this study via machine learning methods outperformed other studies.

Xie et al. [32] achieved an AUC of 91% via linear SVM using several whole-tumor texture features extracted from DCE and DWI-related original images, while we achieved the same AUC values using only two DCE imaging feature, reducing considerably the computational complexity of the Random Forest model. Agner et al. [28] used the morphologic and texture features extracted from the whole tumor on the early postcontrast images in conjunction with an SVM classifier, achieving a lower AUC (of 74%) to detect TN cases. Li at al. [7] also achieved a lower AUC value using quantitative imaging phenotypes of size, shape, and enhancement texture via linear discriminant analysis to predict clinical receptor status, namely ER+ vs ER− (89% AUC), PR+ vs PR− (69% AUC), HER2+ vs HER2− (65%AUC),and TN cases (67% AUC). Yoon et al. [33] used a deep learning approach utilizing imaging data from TCIA to generate prediction of clinical outcomes receptor status. They achieved lower performance to predict ER (82% AUC), PR (75% AUC), HER2 (72% AUC), but they accomplished a slightly higher AUC values using the combination of radiomics and genomics data.

Overall, in this study using robust machine learning methods and employing few radiomic feature to reduce the computational complexity of the ML models, we achieved better AUC values to discriminate clinical receptor status, paving the way to non-invasive disease monitoring using imaging features as potential surrogate markers of underlying molecular activity that may aid in clinical diagnosis and treatment planning.

Most of the radiomic features chosen by the ML methods were normalized using whitening transformation, whereas to detect PR cases the radiomic features were normalized by quantile transformation. These results were expected as quantile and whitening transformation are considered among the best normalizing transformation when compared to other alternatives in machine learning models [52,75]. Both transformation methods reduce the leverage of potentially influential points among candidate predictors and remove redundancy among them. In fact, normalization of the covariates mitigates the leverage and potential influence of these covariates to an extent, which in some cases, will allow for more robust model selection.

However, this study presents some limitations. The MR images used in this study were acquired by different institutions more than 10 years ago. These may have had different acquisition protocols, different weight-based dosing regimen for contrast agents, and different time resolution of post-contrast sequences, and therefore, these images may not reflect current MRI technology, which has advanced considerably during the past decade. Consequently, our results can only be generalized to this population. However, the bias was limited by performing several normalization methods on the extracted radiomic features. Another limitation of our study was that the patient sample was relatively small and unbalanced, but by performing a cross validation for each molecular classification assessment (e.g., between ER+ and ER− cases) and applying balancing methods (SMOTE) to the developed model, the overall bias was reduced. In addition, our study lacks further validation on internal cohort, for which patient recruitment is ongoing.

Therefore, after this pilot study, which helped us establishing a robust framework of analysis, upcoming work will include studies on a larger and more recent clinically annotated data set to verify and validate the results from this preliminary study. We will further assess the role of the MRI phenotypes in combination with genomic and clinical information to improve the prediction power of the machine learning-based models. Furthermore, molecular breast cancer intrinsic subtypes will be also investigated.

5. Conclusions

In this study, our results demonstrate that there are statistically significant associations between radiomic tumor features and breast cancer molecular receptor status. Breast tumor characterization, including the ER, PR, and HER2 molecular receptor status, represents a primary goal to direct treatment options and targeted chemotherapies. Thus, in order to achieve a more accurate and early diagnosis is relevant to identify non-invasive diagnostic imaging biomarker associated to the molecular receptor status. This study investigated several statistical approaches to identify the relationship between medical imaging quantitative descriptors of clinical phenotypes and molecular tumor characteristics. Moreover, the prediction power of each radiomic feature normalization method was assessed by three advanced machine learning algorithms. The results from this study offer a better understanding into the underlying tumor biology including tumor enhancement texture. Identifying receptor status via imaging phenotypes may aid in clinical diagnosis and treatment planning. At the same time, we aware researchers to implement in radiomic analysis framework different radiomic feature normalization approaches and standards for post-acquisition data processing, in order to ensure more robust findings.

Another important advantage of our approach is that opens the door to the identification of non-invasive in vivo imaging surrogate markers that could reflect the underlying tumor biology.

Supplementary Materials: The following are available online at http://www.mdpi.com/2072-6694/12/2/518/s1, Figure S1: Relationship between breast cancer miRNAs expression and ER receptor status; Figure S2: Relationship between breast cancer miRNAs expression and PR receptor status; Figure S3: Relationship between breast cancer miRNAs expression and HER2 receptor status; Figure S4: Relationship between breast cancer miRNAs expression and TN cases; Figure S5. Box plots of radiomic features chosen by the machine learning methods to automatically detect ER status; Figure S6: Box plots of radiomic features chosen by the machine learning methods to automatically detect PR status; Figure S7: Box plots of radiomic features chosen by the machine learning methods to automatically detect HER2 receptor; Figure S8: Box plots of radiomic features chosen by the machine learning methods to automatically detect TN cases. Table S1: Additional Clinical Parameters; Table S2: Radiomic Features; Table S3: Correlation Analysis on the Whole Dataset between Non-Normalized and Normalized Radiomic Features; Table S4: Imaging-genomic associations; Table S5: Support Vector Machine Performance on Testing dataset ER+ vs ER−; Table S6: Random Forest Performance on Testing dataset ER+ vs ER−; Table S7: Naïve Bayesian Performance on Testing dataset ER+ vs ER−; Table S8: Support Vector Machine Performance on Testing dataset PR+ vs PR−; Table S9: Random Forest Performance on Testing dataset PR+ vs PR−; Table S10: Naïve Bayesian Performance on Testing dataset PR+ vs PR−; Table S11: Support Vector Machine Performance on Testing dataset TN vs Others; Table S12: Random Forest Performance on Testing dataset TN vs Others; Table S13: Naïve Bayesian Performance on Testing dataset TN vs Others.

Author Contributions: R.C. and K.P. wrote the manuscript, designed the analysis framework for radiomics and genomics, contributing equally to this work. M.F. contributed to conception and design and supported data analysis. E.N. interpreted data and validated the results. M.S. revised the manuscript critically and approved the version to be published. All authors have read and agreed to the published version of the manuscript.

Funding: This research received no external funding.

Conflicts of Interest: The authors declare no conflict of interest.

References

1. Siegel, R.; Ma, J.; Zou, Z.; Jemal, A. Cancer statistics, 2014. *CA Cancer J. Clin.* **2014**, *64*, 9–29. [CrossRef] [PubMed]
2. Fiordelisi, M.; Auletta, L.; Meomartino, L.; Basso, L.; Fatone, G.; Salvatore, M.; Mancini, M.; Greco, A. Preclinical Molecular Imaging for Precision Medicine in Breast Cancer Mouse Models. *Contrast Media Mol. Imaging* **2019**, *2019*, 8946729. [CrossRef] [PubMed]
3. Carey, L.A.; Perou, C.M.; Livasy, C.A.; Dressler, L.G.; Cowan, D.; Conway, K.; Karaca, G.; Troester, M.A.; Tse, C.K.; Edmiston, S. Race, breast cancer subtypes, and survival in the Carolina Breast Cancer Study. *JAMA* **2006**, *295*, 2492–2502. [CrossRef] [PubMed]
4. Voduc, K.D.; Cheang, M.C.; Tyldesley, S.; Gelmon, K.; Nielsen, T.O.; Kennecke, H. Breast cancer subtypes and the risk of local and regional relapse. *J. Clin. Oncol.* **2010**, *28*, 1684–1691. [CrossRef] [PubMed]
5. Metzger-Filho, O.; Sun, Z.; Viale, G.; Price, K.N.; Crivellari, D.; Snyder, R.D.; Gelber, R.D.; Castiglione-Gertsch, M.; Coates, A.S.; Goldhirsch, A. Patterns of recurrence and outcome according to breast cancer subtypes in lymph node–negative disease: Results from International Breast Cancer Study Group Trials VIII and IX. *J. Clin. Oncol.* **2013**, *31*, 3083. [CrossRef]
6. Arvold, N.D.; Taghian, A.G.; Niemierko, A.; Raad, R.F.A.; Sreedhara, M.; Nguyen, P.L.; Bellon, J.R.; Wong, J.S.; Smith, B.L.; Harris, J.R. Age, breast cancer subtype approximation, and local recurrence after breast-conserving therapy. *J. Clin. Oncol.* **2011**, *29*, 3885. [CrossRef]
7. Li, H.; Zhu, Y.; Burnside, E.S.; Huang, E.; Drukker, K.; Hoadley, K.A.; Fan, C.; Conzen, S.D.; Zuley, M.; Net, J.M. Quantitative MRI radiomics in the prediction of molecular classifications of breast cancer subtypes in the TCGA/TCIA data set. *NPJ Breast Cancer* **2016**, *2*, 16012. [CrossRef]
8. Goldhirsch, A.; Wood, W.C.; Coates, A.S.; Gelber, R.D.; Thürlimann, B.; Senn, H.-J.; Members, P. Strategies for subtypes—dealing with the diversity of breast cancer: Highlights of the St Gallen International Expert Consensus on the Primary Therapy of Early Breast Cancer 2011. *Ann. Oncol.* **2011**, *22*, 1736–1747. [CrossRef]
9. Gnant, M.; Harbeck, N.; Thomssen, C. St. Gallen/Vienna 2017: A brief summary of the consensus discussion about escalation and de-escalation of primary breast cancer treatment. *Breast Care* **2017**, *12*, 101–106. [CrossRef]
10. Aerts, H.J. The potential of radiomic-based phenotyping in precision medicine: A review. *JAMA Oncol.* **2016**, *2*, 1636–1642. [CrossRef]

11. Wu, J.; Tha, K.K.; Xing, L.; Li, R. Radiomics and radiogenomics for precision radiotherapy. In *J. Radiat. Res.*; 2018; Volume 59, (Suppl_1), pp. i25–i31.
12. Gillies, R.J.; Kinahan, P.E.; Hricak, H. Radiomics: Images are more than pictures, they are data. *Radiology* **2015**, *278*, 563–577. [CrossRef] [PubMed]
13. Wu, J.; Li, B.; Sun, X.; Cao, G.; Rubin, D.L.; Napel, S.; Ikeda, D.M.; Kurian, A.W.; Li, R. Heterogeneous enhancement patterns of tumor-adjacent parenchyma at MR imaging are associated with dysregulated signaling pathways and poor survival in breast cancer. *Radiology* **2017**, *285*, 401–413. [CrossRef] [PubMed]
14. Mazurowski, M.A. Radiogenomics: What it is and why it is important. *J. Am. Coll. Radiol.* **2015**, *12*, 862–866. [CrossRef] [PubMed]
15. Network, C.G.A. Comprehensive molecular portraits of human breast tumours. *Nature* **2012**, *490*, 61. [CrossRef] [PubMed]
16. Clark, K.; Vendt, B.; Smith, K.; Freymann, J.; Kirby, J.; Koppel, P.; Moore, S.; Phillips, S.; Maffitt, D.; Pringle, M. The Cancer Imaging Archive (TCIA): Maintaining and operating a public information repository. *J. Digit. Imag.* **2013**, *26*, 1045–1057. [CrossRef]
17. Zanfardino, M.; Pane, K.; Mirabelli, P.; Salvatore, M.; Franzese, M. TCGA-TCIA Impact on Radiogenomics Cancer Research: A Systematic Review. *Intl. J. Mol. Sci.* **2019**, *20*, 6033. [CrossRef]
18. Zanfardino, M.; Franzese, M.; Pane, K.; Cavaliere, C.; Monti, S.; Esposito, G.; Salvatore, M.; Aiello, M. Bringing radiomics into a multi-omics framework for a comprehensive genotype–phenotype characterization of oncological diseases. *J. Translat. Med.* **2019**, *17*, 337. [CrossRef]
19. Schiano, C.; Franzese, M.; Pane, K.; Garbino, N.; Soricelli, A.; Salvatore, M.; de Nigris, F.; Napoli, C. Hybrid 18F-FDG-PET/MRI Measurement of Standardized Uptake Value Coupled with Yin Yang 1 Signature in Metastatic Breast Cancer. A Preliminary Study. *Cancers* **2019**, *11*, 1444. [CrossRef]
20. Bhooshan, N.; Giger, M.L.; Jansen, S.A.; Li, H.; Lan, L.; Newstead, G.M. Cancerous breast lesions on dynamic contrast-enhanced MR images: Computerized characterization for image-based prognostic markers. *Radiology* **2010**, *254*, 680–690. [CrossRef]
21. Guo, W.; Li, H.; Zhu, Y.; Lan, L.; Yang, S.; Drukker, K.; Morris, E.A.; Burnside, E.S.; Whitman, G.J.; Giger, M.L. Prediction of clinical phenotypes in invasive breast carcinomas from the integration of radiomics and genomics data. *J. Med. Imag.* **2015**, *2*, 041007. [CrossRef]
22. Zhu, Y.; Li, H.; Guo, W.; Drukker, K.; Lan, L.; Giger, M.L.; Ji, Y. Deciphering genomic underpinnings of quantitative MRI-based radiomic phenotypes of invasive breast carcinoma. *Sci. Rep.* **2015**, *5*, 17787. [CrossRef] [PubMed]
23. Giger, M.L.; Karssemeijer, N.; Schnabel, J.A. Breast image analysis for risk assessment, detection, diagnosis, and treatment of cancer. *Annu. Rev. Biomed. Eng.* **2013**, *15*, 327–357. [CrossRef] [PubMed]
24. Bhooshan, N.; Giger, M.; Edwards, D.; Yuan, Y.; Jansen, S.; Li, H.; Lan, L.; Sattar, H.; Newstead, G. Computerized three-class classification of MRI-based prognostic markers for breast cancer. *Phys. Med. Biol.* **2011**, *56*, 5995.
25. Grimm, L.J.; Zhang, J.; Mazurowski, M.A. Computational approach to radiogenomics of breast cancer: Luminal A and luminal B molecular subtypes are associated with imaging features on routine breast MRI extracted using computer vision algorithms. *J. Magnet. Resonance Imag.* **2015**, *42*, 902–907. [CrossRef]
26. Wu, J.; Cui, Y.; Sun, X.; Cao, G.; Li, B.; Ikeda, D.M.; Kurian, A.W.; Li, R. Unsupervised clustering of quantitative image phenotypes reveals breast cancer subtypes with distinct prognoses and molecular pathways. *Clin. Cancer Res.* **2017**, *23*, 3334–3342. [CrossRef]
27. Burnside, E.S.; Drukker, K.; Li, H.; Bonaccio, E.; Zuley, M.; Ganott, M.; Net, J.M.; Sutton, E.J.; Brandt, K.R.; Whitman, G.J. Using computer-extracted image phenotypes from tumors on breast magnetic resonance imaging to predict breast cancer pathologic stage. *Cancer* **2016**, *122*, 748–757. [CrossRef]
28. Agner, S.C.; Rosen, M.A.; Englander, S.; Tomaszewski, J.E.; Feldman, M.D.; Zhang, P.; Mies, C.; Schnall, M.D.; Madabhushi, A. Computerized image analysis for identifying triple-negative breast cancers and differentiating them from other molecular subtypes of breast cancer on dynamic contrast-enhanced MR images: A feasibility study. *Radiology* **2014**, *272*, 91–99. [CrossRef]
29. Yamaguchi, K.; Abe, H.; Newstead, G.M.; Egashira, R.; Nakazono, T.; Imaizumi, T.; Irie, H. Intratumoral heterogeneity of the distribution of kinetic parameters in breast cancer: Comparison based on the molecular subtypes of invasive breast cancer. *Breast Cancer* **2015**, *22*, 496–502. [CrossRef]

30. Fiordelisi, M.F.; Cavaliere, C.; Auletta, L.; Basso, L.; Salvatore, M. Magnetic Resonance Imaging for Translational Research in Oncology. *J. Clin. Med.* **2019**, *8*, 1883. [CrossRef]
31. Blaschke, E.; Abe, H. MRI phenotype of breast cancer: Kinetic assessment for molecular subtypes. *J. Magnet. Resonance Imag.* **2015**, *42*, 920–924. [CrossRef]
32. Xie, T.; Wang, Z.; Zhao, Q.; Bai, Q.; Zhou, X.; Gu, Y.; Peng, W.; Wang, H. Machine Learning-based Analysis of MR Multiparametric Radiomics for the Subtype Classification of Breast Cancer. *Fron. Oncol.* **2019**, *9*, 505. [CrossRef] [PubMed]
33. Yoon, H.-J.; Ramanathan, A.; Alamudun, F.; Tourassi, G. Deep radiogenomics for predicting clinical phenotypes in invasive breast cancer. In In Proceedings of the 14th International Workshop on Breast Imaging (IWBI 2018), Atlanta, GA, USA, 8–11 July 2018; International Society for Optics and Photonics: Bellingham, WA, USA, 2018; p. 107181H.
34. Parmar, C.; Barry, J.D.; Hosny, A.; Quackenbush, J.; Aerts, H. Data Analysis Strategies in Medical Imaging. *Clin. Cancer Res.* **2018**, *24*, 3492–3499. [CrossRef] [PubMed]
35. Kotsiantis, S.; Kanellopoulos, D.; Pintelas, P. Data preprocessing for supervised leaning. *Intl. J. Comput. Sci.* **2006**, *1*, 111–117.
36. Rizzo, S.; Botta, F.; Raimondi, S.; Origgi, D.; Fanciullo, C.; Morganti, A.G.; Bellomi, M. Radiomics: The facts and the challenges of image analysis. *Eur. Radiol. Exp.* **2018**, *2*, 1–8. [CrossRef]
37. Madabhushi, A.; Udupa, J.K. New methods of MR image intensity standardization via generalized scale. *Med. Phys.* **2006**, *33*, 3426–3434. [CrossRef]
38. Nyúl, L.G.; Udupa, J.K. On standardizing the MR image intensity scale. *Magnet. Resonance Med.* **1999**, *42*, 1072–1081.
39. Nyúl, L.G.; Udupa, J.K.; Zhang, X. New variants of a method of MRI scale standardization. *IEEE Trans. Med. Imag.* **2000**, *19*, 143–150. [CrossRef]
40. Ge, Y.; Udupa, J.K.; Nyul, L.G.; Wei, L.; Grossman, R.I. Numerical tissue characterization in MS via standardization of the MR image intensity scale. *J. Magnet. Resonance Imag.* **2000**, *12*, 715–721. [CrossRef]
41. Li, H.; Zhu, Y.; Burnside, E.S.; Drukker, K.; Hoadley, K.A.; Fan, C.; Conzen, S.D.; Whitman, G.J.; Sutton, E.J.; Net, J.M. MR imaging radiomics signatures for predicting the risk of breast cancer recurrence as given by research versions of MammaPrint, Oncotype DX, and PAM50 gene assays. *Radiology* **2016**, *281*, 382–391. [CrossRef]
42. R Core Team. *R: A Language and Environment for Statistical Computing*; R Foundation for Statistical Computing: Vienna, Austria, 2012. Available online: http://www.R-project.org (accessed on 2 January 2020).
43. Colaprico, A.; Silva, T.C.; Olsen, C.; Garofano, L.; Cava, C.; Garolini, D.; Sabedot, T.S.; Malta, T.M.; Pagnotta, S.M.; Castiglioni, I. TCGAbiolinks: An R/Bioconductor package for integrative analysis of TCGA data. *Nucl. Acids Res.* **2015**, *44*, e71. [CrossRef]
44. Incoronato, M.; Grimaldi, A.M.; Mirabelli, P.; Cavaliere, C.; Parente, C.A.; Franzese, M.; Staibano, S.; Ilardi, G.; Russo, D.; Soricelli, A. Circulating miRNAs in Untreated Breast Cancer: An Exploratory Multimodality Morpho-Functional Study. *Cancers* **2019**, *11*, 876. [CrossRef] [PubMed]
45. Shapiro, S.S.; Wilk, M.B. An analysis of variance test for normality (complete samples). *Biometrika*, 1965; *52*, 3/4, 591–611.
46. Abdi, H. Z-scores. *Encyclopedia of Measurement and Statistics* **2007**, *3*, 1055–1058.
47. Huynh, H.; Meyer, P. Use of robust z in detecting unstable items in item response theory models. *Pract. Assess. Res. Eval.* **2010**, *15*, 1–8.
48. Feng, C.; Wang, H.; Lu, N.; Tu, X.M. Log transformation: Application and interpretation in biomedical research. *Stat. Med.* **2013**, *32*, 230–239. [CrossRef] [PubMed]
49. Bullard, J.H.; Purdom, E.; Hansen, K.D.; Dudoit, S. Evaluation of statistical methods for normalization and differential expression in mRNA-Seq experiments. *BMC Bioinf.* **2010**, *11*, 94. [CrossRef]
50. Bolstad, B.M.; Irizarry, R.A.; Åstrand, M.; Speed, T.P. A comparison of normalization methods for high density oligonucleotide array data based on variance and bias. *Bioinformatics* **2003**, *19*, 185–193. [CrossRef]
51. Hicks, S.C.; Irizarry, R.A. When to use quantile normalization? *BioRxiv* **2014**, 012203.
52. Kessy, A.; Lewin, A.; Strimmer, K. Optimal whitening and decorrelation. *Am. Statist.* **2018**, *72*, 309–314. [CrossRef]
53. Bland, J.M.; Altman, D. Statistical methods for assessing agreement between two methods of clinical measurement. *Lancet* **1986**, *327*, 307–310. [CrossRef]

54. Castaldo, R.; Melillo, P.; Bracale, U.; Caserta, M.; Triassi, M.; Pecchia, L. Acute mental stress assessment via short term HRV analysis in healthy adults: A systematic review with meta-analysis. *Biomed. Signal Process. Control* **2015**, *18*, 370–377. [CrossRef]
55. Castaldo, R.; Melillo, P.; Izzo, R.; Luca, N.D.; Pecchia, L. Fall Prediction in Hypertensive Patients via Short-Term HRV Analysis. *IEEE J. Biomed. Health Inf.* **2017**, *21*, 399–406. [CrossRef] [PubMed]
56. Castaldo, R.; Montesinos, L.; Melillo, P.; James, C.; Pecchia, L. Ultra-short term HRV features as surrogates of short term HRV: A case study on mental stress detection in real life. *BMC Med. Inform. Decis. Making* **2019**, *19*, 12. [CrossRef] [PubMed]
57. Robinson, M.D.; Smyth, G.K. Moderated statistical tests for assessing differences in tag abundance. *Bioinformatics* **2007**, *23*, 2881–2887. [CrossRef] [PubMed]
58. Foster, K.R.; Koprowski, R.; Skufca, J.D. Machine learning, medical diagnosis, and biomedical engineering research-commentary. *BioMed. Eng. OnLine* **2014**, *13*, 10.1186. [CrossRef]
59. Chawla, N.V.; Bowyer, K.W.; Hall, L.O.; Kegelmeyer, W.P. SMOTE: Synthetic minority over-sampling technique. *J. Artif. Intell. Res.* **2002**, *16*, 321–357. [CrossRef]
60. Provost, F. Machine learning from imbalanced data sets 101. In *Proceedings of the AAAI'2000 Workshop on Imbalanced Data Sets*; AAAI Press: Menlo Park, CA, USA, 2000; pp. 1–3.
61. Vapnik, V.N. *Statistical Learning Theory*; Wiley: New York, NY, USA, 1998; p. 736.
62. Quinlan, J.R. *C4.5: Programs For Machine Learning*; Morgan Kaufmann Publishers: San Mateo, CA, USA, 1993.
63. Nguyen, C.; Wang, Y.; Nguyen, H.N. Random forest classifier combined with feature selection for breast cancer diagnosis and prognostic. *J. Biomed. Sci. Eng.* **2013**, *6*, 551. [CrossRef]
64. Kononenko, I. *Semi-Naive Bayesian Classifier*; European Working Session on Learning; Springer: Dordrecht, The Netherlands, 1991; pp. 206–219.
65. Kohl, M. Performance measures in binary classification. *Intl. J. Stat. Med. Res.* **2012**, *1*, 79–81. [CrossRef]
66. Loh, H.-Y.; Norman, B.P.; Lai, K.-S.; Rahman, N.M.A.N.A.; Alitheen, N.B.M.; Osman, M.A. The Regulatory Role of MicroRNAs in Breast Cancer. *Intl. J. Mol. Sci.* **2019**, *20*, 4940. [CrossRef]
67. Changyong, F.; Hongyue, W.; Naiji, L.; Tian, C.; Hua, H.; Ying, L. Log-transformation and its implications for data analysis. *Shanghai Arch. Psychiat.* **2014**, *26*, 105.
68. Haga, A.; Takahashi, W.; Aoki, S.; Nawa, K.; Yamashita, H.; Abe, O.; Nakagawa, K. Standardization of imaging features for radiomics analysis. *J. Med. Invest.* **2019**, *66*, 35–37. [CrossRef]
69. Panayides, A.S.; Pattichis, M.S.; Leandrou, S.; Pitris, C.; Constantinidou, A.; Pattichis, C.S. Radiogenomics for precision medicine with a big data analytics perspective. *IEEE J. Biomed. Health Inform.* **2018**, *23*, 2063–2079. [CrossRef] [PubMed]
70. Chen, J.H.; Baek, H.M.; Nalcioglu, O.; Su, M.Y. Estrogen receptor and breast MR imaging features: A correlation study. *J. Magnet. Resonance Imag.* **2008**, *27*, 825–833. [CrossRef]
71. Koukourakis, M.I.; Manolas, C.; Minopoulos, G.; Giatromanolaki, A.; Sivridis, E. Angiogenesis relates to estrogen receptor negativity, c-erbB-2 overexpression and early relapse in node-negative ductal carcinoma of the breast. *Intl. J. Surg. Pathol.* **2003**, *11*, 29–34. [CrossRef]
72. Fuckar, D.; Dekanic, A.; Stifter, S.; Mustac, E.; Krstulja, M.; Dobrila, F.; Jonjic, N. VEGF expression is associated with negative estrogen receptor status in patients with breast cancer. *Intl. J. Surg. Pathol.* **2006**, *14*, 49–55. [CrossRef] [PubMed]
73. Arpino, G.; Weiss, H.; Lee, A.V.; Schiff, R.; De Placido, S.; Osborne, C.K.; Elledge, R.M. Estrogen receptor–positive, progesterone receptor–negative breast cancer: Association with growth factor receptor expression and tamoxifen resistance. *J. Nat. Cancer Inst.* **2005**, *97*, 1254–1261. [CrossRef] [PubMed]
74. Youk, J.H.; Son, E.J.; Chung, J.; Kim, J.-A.; Kim, E.-k. Triple-negative invasive breast cancer on dynamic contrast-enhanced and diffusion-weighted MR imaging: Comparison with other breast cancer subtypes. *Eur. Radiol.* **2012**, *22*, 1724–1734. [CrossRef]
75. Peterson, R.A.; Cavanaugh, J.E. Ordered quantile normalization: A semiparametric transformation built for the cross-validation era. *J. Appl. Stat.* **2019**, 1–16. [CrossRef]

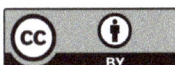

© 2020 by the authors. Licensee MDPI, Basel, Switzerland. This article is an open access article distributed under the terms and conditions of the Creative Commons Attribution (CC BY) license (http://creativecommons.org/licenses/by/4.0/).

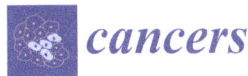

Article

Usefulness of Hybrid PET/MRI in Clinical Evaluation of Head and Neck Cancer Patients

Natalia Samolyk-Kogaczewska [1], Ewa Sierko [1,2,*], Dorota Dziemianczyk-Pakiela [3], Klaudia Beata Nowaszewska [4], Malgorzata Lukasik [5] and Joanna Reszec [5]

1. Department of Radiotherapy, Comprehensive Cancer Center, 15-027 Bialystok, Poland; natalia.samolyk@gmail.com
2. Department of Oncology, Medical University of Bialystok, 15-027 Bialystok, Poland
3. Department of Otolaryngology and Maxillofacial Surgery, Jedrzej Sniadecki Memorial Regional Hospital, 15-950 Bialystok, Poland; dyrka2@wp.pl
4. Department of Maxillofacial and Plastic Surgery, Medical University of Bialystok, 15-276 Bialystok, Poland; beata.nowaszewska@wp.pl
5. Department of Medical Pathology, Medical University of Bialystok, 15-089 Bialystok, Poland; mblukasik@gmail.com (M.L.); joannareszec@gmail.com (J.R.)
* Correspondence: ewa.sierko@iq.pl; Tel.: +48-85-6646827

Received: 31 December 2019; Accepted: 17 February 2020; Published: 22 February 2020

Abstract: (1) Background: The novel hybrid of positron emission tomography/magnetic resonance (PET/MR) examination has been introduced to clinical practice. The aim of our study was to evaluate PET/MR usefulness in preoperative staging of head and neck cancer (HNC) patients (pts); (2) Methods: Thirty eight pts underwent both computed tomography (CT) and PET/MR examination, of whom 21 pts underwent surgical treatment as first-line therapy and were further included in the present study. Postsurgical tissue material was subjected to routine histopathological (HP) examination with additional evaluation of p16, human papillomavirus (HPV), Epstein-Barr virus (EBV) and Ki67 status. Agreement of clinical and pathological T staging, sensitivity, specificity, positive predictive value (PPV), negative predictive value (NPV) of CT and PET/MR in metastatic lymph nodes detection were defined. The verification of dependences between standardized uptake value (SUV value), tumor geometrical parameters, number of metastatic lymph nodes in PET/MR and CT, biochemical parameters, Ki67 index, p16, HPV and EBV status was made with statistical analysis of obtained results; (3) Results: PET/MR is characterized by better agreement in T staging, higher specificity, sensitivity, PPV and NPV of lymph nodes evaluation than CT imaging. Significant correlations were observed between SUVmax and maximal tumor diameter from PET/MR, between SUVmean and CT tumor volume, PET/MR tumor volume, maximal tumor diameter assessed in PET/MR. Other correlations were weak and insignificant; (4) Conclusions: Hybrid PET/MR imaging is useful in preoperative staging of HNC. Further studies are needed.

Keywords: PET/MRI; head and neck cancer; HPV; EBV; p16

1. Introduction

Head and neck cancers (HNC) are the sixth most common cancers worldwide. The vast majority (more than 90%) are squamous cell carcinomas, so that the term HNC is often used to describe all carcinomas arising from the epithelium lining the sinonasal tract, oral cavity, pharynx and larynx and showing microscopic evidence of squamous differentiation. Approximately two-thirds of patients with HNC present with locally advanced disease at the primary site and/or spread to regional lymph nodes. The 5-year survival rate of HNC patients ranges between 40% and 70%, depending on the primary site and stage [1,2]. Positron emission tomography (PET) with fluorine-18 labelled fluorodeoxyglucose

(18F-FDG) as a radiotracer is an established procedure in head and neck squamous cell carcinoma (HNSCC) diagnosis [2]. It is vitally important to the characterization of local, regional and distant disease [3]. PET supports the initial staging of difficult cases, where other imaging methods produce equivocal results. It is useful in the detection of occult primary tumors and synchronous primary cancers. Furthermore, PET aids in assessing tumor response to therapy and helps in detecting cancer recurrence and metastasis during the follow-up period [3–5].

Contrary to anatomical imaging, 18F-FDG-PET takes into account biological differences in metabolism and the radiopharmacological uptake between the tumor and the surrounding normal tissue [6]. PET images are characterized by high contrast but low spatial resolution, which creates a need for combining PET with morphological imaging methods such as cone beam computed tomography (CBCT). A novel hybrid imaging technology, Positron Emission Tomography-Magnetic Resonance Imaging (PET/MRI), has been introduced to clinical practice [7]. The integrated PET/MRI technique combines the benefits of both methods such as superior soft tissue contrast, multiplanar image acquisition and functional imaging capability [8].

A suspicion of head and neck cancer (HNC) is predominantly based on the identification of a primary tumor or the presence of palpable metastatic lymph nodes in the head and neck region during a clinical examination [9]. Accurate, pre-treatment staging is crucial in newly diagnosed HNSCC patients since it enables clinicians to determine patient prognosis and develop an optimal treatment strategy [5]. Precision imaging methods play an integral role in this process [4]. Furthermore, proper imaging is vital to the accurate delineation of target volumes in radiotherapy (RT) planning, particularly when highly conformal RT techniques such as intensity modulated radiotherapy (IMRT) or volumetric arc therapy (VMAT) are utilized [9]. Initial reports have revealed that hybrid 18F-FDG PET/MRI offers higher sensitivity and specificity in the detection of HNC when compared to PET, CT and MRI used separately [10,11]. Moreover, PET/MRI has a higher correlation coefficient with pathological tumor size in comparison to contrast-enhanced CT (CECT), MR and PET/CT [10]. PET/MRI outperformed PET/CT by providing greater tumor conspicuity and higher sensitivity in determining the perineural spread in primary HNSCC. One study has demonstrated PET/MRI sensitivity to be 85% and specificity 92% in the detection of metastatic lymph nodes [3].

In HNSCC patient population, a group of younger, healthier individuals with limited or no tobacco exposure can be distinguished [12]. Prognosis in such cases is excellent as these patients are highly responsive to treatment [13]. Human papillomavirus (HPV)-related oropharyngeal cancers (OPC) are a frequent finding in this group of patients. Presence of HPV is an important prognostic factor, which is reflected in the 8th edition of the American Joint Committee on Cancer (AJCC) TNM (Tumor Nodes Metastases classification) staging system [13,14]. There is a limited number of studies on the relationship between PET imaging and HPV status in HNSCC [3,15–17]. Furthermore, very few studies concern the utility of PET/MRI in the characterization of HPV-related HNC [8,18]. According to our knowledge, there are no literature reports documenting the correlation between Epstein-Barr virus (EBV) status and PET/MRI features. Therefore, the aim of our study was to evaluate the correlation between PET/MR and CT parameters, biochemical parameters, Ki67 index, p16, HPV and EBV status as well as usefulness of PET/MRI in the preoperative staging of HNC patients.

2. Results

This section may be divided by subheadings. It should provide a concise and precise description of the experimental results, their interpretation as well as the experimental conclusions that can be drawn.

2.1. Accuracy of T staging

Agreement between T stages determined with CT, PET/MRI and histopathological (HP) examination, which is the clinical gold-standard technique used for cancer diagnosis, was evaluated. The T stage determined with CT was compatible with the HP stage in 56% of cases. T overstaging was observed in 11% of cases, downstaging in 33% of patients. PET/MRI results corresponded to HP staging in 67% of cases, were overstaged in 11%, downstaged in 22%.

2.2. Specificity, Sensitivity, Positive Predictive Value (PPV) and Negative Predictive Value (NPV) of Lymph Node Evaluation in CT and PET/MRI

The total number of detected lymph nodes in the HP examination of postoperative tissue material was 475, out of which 31 were metastatic. Twenty seven lymph nodes were described as malignant in CT scans and 24 in PET/MRI scans. Based on the CT and PET/MRI scans, lymph nodes of the neck were assigned into appropriate levels [19]. Results of the HP were referenced values. In regard to lymph node detection, PET/MRI sensitivity was 55%, specificity—98%, PPV—71%, NPV—97% and test reliability was 95%. Computed tomography sensitivity was 47%, specificity—97%, PPV—53%, NPV—96% and test reliability—94%.

2.3. Correlations between Clinical, Morphological and Metabolic Parameters

2.3.1. SUV Values in Relation to Tumor Geometrical Parameters, Biochemical Parameters and Ki67 Index

A high, statistically significant correlation between standardized uptake value (SUV)max and maximal tumor diameter determined with PET/MRI ($r = 0.457$, $p = 0.036$) (Figure 1) was revealed in comparison to the measurements obtained from CT images ($r = 0.025$, $p = 0.913$). On the other hand, poor and statistically insignificant correlations were observed between SUVmax values and tumor volume determined with PET/MRI ($r = 0.309$, $p = 0.172$), tumor volume determined with CT ($r = 0.289$, $p = 0.203$), Ki67 index ($r = 0.04$, $p = 0.862$), CRP concentration ($r = 0.069$, $p = 0.764$) and glucose levels ($r = 0.308$, $p = 0.173$).

A significant relationship was observed between SUVmean and CT tumor volume ($r = 0.563$, $p = 0.007$), PET/MRI tumor volume ($r = 0.607$, $p = 0.003$) and maximal tumor diameter determined with PET/MRI ($r = 0.788$, $p = 0.00002$) (Figure 1). Contrary to the aforementioned findings, correlations between SUVmean and maximal tumor diameter in CT ($r = 0.165$, $p = 0.474$), Ki67 index ($r = 0.08$, $p = 0.728$), CRP concentration ($r = 0.138$, $p = 0.549$) and glucose levels ($r = 0.253$, $p = 0.268$) were weak and insignificant.

2.3.2. Presence of p16, HPV and EBV in Relation to SUV Values, Tumor Geometrical Parameters

The average value of SUVmax in p16-positive patients was lower than in p16-negative patients. Despite substantial discrepancies in the obtained results, the difference between the p16-positive and the p16-negative groups was insignificant ($p = 0.37$). Maximal SUV was not significantly correlated with HPV and EBV status, and neither was maximal tumor diameter determined with CT or PET/MRI correlated with the presence of p16, HPV, EBV.

The average values of SUVmean in p16-, HPV- and EBV-positive patients were close to the values in p16-, HPV- and EBV-negative groups.

2.3.3. Number of Metastatic Lymph Nodes in Relation to SUV Values, Tumor Geometrical Parameters, Ki67 Index and Presence of p16, HPV, EBV

The correlation between CT-based tumor volume and the number of metastatic lymph nodes determined with CT was statistically significant ($p = 0.006$). The highest tumor volumes were found in the group of patients with 1 metastatic lymph node and the lowest in those without metastatic lymph nodes ($p = 0.01$). The number of metastatic lymph nodes determined with CT or PET/MRI and SUV values, PET/MRI-based tumor volume, maximal tumor diameter based on CT or PET/MR imaging, Ki67 index were insignificant.

No significant correlations were observed between the presence of p16 ($p = 0.431$, df = 2, Chi2 = 1.68), HPV ($p = 0.623$ df = 2, Chi2 = 0.946), EBV ($p = 0.714$ df = 2, Chi2 = 0.674) and the number of metastatic lymph nodes detected with CT, as well as between the positive status of p16 (p = 0.24 df = 2, Chi2 = 2.854), HPV (p = 0.139 df = 2, Chi2 = 3.94), EBV (p = 0.414 df = 2, Chi2 = 1.763) and the number of metastatic lymph nodes detected with PET/MRI.

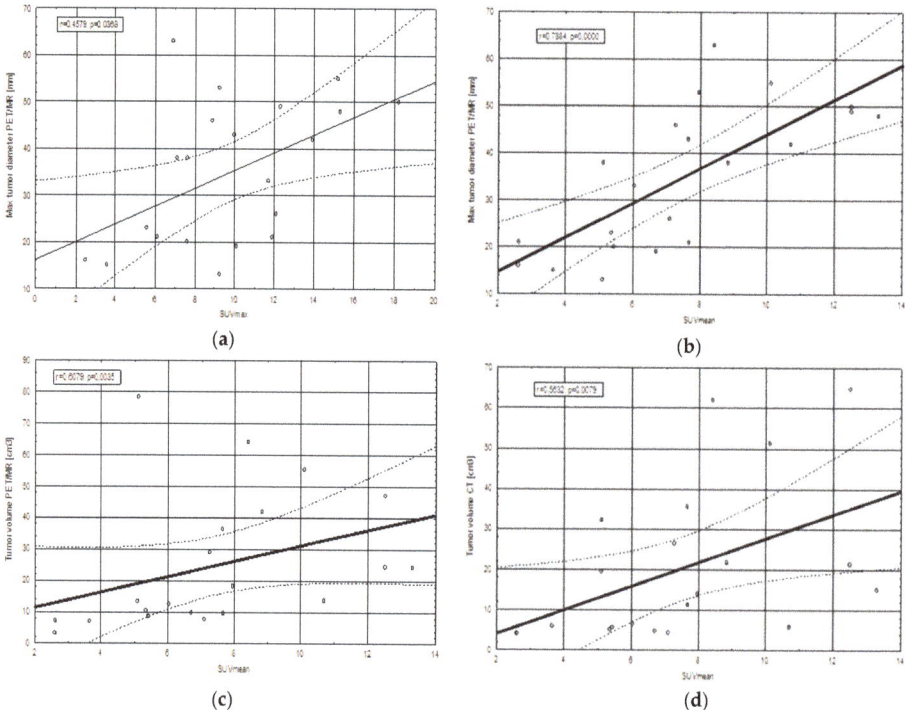

Figure 1. Statistically significant correlation between standardized uptake value (SUV) values and maximal tumor diameter (**a**,**b**) and tumor volume (**c**,**d**) obtained from positron emission tomography/magnetic resonance (PET/MR) or computed tomography (CT). Abbreviations: SUVmax—maximal standardized uptake value, SUVmean—mean standardized uptake value, r—correlation coefficient from Spearman's correlation test, p—statistical significance value.

3. Discussion

Hybrid PET/MRI imaging can play an important role in the initial staging of HNC patients. In our study, we compared the efficacy of PET/MRI with the routinely used CT scanning and HP examination, which is the clinical gold-standard technique used for cancer diagnosis, in primary tumor staging (T features) according to the AJCC TNM classification. Our results demonstrated that T staging based on PET/MRI images was compatible with HP outcomes in a higher number of patients (67%) in comparison with T staging based on CT images alone (56%). Similar results were obtained by other authors - T staging performed with PET/MRI was accurate in 75% of HNC cases compared to 59% with PET/CT and 50% with MRI alone [20]. Chan et al. demonstrated that greater accuracy in defining the extent of primary nasopharyngeal tumors was achieved with PET/MRI in comparison to PET/CT [21]. PET/MRI imaging offers more precision in depicting perineural infiltration, intracranial or inferior orbital fissure involvement. It should be mentioned that our study did not include nasopharyngeal cancer (NPC) patients. Other authors have demonstrated similar results: fused PET and MR imaging delivered more accurate T staging of HNC patients (74%) compared with PET/CT (63%) [22]. Tsujikawa et al. demonstrated that FDG PET/MRI with its greater soft tissue contrast, multiplanar image acquisition and functional imaging capability is useful in the evaluation of stages of oral cavity cancers and the assessment of oropharyngeal cancer patients based on the new AJCC TNM staging system [8].

Regional metastasis to the lymph nodes is one of the most important predictors of poor prognosis in HNC [23]. Based on the results of CT and PET/MRI scans, we calculated the sensitivity, specificity, PPV and NPV of both diagnostic tests. Positive predictive value expresses the probability that a positive diagnostic test result is reliable. Similarly, NPV determines the probability that a negative test result is reliable [24]. Our study revealed relatively low sensitivity of PET/MRI in metastatic lymph node detection. This could be associated with the fact that detecting small nodes with micrometastases remains a challenge for currently available diagnostic modalities, including PET/MRI [2]. Metastases can be present in unenlarged lymph nodes and not all enlarged nodes are malignant [25]. Another explanation for such results may be limited radiological expertise in interpreting PET/MRI images as this is a novel hybrid imaging technique. Our study has found that specificity, NPV and test reliability of PET/MR is marginally better than in CT results. On the other hand, PET/MR has 8% higher sensitivity and 18% higher PPV compared with CT. In a different study, the sensitivity, specificity and accuracy of PET/MRI-based evaluation of regional node status achieved a 99% rate each [21]. Based on lymph node levels, Schaarschmidt et al. demonstrated sensitivity, specificity, NPV and PPV of 81%, 99%, 98% and 89%, respectively, for PET/MRI [20]. On the other hand, Platzek et al. found that PET/MRI is capable of detecting 64% more metastatic lymph nodes, partly due to the fact that PET/MRI scans were performed following PET/CT scans without the additional FDG injection and the time interval between the FDG injection and PET/MR was longer, which contributed to an increase in FDG uptake by the lymph nodes [26]. Another study has highlighted a better diagnostic value of PET/MRI staging in primary tumors compared with cervical node classification in head and neck malignancies with 94% of primary tumors and 82% of regional nodes correctly classified in comparison to histopathology results [27].

Positron emission tomography with FDG as a radiotracer reflects the metabolic activity of tumor tissue which is expressed in SUV values [28]. Our study revealed a stronger correlation between SUVmean and tumor geometry, such as volume and maximal diameter, than between SUVmax and tumor geometry. PET complements anatomical imaging modalities, particularly in tumor volume determination. Therefore, our study demonstrated stronger correlations between SUV values and PET/MRI than between those values and CT [29]. Tumor volume and SUV values are considered prognostic factors—increased values of both are associated with a higher risk of death [30,31]. Biologically, larger tumors have higher metabolic activity and therefore, higher SUV values indicate a worse prognosis [32]. PET/MRI has an advantage over CT as it enables the measurements of tumor volume and SUV values to be obtained during one examination.

Poor and statistically insignificant correlations were found between SUVmax, SUVmean and KI67, CRP, glycemic parameters in our study. The authors of a meta-analysis concerning correlations between FDG uptake and Ki67 reported significant heterogeneity in HNC cases [33]. Furthermore, pretreatment SUVmax was significantly higher in patients with enhanced Ki67 expression in comparison to those with low Ki67 expression, but the study concerned diffuse large B-cell lymphoma [34]. Surov et al. reported that SUVmax was moderately correlated with Ki67 expression and therefore cannot be used as a surrogate marker for tumor proliferation [35]. A Chinese study on a group of lymphoma patients showed that post-treatment SUVmax values were significantly correlated with post-treatment CRP values [36]. By contrast, a previously mentioned study demonstrated that baseline SUVmax was weakly correlated with CRP ($r = 0.215$, $p = 0.011$) [34].

A recent meta-analysis investigating the effect of blood glucose levels on SUV values assessed with FDG-PET scans revealed positive correlations between glucose levels and SUVmax and SUVmean values in normal tissue such as brain, muscle, liver, but no significant correlations were found between blood glucose levels and SUVmax or SUVmean values in primary malignant tumors [37]. No evidence of a linear relationship between glycaemia and SUV has been reported by other authors [38].

However, it should be emphasized that high plasma glucose levels decrease FDG uptake, which might affect SUV values [39].

In the present study, differences between SUVmax or SUVmean and HPV or p16 presence were insignificant. Comparable results have been obtained in other studies, where no differences in SUVmax values between p16- and HPV-positive, and p16- and HPV-negative patients were reported [40–42]. By contrast, Schouten et al. demonstrated that SUVmax in HPV-positive tumors was significantly lower than in HPV-negative tumors [43]. This finding is in agreement with a study by Surov et al. which revealed that p16-negative tumors showed significantly higher SUVmax and SUVmean values in comparison to p16-positive carcinomas [44].

In our study, no correlation between SUV values and EBV infection status was observed. Literature data confirms our results [45,46].

Similarly, in the present study p16, HPV, EBV did not have a significant impact on the results of CT- or PET/MRI-determined tumor volume and maximal tumor diameter. However, according to the literature, in HNC patients, p16/HPV-positive tumors are usually smaller than p16/HPV-negative tumors [44,47]. Some studies have demonstrated that EBV status and primary tumor volume can be utilized in the prognostic stratification of NPC patients [48,49]. On the other hand, data confirming correlations between primary tumor volume and EBV-positivity is limited [50,51].

Maximal tumor diameter is an important primary tumor feature which is reflected in the TNM classification of HNC (e.g., T1 denotes a tumor size 2 cm or less in its largest dimension) [13]. There are a few studies demonstrating the prognostic value of maximal tumor diameter in OPC [52] and NPC [53], but there are no published papers concerning the influence of p16-, HPV- or EBV-positivity on maximal tumor diameter determined with CT or PET/MRI.

According to our knowledge, there are no literature reports examining the relationship between PET/MRI-based tumor volume and the number of metastatic lymph nodes in HNC patients. Our study did not find any correlations between tumor features obtained from PET/MRI scans and the number of metastatic lymph nodes. By contrast, correlations between tumor volume and the number of metastatic lymph nodes based on CT images were significant. The lowest tumor volumes determined with CT correlated with no metastases in the lymph nodes. This is normally the case in early stage HNC patients. We therefore expected to find significant correlations between the highest tumor volumes determined with CT and multiple metastatic lymph nodes. However, the highest CT-based tumor volumes were observed in patients with 1 metastatic lymph node. This can be explained by the highly inflammatory nature of HNSSC, particularly at advanced stages of the disease [54]. Large tumors investigated in the present study probably consisted not only of neoplastic tissue but also contained peritumoral inflammatory infiltrate. On the other hand, HNC has a high propensity to metastasize through the lymphatic pathway [55]. This could explain the occurrence of multiple metastases in the lymph nodes independently of tumor volumes presented in our study. Research concerning lung adenocarcinoma has demonstrated positive correlations between tumor size and the number of metastatic lymph nodes [56]. By contrast, Miller et al. reported that tumor volume in cervical cancer patients did not correlate with the presence of lymph node metastases [57].

In the present study, the correlation between the number of metastatic lymph nodes determined with PET/MRI and primary tumor SUV values was insignificant. Only few papers have explored this issue but the results obtained were contradictory. Some authors report that in lung cancer patients no statistically significant differences in SUVmax and SUVmean values between individuals with occult lymph nodes and those without have been found [58]. A different study has demonstrated that SUVmax and SUVmean are significantly associated with lymph node involvement in oesophageal cancer patients [59].

Correlations between the presence of HPV, p16 and EBV, and the number of metastatic lymph nodes determined with PET/MRI were insignificant in our study. Other authors have obtained similar results—HPV-positive patients were heterogenous in terms of nodal stages [60]. By contrast, in TROG 02.02 phase III trial, p16-positive patients were included in a more advanced nodal category in comparison with the p16-negative group [47]. The vast majority of NPC is linked to Epstein-Barr virus infection [61,62]. A lack of relationship between EBV status and the number of lymph nodes detected with PET/MRI is most probably associated with the inclusion of oropharyngeal and oral cavity cancer patients in our study.

Based on our results, further studies should include a larger number of HNC pts.

4. Materials and Methods

Thirty eight HNSCC patients underwent both CT and PET/MRI examinations. (Figure 2) Based on the CT and PET/MRI results, 21 patients underwent surgical treatment as first-line therapy and this group was subsequently included in the present study. The remaining patients received radiochemotherapy or palliative RT. Study inclusion criteria were as follows: age over 18 years old, informed consent for study participation, no unmanaged systemic diseases, no hypersensitivity or previous allergic reaction to intravenous iodine contrast or FDG, glucose blood level below 160mg/dL, no metal elements in the body (cardiac pacemakers, metal surgical stitches or clips, intrauterine contraceptive devices, metal shavings in the eyeball, cochlear implants, etc.). Clinical characteristics of the group are presented in Table 1. All pts had squamous cell carcinoma and in about 87% of cases histology grade score (G) was G2. The median age of study participants was 60 years (range of 36–74 years). Twelve of them were female, nine were male. Hypertension and diabetes were the most common comorbidities. In terms of laboratory parameters (Complete Blood Count, renal and liver function parameters, electrolyte blood concentration, thyroid hormones level), the group of patients was homogenous. Discrepancies were observed in C reactive protein (CRP) levels in the blood and its values ranged from 0.3 mg/mL to 120.5 mg/mL.

Prior to surgical treatment, contrast-enhanced (Ultravist 300, 1 mL/kg) CT was routinely performed in all study participants on the 64-detector row CT scanner (Aquilion CX, Canon Medical Systems Corporation, Otawara, Japan). Axial images were obtained with 3 mm slice thickness from the top of the cranium to manubrium sterni. The parameters included a 120 kV tube voltage, tube current 200 mA, 0.5 s rotation time, matrix size, 512 × 512 and a field of view of 250 mm. CT scans were interpreted by a radiologist experienced in the interpretation of head and neck region CT images.

All study participants also underwent PET/MRI scans on the 3 Tesla Siemens Biograph mMR scanner (Siemens Healthcare GmbH, Erlangen, Germany) after an average of 9 days (range 1 to 20 days) from the CT scans. The examination consisted of whole-body, low resolution MRI imaging, followed by a PET scan and a diagnostic MRI scan (T1- and T2-weighted sequences and contrast-enhanced sequences) of the head and neck region. MRI attenuation images were acquired using the Dixon approach with a coronal 2-point 3D T1-weighted volumetric interpolated breath hold examination (VIBE) (3.12 mm slice thickness, 20% interslice gap, integrated parallel acquisition technique factor 2, acquisition time 19s, 192 × 121 matrix, 500mm × 328 mm field of view (FOV), repetition time 3.6ms, echo time 1.23 and 2.46ms, scanning time 4 minutes 10 seconds). PET/MRI scans were obtained simultaneously with the patient remaining in the same position without specific head and neck immobilization (Orfit mask). All patients fasted for at least 6 hours prior to the test. Diagnostic scans were performed 1 hour after the intravenous administration of 18F-FDG (4 MBq/kg, range of 203–417 MBq 18F-FDG per patient). PET/MRI images were evaluated by both a radiologist and nuclear medicine specialist. Maximal and mean SUV of the primary volume were measured. Mean SUV was defined as the average SUV value in the voxel that showed ≥ 40% of SUVmax [63].

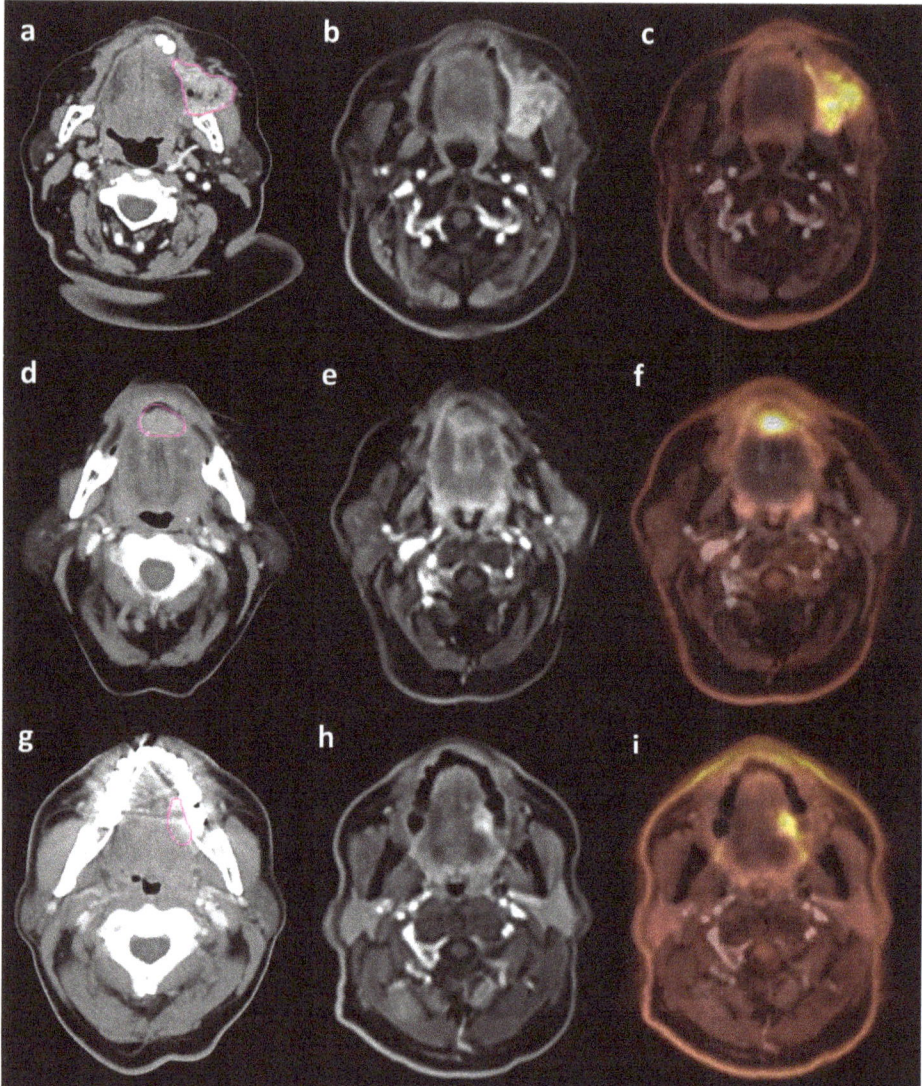

Figure 2. Contrast enhancement computed tomography (CT) (**a**,**d**,**g**), T1-weighted volumetric interpolated breath hold examination (VIBE) magnetic resonance (MR) (**b**,**e**,**h**) and positron emission tomography/MR (PET/MR) (**c**,**f**,**i**) imaging of head and neck cancer patients. (**a**,**b**,**c**)—patient with squamous cell carcinoma of the buccal mucosa in clinical stage T3N2b; (**d**,**e**,**f**)—patient with squamous cell carcinoma of the floor of the mouth in clinical stage T1N0; (**g**,**h**,**i**)—patient with squamous cell carcinoma of the oral tongue in clinical stage T2N0.

Table 1. Characterization of patient with head and neck squamous cell carcinoma (SSC) according to localization of the primary tumor, Ki67 expression, clinical stage (TNM classification, AJCC, ed. 8, 2017) based on postoperative histopathological (HP) examination, status of p16 protein, human papilloma virus (HPV) and Epstein–Barr virus (EBV) positivity, smoking status and biopsy performed before positron emission tomography/magnetic resonance (PET/MR) imaging.

No. of pts.	Localization of Primary Tumor	TNM Stage	Ki67 Index [%]	p16 Status	HPV Status	EBV Status	Smoking	Biopsy before PET/MR (days)
1	OT	T2 N1 M0	30	0	0	0	1	28
2	BM	T2 N1 M0	30	0	0	0	0	25
3	LG	T3 N2b M0	20	0	0	0	1	21
4	BoT	T2 N0 M0	20	0	0	0	1	20
5	BoT	T3 N2c M0	40	1	0	0	0	14
6	BoT	T2 N2c M0	30	0	0	0	1	18
7	OT	T1 N1 M0	50	1	1	1	0	14
8	FoM	T2 N2c M0	30	1	1	0	1	21
9	FoM	T1 N2b M0	20	0	0	0	0	18
10	OT	T2 N1 M0	40	1	1	0	0	16
11	MAR	T3 N0 M0	40	1	1	0	0	23
12	FoM	T3 N0 M0	20	0	0	0	1	20
13	FoM	T2 N2b M0	50	1	0	1	1	30
14	LG	T2 N0 M0	60	1	0	0	0	14
15	SSG	T3 N0 M0	30	0	0	0	0	15
16	OT	T1 N0 M0	30	0	0	0	0	15
17	OT	T3 N2b M0	30	0	0	0	1	21
18	FoM	T1 N0 M0	20	0	0	0	0	17
19	BM	T3 N2b M0	30	0	0	1	1	18
20	BoT	T1 N0 M0	20	0	0	0	0	28
21	FoM	T4a N2c M0	50	1	0	0	1	24

Abbreviations: OT—oral tongue, BM—buccal mucosa, LG—lower gingiva, BoT—base of tongue, FoM—floor of mouth, MAR—maxillary alveolar ridge, SSG—submandibular salivary gland, 0—absence of test feature, 1—presence of test feature.

Surgical treatment was performed an average of 19 days (range of 9 to 28 days) after the CT scans and an average of 13 days (range of 2 to 27 days) after the PET/MRI scans.

Tissue material obtained during surgery was subjected to routine histopathological examination (HP). Additionally, the HP protocol included the immunohistochemical evaluation of p16 protein expression as a surrogate marker for HPV infection, the latent membrane protein 1 (LMP1) expression as a surrogate marker for EVB as well as the detection of Ki67 protein indicating the proliferation rate of cancer cells. The immunohistochemical evaluation of p16 protein expression was conducted using a method described elsewhere [64,65]. Slides were considered positive for p16 protein if the specimen showed continuous staining of at least 50% of tumor cells. For the immunohistochemical detection (Dako, Poland) of EBV presence, antibodies against LMP1—monoclonal mouse anti-LMP protein (clone CS.1-4, Dako, Poland) were used. The expression of Ki67 protein was evaluated with an immunohistochemical method described in the literature [66]. Nuclear accumulation of Ki67 protein in neoplastic cells was assessed semiquantitatively and defined as a percentage of reaction-positive cells.

The presence of HPV genetic material was examined using the PCR method. A positive result (HPV presence in the analyzed material) was determined when at least one of the bands associated with a different HPV subtype was present on the strip along with the developing control line and the positive control. A negative result (no HPV presence) was determined when no bands associated with HPV were developed while the developing control line and the positive control band were both present.

Clinical and pathological stages of the disease were determined according to the 8th ed. of AJCC TNM classification [8]. Based on imaging tests, only round-shaped lymph nodes or nodes exceeding 10mm in the smallest transverse dimension with contrast enhancement on CT or MRI and/or increased 18F-FDG uptake in PET scans were taken into consideration. The results obtained from CECT, PET/MRI and HP were compared. HP results were referenced.

Agreement between CT- and PET/MRI-based T staging, sensitivity, specificity, PPV, NPV in metastatic lymph node detection were defined. Sensitivity was the proportion of patients with positive diagnostic test results (CT or PET/MRI scanning) who were correctly diagnosed in relation to referenced HP results. Specificity was the proportion of patients with negative imaging test results who were correctly diagnosed [67]. Positive predictive value is a proportion of true positive results among all positive findings (true positives and false positives). Similarly, negative predictive value is a proportion of true negative results among all negative results (true negatives and false negatives) [22].

Dependences between SUVmax and SUVmean values, the size and maximal diameter of the primary tumor, the number of metastatic lymph nodes detected with PET/MRI, HPV and EBV status, Ki67 index, glucose level and CRP concentration status were verified in the statistical analysis of the obtained results (Table 2). Considering the number of lymph nodes, study participants were divided into 3 groups: those without metastatic lymph nodes, those with 1 metastatic lymph node and those with 2 or more metastatic lymph nodes. The division was based on the 8th ed. of AJCC TNM classification of HNC, where N0 means no lymph node metastasis, N1–metastasis in single small lymph node and N2–among others, metastasis in multiple lymph nodes.

Table 2. Measurements of standardized uptake value (SUV) values, tumor geometrical parameters and number of metastatic lymph nodes obtained from positron emission tomography/magnetic resonance (PET/MR) and computed tomography (CT), as well as biochemical parameters in pts (patients) with head and neck squamous cell carcinoma.

No of pts	SUVmax [g/mL]	SUVmean [g/mL]	Maximal Tumor Diameter CT [mm]	Maximal Tumor Diameter PET/MR [mm]	Tumor Volume PET/MR [cm³]	Tumor Volume CT [cm³]	No of mts Lymph Nodes in CT	No of mts Lymph Nodes in PET/MR	CRP [mg/L]	Glucose [mg/dL]
1	11.7	6.03	34	33	12.63	6.65	0	1	1.9	92
2	11.9	7.68	15	21	9.62	11.24	2≤	0	0.5	110
3	9.25	7.96	45	53	18.23	13.97	2≤	2≤	3.1	99
4	12.1	7.09	27	26	7.76	4.35	0	1	9.1	139
5	15.2	10.1	50	55	55.48	51.26	2≤	2≤	1.1	88
6	9.26	5.09	28	13	13.38	19.51	2≤	2≤	0.9	99
7	10.1	6.7	24	19	9.76	4.78	0	1	0.4	93
8	7.08	5.1	51	38	78.35	32.12	2≤	2≤	1.1	117
9	15.3	13.3	10	48	24.27	15.06	0	2≤	4.2	122
10	5.59	5.35	25	23	10.31	5.09	0	1	1.2	104
11	7.59	8.84	35	38	41.97	21.82	2≤	2≤	44.4	91
12	10	7.65	41	43	36.2	35.65	0	0	0.9	83
13	3.62	3.64	18	15	6.91	6.07	2≤	2≤	0.7	92
14	13.9	10.7	18	42	13.79	5.89	2≤	1	3.6	118
15	12.3	12.5	39	49	47.08	64.8	1	0	0.3	93
16	6.11	2.61	25	21	7.16	4.08	0	0	16	85
17	8.9	7.26	0	46	28.85	26.4	2≤	2≤	120.5	98
18	7.59	5.43	19	20	8.71	5.66	0	0	17.4	122
19	18.2	12.5	39	50	24.37	21.34	2≤	2≤	2.1	104
20	2.5	2.6	20	16	3.28	4.12	0	0	0.6	87
21	6.9	8.41	60	63	64.14	62.03	1	0	5.1	101

Statistical analysis was performed using Microsoft Excel (version 2019, Microsoft Corporation, Washington, DC, USA) and Statistica 10 (Statsoft Inc., Tulsa, OK, USA). The level of statistical significance was established at $p < 0.05$. The Spearman's correlation test was used to analyze correlations between SUVmax/SUVmean values and maximal tumor diameter determined with CT or PET/MRI, CT or PET/MRI tumor volume, Ki67 index, CRP concentration, glucose level. The correlations between SUVmax, SUVmean, maximal tumor diameter determined with CT or PET/MRI and p16, HPV, EBV presence were analyzed using the t test. Correlation analysis between CT or PET/MRI tumor volume, Ki67 index, CRP concentration and p16, HPV, EBV status was performed with the Mann–Whitney U test. Correlations between the number of metastatic lymph nodes determined with CT or PET/MRI and features such as SUV values, maximal tumor diameter and tumor volume determined with CT or PET/MRI, KI67 index were established with the Kruskal–Wallis test. The Ch2 test was used to analyze the relationship between the number of metastatic lymph nodes determined with CT or PET/MRI and the positivity of p16, HPV and EBV.

5. Conclusions

Hybrid PET/MRI imaging is useful in the preoperative staging of HNC patients. Compared with CT scanning, the outcomes obtained using this imaging modality are more consistent with histopathology results, the gold-standard technique in cancer diagnosis, in regard to T staging. This novel imaging tool also offers higher specificity, sensitivity, PPV and NPV of lymph node evaluation in comparison with CT scanning. Statistically important correlations between SUVmax and maximal tumor diameter as well as between SUV mean and tumor volume and maximal tumor diameter evaluated with PET/MRI were revealed in the present study, which suggests that these parameters may be useful in clinical practice. The presence of p16, HPV, EBV did not correlate with SUV values, geometrical parameters of the tumor or the number of metastatic lymph nodes. Further studies on a larger group of patients are required.

Author Contributions: N.S.-K.—conceptualization, data curation, formal analysis, investigation, methodology, project administration, resources, visualization, writing-original draft, writing—review and editing, E.S.—conceptualization, data curation, funding acquisition, investigation, methodology, project administration, supervision, writing-original draft, writing—review and editing, D.D.-P.—investigation, methodology, K.B.N.—data curation, investigation, methodology, M.L.—formal analysis, investigation, methodology, J.R.—investigation, methodology, project administration, supervision, visualization. All authors have read and agreed to the published version of the manuscript.

Funding: This research was funded by Leading National Research Centre (KNOW, Krajowy Naukowy Ośrodek Wiodący), Medical University of Bialystok, Poland; grant number KNOW-0600-SD63-1/2016 and Medical University of Bialystok internal grant to E.S.

Acknowledgments: The authors would like to express their thanks for fruitful help for Dorota Jurgilewicz, Malgorzata Mojsak, Piotr Szumowski, Marcin Hladunski, from Laboratory of Molecular Imaging, Medical University of Bialystok, Poland.

Conflicts of Interest: The authors declare no conflict of interest.

References

1. Burela, N.; Soni, T.; Patni, N.; Bhagat, J.; Kumar, T.; Natarajan, T. A quantitative comparison of gross tumor volumes delineated on [18F]-FDG-PET/CT scan and contrast-enhanced computed tomography scan in locally advanced head and neck carcinoma treated with intensity modulated radiotherapy. *Adv. Mod. Oncol. Res.* **2017**, *3*, 143–151. [CrossRef]
2. Kim, S.G.; Friedman, K.; Patel, S.; Hagiwara, M. Potential role of PET/MRI for imaging metastatic lymph nodes in head and neck cancer. *Am. J. Roentgenol.* **2016**, *207*, 248–256. [CrossRef] [PubMed]
3. Szyszko, T.A.; Cook, G.J.R. PET/CT and PET/MRI in head and neck malignancy. *Clin. Radiol.* **2018**, *73*, 60–69. [CrossRef] [PubMed]
4. Goel, R.; Moore, W.; Sumer, B.; Khan, S.; Sher, D.; Subramaniam, R.M. Clinical practice in PET/CT for the management of head and neck squamous cell cancer. *Am. J. Roentgenol.* **2017**, *209*, 289–303. [CrossRef]

5. Zheng, E.; Khariwala, S.S. Do All Patients with Head and Neck Cancer Require a Positron Emission Tomography Scan at Diagnosis? *Laryngoscope* **2018**. [CrossRef]
6. Leclerc, M.; Lartigau, E.; Lacornerie, T.; Daisne, J.F.; Kramar, A.; Grégoire, V. Primary tumor delineation based on 18FDG PET for locally advanced head and neck cancer treated by chemo-radiotherapy. *Radiother. Oncol.* **2015**, *116*, 87–93. [CrossRef]
7. Ligtenberg, H.; Jager, E.A.; Caldas-Magalhaes, J.; Schakel, T.; Pameijer, F.A.; Kasperts, N.; Philippens, M.E. Modality-specific target definition for laryngeal and hypopharyngeal cancer on FDG-PET, CT and MRI. *Radiother. Oncol.* **2017**, *123*, 63–70. [CrossRef]
8. Tsujikawa, T.; Narita, N.; Kanno, M.; Takabayashi, T.; Fujieda, S.; Okazawa, H. Role of PET/MRI in oral cavity and oropharyngeal cancers based on the 8th edition of the AJCC cancer staging system: A pictorial essay. *Ann. Nucl. Med.* **2018**, *32*, 239–249. [CrossRef]
9. Differding, S.; Hanin, F.X.; Grégoire, V. PET imaging biomarkers in head and neck cancer. *Eur. J. Nucl. Med. Mol. Imaging* **2015**, *42*, 613–622. [CrossRef]
10. Huang, S.H.; Chien, C.Y.; Lin, W.C.; Fang, F.M.; Wang, P.W.; Lui, C.C.; Chang, C.C. A comparative study of fused FDG PET/MRI, PET/CT, MRI, and CT imaging for assessing surrounding tissue invasion of advanced buccal squamous cell carcinoma. *Clin. Nucl. Med.* **2011**, *36*, 518–525. [CrossRef]
11. Loeffelbein, D.J.; Souvatzoglou, M.; Wankerl, V.; Dinges, J.; Ritschl, L.M.; Mücke, T.; Beer, A.J. Diagnostic value of retrospective PET-MRI fusion in head-and-neck cancer. *BMC Cancer* **2014**, *14*, 846. [CrossRef] [PubMed]
12. Mehanna, H.; Jones, T.M.; Gregoire, V.; Ang, K.K. Oropharyngeal carcinoma related to human papillomavirus. *BMJ Br. Med. J.* **2010**, *340*. [CrossRef] [PubMed]
13. Lydiatt, W.M.; Patel, S.G.; O'Sullivan, B.; Brandwein, M.S.; Ridge, J.A.; Migliacci, J.C.; Shah, J.P. Head and neck cancers—Major changes in the American Joint Committee on cancer eighth edition cancer staging manual. *CA Cancer J. Clin.* **2017**, *67*, 122–137. [CrossRef] [PubMed]
14. O'Sullivan, B.; Huang, S.H.; Su, J.; Garden, A.S.; Sturgis, E.M.; Dahlstrom, K.; Adelstein, D. Development and validation of a staging system for HPV-related oropharyngeal cancer by the International Collaboration on Oropharyngeal cancer Network for Staging (ICON-S): A multicentre cohort study. *Lancet Oncol.* **2016**, *17*, 440–451. [CrossRef]
15. Tahari, A.K.; Alluri, K.; Quon, H.; Koch, W.; Wahl, R.L.; Subramaniam, R.M. FDG PET/CT imaging of Oropharyngeal SCC: Characteristics of HPV positive and negative tumors. *Clin. Nucl. Med.* **2014**, *39*, 225–231. [CrossRef]
16. Sharma, S.J.; Wittekindt, C.; Knuth, J.; Steiner, D.; Wuerdemann, N.; Laur, M.; Klussmann, J.P. Intraindividual homogeneity of 18F-FDG PET/CT parameters in HPV-positive OPSCC. *Oral Oncol.* **2017**, *73*, 166–171. [CrossRef]
17. Nesteruk, M.; Lang, S.; Veit-Haibach, P.; Studer, G.; Stieb, S.; Glatz, S.; Guckenberger, M. Tumor stage, tumor site and HPV dependent correlation of perfusion CT parameters and [18F]-FDG uptake in head and neck squamous cell carcinoma. *Radiother. Oncol.* **2015**, *117*, 125–131. [CrossRef]
18. Kim, Y.I.; Cheon, G.J.; Kang, S.Y.; Paeng, J.C.; Kang, K.W.; Lee, D.S.; Chung, J.K. Prognostic value of simultaneous 18 F-FDG PET/MRI using a combination of metabolo-volumetric parameters and apparent diffusion coefficient in treated head and neck cancer. *EJNMMI Res.* **2018**, *8*, 2. [CrossRef]
19. Grégoire, V.; Ang, K.; Budach, W.; Grau, C.; Hamoir, M.; Langendijk, J.A.; Lee, A.; Le, Q.T.; Maingon, P.; Nutting, C.; et al. Delineation of the neck node levels for head and neck tumors: A 2013 update. DAHANCA, EORTC, HKNPCSG, NCIC CTG, NCRI, RTOG, TROG consensus guidelines. *Radiother. Oncol.* **2014**, *110*, 172–181. [CrossRef]
20. Schaarschmidt, B.M.; Heusch, P.; Buchbender, C.; Ruhlmann, M.; Bergmann, C.; Ruhlmann, V.; Schlamann, M.; Antoch, G.; Forsting, M.; Wetter, A. Locoregional tumour evaluation of squamous cell carcinoma in the head and neck area: A comparison between MRI, PET/CT and integrated PET/MRI. *Eur. J. Nucl. Med. Mol. Imaging* **2016**, *43*, 92–102. [CrossRef]
21. Chan, S.C.; Yeh, C.H.; Yen, T.C.; Ng, S.H.; Chang, J.T.; Lin, C.Y.; Yen-Ming, T.; Fan, K.H.; Huang, B.S.; Hsu, C.L.; et al. Clinical utility of simultaneous whole-body 18 F-FDG PET/MRI as a single-step imaging modality in the staging of primary nasopharyngeal carcinoma. *Eur. J. Nucl. Med. Mol. Imaging* **2018**, *45*, 1297–1308. [CrossRef] [PubMed]

22. Sekine, T.; de Galiza Barbosa, F.; Kuhn, F.P.; Burger, I.A.; Stolzmann, P.; Huber, G.F.; Kollias, S.S.; von Schulthess, G.K.; Veit-Haibach, P.; Huellner, M.W. PET+ MR versus PET/CT in the initial staging of head and neck cancer, using a trimodality PET/CT+ MR system. *Clin. Imaging* **2017**, *42*, 232–239. [CrossRef] [PubMed]
23. De Bondt, R.B.; Nelemans, P.J.; Hofman, P.A.; Casselman, J.W.; Kremer, B.; van Engelshoven, J.M.; Beets-Tan, R.G. Detection of lymph node metastases in head and neck cancer: A meta-analysis comparing US, USgFNAC, CT and MR imaging. *Eur. J. Radiol.* **2007**, *64*, 266–272. [CrossRef] [PubMed]
24. Altman, D.G.; Bland, J.M. Statistics Notes: Diagnostic tests 2: Predictive values. *BMJ* **1994**, *309*, 102. [CrossRef]
25. Torabi, M.; Aquino, S.L.; Harisinghani, M.G. Current concepts in lymph node imaging. *J. Nucl. Med.* **2004**, *45*, 1509–1518.
26. Platzek, I.; Beuthien-Baumann, B.; Schneider, M.; Gudziol, V.; Langner, J.; Schramm, G.; Laniado, M.; Kotzerke, J.; van den Hoff, J. PET/MRI in head and neck cancer: Initial experience. *Eur. J. Nucl. Med. Mol. Imaging* **2013**, *40*, 6–11. [CrossRef]
27. Geraldine, B.E.; Pyatigorskaya, N.; De Laroche, R.; Herve, G.; Zaslavsky, C.; Bertaux, M.; Giron, A.; Soret, M.; Bertolus, C.; Sahli-Amor, M.; et al. Diagnostic performance of 18F-FDG PET/MR in head and neck malignancies. *J. Nucl. Med.* **2017**, *58*, 280.
28. Grégoire, V.; Thorwarth, D.; Lee, J. Molecular imaging-guided radiotherapy for the treatment of head-and-neck squamous cell carcinoma: Does it fulfill the promises? *Semin. Radiat. Oncol.* **2018**, *28*, 35–45. [CrossRef]
29. Samołyk-Kogaczewska, N.; Sierko, E.; Zuzda, K.; Gugnacki, P.; Szumowski, P.; Mojsak, M.; Burzyńska-Śliwowska, J.; Wojtukiewicz, M.Z.; Szczecina, K.; Jurgilewicz, D.H. PET/MRI-guided GTV delineation during radiotherapy planning in patients with squamous cell carcinoma of the tongue. *Strahlenther. Onkol.* **2019**, *195*, 780–791. [CrossRef]
30. Kocher, M.R.; Sharma, A.; Garrett-Mayer, E.; Ravenel, J.G. Pretreatment 18F-Fluorodeoxyglucose Positron Emission Tomography Standardized Uptake Values and Tumor Size in Medically Inoperable Nonsmall Cell Lung Cancer Is Prognostic of Overall 2-Year Survival after Stereotactic Body Radiation Therapy. *J. Comput. Assist. Tomo.* **2018**, *42*, 146–150. [CrossRef]
31. Rutkowski, T. The role of tumor volume in radiotherapy of patients with head and neck cancer. *Radiat. Oncol.* **2014**, *9*, 23. [CrossRef] [PubMed]
32. Paul, A.G.; Heilbrun, L.K.; Smith, D.W.; Miller, S.R. Association of 18F-FDG-PET SUV and Tumor Size in Cervical Cancer. *Int. J. Radiat. Oncol.* **2018**, *102*, e632. [CrossRef]
33. Deng, S.M.; Zhang, W.; Zhang, B.; Chen, Y.Y.; Li, J.H.; Wu, Y.W. Correlation between the uptake of 18F-fluorodeoxyglucose (18F-FDG) and the expression of proliferation-associated antigen Ki-67 in cancer patients: A meta-analysis. *PLoS ONE* **2015**, *10*. [CrossRef]
34. Huang, H.; Xiao, F.; Han, X.; Zhong, L.; Zhong, H.; Xu, L.; Zhu, J.; Ni, B.; Liu, J.; Fang, Y.; et al. Correlation of pretreatment 18F-FDG uptake with clinicopathological factors and prognosis in patients with newly diagnosed diffuse large B-cell lymphoma. *Nucl. Med. Commun.* **2016**, *37*, 689–698. [CrossRef] [PubMed]
35. Surov, A.; Meyer, H.J.; Wienke, A. Associations between PET parameters and expression of Ki-67 in breast cancer. *Transl. Oncol.* **2019**, *12*, 375–380. [CrossRef] [PubMed]
36. Ucar, E.; Yalcin, H.; Kavvasoglu, G.H.; Ilhan, G. Correlations between the maximum standard uptake value of positron emission tomography/computed tomography and laboratory parameters before and after treatment in patients with lymphoma. *Chin. Med. J.* **2018**, *131*, 1776–1779. [CrossRef]
37. Eskian, M.; Alavi, A.; Khorasanizadeh, M.; Viglianti, B.L.; Jacobsson, H. Effect of blood glucose level on standardized uptake value (SUV) in 18 F-FDG PET-scan: A systematic review and meta-analysis of 20, 807 individual SUV measurements. *Eur. J. Nucl. Med. Mol. Imaging* **2019**, *46*, 224–237. [CrossRef]
38. Higashi, T.; Saga, T.; Nakamoto, Y.; Ishimori, T.; Fujimoto, K.; Doi, R.; Imamura, M.; Konishi, J. Diagnosis of pancreatic cancer using fluorine-18 fluorodeoxyglucose positron emission tomography (fdg pet)—Usefulness and limitations in "clinical reality". *Ann. Nucl. Med.* **2003**, *17*, 261–279. [CrossRef]
39. Westerterp, M.; Sloof, G.W.; Hoekstra, O.S.; ten Kate, F.J.; Meijer, G.A.; Reitsma, J.B.; Boellaard, R.; van Lanschot, J.J.; Molthoff, C.F. 18 FDG uptake in oesophageal adenocarcinoma: Linking biology and outcome. *J. Cancer Res. Clin.* **2008**, *134*, 227–236.
40. Fleming, J.C.; Woo, J.; Moutasim, K.; Mellone, M.; Frampton, S.J.; Mead, A.; Woelk, C.H. HPV, tumour metabolism and novel target identification in head and neck squamous cell carcinoma. *Br. J. Cancer* **2019**, *120*, 356–367. [CrossRef]

41. Han, M.; Lee, S.J.; Lee, D.; Kim, S.Y.; Choi, J.W. Correlation of human papilloma virus status with quantitative perfusion/diffusion/metabolic imaging parameters in the oral cavity and oropharyngeal squamous cell carcinoma: Comparison of primary tumour sites and metastatic lymph nodes. *Clin. Radiol.* **2018**, *73*, 757.e21–757.e27. [CrossRef]
42. Noij, D.P.; Martens, R.M.; Zwezerijnen, B.; Koopman, T.; de Bree, R.; Hoekstra, O.S.; Castelijns, J.A. Diagnostic value of diffusion-weighted imaging and 18F-FDG-PET/CT for the detection of unknown primary head and neck cancer in patients presenting with cervical metastasis. *Eur. J. Radiol.* **2018**, *107*, 20–25. [CrossRef]
43. Schouten, C.S.; Hakim, S.; Boellaard, R.; Bloemena, E.; Doornaert, P.A.; Witte, B.I.; de Bree, R. Interaction of quantitative 18F-FDG-PET-CT imaging parameters and human papillomavirus status in oropharyngeal squamous cell carcinoma. *Head Neck* **2016**, *38*, 529–535. [CrossRef] [PubMed]
44. Surov, A.; Meyer, H.J.; Höhn, A.K.; Winter, K.; Sabri, O.; Purz, S. Associations between [18 F] FDG-PET and complex histopathological parameters including tumor cell count and expression of KI 67, EGFR, VEGF, HIF-1α, and p53 in head and neck squamous cell carcinoma. *Mol. Imaging Biol.* **2019**, *21*, 368–374. [CrossRef] [PubMed]
45. Ahmedova, A.; Ozkaya, K.; Tambas, M.; Gezer, U.; Ozgur, E.; Sahin, D.; Altun, M. Is there a correlation between serum Epstein-Barr virus DNA level and tumor metabolic activity, TNM staging and tumor load in nasopharyngeal cancer patients? *J. Clin. Oncol.* **2017**, *35*, e17543. [CrossRef]
46. Alessi, A.; Lorenzoni, A.; Cavallo, A.; Padovano, B.; Iacovelli, N.A.; Bossi, P.; Alfieri, S.; Serafini, G.; Colombo, C.B.; Cicchetti, A.; et al. Role of pretreatment 18F-FDG PET/CT parameters in predicting outcome of non-endemic EBV DNA-related nasopharyngeal cancer (NPC) patients treated with IMRT and chemotherapy. *La Radiologia Medica* **2019**, *124*, 414–421. [CrossRef] [PubMed]
47. Rischin, D.; Young, R.J.; Fisher, R.; Fox, S.B.; Le, Q.T.; Peters, L.J.; Solomon, B.; Choi, J.; O'Sullivan, B.; Kenny, L.M.; et al. Prognostic significance of p16INK4A and human papillomavirus in patients with oropharyngeal cancer treated on TROG 02.02 phase III trial. *J. Clin. Oncol.* **2010**, *28*, 4142–4148. [CrossRef] [PubMed]
48. Chen, Q.Y.; Guo, S.Y.; Tang, L.Q.; Lu, T.Y.; Chen, B.L.; Zhong, Q.Y.; Liu, L.T. Combination of tumor volume and Epstein-Barr virus DNA improved prognostic stratification of stage II nasopharyngeal carcinoma in the intensity modulated radiotherapy era: A large-scale cohort study. *Cancer Res. Treat.* **2018**, *50*, 861–871. [CrossRef]
49. Lu, L.; Li, J.; Zhao, C.; Xue, W.; Han, F.; Tao, T.; Lu, T. Prognostic efficacy of combining tumor volume with Epstein-Barr virus DNA in patients treated with intensity-modulated radiotherapy for nasopharyngeal carcinoma. *Oral. Oncol.* **2016**, *60*, 18–24. [CrossRef]
50. Peng, L.; Yang, Y.; Guo, R.; Mao, Y.P.; Xu, C.; Chen, Y.P.; Tang, L.L. Relationship between pretreatment concentration of plasma Epstein-Barr virus DNA and tumor burden in nasopharyngeal carcinoma: An updated interpretation. *Cancer Med.* **2018**, *7*, 5988–5998. [CrossRef]
51. Zhong, Q.; Xiao, Z.Y.; Wu, R.R. The correlation of EBV in plasma and primary tumor volume of NPC. *J. Gannan Med Univ.* **2010**, *4*, 5–11.
52. Gletsou, E.; Papadas, T.A.; Baliou, E.; Tsiambas, E.; Ragos, V.; Armata, I.E.; Fotiades, P.P. HPV infection in oropharyngeal squamous cell carcinomas: Correlation with tumor size. *J. BUON* **2018**, *23*, 433–438. [PubMed]
53. Liang, S.B.; Deng, Y.M.; Zhang, N.; Lu, R.L.; Zhao, H.; Chen, H.Y.; Chen, Y. Prognostic significance of maximum primary tumor diameter in nasopharyngeal carcinoma. *BMC Cancer* **2013**, *13*, 260. [CrossRef] [PubMed]
54. Kågedal, Å.; Rydberg Millrud, C.; Häyry, V.; Kumlien Georén, S.; Lidegran, M.; Munck-Wikland, E.; Cardell, L.O. Oropharyngeal squamous cell carcinoma induces an innate systemic inflammation, affected by the size of the tumour and the lymph node spread. *Clin. Otolaryngol.* **2018**, *43*, 1117–1121. [CrossRef] [PubMed]
55. De Bree, R.; Takes, R.P.; Castelijns, J.A.; Medina, J.E.; Stoeckli, S.J.; Mancuso, A.A.; Hunt, J.L.; Rodrigo, J.P.; Triantafyllou, A.; Teymoortash, A.; et al. Advances in diagnostic modalities to detect occult lymph node metastases in head and neck squamous cell carcinoma. *Head Neck* **2015**, *37*, 1829–1839. [CrossRef] [PubMed]
56. Chen, C.; Chen, Z.; Cao, H.; Yan, J.; Wang, Z.; Le, H.; Weng, J.; Zhang, Y. A retrospective clinicopathological study of lung adenocarcinoma: Total tumor size can predict subtypes and lymph node involvement. *Clin. Imaging* **2018**, *47*, 52–56. [CrossRef] [PubMed]

57. Miller, T.R.; Grigsby, P.W. Measurement of tumor volume by PET to evaluate prognosis in patients with advanced cervical cancer treated by radiation therapy. *Int. J. Radiat. Oncol.* **2002**, *53*, 353–359. [CrossRef]
58. Ouyang, M.L.; Xia, H.W.; Xu, M.M.; Lin, J.; Wang, L.L.; Zheng, X.W.; Tang, K. Prediction of occult lymph node metastasis using SUV, volumetric parameters and intratumoral heterogeneity of the primary tumor in T1-2N0M0 lung cancer patients staged by PET/CT. *Ann. Nucl. Med.* **2019**, *33*, 671–680. [CrossRef]
59. Kim, S.J.; Pak, K.; Chang, S. Determination of regional lymph node status using 18F-FDG PET/CT parameters in oesophageal cancer patients: Comparison of SUV, volumetric parameters and intratumoral heterogeneity. *Br. J. Radiol.* **2016**, *89*. [CrossRef]
60. Raman, A.; Sen, N.; Ritz, E.; Fidler, M.J.; Revenaugh, P.; Stenson, K.; Al-khudari, S. Heterogeneity in the clinical presentation, diagnosis, and treatment initiation of p16-positive oropharyngeal cancer. *Am. J. Otol.* **2019**, *40*, 626–630. [CrossRef]
61. Mirzamani, N.; Salehian, P.; Farhadi, M.; Amin Tehran, E. Detection of EBV and HPV in nasopharyngeal carcinoma by in situ hybridization. *Exp. Mol. Pathol.* **2007**, *81*, 231–234. [CrossRef] [PubMed]
62. Niedobitek, G. Epstein-Barr virus infection in the pathogenesis of nasopharyngeal carcinoma. *Mol. Pathol.* **2000**, *53*, 248–254. [CrossRef] [PubMed]
63. Higuchi, T.; Fujimoto, Y.; Ozawa, H.; Bun, A.; Fukui, R.; Miyagawa, Y.; Imamura, M.; Kitajima, K.; Yamakado, K.; Miyoshi, Y. Significance of Metabolic Tumor Volume at Baseline and Reduction of Mean Standardized Uptake Value in 18 F-FDG-PET/CT Imaging for Predicting Pathological Complete Response in Breast Cancers Treated with Preoperative Chemotherapy. *Ann. Surg. Oncol.* **2019**, *26*, 2175–2183. [CrossRef] [PubMed]
64. Śnietura, M.; Jaworska, M.; Pigłowski, W.; Goraj-Zając, A.; Woźniak, G.; Lange, D. High-risk HPV DNA status and p16 (INK4a) expression as prognostic markers in patients with squamous cell cancer of oral cavity and oropharynx. *Pol. J. Pathol.* **2010**, *61*, 133–139. [PubMed]
65. Begum, S.; Gillison, M.L.; Ansari-Lari, M.A.; Shah, K.; Westra, W.H. Detection of human papillomavirus in cervical lymph nodes: A highly effective strategy for localizing site of tumor origin. *Clin. Cancer Res.* **2003**, *9*, 6469–6475. [PubMed]
66. Guzińska-Ustymowicz, K.; Pryczynicz, A.; Kemona, A.; Czyżewska, J. Correlation between proliferation markers: PCNA, Ki-67, MCM-2 and antiapoptotic protein Bcl-2 in colorectal cancer. *Anticancer Res.* **2009**, *29*, 3049–3052.
67. Altman, D.G.; Bland, J.M. Diagnostic tests. 1: Sensitivity and specificity. *BMJ Br. Med. J.* **1994**, *308*, 1552. [CrossRef]

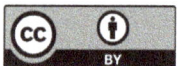

© 2020 by the authors. Licensee MDPI, Basel, Switzerland. This article is an open access article distributed under the terms and conditions of the Creative Commons Attribution (CC BY) license (http://creativecommons.org/licenses/by/4.0/).

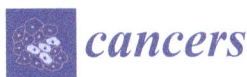

Article

Circulating Tumor Cells and Metabolic Parameters in NSCLC Patients Treated with Checkpoint Inhibitors

Angelo Castello [1], Francesco Giuseppe Carbone [2], Sabrina Rossi [3], Simona Monterisi [4], Davide Federico [5], Luca Toschi [3] and Egesta Lopci [1,*]

[1] Nuclear Medicine, Humanitas Clinical and Research Center-IRCCS, 20089 Rozzano, Italy; angelo.castello@cancercenter.humanitas.it
[2] Anatomy and Histopathology, Santa Chiara Hospital, 38122 Trento, Italy; francesco.gcarbone@gmail.com
[3] Oncology and Hematology, Humanitas Clinical and Research Center-IRCCS, 20089 Rozzano, Italy; sabrina.rossi@cancercenter.humanitas.it (S.R.); luca.toschi@cancercenter.humanitas.it (L.T.)
[4] Immunology and Inflammation, Humanitas Clinical and Research Center-IRCCS, 20089 Rozzano, Italy; simonterisi@gmail.com
[5] Pathology, Humanitas Clinical and Research Center-IRCCS, 20089 Rozzano, Italy; davide.federico@humanitas.it
* Correspondence: egesta.lopci@gmail.com; Tel.: +39-0282247542; Fax: +39-0282246693

Received: 27 November 2019; Accepted: 17 February 2020; Published: 19 February 2020

Abstract: Circulating tumor cells (CTC) count and characterization have been associated with poor prognosis in recent studies. Our aim was to examine CTC count and its association with metabolic parameters and clinical outcomes in non-small cell lung carcinoma (NSCLC) patients treated with immune checkpoint inhibitors (ICI). For this prospective study, data from 35 patients (23 males, 12 females) were collected and analyzed. All patients underwent an 18F-fluorodeoxyglucose positron emission tomography/computed tomography (18F-FDG-PET/CT) scan and CTC detection through Isolation by Size of Tumor/Trophoblastic Cells (ISET) from peripheral blood samples obtained at baseline and 8 weeks after ICI initiation. Association of CTC count with clinical and metabolic characteristics was studied. Progression-free survival (PFS) and overall survival (OS) were analyzed using the Kaplan–Meier method and the log-rank test. Median follow-up was 13.2 months (range of 4.9–21.6). CTC were identified in 16 out of 35 patients (45.7%) at baseline and 10 out of 24 patients at 8 weeks (41.7%). Mean CTC numbers before and after 8 weeks were 15 ± 28 and 11 ± 19, respectively. Prior to ICI, the mean CTC number was significantly higher in treatment-naïve patients (34 ± 39 vs. 9 ± 21, $p = 0.004$). CTC count variation (ΔCTC) was significantly associated with tumor metabolic response set by European Organization for Research and Treatment of Cancer (EORTC) criteria ($p = 0.033$). At the first restaging, patients with a high tumor burden, that is, metabolic tumor volume (MTV) and total lesion glycolysis (TLG), had a higher CTC count ($p = 0.009$). The combination of mean CTC and median MTV at 8 weeks was associated with PFS ($p < 0.001$) and OS ($p = 0.024$). Multivariate analysis identified CTC count at 8 weeks as an independent predictor for PFS and OS, whereas ΔMTV and maximum standardized uptake value variation (ΔSUVmax) was predictive for PFS and OS, respectively. Our study confirmed that CTC number is modulated by previous treatments and correlates with metabolic response during ICI. Moreover, elevated CTC count, along with metabolic parameters, were found to be prognostic factors for PFS and OS.

Keywords: non-small-cell lung cancer; circulating tumor cells; PET/CT; immunotherapy; response to treatment

1. Introduction

The introduction of antibodies against programmed cell death protein-1 (PD-1) and its ligand (PD-L1), a crucial axis involved in the immune surveillance, has prompted encouraging results in the treatment of advanced non-small cell lung carcinoma (NSCLC), although only a minority of patients show clinical response [1]. As a consequence, there is a compelling need to understand the molecular basis of cancer growth and identify potential biomarkers of response, in order to better select patients who will benefit from such new agents.

In the last years, circulating tumor cells' (CTC) count and characterization have become of great interest in the scientific community [2,3]. Some studies have demonstrated that CTC enumeration is related to poor prognosis in different metastatic malignancies, including lung, breast, colorectal, prostate, and gastric cancer. Furthermore, molecular characterization of CTC might expand our knowledge on tumor heterogeneity, especially in patients for whom tissue biopsies are difficult to perform [4–8].

Molecular imaging, using 18F-fluorodeoxyglucose (18F-FDG) with positron emission tomography/computed tomography (PET/CT), is widely applied in oncology as a useful marker of tumor biology. Indeed, by differentiating higher versus less-active metabolic tumor tissues, semi-quantitative metabolic parameters can offer the possibility for non-invasive, in vivo tumor characterization and for correct evaluation of tumor response [9–11]. However, available studies analyzing the association between 18F-FDG PET/CT and CTC in NSCLC are limited to chemotherapy-naïve patients or those treated with "traditional" antitumor drugs [12–15].

On the basis of these premises, our aim was to examine CTC count in NSCLC patients treated with immune checkpoint inhibitors (ICI) and determine its relationship with metabolic parameters by 18F-FDG PET/CT and clinical outcomes.

2. Results

2.1. Patients' Characteristics

A total of 20 patients (57.1%) received nivolumab, 12 (34.3%) pembrolizumab, 2 patients (5.7%) had a combination of nivolumab and ipilimumab, and only 1 (2.9%) patient was treated with atezolizumab. The median number of immunotherapy cycles was 8 (range of 1–47). Median follow-up was 13.2 months (range of 4.9–21.6 months).

2.2. CTC and Clinic-Pathologic Features

CTC were identified (CTC ≥ 1) in 16 out of 35 patients (45.7%) at baseline prior to ICI therapy, and the CTC count ranged between 0 and 130 (mean ± standard deviation (SD), 15 ± 28). The minimum number of CTC detected was 5, in particular 8 patients had a CTC count between 5 and 20, whereas the other 8 patients had CTC from 25 to 130.

At the first restaging, peripheral blood samples were available for 24 patients because of progression of disease or a worsening of clinical conditions in the other cases. CTC were detected in 10 out of 24 patients (41.7%). The median number of CTC was 11 ± 19 in 10 mL of blood. CTC count ranged between 5 and 20 in six patients, and between 30 and 60 in the other four patients. In addition, we demonstrated a reduction of CTC in nine patients (37.5%), unchanged in eight patients (33.3%), and increased in seven patients (29.2%). Although a reduction in the mean number of CTC before and after 8 weeks of treatment was detected, this decrease was not statistically significant.

The association between CTC count and patient characteristics was explored, both before treatment and at the first restaging. There was a statistically significant association between CTC count and previous treatments. Of note, patients who underwent ICI as first-line treatment had a mean number of CTC at baseline higher than patients who started ICI after more lines of treatment (34 ± 39 vs. 9 ± 21, $p = 0.004$) (Figure 1A). Likewise, a trend was observed with high baseline CTC count and pembrolizumab ($p = 0.09$); indeed, the latter is often used in first-line settings. No further association was found between CTC counts, as well as the other clinical variables, such as age, gender, smoking history, and tumor type.

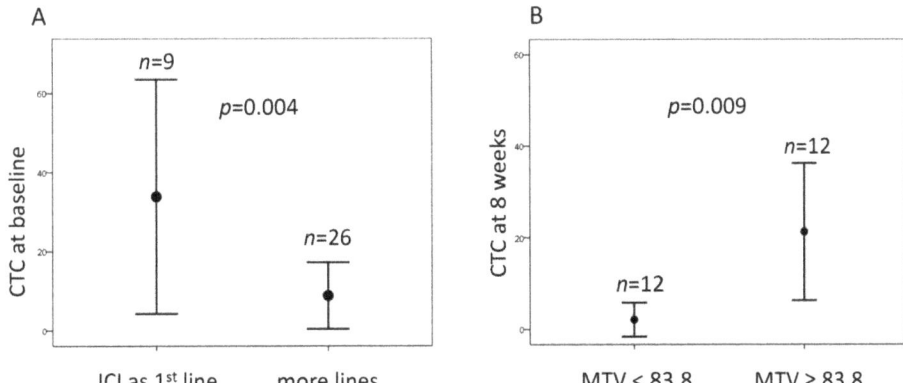

Figure 1. Association of circulating tumor cells (CTC) count with clinical-metabolic features. (**A**) Mean number of CTC at baseline according to the number of previous lines of treatment. (**B**) Mean number of CTC at the first restaging (about 8 weeks) and the median value of metabolic tumor volume (MTV).

2.3. Relationship of CTC and Tumor Response

Of the 35 patients enrolled, 31 patients underwent tumor assessment by computed tomography (CT), whereas 18F-FDG PET/CT scans were available from 28 patients at the first response assessment. According to Response Evaluation Criteria In Solid Tumors (RECIST) 1.1, partial response (PR) was observed in 6 patients, stable disease (SD) was observed in 12, and progressive disease (PD) in 13. We found that patients with PD showed a trend toward higher baseline CTC count (26 ± 36) compared with patients with partial response (14 ± 14) or stable disease (9 ± 26) ($p = 0.076$). There was no significant difference in the CTC count after 8 weeks among the three groups of response.

According to the European Organization for Research and Treatment of Cancer (EORTC) criteria, partial metabolic response (PMR), stable metabolic disease (SMD), and progressive metabolic disease (PMD) were observed in 10, 6, and 12 patients, respectively. There was no significant difference in the baseline CTC count, as well as after 8 weeks, among the three groups. However, considering CTC changes (ΔCTC) within individual patients, among the 24 patients that had their CTC analyzed after 8 weeks of treatment, we found that the increase of CTC count was associated with poor response to ICI by means 18F-FDG PET/CT, as PMD rates were significantly different between patients with CTC increase at 8 weeks and patients with stable or decreased number of CTC (71.4% vs. 28.6% vs. 0%, respectively, $p = 0.033$) (Table 1).

Table 1. Association between circulating tumor cells (CTC) count and response to immune checkpoint inhibitors (ICI).

Parameter	EORTC		
	CMR/PMR	SMD	PMD
Baseline CTC count			
CTC ≤ 15 ($n = 18$)	27.8% (5)	33.3% (6)	38.9% (7)
CTC > 15 ($n = 10$)	50% (5)	0% (0)	50% (5)
p-value	ns	ns	ns
ΔCTC count after 8 weeks			
decreased ($n = 9$)	66.7% (6)	11.1% (1)	22.2% (2)
stable ($n = 8$)	12.5% (1)	37.5% (3)	50% (4)
increased ($n = 7$)	0% (0)	28.6% (2)	71.4% (5)
p-value	ns	ns	0.033

CMR/PMR, complete metabolic response/partial metabolic response; SMD, stable metabolic disease; PMD, progressive metabolic disease. ns: not significant.

2.4. CTC and Semi-Quantitative 18F-FDG Parameters

The median maximum standardized uptake value (SUVmax), average SUV (SUVmean), metabolic tumor volume (MTV), and total lesion glycolysis (TLG) before the initiation of treatment were 13.5 (range of 4.9–35.7), 5.9 (3.2–9.8), 68 (8–1772), and 362.8 (31–2504), respectively. Median SUVmax, SUV mean, MTV, and TLG after 8 weeks were 12.1 (3.6–38.4), 5.6 (3–13.8), 83.8 (2.5–623.3), and 511.2 (7.6–4332.7), respectively. Median ΔSUVmax, ΔSUVmean, ΔTLG, and ΔMTV were −12.9% (−75.5–107.1%), −0.88% (−61.3–130%), 47.8% (−99.4–1295%), and 30.4% (−98–1245%). At baseline, the number of CTC did not correlate with metabolic parameters, and only a trend for SUVmax was observed ($p = 0.072$). Conversely, after 8 weeks of treatment, CTC count was significantly associated with metabolic volume, expressed by MTV and TLG. Indeed, patients with MTV and TLG above the median values had higher mean number of CTC than patients with low metabolic tumor burden (both MTV and TLG $p = 0.009$) (Figure 1B). No difference was found between CTC and percentage changes of metabolic parameters.

2.5. Relationship between CTC Count, 18F-FDG PET Parameters, and Survival

The median progression-free survival (PFS) and overall survival (OS) of patients with CTC counts ≤ 11 after 8 weeks were 6.5 months (range of 5.1–7.9 months) and 18 months (range of 12–24 months), respectively. The median PFS and OS of patients with CTC counts > 11 were 1.8 months (range of 1.7–1.8 months) and 4 months (range of 2.7–5.3 months), respectively. The differences in PFS and OS were both statistically significant ($p < 0.001$, $p = 0.019$ for PFS and OS, respectively) (Figure 2A,B).

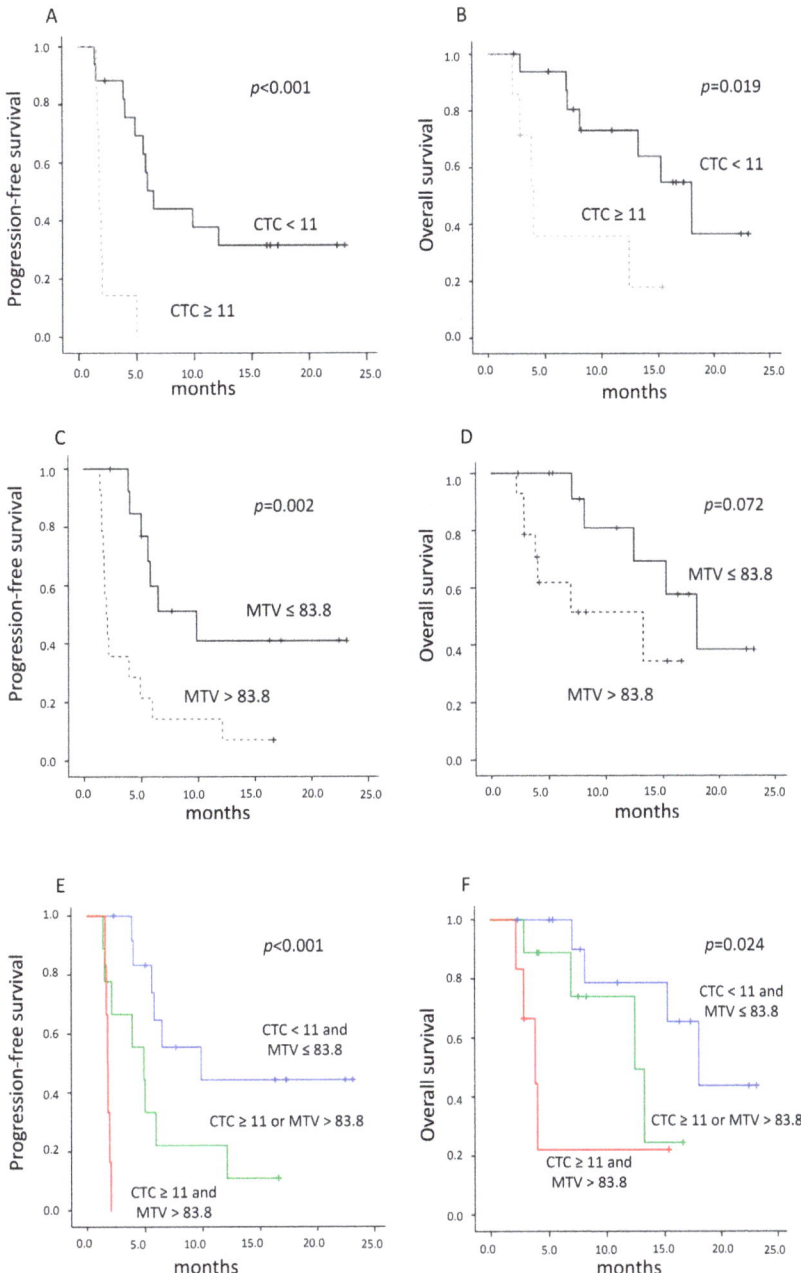

Figure 2. Kaplan–Meier curves according to CTC count and metabolic parameters. (**A,B**) Progression-free survival (PFS) and overall survival (OS) according to CTC count at 8 weeks, below or above the mean value. (**C,D**) PFS and OS of patients with MTV at 8 weeks greater or lower than median value. (**E,F**) PFS and OS according to the combination of mean number of CTC and median MTV after 8 weeks of treatment.

The median PFS and OS of patients with median MTV ≤ 83.8 were 9.9 months (range of 3.6–16.1 months) and 18 months (range of 12.6–23.4 months), respectively. The median PFS and OS of patients with median MTV > 83.8 were 1.9 months (range of 1.5–2.4 months) and 13.2 months (range of 2–24.5 months), respectively. The difference for PFS was statistically significant ($p = 0.002$), whereas for OS it showed only a trend ($p = 0.072$) (Figure 2C,D). Furthermore, we tested whether the combination of CTC count and MTV at 8 weeks could provide further discriminatory value in predicting clinical outcomes. Of note, all patients with MTV ≤ 83.8 and CTC ≤ 11 had the longest PFS and OS. Among patients with median MTV greater than 83.8, those with CTC count ≤ 11 were associated with longer PFS and OS than patients whose CTC were above the mean value (Figure 3E,F) ($p < 0.001$ and $p = 0.024$ for PFS and OS, respectively). Regarding percentage changes of metabolic parameters, we found that ΔMTV and ΔTLG were associated with PFS (both 9.9 vs. 2.1 months, $p = 0.010$ and $p = 0.009$, respectively), whereas ΔSUVmax was prognostic for OS (median not reached vs. 12.4 months, $p = 0.013$).

Finally, due to the low number of events, only three parameters were included in the multivariate Cox analysis. Of note, the number of CTC at the first restaging was confirmed as a predictive factor for PFS and OS, along with ΔMTV for PFS and ΔSUVmax for OS (Table 2).

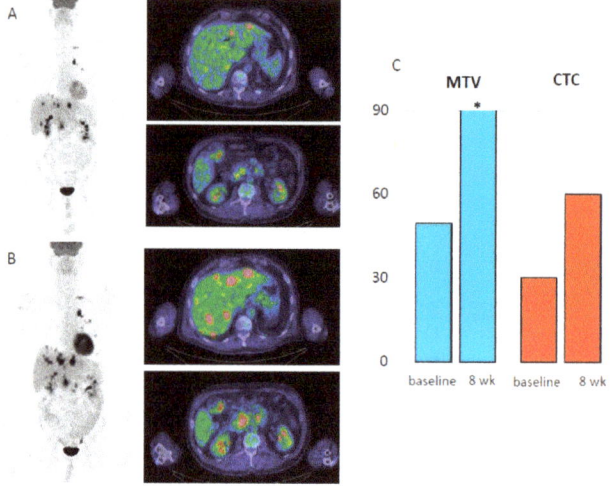

Figure 3. *Cont.*

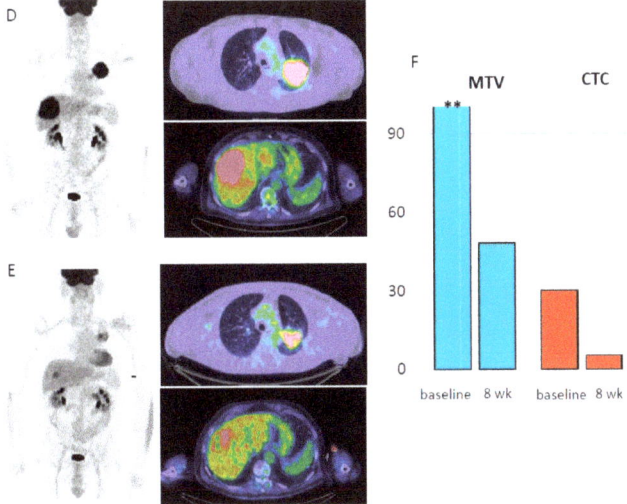

Figure 3. Two cases of progression (**A–C**) and response (**D–F**) to ICI according to metabolic parameters and CTC evaluation. (**A**) Maximum intensity projection (MIP) with two axial slices of liver and celiac node metastases at baseline. (**B**) Increase of tumor burden and appearance of further metastatic sites within the liver and in the abdominal nodes at the first restaging. (**C**) Bar graph representation of MTV (blue bars) between the baseline (49.4 mL) and the first restaging (97.2 mL). Likewise, CTC count (red bars) increased from 30 to 60. (**C**) MIP with two large lesions within the lung and liver at baseline. (**D**) 18F-fluorodeoxyglucose positron emission tomography/computed tomography (18F-FDG PET/CT) at 8 weeks, which demonstrated a decrease of overall tumor burden. (**F**) Bar graph representation of MTV (blue bars) at baseline (256.5 mL) and at 8 weeks (48 mL). Likewise CTC count (red bars) decreased from 30 to 5, * MTV= 97.2 mL; ** MTV= 256.5 mL.

Table 2. Uni- and multivariate Cox proportional hazard regression analyses for the prediction of PFS and OS.

Parameters	PFS			OS		
	Hazard Ratio	95% IC	p-Value	Hazard Ratio	95% IC	p-Value
Age (median)	1.233	0.564–2.694	ns	1.009	0.423–2.910	ns
Gender	0.346	0.156–0.768	0.009	0.329	0.119–0.905	0.031
Smoking history	1.407	0.480–4.129	ns	3.518	1.050–11.790	0.041
Histology	0.828	0.345–1.990	ns	0.907	0.291–2.822	ns
PD-L1 status	0.736	0.255–2.128	ns	0.659	0.147–2.957	ns
CTC baseline (median)	1.089	0.472–2.512	ns	1.869	0.607–5.759	ns
CTC at 8 weeks (median)	0.135	0.040–0.458	0.001	0.260	0.77–0.871	0.029
SUVmax baseline (median)	1.049	0.483–2.276	ns	0.996	0.383–2.654	ns
SUVmean baseline (median)	0.701	0.320–1.534	ns	0.839	0.312–2.257	ns
TLG baseline (median)	0.998	0.459–2.171	ns	1.016	0.389–1.534	ns
MTV baseline (median)	1.601	0.739–3.468	ns	2.473	0.934–6.551	ns
ΔSUVmax (median)	2.409	0.954–6.085	ns	0.179	0.039–0.825	0.027
ΔSUVmean (median)	1.498	0.611–3.671	ns	0.375	0.100–1.402	ns
ΔTLG (median)	0.310	0.122–787	0.014	0.751	0.241–2.346	ns
ΔMTV (median)	0.312	0.123–792	0.014	0.481	0.151–1.532	ns
Multivariate Cox proportional hazards regression analysis						
CTC at 8 weeks (median)	0.115	0.030–0.434	0.001 *	0.178	0.045–0.707	0.014 *
ΔMTV (median)	0.357	0.130–0.984	0.046 *			
ΔSUVmax (median)				0.144	0.028–0.736	0.02 *

* $p < 0.05$.

Figure 4A,B shows two cases with metabolic response by 18F-FDG PET/CT and CTC assessment before and after 8 weeks of ICI.

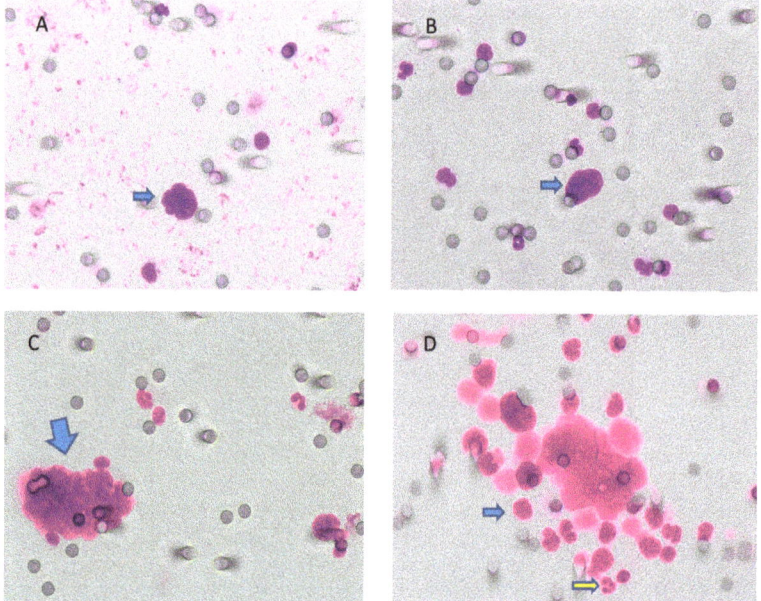

Figure 4. Comparison of positive (**A–C**) and negative findings (**D**) for CTC visualized by May–Grünwald–Giemsa (MGG) staining at 40× magnification. (**A**) Naked nucleus (without cytoplasm), intensely stained (hypercromatic), with irregular shape and scalloped borders, suspect for carcinoma. The absence of a clearly visible cytoplasm did not permit the evaluation of the nuclear/cytoplasmic ratio. (**B**) The same as the previous image; herein, we can compare the size of the naked nucleus (arrow) with the size of neighboring leukocytes (around 3–4 times bigger). (**C**) A cluster of cells with a high nucleus/cytoplasm ratio, hypercromasia, and irregular shape of nuclei. Additionally, cells were bigger than leukocytes. (**D**) Some of the cells in this sample were degenerated. We did not take into account these cells. The remaining population (for example, the cell indicated by the blue arrow) had a nuclear size somewhat similar to that of leukocytes (yellow arrow). Where cytoplasm was present, it was granular. Thus, all of these cells were probably leukocytes. * CTC = circulating tumor cells; MGG = May–Grünwald–Giemsa.

3. Discussion

Several studies have investigated the prevalence and the prognostic role of CTC in different cancer types, including NSCLC, but only a limited number have analyzed their relationship to 18F-FDG PET/CT parameters [13,16–18]. On the other side, only a few studies have assessed the role of CTC in patients with advanced NSCLC treated with checkpoint inhibitors [19,20]. If we exclude our preliminary data [21], to the best of our knowledge, this research is the first to report a significant association between the CTC count and the tumor 18F-FDG uptake in a similar patient cohort treated with immunotherapy.

In our analysis, CTC were detected in 46% of the patients before the initiation of ICI and in 42% at the first assessment. Our detection rate was superior compared to Tamminga' study [20], that being 32% before ICI and 27% after 4 weeks, where CTC identification was performed by epithelial marker-dependent (CellSearch) technology. Moreover, our finding is consistent with previous studies in lung cancer patients, which demonstrated an overall sensitivity higher for cell size rather than marked-based approaches, although not in an ICI setting [22–26]. Nevertheless, in the abovementioned study from the Italian group [19], using another system based on cell size (i.e., Screencells Cyto), the prevalence of CTC was almost double that of our study (91% vs. 46%) in a larger population ($n = 89$). This discrepancy by the two techniques, although based on the same filter diameter, might suggest a high inter-reader variability due to both readers' skills and the lack of uniformly accepted criteria for CTC definition. Therefore, further and larger studies are needed.

Similar to Krebs et al., in our study, the presence and the number of CTC were influenced by previous lines of therapy. Indeed, patients with a positive history for previous therapy had a mean number of CTC lower than those who underwent ICI as first-line therapy ($p = 0.004$) [7]. As a consequence, the presence of CTC in the peripheral blood after chemotherapy might suggest the grade of response to treatment or, in other words, the aggressiveness of the tumor determining how fast cancer can return after a macroscopic response. Hence, residual CTC after chemotherapy could be characterized in order to identify those morphological or genetic modification-inducing expression of genes and proteins conferring drug-resistance, such as the endothelial to mesenchymal transition observed in cancer stem cells [27,28]. In line with previous studies, we did not find a significant association between CTC and clinicopathological characteristics (e.g., age, gender, tobacco exposure, tumor size, and histologic subtype) in patients with advanced NSCLC [14,29,30]. Moreover, CTC count both at baseline and after 8 weeks, as well as their change during treatment, was not associated with tumor response according to morphologic criteria (RECIST 1.1), although a trend of significance with higher mean number of CTC for the PD group ($p = 0.076$) was evident. Such a finding was consistent with the two abovementioned studies in NSCLC patients treated with ICI [19,20]. Of note, CTC were associated with durable response, defined as no progression for at least 6 months measured by RECIST 1.1, more pronounced than early tumor response at 4–6 weeks [20]. Likewise, Nair et al., prior to any therapeutic intervention for NSCLC, reported no correlation for CTC and tumor diameter [13]. On the other hand, considering EORTC criteria, we showed a significant association between patients with increased CTC and poor metabolic response by 18F-FDG PET/CT at first assessment after 8 weeks of treatment. Similarly, Punnoose and colleagues [15] demonstrated higher levels of CTC in patients classified as non-responders by metabolic criteria, although this was performed in a cohort treated with erlotinib and pertuzumab. Hence, our results confirm on one hand the prevailing cytostatic effect of ICI compared to cytocidal and, on the other, the precocious metabolic changes detected by 18F-FDG that occur earlier than morphologic changes.

We also investigated the relationship between CTC and metabolic 18F-FDG positron emission tomography (PET)-based indexes. Interestingly, we detected a significant association between higher densities of CTC after 8 weeks and metabolic tumor burden, expressed by MTV and TLG (both $p = 0.009$). A significant difference was also found between the number of CTC at 8 weeks and the percentage changes of metabolic volume (i.e., ΔMTV and ΔTLG). These findings suggest, as already stated previously, that the CTC count in the peripheral blood can reflect the entity of the tumor burden and provide valuable information on the metabolic activity, which may serve as a marker of tumor aggressiveness in advanced NSCLC. Hence, as CTC count is a marker of poor response, if our results were confirmed in a larger cohort, CTC along with metabolic indexes would be useful for monitoring disease, allowing for early cessation of treatment with checkpoint inhibitors, and switching to an alternative therapeutic regimen. Because our paper is the first in the era of checkpoint inhibitors investigating CTC and 18F-FDG PET parameters, comparison with other reports is not well applicable. Previously, some studies demonstrated a significant correlation between CTC and SUV value in patients with chemotherapy-naïve lung cancer [12–14,31]. On the contrary, Nygaard et al. did not find any association between metabolic parameters and cell-free (cf) DNA, another tumor-derived biomarker [32].

The presence of CTC is related with survival and is predictive of disease progression and death in NSCLC during chemotherapy and targeted therapies [15,23,29,33–37]. In the present study, CTC count after 8 weeks was significantly associated with PFS and OS, whereas MTV at first restaging was prognostic only for PFS, and showed a trend for OS ($p = 0.072$), in our opinion due to limited sample size. In addition, CTC and MTV were also prognostic factors when considered in conjunction. In this regard, we identified a group characterized by poor PFS presenting with high CTC and high MTV at 8 weeks. Our findings are consistent with the only two abovementioned studies, which explored the prognostic role of CTC in patients receiving ICI [19,20]. Interestingly, Tamminga et al. showed that CTC and cell-free DNA (cfDNA), although at baseline, separately and in conjunction, were significantly associated with OS in NSCLC patients receiving nivolumab [20]. Moreover, CTC count after 8 weeks was predictive for both PFS and OS, along with ΔMTV and ΔSUVmax for PFS and OS, respectively, suggesting that large and highly metabolic tumors could have the potential of shedding a high number of CTC in the bloodstream, increasing the possibility to metastasize at distant sites.

These findings may be particularly interesting for patients in whom no tumor tissue is available for other predictive analysis. On the same line, Fiorelli et al. identified SUVmax as an independent predictor for CTC presence after surgery in NSCLC patients [31].

Nevertheless, our study had some shortcomings. First, a limited sample size, and second, we did not evaluate PD-L1 expression on CTC. Recently, Ilié et al. demonstrated that patients who had PD-L1-negative CTC 6 months after the start of checkpoint inhibitors benefitted from immunotherapy, highlighting CTC as a heterogeneous population worthy of further investigation [33]. Third, we did not investigate the genetic features of CTC, which could open a new frontier in the understanding of therapy resistance. Finally, we did not collect other circulating markers, such as cfDNA, known as potential biomarkers in cancer patients.

4. Materials and Methods

4.1. Patients and Study Design

The current study was conducted following the approval of the local institutional review board and in accordance with the Declaration of Helsinki and Good Clinical Practice guidelines (Prot. Nr. CE Humanitas ex D.M. 8/2/2013 335/17). Written informed consent was obtained in all cases. The trial was registered at www.clinicaltrials.gov (NCT03563482). Between April 2017 and March 2019, 35 patients (23 males, 12 females) affected by metastatic or relapsed NSCLC were referred to our hospital, Humanitas Clinical and Research Center, for treatment with ICI, and were prospectively enrolled. ICI therapy was administered intravenously at a dose of 3 mg/kg every 2 weeks for nivolumab or at a fixed dose of 200 mg every 3 weeks for pembrolizumab.

All patients performed whole-body contrast-enhanced CT, 18F-FDG PET/CT scan, and peripheral blood sample for CTC isolation at baseline and at the first restaging after approximately 8 weeks (after three cycles for pembrolizumab and atezolizumab, and after four cycles for nivolumab). The patients' epidemiologic and clinical characteristics are reported in Table 3.

Table 3. Patients' characteristics at baseline.

Characteristics	N (%)
Patients	35
Median age (range)	77 (51–86)
Gender	
Male	23 (65.7)
Female	12 (34.3)
Smoking status	
Never	5 (14.3)
Former	19 (54.3)
Smoker	11 (31.4)
ECOG PS	
0	18 (51.4)
≥1	17 (48.6)

Table 3. Cont.

Characteristics	N (%)
Therapy line	
0	9 (25.7)
1	14 (40)
≥2	12 (34.3)
Metastatic sites	
1–2	16 (45.7)
>2	19 (54.3)
Histology	
Adeno	24 (68.6)
Squamous	7 (20)
Poorly differentiated	34 (8.6)
Sarcomatoid	1 (2.8)
Tumor PD-L1 status	
Negative	7 (20)
Positive	14 (40)
Not evaluable *	14 (40)

* Programmed cell death ligand 1 (PD-L1) could not be evaluated in 14 patients as biopsied material was of insufficient quality or quantity.

4.2. CTC Isolation and Enumeration

For CTC detection, 10 mL of blood was collected in EDTA (ethylenediaminetetraacetic acid) tubes and processed within 2 h on the Isolation by Size of Tumor/Trophoblastic Cells (ISET) platform (Rarecells, Paris, France). Peripheral blood was filtered through the ISET polycarbonate membrane containing 10 filter-spots with calibrated 8 μm diameter cylindrical pores, each spot representing the filtration of 1 mL of blood. The membrane was cut into two parts containing four and six spots per part. Four spots were stained using a freshly made May–Grünwald–Giemsa (MGG) solution according to the technique described by Hofman and colleagues [29] for 5 min with undiluted May–Grünwald, and subsequently for 5 min with 50% diluted May–Grünwald and 40 min in 10% diluted Giemsa, followed by rinsing with water. Membranes were then air-dried and mounted with limonene mounting medium (Sigma-Aldrich, St. Louis, MO, USA) and kept in the dark at room temperature. Stained spots were examined under a light microscopy (Olympus BX51, Olympus Corporation, Shinjuku, Tokyo, Japan) at 10× and subsequently digitized at 40× magnification. All images were analyzed by two cytopathologists blinded to the study data. CTC were recognized on the basis of four cytopathological features: (a) nuclear hyperchromatism, (b) increased nuclear volume, (c) irregular nuclear borders, and (d) increased nucleus-to-cytoplasm ratio. Cells were defined as CTC when all four abovementioned criteria were fulfilled, as previously described by Hofman and colleagues [29]. A dedicated pathologist analyzed and counted CTC present in the membranes (four spots per patient). A panel of features obtainable after magnification is illustrated in Figure 3.

4.3. 18F-FDG PET/CT and Image Analysis

Patients fasted at least 6 h before intravenous administration of 250–500 MBq of fluorodeoxyglucose (FDG) in a quiet room. Images were acquired 60 min after tracer injection using two scanners accredited by EANM Research Ltd. (EARL) program [38]: (a) Siemens Biograph LSO (lutetium oxyorthosilicate) 6 scanner (Siemens Erlangen, Munich, Germany), with an integrated 6-slice CT; and (b) GE Discovery PET/CT 690 (General Electric Healthcare, Waukesha, WI, USA), with an integrated 64-slice CT. Attenuation-correction images were obtained with a low-dose CT (120 kV, 30 mA). Unenhanced low-dose CT was performed at 140 kV and 40 mA for attenuation correction of emission data and anatomic localization of the PET dataset. PET sinograms were reconstructed by means of an ordered-subset expectation maximization iterative reconstruction algorithm (three iterations; eight subsets). Images were displayed on a GE ADW4.6 workstation (GE Healthcare, Waukesha,

WI, USA) and interpreted by two experienced nuclear medicine physicians. From 18F-FDG PET/CT images, the following parameters were measured: SUVmax, SUVmean, MTV, and TLG; MTV was assessed using a PETVCAR (GE Healthcare, Waukesha, WI, USA) workstation and was computed using an SUVmax threshold of 41%; TLG was computed as MTV × SUVmean. Percentage reduction between baseline and restaging was calculated using the formula: [(8 weeks SUVmax − pretreatment SUVmax)/pretreatment SUVmax] × 100 for SUVmax; similarly for the other metabolic parameters.

4.4. Tumor Response Assessment

Early tumor response, after approximately 8 weeks of treatment, was measured using the revised RECIST 1.1 criteria [39]. Four categories were identified: complete response (CR), disappearance of all target lesions; PR, reduction of at least 30% in the sum of diameters of target lesions; PD, increase of at least 20% in the sum of diameters of target lesions or appearance of new lesions; SD, neither CR, nor PR or PD.

Metabolic response was evaluated according to EORTC criteria with the following categories: complete metabolic response (CMR), complete resolution of 18F-FDG uptake within all lesions; PMR, reduction of at least 25% in the sum of SUVmax; PMD, increase of at least 25% in the sum of SUVmax or appearance of new 18F-FDG avid lesions that are typical of cancer and not related to inflammation or infection; SMD, neither CMR, nor PMR or PMD [40].

4.5. Statistical Analysis

Descriptive statistics for clinical, imaging, and pathologic variables were determined using the median (range) or media with SD as appropriate.

Associations of CTC with clinical and metabolic characteristics were studied by means of t-tests and Mann–Whitney U tests for continuous variables and χ^2 tests or Fisher's exact test for categorical variables.

Clinical outcomes were evaluated in terms of PFS, defined as the interval from the date of initiation of ICI to the date of either disease progression or death, and OS calculated as the duration between the date of initiation of immunotherapy and the date of death. For the univariate and multivariate analyses of survival, Cox's proportional hazard model was employed as well as the log-rank test with Kaplan–Meier analysis. All statistical analyses were carried out using the Statistical Package for Social Sciences, version 23.0, for Windows (SPSS, Chicago, IL, USA), and p-values < 0.05 were considered as being statistically significant.

5. Conclusions

In our study, analyzing for the first-time concomitant CTC and metabolic parameters in NSCLC patients receiving ICI, we observed that CTC number was modulated by previous therapeutic interventions. Moreover, the presence of elevated CTC count was an additional prognostic and predictor factor along with metabolic tumor burden. Further large-scaled studies confirming the clinical utility of CTC in combination with metabolic PET-based parameters in this setting are now warranted.

Author Contributions: Conceptualization, E.L., L.T. and A.C.; methodology, A.C., E.L., S.M., F.G.C., S.R., D.F. and L.T.; software, E.L., A.C.; formal analysis, A.C., S.M., F.G.C., D.F.; investigation, E.L., A.C.; resources, E.L., L.T.; data curation, E.L.; writing—original draft preparation, A.C.; writing—review and editing, A.C., E.L., S.M., F.G.C., S.R., D.F. and L.T.; supervision, E.L.; project administration, E.L.; funding acquisition, E.L. All authors have read and agreed to the published version of the manuscript.

Funding: This study is supported by Fondazione AIRC (Associazione Italiana per la Ricerca sul Cancro) with the grant no. 18923.

Acknowledgments: The Italian Association for Research on Cancer (AIRC—Associazione Italiana per la Ricerca sul Cancro) is acknowledged for the support on this research. ISET machine is available thanks to a grant from LILT (Lega Italiana per la Lotta contro i Tumori). The authors are particularly grateful to the Immunology Research Lab (D. Qehajaj, F. Grizzi) and to the Thoracic Surgery of Humanitas (G. Veronesi, E. Dieci, P. Novellis) for the support on research.

Conflicts of Interest: E.L. is winner of the individual grant no. 18923 provided by AIRC. A.C. is supported with fellowships related to the grant no. 18923. S.M. reports fellowship support from Fondazione Umberto Veronesi. No other potential conflicts of interest relevant to this article exist.

References

1. Chen, D.S.; Mellman, I. Oncology meets immunology: The cancer immunity cycle. *Immunity* **2013**, *39*, 1–10. [CrossRef] [PubMed]
2. Tanaka, F.; Yoneda, K.; Kondo, N.; Hashimoto, M.; Takuwa, T.; Matsumoto, S.; Okumura, Y.; Rahman, S.; Tsubota, N.; Tsujimura, T.; et al. Circulating tumor cell as a diagnostic marker in primary lung cancer. *Clin. Cancer Res.* **2009**, *15*, 6980–6986. [CrossRef] [PubMed]
3. Krebs, M.G.; Metcalf, R.L.; Carter, L.; Brady, G.; Blackhall, F.H.; Dive, C. Molecular analysis of circulating tumour cells-biology and biomarkers. *Nat. Rev. Clin. Oncol.* **2014**, *11*, 129–144. [CrossRef] [PubMed]
4. Hayes, D.F.; Cristofanilli, M.; Budd, G.T.; Ellis, M.J.; Stopeck, A.; Miller, M.C.; Matera, J.; Allard, W.J.; Doyle, G.V.; Terstappen, L.W. Circulating tumor cells at each follow-up time point during therapy of metastatic breast cancer patients predict progression-free and overall survival. *Clin. Cancer Res.* **2006**, *12*, 4218–4224. [CrossRef] [PubMed]
5. Cohen, S.J.; Punt, C.J.; Iannotti, N.; Saidman, B.H.; Sabbath, K.D.; Gabrail, N.Y.; Picus, J.; Morse, M.; Mitchell, E.; Miller, M.C.; et al. Relationship of circulating tumor cells to tumor response, progression-free survival, and overall survival in patients with metastatic colorectal cancer. *J. Clin. Oncol.* **2008**, *26*, 3213–3221. [CrossRef]
6. de Bono, J.S.; Scher, H.I.; Montgomery, R.B.; Parker, C.; Miller, M.C.; Tissing, H.; Doyle, G.V.; Terstappen, L.W.; Pienta, K.J.; Raghavan, D. Circulating tumor cells predict survival benefit from treatment in metastatic castration-resistant prostate cancer. *Clin. Cancer Res.* **2008**, *14*, 6302–6309. [CrossRef]
7. Frick, M.A.; Feigenberg, S.J.; Jean-Baptiste, S.R.; Aguarin, L.A.; Mendes, A.; Chinniah, C.; Swisher-McClure, S.; Berman, A.; Levin, W.; Cengel, K.; et al. Circulating tumor cells are associated with recurrent disease in patients with early stage non-small cell lung cancer. *Clin. J. Cancer Res.* **2020**. [CrossRef]
8. Hofman, V.; Ilie, M.; Long, E.; Guibert, N.; Selva, E.; Washetine, K.; Mograbi, B.; Mouroux, J.; Vénissac, N.; Reverso-Meinietti, J.; et al. Detection of circulating tumour cells from lung cancer patients in the era of targeted therapy: Promises, drawbacks and pitfalls. *Curr. Mol. Med.* **2014**, *14*, 440–456. [CrossRef]
9. Paesmans, M.; Berghmans, T.; Dusart, M.; Garcia, C.; Hossein-Foucher, C.; Lafitte, J.J.; Mascaux, C.; Meert, A.P.; Roelandts, M.; Scherpereel, A.; et al. Primary tumor standardized uptake value measured on fluorodeoxyglucose positron emission tomography is of prognostic value for survival in non-small cell lung cancer: Update of a systematic review and meta-analysis by the European Lung Cancer Working Party for the International Association for the Study of Lung Cancer Staging Project. *J. Thorac. Oncol.* **2010**, *5*, 612–619.
10. Sharma, A.; Mohan, A.; Bhalla, A.S.; Vishnubhatla, S.; Pandey, A.K.; Bal, C.S.; Kumar, R. Role of various semiquantitative parameters of 18F-FDG PET/CT studies for interim treatment response evaluation in non-small-cell lung cancer. *Nucl. Med. Commun.* **2017**, *38*, 858–867. [CrossRef]
11. Huang, W.; Fan, M.; Liu, B.; Fu, Z.; Zhou, T.; Zhang, Z.; Gong, H.; Li, B. Value of metabolic tumor volume on repeated 18F-FDG PET/CT for early prediction of survival in locally advanced non-small cell lung cancer treated with concurrent chemoradiotherapy. *J. Nucl. Med.* **2014**, *55*, 1584–1590. [CrossRef] [PubMed]
12. Morbelli, S.; Alama, A.; Ferrarazzo, G.; Coco, S.; Genova, C.; Rijavec, E.; Bongioanni, F.; Biello, F.; Dal Bello, M.G.; Barletta, G.; et al. Circulating Tumor DNA Reflects Tumor Metabolism Rather Than Tumor Burden in Chemotherapy-Naive Patients with Advanced Non-Small Cell Lung Cancer: 18F-FDG PET/CT Study. *J. Nucl. Med.* **2017**, *58*, 1764–1769. [CrossRef] [PubMed]
13. Nair, V.S.; Keu, K.V.; Luttgen, M.S.; Kolatkar, A.; Vasanawala, M.; Kuschner, W.; Iagaru, A.H.; Hoh, C.; Shrager, J.B.; Loo, B.W., Jr.; et al. An observational study of circulating tumor cells and 18F-FDG PET uptake in patients with treatment-naive non-small cell lung cancer. *PLoS ONE* **2013**, *8*, e67733. [CrossRef] [PubMed]
14. Bayarri-Lara, C.I.; de Miguel Pérez, D.; Cueto Ladrón de Guevara, A.; Rodriguez Fernández, A.; Puche, J.L.; Sánchez-Palencia Ramos, A.; Ruiz Zafra, J.; Giraldo Ospina, C.F.; Delgado-Rodríguez, M.; Expósito Ruiz, M.; et al. Association of circulating tumour cells with early relapse and 18F-fluorodeoxyglucose positron emission tomography uptake in resected non-small-cell lung cancers. *Eur. J. Cardiothorac. Surg.* **2017**, *52*, 55–62. [CrossRef]

15. Punnoose, E.A.; Atwal, S.; Liu, W.; Raja, R.; Fine, B.M.; Hughes, B.G.; Hicks, R.J.; Hampton, G.M.; Amler, L.C.; Pirzkall, A.; et al. Evaluation of circulating tumor cells and circulating tumor DNA in non-small cell lung cancer: Association with clinical endpoints in a phase II clinical trial of pertuzumab and erlotinib. *Clin. Cancer Res.* **2012**, *18*, 2391–2401. [CrossRef]
16. Cristofanilli, M.; Budd, G.T.; Ellis, M.J.; Stopeck, A.; Matera, J.; Miller, M.C.; Reuben, J.M.; Doyle, G.V.; Allard, W.J.; Terstappen, L.W.; et al. Circulating tumor cells, disease progression, and survival in metastatic breast cancer. *N. Engl. J. Med.* **2004**, *351*, 781–791. [CrossRef]
17. Huang, X.; Gao, P.; Song, Y.; Sun, J.; Chen, X.; Zhao, J.; Xu, H.; Wang, Z. Meta-analysis of the prognostic value of circulating tumor cells detected with the CellSearch System in colorectal cancer. *BMC Cancer* **2015**, *15*, 202. [CrossRef]
18. Scher, H.I.; Heller, G.; Molina, A.; Attard, G.; Danila, D.C.; Jia, X.; Peng, W.; Sandhu, S.K.; Olmos, D.; Riisnaes, R.; et al. Circulating tumor cell biomarker panel as an individual-level surrogate for survival in metastatic castration-resistant prostate cancer. *J. Clin. Oncol.* **2015**, *33*, 1348–1355. [CrossRef]
19. Alama, A.; Coco, S.; Genova, C.; Rossi, G.; Fontana, V.; Tagliamento, M.; Giovanna Dal Bello, M.; Rosa, A.; Boccardo, S.; Rijavec, E.; et al. Prognostic Relevance of Circulating Tumor Cells and Circulating Cell-Free DNA Association in Metastatic Non-Small Cell Lung Cancer Treated with Nivolumab. *J. Clin. Med.* **2019**, *8*, 1011. [CrossRef]
20. Tamminga, M.; de Wit, S.; Hiltermann, T.J.N.; Timens, W.; Schuuring, E.; Terstappen, L.W.M.M.; Groen, H.J.M. Circulating tumor cells in advanced non-small cell lung cancer patients are associated with worse tumor response to checkpoint inhibitors. *J. Immunother. Cancer.* **2019**, *7*, 173. [CrossRef]
21. Monterisi, S.; Castello, A.; Toschi, L.; Federico, D.; Rossi, S.; Veronesi, G.; Lopci, E. preliminary data on circulating tumor cells in metastatic NSCLC patients candidate to immunotherapy. *Am. J. Nucl. Med. Mol. Imaging* **2019**, *9*, 282–295. [PubMed]
22. Hofman, V.; Ilie, M.I.; Long, E.; Selva, E.; Bonnetaud, C.; Molina, T.; Vénissac, N.; Mouroux, J.; Vielh, P.; Hofman, P. Detection of circulating tumor cells as a prognostic factor in patients undergoing radical surgery for non-small-cell lung carcinoma: Comparison of the efficacy of the CellSearch Assay™ and the isolation by size of epithelial tumor cell method. *Int. J. Cancer* **2011**, *129*, 1651–1660. [CrossRef] [PubMed]
23. Krebs, M.G.; Hou, J.M.; Sloane, R.; Lancashire, L.; Priest, L.; Nonaka, D.; Ward, T.H.; Backen, A.; Clack, G.; Hughes, A. Analysis of circulating tumor cells in patients with non-small cell lung cancer using epithelial marker-dependent and -independent approaches. *J. Thorac. Oncol.* **2012**, *7*, 306–315. [CrossRef]
24. Pailler, E.; Adam, J.; Barthélémy, A.; Oulhen, M.; Auger, N.; Valent, A.; Ward, T.H.; Backen, A.; Clack, G.; Hughes, A.; et al. Detection of circulating tumor cells harboring a unique ALK rearrangement in ALK-positive non-small-cell lung cancer. *J. Clin. Oncol.* **2013**, *31*, 2273–2281. [CrossRef]
25. Farace, F.; Massard, C.; Vimond, N.; Drusch, F.; Jacques, N.; Billiot, F.; Laplanche, A.; Chauchereau, A.; Lacroix, L.; Planchard, D.; et al. A direct comparison of CellSearch and ISET for circulating tumour-cell detection in patients with metastatic carcinomas. *Br. J. Cancer* **2011**, *105*, 847–853. [CrossRef] [PubMed]
26. Illie, M.; Szafer-Glusman, E.; Hofman, V.; Long-Mira, E.; Suttmann, R.; Darbonne, W.; Butori, C.; Lalvée, S.; Fayada, J.; Selva, E.; et al. Expression of MET in circulating tumor cells correlates with expression in tumor from advanced-stage lung cancer patients. *Oncotarget* **2017**, *8*, 26112–26121. [CrossRef] [PubMed]
27. Shibue, T.; Weinberg, R.A. EMT, CSCs, and drug resistance: The mechanistic link and clinical implications. *Nat. Rev. Clin. Oncol.* **2017**, *14*, 611–629. [CrossRef]
28. Lecharpentier, A.; Vielh, P.; Perez-Moreno, P.; Planchard, D.; Soria, J.C.; Farace, F. Detection of circulating tumour cells with a hybrid (epithelial/mesenchymal) phenotype in patients with metastatic non-small cell lung cancer. *Br. J. Cancer* **2011**, *105*, 1338–1341. [CrossRef]
29. Hofman, V.; Bonnetaud, C.; Ilie, M.I.; Vielh, P.; Vignaud, J.M.; Fléjou, J.F.; Lantuejoul, S.; Piaton, E.; Mourad, N.; Butori, C.; et al. Preoperative circulating tumor cell detection using the isolation by size of epithelial tumor cell method for patients with lung cancer is a new prognostic biomarker. *Clin. Cancer Res.* **2011**, *17*, 827–835. [CrossRef]
30. Zhang, Z.; Xiao, Y.; Zhao, J.; Chen, M.; Xu, Y.; Zhong, W.; Xing, J.; Wang, M. Relationship between circulating tumour cell count and prognosis following chemotherapy in patients with advanced non-small-cell lung cancer. *Respirology* **2016**, *21*, 519–525. [CrossRef]

31. Fiorelli, A.; Accardo, M.; Carelli, E.; Angioletti, D.; Santini, M.; Di Domenico, M. Circulating tumor cells in diagnosing lung cancer: Clinical and mophological analysis. *Ann. Thorac. Surg.* **2015**, *99*, 1899–1905. [CrossRef] [PubMed]
32. Nygaard, A.D.; Holdgaard, P.C.; Spindler, K.L.; Pallisgaard, N.; Jakobsen, A. The correlation between cell-free DNA and tumour burden was estimated by PET/CT in patients with advanced NSCLC. *Br. J. Cancer* **2014**, *110*, 363–368. [CrossRef] [PubMed]
33. Ilié, M.; Szafer-Glusman, E.; Hofman, V.; Chamorey, E.; Lalvée, S.; Selva, E.; Leroy, S.; Marquette, C.H.; Kowanetz, M.; Hedge, P.; et al. Detection of PD-L1 in circulating tumor cells and white blood cells from patients with advanced non-small-cell lung cancer. *Ann. Oncol.* **2018**, *29*, 193–199. [CrossRef] [PubMed]
34. de Wit, S.; van Dalum, G.; Lenferink, A.T.M.; Tibbe, A.G.J.; Hiltermann, T.J.N.; Groen, H.J.M.; van Rijn, C.J.; Terstappen, L.W. The detection of EpCAM+ and EpCAM– circulating tumor cells. *Sci. Rep.* **2015**, *5*, 12270. [CrossRef] [PubMed]
35. Muinelo-Romay, L.; Vieito, M.; Abalo, A.; Nocelo, M.A.; Barón, F.; Anido, U.; Brozos, E.; Vázquez, F.; Aguín, S.; Abal, M. Evaluation of circulating tumor cells and related events as prognostic factors and surrogate biomarkers in advanced NSCLC patients receiving first-line systemic treatment. *Cancers* **2014**, *6*, 153–165. [CrossRef] [PubMed]
36. Juan, O.; Vidal, J.; Gisbert, R.; Muñoz, J.; Maciá, S.; Gómez-Codina, J. Prognostic significance of circulating tumor cells in advanced non-small cell lung cancer patients treated with docetaxel and gemcitabine. *Clin. Transl. Oncol.* **2014**, *16*, 637–643. [CrossRef]
37. Krebs, M.G.; Sloane, R.; Priest, L.; Lancashire, L.; Hou, J.-M.J.M.; Greystoke, A.; Ward, T.H.; Ferraldeschi, R.; Hughes, A.; Clack, G.; et al. Evaluation and prognostic significance of circulating tumor cells in patients with non-small-cell lung cancer. *J. Clin. Oncol.* **2011**, *29*, 1556–1563. [CrossRef]
38. Boellaard, R.; Delgado-Bolton, R.; Oyen, W.J.; Giammarile, F.; Tatsch, K.; Eschner, W.; Verzijlbergen, F.J.; Barrington, S.F.; Pike, L.C.; Weber, W.A.; et al. FDG PET/CT: EANM procedure guidelines for tumour imaging: Version 2.0. *Eur. J. Nucl. Med. Mol. Imaging* **2015**, *42*, 328–354. [CrossRef]
39. Eisenhauer, E.; Therasse, P.; Bogaerts, J.; Schwartz, L.H.; Sargent, D.; Ford, R.; Dancey, J.; Arbuck, S.; Gwyther, S.; Mooney, M.; et al. New response evaluation criteria in solid tumours: Revised RECIST guideline (version 1.1). *Eur. J. Cancer* **2009**, *45*, 228–247. [CrossRef]
40. Young, H.; Baum, R.; Cremerius, U.; Herholz, K.; Hoekstra, O.; Lammertsma, A.A.; Pruim, J.; Price, P. Measurement of clinical and subclinical tumour response using [18F]-fluorodeoxyglucose and positron emission tomography: Review and 1999 EORTC recommendations. European Organization for Research and Treatment of Cancer (EORTC) PET Study Group. *Eur. J. Cancer* **1999**, *35*, 1773–1782. [CrossRef]

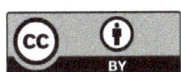 © 2020 by the authors. Licensee MDPI, Basel, Switzerland. This article is an open access article distributed under the terms and conditions of the Creative Commons Attribution (CC BY) license (http://creativecommons.org/licenses/by/4.0/).

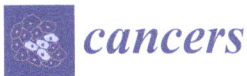

Article

PSA and PSA Kinetics Thresholds for the Presence of ^{68}Ga-PSMA-11 PET/CT-Detectable Lesions in Patients with Biochemical Recurrent Prostate Cancer

Manuela Andrea Hoffmann [1,2,*], Hans-Georg Buchholz [2], Helmut J. Wieler [3], Matthias Miederer [2], Florian Rosar [2,4], Nicolas Fischer [5], Jonas Müller-Hübenthal [6], Ludwin Trampert [7], Stefanie Pektor [2] and Mathias Schreckenberger [2]

1. Department of Occupational Health & Safety, Federal Ministry of Defense, 53123 Bonn, Germany
2. Clinic of Nuclear Medicine, Johannes Gutenberg-University, 55101 Mainz, Germany; hans-georg.buchholz@unimedizin-mainz.de (H.-G.B.); matthias.miederer@unimedizin-mainz.de (M.M.); florian.rosar@uks.eu (F.R.); stefanie.pektor@unimedizin-mainz.de (S.P.); mathias.schreckenberger@unimedizin-mainz.de (M.S.)
3. Clinic of Nuclear Medicine, Bundeswehr Central Hospital, 56072 Koblenz, Germany; helmut.wieler@web.de
4. Department of Nuclear Medicine, Saarland University Medical Center, 66421 Homburg, Germany
5. Department of Urology, Helios Kliniken Krefeld, 47805 Krefeld, Germany; simplissimus@gmx.de
6. Practice of Radiology and Nuclear Medicine, Praxis im KölnTriangle, 50679 Köln, Germany; jmh@praxis-im-koelntriangle.de
7. Clinic of Nuclear Medicine, Klinikum Mutterhaus der Borromäerinnen, 54290 Trier, Germany; ludwin.trampert@mutterhaus.de
* Correspondence: manuhoffmann@web.de

Received: 31 December 2019; Accepted: 4 February 2020; Published: 8 February 2020

Abstract: ^{68}Ga-PSMA-11 positron-emission tomography/computed tomography (PET/CT) is commonly used for restaging recurrent prostate cancer (PC) in European clinical practice. The goal of this study is to determine the optimum time for performing these PET/CT scans in a large cohort of patients by identifying the prostate-specific-antigen (PSA) and PSA kinetics thresholds for detecting and localizing recurrent PC. This retrospective analysis includes 581 patients with biochemical recurrence (BC) by definition. The performance of ^{68}Ga-PSMA-11 PET/CT in relation to the PSA value at the scan time as well as PSA kinetics was assessed by the receiver-operating-characteristic-curve (ROC) generated by plotting sensitivity versus 1-specificity. Malignant prostatic lesions were identified in 77%. For patients that were treated with radical prostatectomy (RP) a PSA value of 1.24 ng/mL was found to be the optimal cutoff level for predicting positive and negative scans, while for patients previously treated with radiotherapy (RT) it was 5.75 ng/mL. In RP-patients with PSA value <1.24 ng/mL, 52% scans were positive, whereas patients with PSA ≥1.24 ng/mL had positive scan results in 87%. RT-patients with PSA <5.75 ng/mL had positive scans in 86% and for those with PSA ≥5.75 ng/mL 94% had positive scans. This study identifies the PSA and PSA kinetics threshold levels for the presence of ^{68}Ga-PSMA-11 PET/CT-detectable PC-lesions in BC patients.

Keywords: ^{68}Gallium-PSMA PET/CT; prostate-specific-antigen; prostate cancer; PSA kinetics thresholds; biochemical recurrence; optimal cutoff level

1. Introduction

Prostate cancer (PC) is the second most common type of malignant cancers and it accounts for 55% of global cancer incidence, together with lung, stomach, and breast cancer [1]. The global incidence of PC in 2012 is 1.1 million per year and accounts for approximately 7% of deaths in men [2]. PC incidence has increased to 95–116 per 10,000 persons and the incidence of death related to PC is 2 per 10,000 per person years since the introduction of prostate-specific-antigen (PSA)-screening [3].

Most patients with BC of PC are diagnosed at an early tumor stage with local disease. The primary treatment of choice for localized PC is radical prostatectomy (RP) or radiation therapy (RT). In recent years, several alternative treatment options have been approved, especially for the therapy of aggressive PC and/or metastatic spread [4,5]. BC occurs in about 30% of the patients treated, in spite of radical therapy [5,6]. BC is defined as a PSA is > 0.2 ng/mL after radical prostatectomy (RP) or > 2 ng/mL above the nadir following radiotherapy (RT) [7]. The shorter the time between primary treatment and BC is, the greater the risk for metastatic recurrence and clinical progression will be. In comparison, the longer the timeline, the higher the association of localized recurrence [4]. In this setting, PSA and PSA kinetics (i.e., PSA doubling time (PSAdt)—"which measures the exponential increase in serum PSA over time" [8] and PSA velocity (PSAvel)—an indication of the "absolute annual increase in serum PSA (ng/mL/year)" [8]) are valuable for the forecast of recurrent PC [4,9]. However the PSA alone does not indicate the localization of malignant lesions.

Cornford et al. shows imaging guidelines and salvage therapy protocols after primary treatment [7]. In patients with presumptive cancer after initial curative treatment, diagnostic imaging is challenging in the evaluation of patients with recurrent PC and/or distant metastases. Current standard imaging techniques for restaging include transrectal ultrasonography (TRUS), ^{99m}Tc-diphosphonate bone scintigraphy, computed tomography (CT), and magnetic resonance imaging (MRI). Morphological imaging modalities, such as CT and MRI, often fail to visualize cancer lesions. Therefore, their accuracy is limited, especially for the detection of lymph node metastases (LNM). Other diagnostic methods, such as positron-emission tomography (PET) (with various tracers) or MR spectroscopy, which show metabolic activity, will be used, in order to minimize this limitation [10].

Hybrid PET/CT has been favored for several years and has been applied according to international guidelines to improve the diagnostic accuracy [8,11]. ^{68}Gallium (Ga)-prostate specific membrane antigen (PSMA) is currently one of the most successful tracers for PC imaging due to its clinical specificity [12,13]. PSMA is a transmembrane protein that is overexpressed in 95% of PC cells, especially in higher grade PC, recurrent PC and metastatic disease [14]. In benign prostate tissue, it is only weakly or not expressed. PSMA provides an optimal target for the diagnosis of PC as well as the treatment of PC [15]. Different ^{68}Ga-labelled PSMA inhibitors have been studied regarding their sensitivity and specificity to diagnose recurrence of PC such as HBED-CC, which is an efficient ^{68}Ga-chelator [13,16]. A German group has developed Glu-NH-CO-NH-Lys(Ahx)-{^{68}Ga-(N,N'-bis-[2-hydroxy-5-(carboxyethyl)benzyl]ethylen-ediamine-N,N' -diacetic acid)}(^{68}Ga-HBED-CC-PSMA or ^{68}Ga-PSMA-11), a small-molecule inhibitor for PSMA [6,16]. The HBED-CC ligand has a fast blood and organ clearance and little of the ligand is taken up into the liver. ^{68}Ga-PSMA-11 PET/CT is a favorable diagnostic tool due to its excellent contrast-to-noise ratio and the improved detection of lesions. The HBED-CC conjugated PSMA inhibitor ^{68}Ga-PSMA-11 precisely binds to PSMA-positive cells and it is more specifically internalized into PSMA expressing tumor cells and PSMA-positive metastatic lesion cells of PC [13,16,17]. In recent years, several other PSMA ligands have been developed for labelling with ^{68}Ga and ^{18}F. In particular, the ^{18}F-labelled PSMA ligands continue to be researched [6,18,19]. To date, thousands of patients have been scanned with ^{68}Ga-PSMA, while ^{18}F-PSMA has only been used in a few hundred patients.

The current research is directed toward the development of more sensitive PET molecules for detection of BC at low PSA levels to allow for a personalized treatment planning at an early stage of recurrent disease. PSA kinetics has been proposed to supplement other diagnostic modalities in patient selection, especially with low PSA [9].

The goal of this study is to determine the best time for performing ^{68}Ga-PSMA-11 PET/CT scans in patients with BC by calculating PSA and PSA kinetics thresholds for the detection and localization of recurrent PC.

2. Results

2.1. Clinical Characteristics

Table 1 summarizes the clinical and pathological characteristics of the 581 study patients. At the time of the scan, the median PSA levels were 2.98 ng/mL, range (0.2–2000). Gleason Score (GS, the grading system for determining the aggressiveness of PC) [8] was for GS ≤ 6 in 37 patients. 303 patients had GS 7 (7a + 7b), 104 patients had GS 8, and 139 patients GS > 8. 36% of the patients were treated with systemic androgen deprivation therapy (ADT). The primary treatment of most patients (493) was radical prostatectomy (85%). 88 patients (15%) were primarily treated with radiotherapy (Table 1).

Table 1. Patient characteristics.

Characteristics (n)	Parameters
Number of patients	581
Age (y) (581)	
Median	71
Range	49–88
Mean ± SD	71.3 ± 7.5
Gleason Score (581)	
≤ 6 (low risk + grade group 1)	37
7 (intermediate risk + grade group 2+3)	303
8 (high risk + grade group 4)	104
> 8 (high risk + grade group 5)	139
PSA (ng/mL) (581)	
Median	2.98
Range	0.2–2000
Mean ± SD	18.21 ± 101.91
PSAvel (ng/mL/y) (196)	
Median	1.24
Range	0–620.1
Mean ± SD	10.89 ± 54.25
PSAdt (months) (581)	
Median	10.35
Range	0–628.2
Mean ± SD	22.1 ± 48.8
Prior treatment of primary tumor (581)	
Surgery (radical prostatectomy)	493
Radiotherapy and other	88
Further treatment	
Anti-androgen therapy	209
Positivity rate	
Total/PET/CT positive patients	450/581

Abbreviations: PSA, prostate-specific-antigen; vel, velocity; dt, doubling time; SD, standard deviation; n, number of patients; y, year.

2.2. Overall Positivity Rate of ^{68}Ga-PSMA-11 PET/CT

^{68}Ga-PSMA-11 PET/CT showed a positivity rate in 450 out of 581 patients (77%) (mean PSA 18.21 ± 101.91 ng/mL). The discrimination of the PSA values between patients with a PSMA-positive scan and those with a PSMA-negative scan was statistically significant ($p < 0.001$). The mean PSA levels of patients with positive scans were significantly higher than those of patients with negative scan results (22.94 ± 115.38 ng/mL versus 1.95 ± 3.28 ng/mL, $p < 0.001$, Mann-Whitney-U test) (Table 2).

Table 2. ^{68}Ga-PSMA-11 positron-emission tomography/computed tomography (PET/CT)-11 positive and negative scan results in relation to prostate-specific-antigen (PSA).

PET/CT Results	PSA (ng/mL)		
	Mean ± SD	Median (range)	p Value
Positive (450/581)	22.94 ± 115.38	4.01 (0.2-2000)	
Negative (131/581)	1.95 ± 3.28	0.8 (0.2-25.67)	
Total	18.21 ± 101.91	2.98 (0.2-2000)	$p < 0.001$ *

* Mann-Whitney-U test. Abbreviations: PSA, prostate-specific-antigen; SD, standard deviation; $p < 0.05$ is considered significant.

This retrospective analysis includes 581 patients with a BC. We looked at the two groups of patients with different BC by definition (patient-group RP and patient-group RT) separately to ensure proper statistics and a homogeneous patient collective.

2.3. Positivity Rate of ^{68}Ga-PSMA-11 PET/CT in Detecting Clinical Recurrence Post-Prostatectomy

^{68}Ga-PSMA-11 PET/CT revealed malignant prostatic lesions in 370 of 493 patients (75%). A statistically significant demarcation in PSA values was shown ($p < 0.001$) between patients with a positive (3.20 ng/mL) and a negative (0.70 ng/mL) ^{68}Ga-PSMA-11 PET/CT scan.

The detection efficacy of ^{68}Ga-PSMA-11 PET/CT for post-prostatectomy (patient-group RP) was 40% (27) for PSA levels of 0.2 to < 0.5 ng/mL and 62% (48), 70% (61), 84% (99), 94% (135) for PSA levels of 0.5 to < 1 ng/mL, 1 to < 2 ng/mL, 2 to < 5 ng/mL, and ≥ 5 ng/mL, respectively ($p < 0.001$) (Table 3A).

Table 3A shows the sites of lesions that were detected by ^{68}Ga-PSMA-11 PET/CT scans in patient-group RP. Local recurrence was evident in 29% (109/370) of the patients with a positive scan. Out of all patients with positive scans, 85% showed metastases. 54% of these patients exhibited local metastases and 23% distant metastases. Multiple metastases were observed in 66% of these patients. Lymph node (LN) metastases (LNM) were evident in 78% of the patients, 75% of which were local, 8% distant LNM, and 18% were local and distant LNM. Bone metastases were revealed in 43% of the patients with positive ^{68}Ga-PSMA-11 PET/CT scans. Visceral metastases rarely occurred in 7% (Table 3A). Single metastases were detected in 28% of the patients ($n = 105$) with positive ^{68}Ga-PSMA-11 PET/CT results and 56% of the patients ($n = 208$) showed multiple PC metastases (Table 4).

Table 3. (**A**) Prostate cancer (PC) recurrence (patient-group radical prostatectomy (RP)) location related to different PSA values. (**B**) PC recurrence (patient-group RT) location related to different PSA values.

(A) Prostate cancer (PC) recurrence (patient-group radical prostatectomy (RP)) location related to different PSA values.						
PSA (ng/mL)	0.2–<0.5	0.5–<1.0	1.0–<2.0	2.0–<5.0	≥5.0	Chi^2, p
Number (x/493) patient-group RP	67	78	87	118	143	
PET/CT positive	27	48	61	99	135	$r = 0.413$; $p < 0.001$
Positivity rate	40.3%	61.5%	70.1%	83.9%	94.4%	
Androgen deprivation therapy	15	13	21	31	77	$r = 0.252$; $p < 0.001$
Regions:						
Local recurrence	6	14	19	29	41	$r = 0.149$; $p = 0.02$
Metastases	22	39	49	80	123	$r = 0.365$; $p < 0.001$
Site of metastases:						$r = 0.402$; $p < 0.001$
Local metastases	16	28	32	43	50	
Distant metastases	3	7	12	18	31	
Local + distant metastases	3	4	5	19	42	
Number of metastases:						$r = 0.397$; $p < 0.001$
Single metastases	14	14	23	25	29	
Multiple metastases	8	25	26	55	94	
Lymph node metastases (LNM)	19	30	38	61	97	$r = 0.266$; $p < 0.001$
Site of LNM:						$r = 0.344$; $p < 0.001$
Local LNM	18	28	34	51	52	
Distant LNM	0	0	2	4	13	
Local + distant LNM	1	2	2	6	32	
Bone metastases	8	11	12	33	72	$r = 0.315$; $p < 0.001$
Visceral metastases	1	1	2	5	12	$r = 0.128$; $p = 0.075$ *

(B) PC recurrence (patient-group RT) location related to different PSA values.			
PSA (ng/mL)	2.0–<5.0	≥5.0	Chi^2, p
Number (x/88) patient-group RT	33	55	
PET/CT positive	29	51	$r = 0.08$; $p = 0.44$
Positivity rate	87.9%	92.7%	
Androgen deprivation therapy	11	41	$r = 0.406$; $p = 0.001$
Regions:			
Local recurrence	21	29	$r = -0.107$; $p = 0.317$
Metastases	14	37	$r = 0.244$; $p = 0.022$
Site of metastases:			$r = 0.306$; $p = 0.011$
Local metastases	10	12	
Distant metastases	1	13	
Local + distant metastases	3	12	
Number of metastases:			$r = 0.289$; $p = 0.022$

Table 3. Cont.

Single metastases	6	7	
Multiple metastases	8	30	
Lymph node metastases (LNM)	12	23	$r = 0.054$; n.s.
Site of LNM:			$r = 0.076$; n.s.
Local LNM	9	17	
Distant LNM	2	1	
Local + distant LNM	1	5	
Bone metastases	5	22	$r = -0.261$; $p = 0.014$
Visceral metastases	2	1	$r = -0.113$; n.s.

* Fisher exact test. Abbreviations: PSA, prostate-specific-antigen; LNM, lymph node metastases; $p < 0.05$ is considered significant; r, Pearson correlation coefficient.

Table 4. Tumor location and positivity rate of detected lesions.

Tumor Location	n (493)	% (370)	n (88)	% (80)
PET/CT positive patients	370		80	
Local recurrence	109	29.5%	50	62.5%
Metastases	313	84.6%	51	63.8%
local	169	45.7%	22	27.5%
distant	71	19.2%	14	17.5%
local and distant	73	19.7%	15	18.8%
single	105	28.4%	13	16.3%
multiple	208	56.2%	38	47.5%
Lymph node metastases	245	66.2%	35	43.8%
Local/regional	183	49.6%	26	32.5%
Distant	19	5.1%	3	3.8%
Local and distant	43	11.6%	6	7.5%
Bone metastases	136	36.8%	27	33.8%
Visceral metastases (lung, liver, adrenals, soft tissue, spleen, thyroid)	21	5.7%	3	7.5%

Abbreviation: n, number of patients.

2.4. Positivity Rate of ^{68}Ga-PSMA-11 PET/CT in Detecting Clinical Recurrence Post-Radiotherapy

Overall, 80 of 88 patients had a positive ^{68}Ga-PSMA-11 PET/CT scan (91%). The discrimination in PSA values between the patients with a positive (7.15 ng/mL) and a negative (5.25 ng/mL) scan was not statistically significant ($p = 0.384$).

For patients that were treated with RT, the detection efficacy of ^{68}Ga-PSMA-11 PET/CT was 88% (29) for PSA levels of 2 to < 5 ng/mL and 93% (51) for PSA levels of ≥ 5 ng/mL, respectively ($p = 0.44$) (Table 3B).

Table 3B shows the sites of lesions that were detected by ^{68}Ga-PSMA-11 PET/CT scans in patient-group RT. In 63% (50/80) of the patients with a positive scan, local recurrence was detected. Of the positive scans, 64% showed metastases and 43% of these patients exhibited local metastases, whereas 27% showed at least one distant finding (extra pelvic LN and/or bone and/or visceral metastases). Multiple metastases were demonstrated in 75% of these patients. A total of 69% of the patients showed LNM (74% of them local, 9% distant, and 17% local and distant LNM). Bone metastases were revealed in 34% of the patients with positive ^{68}Ga-PSMA-11 PET/CT scans. Visceral metastases were detected in only 4% of the positive scans (Table 3B). Multimetastatic disease was shown in 48% of the PSMA-positive patients ($n = 38$), whereas in 16% of the patients ($n = 13$) single PC metastases were detected (Table 4).

2.5. PSA and PSA Kinetics Threshold Levels

The performance of ^{68}Ga-PSMA-11 PET/CT in relation to the PSA value at the time of the scans, as well as PSA kinetics, were assessed by receiver-operating-characteristic-curve (ROC) generated by plotting sensitivity versus 1-specificity. A PSA value of 1.24 ng/mL was found to be the optimal cutoff level for predicting positive and negative scans by means of ROC analysis (AUC = 0.788; 95% CI 0.746–0.831) in all the patients primarily treated with RP and with RT (the cohort of 581 patients).

2.6. PSA and PSA Kinetics Threshold Levels Post-Prostatectomy

The optimal cutoff level was also 1.24 ng/mL for patients that were treated with radical prostatectomy (370/493 patient-group RP) (AUC = 0.784; 95% CI 0.740–0.828) (Figure 1).

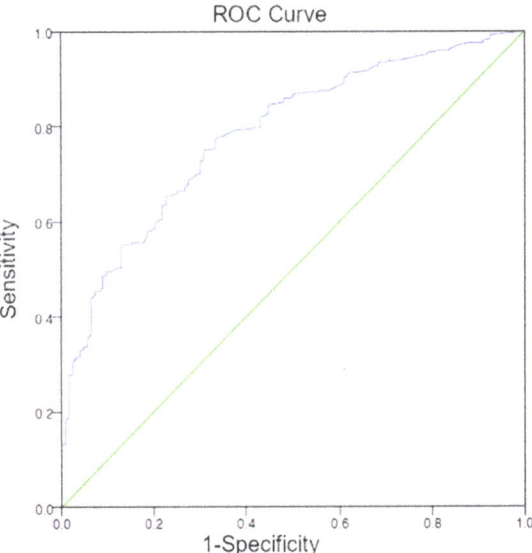

Figure 1. Receiver-operating-characteristic-curve (ROC) curve for PSA (patient-group RP) with an optimal cutoff level of 1.24 ng/mL.

In patients with a PSA value <1.24 ng/mL, 52% (92/177) ^{68}Ga-PSMA-11 PET/CT scans were positive, whereas patients with a PSA ≥1.24 ng/mL exhibited positive scan results in 87% (278/316) ($p < 0.001$). Local recurrence in the prostate bed was noted in 13% vs. 27% of the patients with PSA levels below and above the cutoff. Multimetastatic disease was determined in 21% of the patients with PSA values that were below cutoff level vs. 79% of patients with PSA above cutoff ($p < 0.001$, r 0.315) (Table 5A). The local and distant metastases were determined in 6% (11/177) of patients with PSA values below the cutoff level vs. 20% (62/316) of patients with PSA above cutoff ($p < 0.001$) (Table 5A). Local metastases were detected in 51 patients (29%) below and in 118 patients (37%) above cutoff PSA values ($p < 0.001$). Distant lesions were identified in 9% below vs. 18% above cutoff levels, respectively ($p < 0.001$; Table 5A). As compared to patients with PSA values that were below the optimal cutoff level, patients with PSA levels ≥ 1.24 more frequently exhibited LNM (25% vs. 75%, $p < 0.001$, r 0.228) and bone metastases (18% vs. 82%, $p < 0.001$, r 0.235).

Table 5. (**A**) ^{68}Ga-PSMA-11 PET/CT positivity rate (RP) of different subgroups related to PSA levels. (**B**) 68Ga-PSMA-11 PET/CT positivity rate (RT) of different subgroups that were related to PSA levels.

(A) ^{68}Ga-PSMA-11 PET/CT positivity rate (RP) of different subgroups related to PSA levels.						
PSA Range (ng/mL)	Overall Positivity	p/r Value	Single Metastases	Multiple Metastases		p/r Value
0.2 to <1 (145)	75 (51.7%)		28 (19.3%)	33 (22.8%)		
<1.24 (177)	92 (52%)		33 (31%)	44 (21%)		
≥1.24 (316)	278 (87.4%)		72 (69%)	164 (79%)		
Total (493)	370 (75%)	$p < 0.001$: r 0.400	105	208		$p < 0.001$: r 0.315
PSA Range (ng/mL)	Local Recur-Rence	p/r Value	Local Metastases	Distant Metastases	Local + Distant Metastases	p/r Value
0.2 to <1 (145)	20 (13.8%)		44 (30.3%)	10 (6.9%)	7 (4.8%)	
<1.24 (177)	23 (13%)		51 (28.8%)	15 (8.5%)	11 (6.2%)	
≥1.24 (316)	86 (27.2%)		118 (37.3%)	56 (17.7%)	62 (19.6%)	
Total (493)	109	$p < 0.001$; r 0.164	169	71	73	$p < 0.001$; r 0.308
(B) ^{68}Ga-PSMA-11 PET/CT positivity rate (RT) of different subgroups that were related to PSA levels.						
PSA Range (ng/mL)	Overall Positivity	p/r Value	Single Metastases	Multiple Metastases		p/r Value
<5.75 (36)	31 (86.1%)		15 (41.7%)	19 (52.8%)		
≥5.75 (52)	49 (94.2%)		7 (13.5%)	29 (55.8%)		
Total (88)	80 (91%)	$p = 0.19$; r 0.139	22	48		$p = 0.008$; r 0.255
PSA Range (ng/mL)	Local Recur-Rence	p/r Value	Local Metastases	Distant Metastases	Local + Distant Metastases	p/r Value
<5.75 (36)	22 (61.1%)		11 (30.6%)	1 (2.8%)	4 (11.1%)	
≥5.75 (52)	28 (53.8%)		11 (21.2%)	13 (25%)	11 (21.2%)	
Total (88)	50	$p = 0.5$; r −0.07	22	14	15	$p = 0.01$; r 0.286

Abbreviations: PSA, prostate-specific-antigen; $p < 0.05$ is considered significant; r, Pearson correlation coefficient.

The optimal PSAvel threshold from ROC analysis for the detection of recurrent PC-lesions (patient-group RP) was 1.32 ng/mL/year (AUC = 0.777; 95% CI 0.709–0.845) (Figure 2), which showed significant differences between the PET-positive and PET-negative scans ($p < 0.001$).

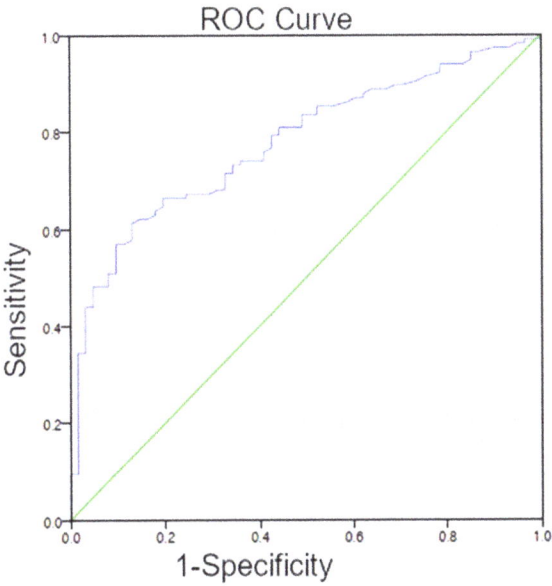

Figure 2. ROC curve for PSAvel (patient-group RP) with an optimal cutoff level of 1.32 ng/mL/year.

The ROC curve analysis showed that PSAdt was not useful in distinguishing between patients with positive and negative ^{68}Ga-PSMA-11 PET/CT scan results with an AUC of 0.450.

2.7. PSA and PSA Kinetics Threshold Levels Post-Radiotherapy

The optimal cutoff level for patients that were previously been treated with RT (80/88 patient-group RT) was 5.75 ng/mL (AUC = 0.594; 95% CI 0.400–0.788) (Figure 3). In patients with a PSA value <5.75 ng/mL, 86% (31/36) ^{68}Ga-PSMA-11 PET/CT scans were positive, whereas patients with a PSA ≥5.75 ng/mL exhibited positive scan results in 94% (49/52) ($p = 0.19$, r 0.139). Local recurrence in the prostate appeared in 61% vs. 54% of the patients with PSA levels that were below and above cutoff, respectively. Multimetastatic disease was determined in 53% of the patients with PSA values that were below cutoff level vs. 56% of patients with PSA above cutoff ($p = 0.008$, r 0.255) (Table 5B). Local and distant metastases were found in 11% (4/36) of patients with PSA values below cutoff level vs. 21% (11/52) of patients with PSA above cutoff ($p = 0.01$, r 0.286) (Table 5B). Patients with PSA levels ≥ 5.75 more frequently exhibited LNM (33% vs. 41%, $p = 0.393$, r 0.076) and bone metastases (26% vs. 41%, $p = 0.089$, r 0.152) as compared to patients with PSA values below the optimal cutoff level.

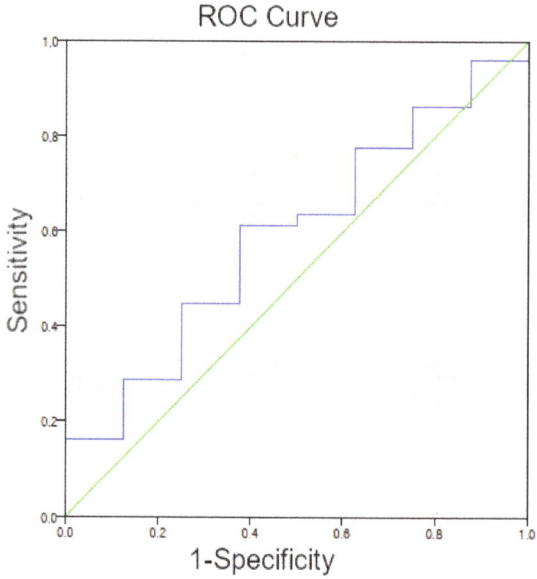

Figure 3. ROC curve for PSA (patient-group RT) with an optimal cutoff level of.5.75 ng/mL.

An optimal PSAvel threshold from ROC analysis for the detection of recurrent PC-lesions (patient-group RT) could not be ascertained, since only 19 patient data sets were available for the calculation of the value, of which a positive scan result was obtained in 18 patients.

ROC curve analysis revealed a PSAdt threshold of 10.6 months (AUC = 0.600; 95% CI 0.366–0.834) to distinguish patients with positive and negative ^{68}Ga-PSMA-11 PET/CT, but without significance ($p = 0.353$).

2.8. Maximum Standardized Uptake Value (SUV_{max})

As evidenced by the Kolmogorov-Smirnov-Test, the SUV_{max} of the detected sites of malignant lesions were not normally distributed. SUV_{max} was the highest in bone metastases (mean and standard deviation/SD: 22.14 ± 22.98, median: 15) and lowest in lung metastases (mean and SD: 9.84 ± 9.31, median: 6). SUV_{max} of LNM and visceral metastases showed values in between.

2.9. GS

4% of patients with a positive ^{68}Ga-PSMA-11 PET/CT scan were categorized as being low risk PC (International Society of Urological Pathology (ISUP) grade 1; GS < 7), whereas 12% of PSMA-positive patients were categorized GS 7a (ISUP grade 2; intermediate risk), 35% GS 7b (ISUP grade 3; intermediate risk), 22% GS 8 (ISUP grade 4; high risk), and 26% GS > 8 (ISUP grade 5; high risk) [8] (Table 6). High risk (GS 8, GS > 8) as compared to low risk patients (GS < 7) showed a high frequency of positive scan results ($p < 0.001$) and metastases (52% vs. 2%) ($p < 0.001$). When considering local recurrence, the results are similar, but not statistically significant. With regard to the subgroups (GS 7a vs. GS 7b), there is an important distinction between patients with intermediate risk and grade group 2 (GS 7a also called 7 (3 + 4)) (10%) when compared to patients with intermediate risk and grade group 3 (GS 7b also called 7 (4 + 3)) (36%) for PSMA-positive metastases ($p < 0.001$) (Table 6).

Table 6. Gleason Score in relation to ^{68}Ga-PSMA-11 PET/CT-11 positive scan results.

$n = 581$	GS < 7 (37)	GS 7a (97)	GS 7b (204)	GS 8(104)	GS > 8(139)	Chi^2 r, p Value
PET/CT positive (450/581)	16	52	158	97	117	0.288; $p < 0.001$
Local recurrence (159/581)	9	24	56	32	38	0.027; n.s.
Metastases (364/581)	8	36	132	83	105	0.324; $p < 0.001$

Abbreviations: GS, Gleason Score; n, number of patients; $p < 0.05$ is considered significant; r, Pearson correlation coefficient.

2.10. ADT

ADT was significantly associated with increased probability of a positive ^{68}Ga-PSMA-11 PET/CT scan ($p < 0.001$). 37% of PSMA PET/CT-positive and 18% of PSMA PET/CT-negative patients were treated with ADT ($p < 0.001$, r 0.173) in the patient-group RP. For the patient-group RT, 59% of the patients with a positive PSMA scan and 63% with a negative scan were treated with androgens ($p = 0.837$, $r = ™0.022$).

2.11. Alkaline Phosphatase (AP)

AP has been described as an efficient and functional biomarker for the prognosis of PC (43). We wanted to verify whether AP is a predictor for bone involvement of PC. In our study, AP levels of patients with positive ^{68}Ga-PSMA-11 PET/CT scan results were higher than those of patients with negative scans (93 ± 53 IU/L vs. 74 ± 24 IU/L, $p < 0.001$, Mann-Whitney-U test). Patients exhibiting bone metastases showed higher AP than patients without bone metastases (108 ± 70 IU/L vs. 76 ± 23 IU/L; $p < 0.001$).

2.12. Subpopulation

EAU guidelines suggest PSMA PET/CT for restaging PC in the case of patients that were treated with RP, if the PSA level is > 0.2 ng/mL and if the results would influence subsequent treatment decisions [8]. In the event that PSMA PET/CT is not available and the PSA level is ≥ 1 ng/mL, PET/CT with other tracers (Fluciclovine or Choline) has been suggested, if the results could influence subsequent treatment decisions [8]. For PSA recurrence after RT, EAU guidelines recommend performing PSMA PET/CT (if available) or fluciclovine PET/CT or choline PET/CT in patients that qualified for curative salvage treatment [8]. Therefore, we analyzed the PSA range from 0.2 ng/mL to < 1 ng/mL for post-prostatectomy patients. We did not form a separate subgroup for the irradiated patients, as no PSA threshold was stated in the EAU guidelines with regard to them.

All of the prostatectomized patients, 29% (145/493) exhibited PSA levels between 0.2 and < 1 ng/mL and 52% of these patients showed positive PET/CT scans (positive: 0.2 to < 0.5 ng/mL 40% and 0.5 to < 1 ng/mL 62%; $p < 0.001$, r 0.413) (Table 3A). In this subpopulation (overall positivity rate in scans and PSA levels between 0.2 ng/mL and < 1 ng/mL), ^{68}Ga-PSMA-11 PET/CT showed the presence of local recurrence in the prostate bed in 27% (20 of 75), of local metastases in 59% (44 of 75), of distant metastases in 13% (10 of 75), and of local and distant metastases in 9% (7 of 75). Multimetastatic carcinoma was detected in 44% (33 of 75) (Table 3A). The absolute PSA value at the time of the ^{68}Ga-PSMA-11 scan was associated with an increased probability of a positive scan result ($p < 0.001$).

3. Discussion

We evaluated ^{68}Ga-PSMA-11 PET/CT scans in 581 BC patients after primary curative PC therapy (RP as well as RT) in this retrospective study. A high positivity rate of 77% (450/581 patients) for the detection of malignant prostatic lesions was shown (Figure 4A,B)). Our data reflects the positive results of several other studies and confirms that ^{68}Ga-PSMA-11 PET/CT is a promising method for diagnosing PC [12,20–24]. For restaging prostatectomized BC patients by PSMA PET/CT, the EAU guidelines recommend a PSA level of > 0.2 ng/mL [8]. Patients with low cancer burdens have the best chance of a salvage RT to be curative. For this reason, imaging with subsequent therapy planning at an early stage of recurrent disease makes sense, from the point at which carcinoma foci are detectable, even with low PSA [25]. The EAU guidelines report that salvage RT in BC patients after RP was correlated with a tripling in PC-specific survival when compared to the patients who did not get salvage therapy [8]. The purpose of our study was to determine the best time for performing ^{68}Ga-PSMA-11 PET/CT scans in BC patients. For that reason, we calculated the PSA and PSA kinetics thresholds for the detection and localization of recurrent PC. The PSA levels and PSA kinetics were assessed by ROC generated by plotting sensitivity versus 1-specificity.

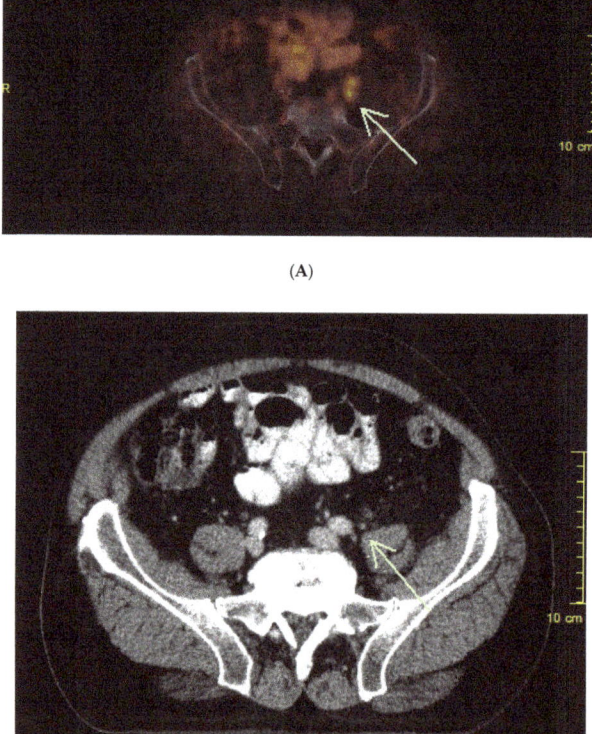

Figure 4. (**A**) History of a patient with prostate cancer followed by radical prostatectomy and lymphadenectomy (pT3, pN0, cM0, G3) in 2012. PSA doubles within three months. ^{68}Ga-PSMA-11 PET/CT scan shows two lymph node metastases with high prostate specific membrane antigen (PSMA)-avidity. (**B**) The two small lymph node metastases are detectable on CT alone, but not suspect of malignancy.

3.1. Overall Positivity Rate

The positivity rate of ^{68}Ga-PSMA-11 PET/CT of the present study was 77% over all patients (mean PSA 22.94 ± 115.38 ng/mL), thereby confirming the results of previous studies where detection rates of 74% to 83% were reported for restaging PET/CT [6,12,26]. There was a statistically significant ability to discriminate PSA values between PSMA-positive and PSMA-negative scans ($p < 0.001$). The overall patient group was divided into the group of patients who were primarily treated with prostatectomy (patient-group RP) and the group of patients who were primarily treated with RT (patient-group RT) to ensure clean statistics.

3.2. Positivity Rate (RP)

In the group of prostatectomized patients, the positivity rate was 75% (370/493 patients) (see Table 3A). Therefore, a clinically relevant percentage of patients with low PSA levels (< 0.5 ng/mL) could be diagnosed with the recurrence of PC, being comparable to the results of other studies [6,12,23,26]. In recent studies of restaging by ^{68}Ga-PSMA PET/CT, the detection rate was 50% at PSA levels of 0.2 to 0.49 ng/mL [6] and, in another study, 57.9% of the patients were ^{68}Ga-PSMA PET/CT-positive at PSA levels from 0.2 to < 0.5 ng/mL [20]. The results from the present study emphasize that ^{68}Ga-PSMA PET/CT is a sensitive tool for restaging PC, even at low PSA values [23]. After early salvage RT (PSA ≤ 0.5 ng/mL), an undetectable PSA level can be reached in 60% of the patients, being associated with a chance of 80% for a progression free five-year survival. This is indicated as second line therapy with curative intent [8,25]. Salvage RT is usually indicated after a persistent increase in PSA after RP, when systemic metastases are not found during staging imaging. If conventional imaging does not show any malignant foci (local and/or distant metastases), only the prostate bed is typically irradiated by Radiation Oncologists. Eiber et al. described that the detection of malignant lesions by PET was extremely important for the final diagnosis in over 50%. They showed lesions that were not detected by computed tomography (CT) [20,23]. Another study demonstrated that, in patients with BC after RP while using the standard procedure, nearly 20% of ^{68}Ga-PSMA PET/CT-positive lesions—suspicious of malignancy—would not have been included in the radiation field. All of these patients belonged to the crucial collective with PSA of < 1 ng/mL. ^{68}Ga-PSMA-11 PET/CT hybrid imaging opens up the possibility of changing the therapy [23,27]. Based on the data, both radiation therapists and urologists should have a more accurate road map for directing therapy. In the end, the radiation therapist should point where to direct his device. If a LN is resectable, a urologist might also resect it.

In comparison to other radiopharmaceuticals (e. g. ^{11}C- and ^{18}F-choline), detection rates of ^{68}Ga-PSMA at low PSA levels were higher [28,29]. PSA levels and ^{11}C-choline scans with positive results were linearly correlated [30–32]. The positivity rate of ^{11}C-choline scans for restaging was 73% at PSA levels of ≥ 3 ng/mL, but at PSA < 1 ng/mL the rate decreased dramatically to 19–36% [4,28]. However, a recent study showed that the second-generation of labelling of PSMA tracers with ^{18}F (e.g., ^{18}F-DCFPyL-PSMA) was superior to ^{68}Ga-PSMA for restaging at PSA levels of 0.5 to 3.5 µg/L with a sensitivity of 88% (15 of 17 patients) vs. 66% (23 of 35 patients). But at PSA values < 0.5 and > 3.5 µg/L, the sensitivity of both methods was comparable. Nevertheless, in 36% of the patients with positive scans, additional lesions were found, while using ^{18}F-PSMA vs. ^{68}Ga-PSMA [18]. Overall, the results of both methods were demonstrated to be similar [18]; this was also shown in a recent study, which compared ^{68}Ga-PSMA-11 and ^{18}F-PSMA-1007 in the case of staging PC [33].

3.3. Positivity Rate (RT)

The positivity rate of RT patients was 91%, but no statistically significant differences could be shown in the distinction of PSA levels between patients with positive and negative scans ($p = 0.384$) (see Table 3B). The EAU Guidelines recommend that PSMA PET/CT can be crucial for PC detection in the setting of BC after RT. However, they suggest that further studies be conducted [8].

3.4. PSA and PSA Kinetics Threshold Levels

We assessed the performance of ^{68}Ga-PSMA-11 PET/CT regarding pre-scan PSA levels by ROC curve separating the two patient-groups RP and RT. Based on the results of previous studies [4,9], which emphasized the importance of PSA kinetics for patient selection and detection, we also calculated PSAvel and PSAdt (see introduction), as they are valuable parameters for the prediction of clinical progression. However, it should also be borne in mind that there are non-PSA-producing tumor masses in metastatic and fully treated PCs.

3.5. PSA and PSA Kinetics Threshold Levels (RP)

In our study, a PSA of 1.24 ng/mL was the optimal cutoff level for distinguishing between positive and negative ^{68}Ga-PSMA-11 PET/CT scans. ^{68}Ga-PSMA-11 PET/CT showed the presence of multimetastatic PC in 21% of the positive lesions in patients with PSA levels below the cutoff value and in 79% in patients with PSA above the cutoff (Table 5A). Thus, we conclude that the cutoff by hybrid imaging with ^{68}Ga-PSMA-11 can be used for patient selection for restaging and also fits well into clinical practice. If you convert 1.24 ng/mL to tumor mass, it might be a small LNM or tissue volume of less than one cubic milliliter.

Significant differences between PET-positive and PET-negative patients were calculated with corresponding optimal PSAvel threshold of 1.32 ng/mL/year ($p < 0.001$). Similarly to other studies, our data show higher positivity rates corresponding to a higher PSAvel, which was also seen in studies with ^{18}F-choline. Like other authors, we propose that in addition to the PSA level, PSAvel could be taken into account in patient selection [9,20,32,34]. On the other hand, a recent study, which assessed a large cohort of patients, did not show significant correlation between ^{68}Ga-PSMA-11 PET/CT positivity and PSAvel [35].

In this study, PSAdt was not significantly associated with ^{68}Ga-PSMA-11 PET/CT positivity. For distinguishing between the positive and negative PSMA-PET findings, no optimal PSAdt cutoff could be determined by ROC analysis (AUC = 0.450). The value of PSA in patient selection is controversial [9]. Verburg et al. recommended combining serum PSA with PSAdt in order to achieve the best PSMA-positive scan result or the detection of distant LNM; in which they emphasized the importance of PSA over that of PSAdt [26]. Ceci et al. demonstrated PSAdt as a valuable predictor of positive ^{68}Ga-PSMA PET/CT scans and pointed out that patients with a short PSAdt and low PSA values showed positive PSMA scans in 85% [36]. Corresponding to the EAU guidelines, these patients were ideal candidates for salvage RT, as salvage RT has been described to be mostly efficient in patients with short PSAdt [8,36]. In contrast, in the same study, 18.7% of patients had low PSA values, but long PSAdt, and also showed positive PSMA-PET/CT findings [36].

3.6. PSA and PSA Kinetics Threshold Levels (RT)

In our study, we calculated an optimal PSA cutoff level from ROC curve of 5.75 ng/mL (Table 5B). We were not able to determine an optimal PSAvel threshold for the irradiated patient-group based on the available data. ROC analysis revealed a PSAdt cutoff of 10.6 months for the identification of RT patients with positive and negative scans, which did not find significance ($p = 0.353$).

At the present time, our cutoff results cannot be compared with the results of other studies in terms of thresholds, since they consider both (the prostatectomized and the irradiated patients) in one common patient group. Otherwise, only the RP-group is analyzed. Radiation groups are rarely examined alone for calculating cutoff levels.

3.7. Subpopulations

The performance of ^{68}Ga-PSMA-11 PET/CT has to be appraised for a therapeutic approach. In particular, the detection of local LNM should be considered, which could lead to a changed therapeutic approach (salvage RP plus LNM dissection or salvage RT with extended radiation field).

We took a closer look at PSA range between 0.2 ng/mL to < 1 ng/mL for post-prostatectomized patients based on the EAU guidelines for performing PSMA PET/CT in different initial situations [8]. The guidelines do not specify a threshold after primary radiation, so we have not formed a subgroup for these patients [8]. In the RP-group, 29% of patients showed PSA values that were between 0.2 and < 1 ng/mL with a PSMA-positivity rate of 52%. There was a significant association between the pre-scan PSA and an increased likelihood of a positive PSMA-scan was proven ($p < 0.001$). In comparison, Eiber et al. demonstrated positive scans in 57.9% for PSA values of 0.2 to < 0.5 ng/mL and even 72.7% at 0.5 to < 1 ng/mL [20]. A published study by Graziani et al. showed that only about 45% of the scans were positive while using hybrid imaging with ^{11}C-choline PET/CT in patients, even with PSA levels between 1 and 2 ng/mL. Multimetastatic disease was detected in 38% of all scans and distant lesions in 19% of the patients with PSA levels between 1–2 ng/mL [37]. In the present study, ^{68}Ga-PSMA-11 PET/CT revealed local metastases in 59%, multimetastatic disease in 44%, and distant lesions were shown in 13% of the subpopulation patients. A clinically relevant number of patients can be selected for salvage therapy due to the effectiveness of ^{68}Ga-PSMA-11 PET/CT for the detection of metastases, which is apparently higher than that of ^{11}C-choline, possibly even for metastatic-directed treatment, which might justify salvage LN dissection rather than systemic therapeutic path, thereby help to avoid unnecessary procedures and complications and also improve the chance of a clinical recurrence-free survival [38,39].

3.8. GS

Histopathological GS was significantly associated with positive ^{68}Ga-PSMA-11 PET/CT results ($p < 0.001$). Patients with GS of 7b (intermediate risk and grade group 3) and > 7 (high risk and grade group 4 or 5) showed an increased incidence of positive ^{68}Ga-PSMA-11 PET/CT scans ($p < 0.001$). Between patients with PSMA-positive scans corresponding to GS 7a (intermediate risk and grade group 2) and PSMA-positive scans corresponding to GS 7b, there was a significant demarcation ($p < 0.001$). Regarding the clinically important, highly significant differentiation between GS 7a (3 + 4) and 7b (4 + 3), patients with GS 7b exhibited more frequent pathologic ^{68}Ga-PSMA-11 PET/CT scans and metastases [8,40]. Therefore, the findings of hybrid imaging with ^{68}Ga-PSMA-11 agree in many cases with higher risk relapses on the basis of histology (frequency and detection of metastases). Our results are in line with other studies, which could possibly be due to the fact that the PSMA expression is usually more intense in higher-grade GS lesions than in lesions with a lower-grade GS [8,12,23,41]. Our results correspond to the immunohistochemical results of PSMA expression in PC [20].

3.9. ADT

The positivity rate of ^{68}Ga-PSMA-11 PET/CT was significantly correlated with accompanying ADT in this study. This is in line with the results of a study, in which the ADT-treated patients revealed positive PET/CT results more often and that was believed to be due to the frequent use of ADT in patients with advanced disease [20]. The same phenomenon has also been described when using ^{11}C-choline [37]. Furthermore, there have been reports of higher PSMA-expression of PC tumor cells as part of ADT [42]. Overall, the scientific knowledge on this issue remains unclear and further studies are needed [12,20].

3.10. AP

In our study, patients with PSMA-positive lesions showed higher AP levels than patients with negative PSMA scans ($p < 0.001$). Additionally, the detection of bone metastases was significantly associated with high AP. Our results corroborate the findings of other studies where serum AP was found to be a predictor for bone involvement of PC and to be an efficient and reliable biomarker for the prognosis of PC [43]. The AP levels were higher in patients with positive ^{68}Ga-PSMA-11 PET/CT scan results, with higher PSA levels, in patients receiving ADT and in patients exhibiting bone metastases in our study. Li et al. suggest that high AP is significantly related to poor overall survival and poor progression-free survival in PC, but there is no apparent association to cancer specific survival [43]. Skeletal AP is prognostic for bone metastases for M-staging of PC, and it is a dependable marker of osteoblastic activity. Another study demonstrated that AP levels were more closely associated with pathological bone scans than with PSA values and that the amount of AP was positively related to bone metastases [44]. From this, we conclude that the term "bone-specific AP" can reasonably be used.

4. Materials and Methods

4.1. Patient Characteristics

581 BC patients that had previously been treated with RP or RT, underwent ^{68}Ga-PSMA-11 (Glu-urea-Lys(Ahx)-HBED-CC) PET/CT between 2015 and 2019 and were retrospectively evaluated. The inclusion criteria for the performance of a ^{68}Ga-PSMA-11 PET/CT scan were: (a) histopathologically proven primary PC; (b) treatment with RP or RT (with or without ADT); and, (c) proven BC by definition (BC is defined as an elevation of the PSA value after primary treatment to > 0.2 ng/mL after RP or > 2 ng/mL above nadir following RT). The data on some of the patients included were already considered in another study with different aim. The PSA levels were available at the time of surgery as well as nadir, interim, and PET/CT scans (BC). Mean relapse PSA levels were 18.21 ng/mL ± 101.91 ng/mL (median 2.98, range 0.2–2000). 209 patients were treated with anti-androgens (Table 1). The patient data were collected from four Nuclear Medicine Institutions (a–d) in Germany. We have classified the patients into the following groups: (1) To obtain a clean statistic, we looked at the patient-group after RP and the patient group after RT separately, as, by definition, they have a different BC. (2) The subgroup of RP-patients was divided into five groups: 0.2 to < 0.5 ng/mL, 0.5 to < 1 ng/mL, 1 to < 2 ng/mL, 2 to < 5 ng/mL, and 5 ng/mL, and above. (3) The RT-patients were divided into two groups: 2 to < 5 ng/mL and 5 ng/mL and above. Additionally, patients were assigned to five-tiered GS groups: < 7, 7a and 7b, 8 and > 8, respectively. The following parameters were evaluated: ^{68}Ga-PSMA PET/CT scan results, PSA values, PSA kinetics, SUV_{max} of the malignant lesions, GS, ADT, AP and local/distant/single/multiple metastases, regional and/or distant LNM, bone metastases, and visceral metastases (e.g., lung). The main limitation of this retrospective study as compared to many other retrospective studies is that most of the patients did not have histopathological confirmation of the lesions. As a result, we use the term positivity rate instead of detection rate in this study. In addition to the histopathological findings (when available), we used a significant increase in PSA or a decrease in PSA after subsequent therapy (e.g. salvage RT) or a confirmation of the pathological focus in follow-up imaging or an increase and/or enlargement of the lesions in follow-up imaging, as indicators. We evaluated the optimal cutoff level by calculating PSA and PSA kinetics thresholds while using the ROC curve to determine the best time to perform ^{68}Ga-PSMA-11 PET/CT scans in patients with BC. The present study was in accordance with the Helsinki Declaration and the German Medicinal Products Act, AMG §13.2b. The retrospective study was conducted in accordance with the Declaration of Helsinki, and the Ethics Committee of Laek Rlp (2018-13390, approval date: 29 October 2018) and Aek No (41/2019, approval date: 22 February 2019) approved the protocol. All of the patients gave their written informed consent for the examination and for inclusion in the study.

4.2. Radiopharmaceuticals

The ^{68}Ga-labelled PSMA ligand, Glu-urea-Lys(Ahx)-HBED-CC (^{68}Ga-PSMA-11), was synthesized while using modification of a method described in 2012 [16]. In short, ^{68}Ga was achieved from a ^{68}Ge/^{68}Ga radionuclide generator (Garching, Germany) to be used to label the PSMA ligand. The labelled tracer without carrier additive was cleaned using a reverse phase cartridge (Sep-Pak C18 Plus Light cartridge, 130 mg Sorbent; Waters) and formulated in 10 mL phosphate-buffered saline with 5% by volume ETOH. Confirmation by radio thin-layer chromatography (TLC) and high-performance liquid chromatography (HPLC) was able to show a radiochemical purification yield of over 98%. ^{68}Ga-PSMA-11 was obtained from the Clinic of Nuclear Medicine of the Medical Center of the University Johannes Gutenberg (Mainz, Germany; b, c), from Advanced Accelerator Applications (Bonn, Germany; b, c), from Eckert & Ziegler (Bonn, Germany; d) or was produced in house (Mainz, Germany; a), depending on the availability.

4.3. Imaging Protocol

Each patient received an intravenous injection of ^{68}Ga-PSMA-11 (mean and SD: 199 ± 61 MBq, median activity: 200 MBq, range: 50–390 MBq). The PET data of tracer distribution were acquired 60 ± 10 min. (whole body) after injection of ^{68}Ga-PSMA-11. The patients were imaged on a PET/CT scanner named Gemini TF16 (Philips Medical Systems, Best, The Netherlands) (a, c) or a PET/CT scanner, named Biograph 64/Z64, R4 (HD and time of flight)/Biograph 64 TruePoint (True V HD; Siemens, Erlangen, Germany) (b, d). Either a mid-inspiratory low-dose CT scan (120 kV, 20–60 mAs, CT transverse scan field 50 cm, 70 cm extended field of view, high contrast resolution 1.0 s, 0.6 mm) without contrast enhancement or a maximum inspiratory venous-phase diagnostic contrast enhanced (Ultravist 300; Bayer AG, Berlin, Germany) CT scan (140 kV, 100–400 mAs, dose modulation) from the head to the upper-thigh was used for anatomical correlation and for attenuation corrections. PET was performed while using a standard technique on a dedicated three-dimensional (3D) system (a, c: matrix 144 × 144; d: 400 × 400; b: 168 × 168), with an acquisition time of 3 min. per bed position (axial field of view d: 13.3 cm; b: 21.8 cm; c: 19 cm; a: 18 cm). Random, scatter, and decay correction were applied to the emission data. Ordered-subsets expectation maximization method (OSEM) (a: three iterations, 33 subsets, Gaussian filtering, 4.3 mm full-width at half-maximum; b, c: two iterations, 14 subsets, Gaussian filtering, 5 mm (c) or 4.2 mm (b) transaxial resolution, full-width at half-maximum; d: three iterations, 24 subsets, Gaussian filtering, 5 mm transaxial resolution, full-width at half-maximum) was used for PET image reconstruction. The CT data were converted to attenuation coefficients at 511 keV and applied for attenuation corrections of the PET images.

4.4. Imaging Analysis

The PET/CT images were first visually assessed by individual specialists (nuclear medicine physician, radiologist) while applying coronal, transaxial, and sagittal layers. Subsequently, all of the images were interpreted in consensus by at least one experienced nuclear medicine physician, and two experienced radiologists, each of them board-certified and with PET/CT experience of more than five years as well as rich experience in interpretation of hybrid imaging with ^{68}Ga-PSMA-11. The final diagnosis was reached by consensus. Any PSMA-avid lesion with a morphological substrate on CT and an uptake above the background (but not correlated with physiological tracer uptake) was considered as being suggestive of PC. The SUV_{max} was measured for all lesions, suspicious of malignancy. PSMA-PET-avid lesions as described above were classified as suspected local recurrence in the prostate or prostate bed, as local/regional LN in the pelvis (iliac and/or pararectal) or as distant/extrapelvic LN (retroperitoneal and/or above the iliac bifurcation), as well as bone metastases and visceral metastases (lung, liver, adrenals, soft tissue, spleen, thyroid). When conflicting interpretations were identified, they were discussed and solved by the panel and consensus was passed between the reviewing physicians.

4.5. Statistical Analysis

Statistical analyses were performed while using SPSS version 24.0 (IBM Corporation, Ehningen, Germany). For continuous metric normally distributed variables, Students t-test was performed to determine differences between two groups. Multivariate variance analysis was used for comparison of more than two groups. We analyzed non-normally distributed continuous variables by Mann-Whitney-U test. The Wilcoxon signed rank test was calculated for determining the changes of PSA levels. For further analysis, we subdivided the metric values (e.g., PSAvel and PSAdt) into categories. We analyzed these nominal and ordinal parameters with Chi-square test and Pearson correlation. The performance of ^{68}Ga-PSMA-11 PET/CT was assessed in relation to these parameters by

ROC curves in order to determine the optimal cutoff of PSA levels and of PSA kinetics to differentiate between positive and negative scan results. The data are presented as mean, SD, and/or median and range. $p < 0.05$ was considered to be significant.

5. Conclusions

This study identifies the PSA and PSA kinetics thresholds for the presence of ^{68}Ga-PSMA-11 PET/CT-detectable PC-lesions in patients with BC. Pre-scan PSA was the main predictor of a positive scan with an optimal cutoff level of 1.24 ng/mL for patients that were primarily treated with RP. In this subgroup, kinetics analysis of PSA calculated a threshold velocity of 1.32 ng/mL/year.

We conclude that the PSA levels and kinetics (PSAvel) are suitable risk markers for optimizing the selection of patients who may benefit from ^{68}Ga-PSMA-11 PET/CT, especially in the subgroup of prostatectomized patients. ^{68}Ga-PSMA-11 PET/CT has a great impact on selecting patients with primary RP for salvage RT with curative intent.

Author Contributions: Conceptualization, M.A.H., H.-G.B., H.J.W., M.M. and M.S.; methodology, M.A.H., H.-G.B., H.J.W., M.M., F.R. and M.S.; software, M.A.H., H.-G.B., N.F., J.M.-H. and L.T.; validation, M.A.H., H.-G.B., H.J.W., M.M., F.R., N.F. and M.S.; formal analysis, M.A.H., H.-G.B., H.J.W., M.M., F.R., N.F. and S.P.; investigation, M.A.H., H.J.W., M.M., J.M.-H., L.T. and S.P.; resources, M.A.H., H.-G.B., H.J.W. and M.M.; data curation, H.J.W., M.M., J.M.-H., L.T. and M.S.; writing—original draft preparation, M.A.H., H.-G.B., H.J.W., M.M. and M.S.; writing—review and editing, H.J.W., M.M., F.R., N.F., S.P. and M.S.; visualization, M.A.H., H.-G.B., S.P., and M.S.; supervision, M.M. and M.S.; project administration, H.J.W., M.M. and M.S. All authors have read and agreed to the published version of the manuscript.

Funding: This research received no external funding.

Acknowledgments: The authors thank Ed Michaelson, MD, Fort Lauderdale, Florida, for language revision and Jennifer Steffens, Germany, for technical assistance.

Conflicts of Interest: The authors declare no conflict of interest.

References

1. Pilleron, S.; Sarfati, D.; Janssen-Heijnen, M.; Vignat, J.; Ferlay, J.; Bray, F.; Soerjomataram, I. Global Cancer Incidence in Older Adults, 2012 and 2035: A population-based study. *Int. J. Cancer* **2019**, *144*, 49–58. [CrossRef]
2. World Health Organization. Healthy Ageing. In *World Report an Ageing and Health*; WHO Press: Geneva, Switzerland, 2015; Available online: https://apps.who.int/iris/bitstream/handle/10665/186463/9789240694811_eng.pdf?sequence=1 (accessed on 15 November 2019).
3. Andriole, G.L.; Crawford, E.D.; Grubb, R.L., 3rd; Buys, S.S.; Chia, D.; Church, T.R.; Fouad, M.N.; Gelmann, E.P.; Kvale, P.A.; Reding, D.J.; et al. Mortality results from a randomized prostate-cancer screening trial. *N. Engl. J. Med.* **2009**, *360*, 1310–1319. [CrossRef] [PubMed]
4. Castellucci, P.; Picchio, M. 11C-choline PET/CT and PSA kinetics. *Eur. J. Nucl. Med. Mol. Imaging* **2013**, *40*, 36–40. [CrossRef] [PubMed]
5. Darwish, O.M.; Raj, G.V. Management of biochemical recurrence after primary localized therapy for prostate cancer. *Front. Oncol.* **2012**, *2*, 48. [CrossRef]
6. Von Eyben, F.E.; Picchio, M.; Von Eyben, R.; Rhee, H.; Bauman, G. ^{68}Ga-Labeled Prostate-specific Membrane Antigen Ligand Positron Emission Tomography/Computed Tomography for Prostate Cancer: A Systematic Review and Meta-analysis. *Eur. Urol. Focus* **2018**, *4*, 686–693. [CrossRef]
7. Cornford, P.; Bellmunt, J.; Bolla, M.; Briers, E.; De Santis, M.; Gross, T.; Henry, A.M.; Joniau, S.; Lam, T.B.; Mason, M.D.; et al. EAU-ESTRO-SIOG Guidelines on Prostate Cancer. Part II: Treatment of Relapsing, Metastatic, and Castration-Resistant Prostate Cancer. *Eur. Urol.* **2017**, *71*, 630–642. [CrossRef]
8. Mottet, N.; Bellmunt, J.; Briers, E.; Bolla, M.; Bourke, L.; Cornford, P.; De Santis, M.; Henry, A.; Joniau, S.; Lam, T. Members of the EAU-ESTRO-ESUR-SIOG Prostate Cancer Guidelines Panel. EAU-ESTRO-ESUR-SIOG Guidelines on Prostate Cancer. Available online: https://uroweb.org/guideline/prostate-cancer/ (accessed on 19 March 2019).

9. Chiaravalloti, A.; Di Biagio, D.; Tavolozza, M.; Calabria, F.; Schillaci, O. PET/CT with (18)F-choline after radical prostatectomy in patients with PSA. *Eur. J. Nucl. Med. Mol. Imaging* **2016**, *43*, 1418–1424. [CrossRef] [PubMed]
10. Pijoan, J.M. Diagnostic methodology for the biochemical recurrence of prostate cancer after radiotherapy. *Arch. Españoles Urol.* **2006**, *59*, 1053–1062.
11. Wayant, C.; Cooper, C.; Turner, D.; Vassar, M. Evaluation of the NCCN guidelines using the RIGHT Statement and AGREE II instrument: A cross-sectional review. *BMJ Evid.-Based Med.* **2019**, *24*, 219–226. [CrossRef] [PubMed]
12. Afshar-Oromieh, A.; Avtzi, E.; Giesel, F.L.; Holland-Letz, T.; Linhart, H.G.; Eder, M.; Eisenhut, M.; Boxler, S.; Hadaschik, B.A.; Kratochwil, C.; et al. The diagnostic value of PET/CT imaging with the ^{68}Ga-labelled PSMA ligand HBED-CC in the diagnosis of recurrent prostate cancer. *Eur. J. Nucl. Med. Mol. Imaging* **2015**, *42*, 197–209. [CrossRef]
13. Banerjee, S.R.; Pullambhatla, M.; Byun, Y.; Nimmagadda, S.; Green, G.; Fox, J.J.; Horti, A.; Mease, R.C.; Pomper, M.G. ^{68}Ga-labeled inhibitors of prostate-specific membrane antigen (PSMA) for imaging prostate cancer. *J. Med. Chem.* **2010**, *53*, 5333–5341. [CrossRef]
14. Mestre, R.P.; Treglia, G.; Ferrari, M.; Pascale, M.; Mazzara, C.; Azinwi, N.C.; Llado', A.; Stathis, A.; Giovanella, L.; Roggero, E. Correlation between PSA kinetics and PSMA-PET in prostate cancer restaging: A meta-analysis. *Eur. J. Clin. Investig.* **2019**, *49*, e13063. [CrossRef]
15. Eder, M.; Neels, O.; Müller, M.; Bauder-Wüst, U.; Remde, Y.; Schäfer, M.; Hennrich, U.; Eisenhut, M.; Afshar-Oromieh, A.; Haberkorn, U.; et al. Novel Preclinical and Radiopharma-ceutical Aspects of [68Ga]Ga-PSMA-HBED-CC: A new PET tracer for imaging of prostate cancer. *Pharmaceuticals* **2014**, *7*, 779–796. [CrossRef]
16. Eder, M.; Schäfer, M.; Bauder-Wüst, U.; Hull, W.-E.; Wängler, C.; Mier, W.; Haberkorn, U.; Eisenhut, M. ^{68}Ga-Complex Lipophilicity and the Targeting Property of a Urea-Based PSMA Inhibitor for PET Imaging. *Bioconjugate Chem.* **2012**, *23*, 688–697. [CrossRef]
17. Mottet, N.; Bellmunt, J.; Bolla, M.; Briers, E.; Cumberbatch, M.G.; De Santis, M.; Fossati, N.; Gross, T.; Henri, A.M.; Henry, A.M.; et al. EAU-ESTRO-SIOG Guidelines on Prostate Cancer. Part I: Screening, Diagnosis, and Local Treatment with Curative Intent. *Eur. Urol.* **2017**, *71*, 618–629. [CrossRef] [PubMed]
18. Dietlein, F.; Kobe, C.; Neubauer, S.; Schmidt, M.; Stockter, S.; Fischer, T.; Schomäcker, K.; Heidenreich, A.; Zlatopolskiy, B.D.; Neumaier, B.; et al. PSA-Stratified Performance of (18)F- and (68)Ga-PSMA PET in Patients with Biochemical Recurrence of Prostate Cancer. *J. Nucl. Med.* **2017**, *58*, 947–952. [CrossRef] [PubMed]
19. Giesel, F.L.; Hadaschik, B.; Cardinale, J.; Radtke, J.; Vinsensia, M.; Lehnert, W.; Kesch, C.; Tolstov, Y.; Singer, S.; Grabe, N.; et al. F-18 labelled PSMA-1007: Biodistribution, radiation dosimetry and histopathological validation of tumor lesions in prostate cancer patients. *Eur. J. Nucl. Med. Mol. Imaging* **2017**, *44*, 678–688. [CrossRef] [PubMed]
20. Eiber, M.; Maurer, T.; Souvatzoglou, M.; Beer, A.J.; Ruffani, A.; Haller, B.; Graner, F.-P.; Kübler, H.; Haberhorn, U.; Eisenhut, M.; et al. Evaluation of Hybrid 68Ga-PSMA Ligand PET/CT in 248 Patients with Biochemical Recurrence After Radical Prostatectomy. *J. Nucl. Med.* **2015**, *56*, 668–674. [CrossRef]
21. Fanti, S.; Oyen, W.; Lalumera, E. Consensus Procedures in Oncological Imaging: The Case of Prostate Cancer. *Cancers* **2019**, *11*, 1788. [CrossRef]
22. Zhao, Z.; Weickmann, S.; Jung, M.; Lein, M.; Kilic, E.; Stephan, C.; Erbersdobler, A.; Fendler, A.; Jung, K. A Novel Predictor Tool of Biochemical Recurrence after Radical Prostatectomy Based on a Five-MicroRNA Tissue Signature. *Cancers* **2019**, *11*, 1603. [CrossRef]
23. Hoffmann, M.A.; Wieler, H.J.; Baues, C.; Kuntz, N.J.; Richardsen, I.; Schreckenberger, M. The impact of ^{68}Ga-PSMA PET/CT and PET/MRT on the management of prostate cancer. *Urology* **2019**, *130*, 1–12. [CrossRef] [PubMed]
24. Hoffmann, M.A.; Miederer, M.; Wieler, H.J.; Ruf, C.; Jakobs, F.M.; Schreckenberger, M. Diagnostic performance of ^{68}Gallium-PSMA-11 PET/CT to detect significant prostate cancer and comparison with 18FEC PET/CT. *Oncotarget* **2017**, *8*, 111073–111083. [CrossRef] [PubMed]
25. Stephenson, A.J.; Scardino, P.T.; Kattan, M.W.; Pisansky, T.M.; Slawin, K.M.; Klein, E.A.; Anscher, M.S.; Michalski, J.M.; Sandler, H.M.; Lin, D.W.; et al. Predicting the Outcome of Salvage Radiation Therapy for Recurrent Prostate Cancer After Radical Prostatectomy. *J. Clin. Oncol.* **2007**, *25*, 2035–2041. [CrossRef]

26. Verburg, F.A.; Pfister, D.; Heidenreich, A.; Vogg, A.; Drude, N.I.; Vöö, S.; Mottaghy, F.M.; Behrendt, F.F. Extent of disease in recurrent prostate cancer determined by [(68)Ga]PSMA-HBED-CC PET/CT in relation to PSA levels, PSA doubling time and Gleason score. *Eur. J. Nucl. Med. Mol. Imaging* **2016**, *43*, 397–403. [CrossRef]
27. Calais, J.; Czernin, J.; Cao, M.; Kishan, A.U.; Hegde, J.V.; Shaverdian, N.; Sandler, K.; Chu, F.I.; King, C.R.; Steinberg, M.L.; et al. 68Ga-PSMA-11 PET/CT mapping of prostate cancer biochemical recurrence after radical prostatectomy in 270 patients with a PSA level of less than 1.0 ng/mL: Impact on salvage radiotherapy planning. *J. Nucl. Med.* **2018**, *59*, 230–237. [CrossRef] [PubMed]
28. Mapelli, P.; Incerti, E.; Ceci, F.; Castellucci, P.; Fanti, S.; Picchio, M. 11C- or 18F-Choline PET/CT for Imaging Evaluation of Biochemical Recurrence of Prostate Cancer. *J. Nucl. Med.* **2016**, *57*, 43–48. [CrossRef] [PubMed]
29. Afshar-Oromieh, A.; Zechmann, C.M.; Malcher, A.; Eder, M.; Eisenhut, M.; Linhart, H.G.; Holland-Letz, T.; Hadaschik, B.A.; Giesel, F.L.; Debus, J.; et al. Comparison of PET imaging with a (68)Ga-labelled PSMA ligand and (18)F-choline-based PET/CT for the diagnosis of recurrent prostate cancer. *Eur. J. Nucl. Med. Mol. Imaging* **2014**, *41*, 11–20. [CrossRef]
30. Krause, B.J.; Souvatzoglou, M.; Treiber, U. Imaging of prostate cancer with PET/CT and radioactively labeled choline derivates. *Urol. Oncol. Semin. Orig. Investig.* **2013**, *31*, 427–435. [CrossRef]
31. Kitajima, K.; Murphy, R.C.; Nathan, M.A. Choline PET/CT for imaging prostate cancer: An update. *Ann. Nucl. Med.* **2013**, *27*, 581–591. [CrossRef]
32. Graute, V.; Jansen, N.; Ubleis, C.; Seitz, M.; Hartenbach, M.; Scherr, M.K.; Thieme, S.; Cumming, P.; Klanke, K.; Tiling, R.; et al. Relationship between PSA kinetics and [18F]fluorocholine PET/CT detection rates of recurrence in patients with prostate cancer after total prostatectomy. *Eur. J. Nucl. Med. Mol. Imaging* **2012**, *39*, 271–282. [CrossRef]
33. Kuten, J.; Fahoum, I.; Savin, Z.; Shamni, O.; Gitstein, G.; Hershkovitz, V.; Mabjeesh, N.J.; Yossepowitch, O.; Mishani, E.; Even-Sapir, E. Head- to head Comparison of 68Ga-PSMA-11 with 18F-PSMA-1007 PET/CT in Staging Prostate Cancer Using Histopathology and Immunohistochemical Analysis as Reference-Standard. *J. Nucl. Med.* **2019**. [CrossRef] [PubMed]
34. Schillaci, O.; Calabria, F.; Tavolozza, M.; Caracciolo, C.R.; Agrò, E.F.; Miano, R.; Orlacchio, A.; Danieli, R.; Simonetti, G. Influence of PSA, PSA velocity and PSA doubling time on contrast-enhanced 18F-choline PET/CT detection rate in patients with rising PSA after radical prostatectomy. *Eur. J. Nucl. Med. Mol. Imaging* **2012**, *39*, 589–596. [CrossRef] [PubMed]
35. Afshar-Oromieh, A.; Holland-Letz, T.; Giesel, F.L.; Kratochwil, C.; Mier, W.; Haufe, S.; Debus, N.; Eder, M.; Eisenhut, M.; Schäfer, M.; et al. Diagnostic performance of 68Ga-PSMA-11 (HBED-CC) PET/CT in patients with recurrent prostate cancer: Evaluation in 1007 patients. *Eur. J. Nucl. Med. Mol. Imaging* **2017**, *44*, 1258–1268. [CrossRef] [PubMed]
36. Ceci, F.; Uprimny, C.; Nilica, B.; Geraldo, L.; Kendler, D.; Kroiss, A.; Bektic, J.; Horninger, W.; Lukas, P.; Decristoforo, C.; et al. 68Ga-PSMA PET/CT for restaging recurrent prostate cancer: Which factors are associated with PET/CT detection rate? *Eur. J. Nucl. Med. Mol. Imaging* **2015**, *42*, 1284–1294. [CrossRef]
37. Graziani, T.; Ceci, F.; Castellucci, P.; Polverari, G.; Lima, G.M.; Lodi, F.; Morganti, A.G.; Ardizzoni, A.; Schiavina, R.; Fanti, S. 11C-Choline PET/CT for restaging prostate cancer. Results from 4,426 scans in a single-centre patient series. *Eur. J. Nucl. Med. Mol. Imaging* **2016**, *43*, 1971–1979. [CrossRef]
38. Suardi, N.; Gandaglia, G.; Gallina, A.; Di Trapani, E.; Scattoni, V.; Vizziello, D.; Cucchiara, V.; Bertini, R.; Colombo, R.; Picchio, M.; et al. Long-term Outcomes of Salvage Lymph Node Dissection for Clinically Recurrent Prostate Cancer: Results of a Single-institution Series with a Minimum Follow-up of 5 Years. *Eur. Urol.* **2015**, *67*, 299–309. [CrossRef]
39. Ost, P.; Bossi, A.; Decaestecker, K.; De Meerleer, G.; Giannarini, G.; Karnes, R.J.; Roach, M.; Briganti, A. Metastasis-directed Therapy of Regional and Distant Recurrences After Curative Treatment of Prostate Cancer: A Systematic Review of the Literature. *Eur. Urol.* **2015**, *67*, 852–863. [CrossRef]
40. Kane, C.J.; Eggener, S.E.; Shindel, A.W.; Andriole, G.L. Variability in Outcomes for Patients with Intermediate-risk Prostate Cancer (Gleason Score 7, International Society of Urological Pathology Gleason Group 2–3) and Implications for Risk Stratification: A Systematic Review. *Eur. Urol. Focus* **2017**, *3*, 487–497. [CrossRef]

41. Kasperzyk, J.L.; Finn, S.P.; Flavin, R.; Fiorentino, M.; Lis, R.; Hendrickson, W.K.; Clinton, S.K.; Sesso, H.D.; Giovannucci, E.L.; Stampfer, M.J.; et al. Prostate-specific membrane antigen protein expression in tumor tissue and risk of lethal prostate cancer. *Cancer Epidemiol. Biomark. Prev.* **2013**, *22*, 2354–2363. [CrossRef]
42. Mostaghel, E.A.; Page, S.T.; Lin, D.W.; Fazli, L.; Coleman, I.M.; True, L.D.; Knudsen, B.; Hess, D.L.; Nelson, C.C.; Matsumoto, A.M.; et al. Intraprostatic Androgens and Androgen-Regulated Gene Expression Persist after Testosterone Suppression: Therapeutic Implications for Castration-Resistant Prostate Cancer. *Cancer Res.* **2007**, *67*, 5033–5041. [CrossRef]
43. Li, N.; Lv, H.; Hao, X.; Hu, B.; Song, Y. Prognostic value of serum alkaline phosphatase in the survival of prostate cancer: Evidence from a meta-analysis. *Cancer Manag. Res.* **2018**, *10*, 3125–3139. [CrossRef] [PubMed]
44. Wymenga, L.; Boomsma, J.; Groenier, K.; Piers, D.; Mensink, H. Routine bone scans in patients with prostate cancer related to serum prostate-specific antigen and alkaline phosphatase. *BJU Int.* **2001**, *88*, 226–230. [CrossRef] [PubMed]

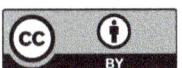

© 2020 by the authors. Licensee MDPI, Basel, Switzerland. This article is an open access article distributed under the terms and conditions of the Creative Commons Attribution (CC BY) license (http://creativecommons.org/licenses/by/4.0/).

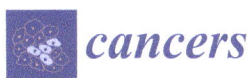

Article

Multiparametric MRI for Prostate Cancer Detection: New Insights into the Combined Use of a Radiomic Approach with Advanced Acquisition Protocol

Serena Monti [1], Valentina Brancato [1,*], Giuseppe Di Costanzo [2], Luca Basso [1], Marta Puglia [2], Alfonso Ragozzino [2], Marco Salvatore [1] and Carlo Cavaliere [1]

1. IRCCS SDN, 80143 Naples, Italy; smonti@sdn-napoli.it (S.M.); lbasso@sdn-napoli.it (L.B.); direzionescientifica@sdn-napoli.it (M.S.); ccavaliere@sdn-napoli.it (C.C.)
2. Ospedale S. Maria delle Grazie, 80078 Pozzuoli, Italy; giupe7700@yahoo.it (G.D.C.); martapuglia@alice.it (M.P.); alfonsoragozzino@gmail.com (A.R.)
* Correspondence: vbrancato@sdn-napoli.it; Tel.: +39-081-2408-299

Received: 19 December 2019; Accepted: 5 February 2020; Published: 7 February 2020

Abstract: Prostate cancer (PCa) is a disease affecting an increasing number of men worldwide. Several efforts have been made to identify imaging biomarkers to non-invasively detect and characterize PCa, with substantial improvements thanks to multiparametric Magnetic Resonance Imaging (mpMRI). In recent years, diffusion kurtosis imaging (DKI) was proposed to be directly related to tissue physiological and pathological characteristic, while the radiomic approach was proven to be a key method to study cancer imaging phenotypes. Our aim was to compare a standard radiomic model for PCa detection, built using T2-weighted (T2W) and Apparent Diffusion Coefficient (ADC), with an advanced one, including DKI and quantitative Dynamic Contrast Enhanced (DCE), while also evaluating differences in prediction performance when using 2D or 3D lesion segmentation. The obtained results in terms of diagnostic accuracy were high for all of the performed comparisons, reaching values up to 0.99 for the area under a receiver operating characteristic curve (AUC), and 0.98 for both sensitivity and specificity. In comparison, the radiomic model based on standard features led to prediction performances higher than those of the advanced model, while greater accuracy was achieved by the model extracted from 3D segmentation. These results provide new insights into active topics of discussion, such as choosing the most convenient acquisition protocol and the most appropriate postprocessing pipeline to accurately detect and characterize PCa.

Keywords: prostate cancer; PI-RADS; radiomics; magnetic resonance imaging; diffusion kurtosis imaging; dynamic contrast-enhanced magnetic resonance imaging

1. Introduction

Prostate cancer (PCa) is the second most common malignant neoplasm among men [1]. The early detection and grading of PCa are crucial for patient management and long-term survival evaluation.

The prostate cancer screening paradigm commonly consists of a serum prostate-specific antigen (PSA) test, a digital rectal examination, a transrectal ultrasound, and prostatic biopsies, but each of these methods has its disadvantages, spanning from low accuracy, i.e., when PSA is used alone, to invasiveness, i.e., in transrectal examinations or biopsies.

Recently, the use of a multiparametric Magnetic Resonance Imaging (mpMRI) approach, combining anatomic T1 or T2-weighted (T2W) images with functional MRI methods as Diffusion Weighted Imaging (DWI) and Dynamic Contrast Enhanced (DCE) imaging, provided substantial improvements in non-invasive prostate cancer detection and characterization [2–4]. In fact, the imaging approach, besides its non-invasiveness, can give "in vivo" information on the entire tumor volume, thereby reducing inaccuracies due to sampling errors in histopathological analyses.

The Prostate Imaging-Reporting and Data System (PI-RADS) was developed in 2013, and then updated in 2015 (PI-RADS v2) [5], in order to standardize the use of mpMRI in PCa imaging. This technology provides a scale indicating how likely an mpMRI finding from T2W, DWI, and DCE is related to a clinically significant cancer. The PI-RADS score ranges from one, which indicates a very low probability of malignancy, to five, which indicates a very high probability that a lesion is malignant. Since its introduction, the PI-RADS classification has played a very important role in PCa diagnosis [6], proving to be a useful tool for the detection of prostatic lesions and their characterization in terms of aggressiveness. However, due to its definition, PI-RADS scoring can be affected by subjectivity and inter-/intra-operator variability [7], which are factors that may compromise PCa assessment. Moreover, it is not unusual to find benign and malignant lesions with similar imaging findings, making it challenging to detect the nature of prostatic lesions [8]. It should also be considered that lesions classified as having a PI-RADS score of three are usually lesions termed as "intermediate" or "equivocal on the presence of clinically significant cancer" [9]. The abovementioned limitations of PI-RADS, together with an ever-growing volume of medical images for each patient and the development of increasingly powerful image acquisition and processing techniques, have led to an increasing interest in new quantitative approaches to analyze mpMRI images [10].

In particular, non-Gaussian diffusion models were proposed to better describe diffusion signal behaviors, which are directly related to tissue physiological and pathological characteristics, and to overcome the possible limitation of standard DWI. One of the most used models in the field of prostate cancer is diffusion kurtosis imaging (DKI), although this technique requires more advanced MRI sequences, longer acquisition time, and specific postprocessing tools compared with standard DWI. DKI parameters, namely, the diffusion coefficient D and the deviation from normal distribution coefficient K, proved to be very useful for PCa detection and characterization [11–14].

On the other hand, a radiomic approach proved to be a key method to study cancer imaging phenotypes, reflecting underlying clinical and pathological information, as well as gene expression patterns [15–18]. Radiomics, in fact, refers to the extraction of a large number of quantitative features from medical images [19], thereby revealing heterogeneous tumor metabolism and anatomy [20,21]. This high-throughput extraction is preparatory to a process of data mining [17] for studies of associations with or predictions of different clinical outcomes [22], thereby giving important prognostic information about disease. The potential of radiomics to extensively characterize intratumoral heterogeneity has shown promise regarding the prediction of treatment responses and outcomes, differentiating benign and malignant tumors, and assessing genetic relationships in many cancer types [23,24].

Several radiomic studies were performed to discriminate PCa from noncancerous tissues, to differentiate between cancers with different Gleason scores, and also to compare radiomic diagnostic capabilities with those of PI-RADS scores [8,25–28]. All of these studies computed radiomic features from standard mpMRI acquisition, including T2W, Apparent Diffusion Coefficient (ADC) computed from a classical Gaussian diffusion model, and eventually DCE images. Feature extraction starting from 2D regions of interest (ROIs) was performed in some of these studies, while 3D volumes of interest (VOI) was utilized in others. Only few works, to the best of our knowledge, applied radiomic approach to DKI imaging; Wang et al. [29] investigated whether radiomic features extracted from T2W, ADC, D, K, and the quantitative perfusion parameter K^{trans} could help to improve the diagnostic performance of structured PI-RADS v2 in clinically relevant PCa. In the study by Hectors et al. [30], radiomics features extracted from T2W, ADC, and DKI maps were correlated with Gleason score, gene expression signatures and cancer-related gene expression levels. Toivonen et al. [31] developed and evaluated a classification system for Gleason score predictions using radiomics features from T2W, DWI, and DKI. However, none of these fully investigated the added value of combining the complex radiomic processing approach with the advanced DKI mathematical model for PCa detection.

The aim of our study was to fully investigate this issue. We obtained mpMRI radiomic signatures to discriminate between 4–5 PI-RADS PCa and healthy tissue (HT) in a standard model, computed using T2W and ADC alone, and using more advanced technology, which included using DKI and quantitative DCE pharmacokinetic parameters [32]. Besides comparing the accuracies obtained by these two radiomic signatures, we also evaluated the differences found in prediction performances when using 2D ROIs or 3D VOIs.

2. Results

First and second order radiomic features (described in detail in the Materials and Methods section) were extracted from T2W, ADC, DKI, and quantitative DCE pharmacokinetic parameters (volume transfer constant from the plasma compartment to the extravascular extracellular space, K^{trans}; rate constant for transfer between the extravascular extracellular space and the blood compartment, K_{ep}; volume of extravascular extracellular space per unit volume of tissue, v_e; the initial area under the enhancement curve, iAUC).

The initial sets of features were composed of 120 features for two of the three analyzed classification tasks, i.e., PI-RADS 4–5 vs. HT on 3D VOI in the advanced model (adv3D), which was computed using first order features from T2W, ADC, D, K, and quantitative DCE pharmacokinetic parameters, and PI-RADS 4–5 vs. HT on 2D ROI in the advanced model (adv2D). The third feature set was composed of 44 features for the classification task PI-RADS 4–5 vs. HT on 3D VOI in the standard model (std3D), which was computed using first and second order features from T2W and ADC.

Considering that, for a single patient, more than one segmentation can be obtained, i.e., both lesion and HT can be obtained from the same prostate and more lesions or more healthy regions in the same subject, a total of 118 3D VOIs were segmented (69 PCa and 49 HT); correspondingly, 118 2D ROIs were extracted.

For each classification task, a reduced feature set was computed according to a stepwise forward feature selection scheme. Each feature set, as reported in Table 1, was composed of the 25 top-ranked features in the gain equation.

Table 1. Reduced feature set for each classification task. For each feature, the image from which it was extracted is indicated. For std3D, whether it is a first or second order feature and the feature name are also indicated. Abbreviations: T2W = T2-weighted; ADC = Apparent Diffusion Coefficient; D = diffusion coefficient of Diffusion Kurtosis Imaging (DKI) model; K = deviation from normal distribution coefficient; iAUC = initial area under the enhancement curve; v_e = volume of extravascular extracellular space per unit volume of tissue; K_{ep} = ; K^{trans} = ; Max = maximum; Mad = mean absolute deviation; Min = minimum; Rms = root mean square; Std = standard deviation; GLCM = Gray Level Co-occurrence Matrix.

adv3D	adv2D	std3D
D—Mean	ADC—Rms	ADC—Mean
D—Energy	T2W—Energy	ADC—Energy
iAUC—Median	K^{trans}—Median	ADC—GLCM Auto Correlation
v_e—Min	T2—Std	ADC—Max
T2W—Max	K—Mad	ADC—Min
K—Mad	K—Std	T2W—Max
ADC—Max	D—Max	T2W—Std
ADC—Min	T2W—Max	T2W—Mean
T2W—Std	ADC—Energy	ADC—Rms
K—Std	D—Mean	ADC—Median
ADC—Energy	ADC—Max	T2W—Variance
K—Variance	D—Energy	T2W—Energy

Table 1. Cont.

adv3D	adv2D	std3D
T2W—Variance	T2W—Variance	T2W—Rms
T2W—Rms	K—Variance	ADC—GLCM Sum Average
D—Max	D—Rms	T2W—Median
D—Min	D—Median	T2W—Mad
T2—Mad	ADC—Mean	T2W—GLCM Correlation
K_{ep}—Median	T2W—Mean	ADC—Skewness
T2W—Energy	K—Rms	T2W—GLCM Homogeneity
T2W—Mean	ADC—Median	T2W—Uniformity
D—Rms	T2W—Mad	T2—Entropy
K^{trans}—Min	K^{trans}—Mean	T2—GLCM Dissimilarity
K^{trans}—Mean	T2W—Median	T2—Min
D—Median	iAUC—Median	ADC—Uniformity
ADC—Mean	T2W—Rms	ADC—GLCM Correlation

For each reduced feature set, multivariable logistic regression models of order from 1 to 10 were obtained and their prediction performances for the different classification tasks are reported in Figures 1 and 2, where the comparisons between adv3D/adv2D and adv3D/std3D are shown, respectively.

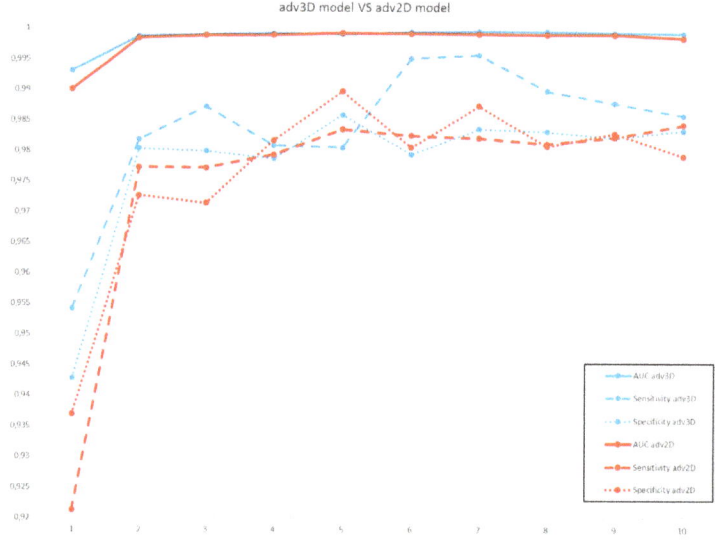

Figure 1. Area under the receiver operating characteristics curve (AUC) (full line), sensitivity (dashed line), and specificity (dotted line) of the multivariable models for adv3D (in blue) and adv2D (in red), for model orders from 1 to 10.

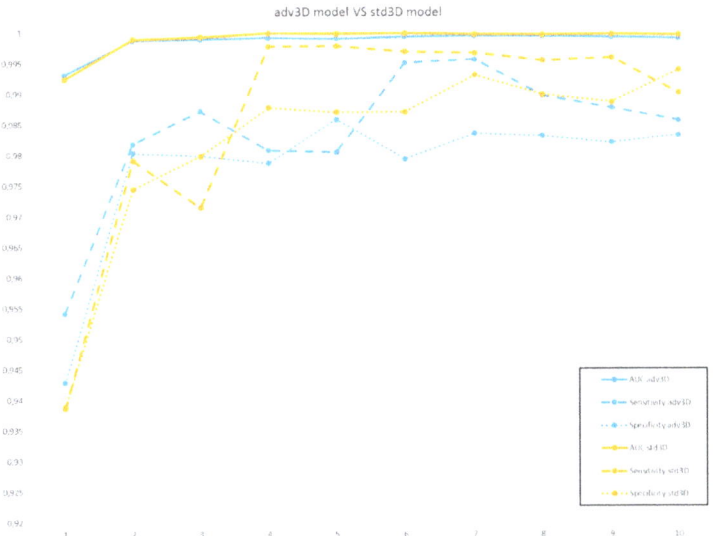

Figure 2. Area under the receiver operating characteristics curve (AUC) (full line), sensitivity (dashed line), and specificity (dotted line) of the multivariable models for adv3D (in blue) and std3D (in yellow), for model orders from 1 to 10.

By inspecting the curves in Figures 1 and 2, very similar and good results were obtained by the three classification models. In more detail, from the comparison between the adv3D and adv2D comparable results in terms of AUC, the sensitivity was higher for adv3D, except for model order 5; this was in contrast with specificity, which was higher on average for adv2D. On the other hand, the comparison between adv3D and std3D highlighted higher results for std3D, except for low order models.

For adv3D, the best model was order 7 based on the T2W mean, Max, Mad, Rms, ADC energy, Min, and K variance. Order 5 was chosen for adv2D based on T2W Mad, ADC mean, median, energy, and K^{trans} median. Finally, order 4 was selected for std3D based on T2W mean and Min, ADC energy, and Min.

3. Discussion

In this work, the added value of combining the radiomic processing approach with the advanced DKI mathematical model for PCa detection was investigated. The main aim was to compare a standard radiomic model built using T2W and ADC with an advanced one which included DKI and quantitative DCE pharmacokinetic parameters in terms of PCa diagnostic accuracy. In addition, we evaluated the differences found in prediction performances when using 2D ROIs or 3D VOIs.

The obtained results of AUC, sensitivity, and specificity were extremely high for all the classification tasks tested (PI-RADS 4–5 vs. HT on adv3D, PI-RADS 4–5 vs. HT on adv2D, and PI-RADS 4–5 vs. HT on std3D), reaching values up to 0.99 for AUC and 0.98 for both sensitivity and specificity. These performances were comparable to those obtained by Chen et al. [27] in their logistic regression model, which was built by incorporating T2W sequences and ADC maps to classify PCa vs. non-PCa tissues. However, in their work, Chen et al. included also shape features, which were deliberately not considered in our models in order to avoid possible biases in feature values introduced by the delineation of HT VOI/ROI which did not follow anatomical boundaries, as in the case of tumor lesions.

Looking at the variables included in the best predictive model chosen for each classification task, the recurrence of ADC energy as a common feature was observed. Interestingly, this index of tumor heterogeneity was previously found to be a promising quantitative imaging biomarker for characterizing cancer imaging phenotypes, since it was associated with tumor gene expression, tumor metabolism, tumor stage, patient prognosis, and treatment response in several studies on different cancer types [33].

To the best of our knowledge, only a few previous works [29–31] performed radiomic studies on prostate cancer, including DKI model parameters, to detect clinically relevant PCa and to evaluate PCa aggressiveness. Even though a direct comparison is not directly applicable, considering the different populations and imaging approaches, some parallels can be carefully drawn with the work by Wang et al. [29], which partially shared our aim and also considered the Toft perfusion model. Those authors found that the best ranked features for PCa detection were extracted from D and K, while pharmacokinetic features were not highly ranked in their classification model. Similarly, in our adv3D model, the majority of the best ranked features (see Table 1) were extracted from DKI and ADC (which was not included in the models by Wang et al. [29]), while few features were derived from the Toft parameters.

In this study, looking in particular at the comparison between standard and advanced models, radiomic approaches based on a standard feature set (T2w and ADC) led to a predictive model with higher AUC, sensitivity, and specificity values than those of the predictive model based on the advanced feature set. It should be noted that the DKI and DCE features, even though they contributed to the features set after the first reduction step, survived only to a minor extent in the final selected models and minimally contributed K variance in the adv3D model and K^{trans} median in the adv2D model. These results suggest that the inclusion of radiomic features derived from DCE and DKI models does not provide a clear added value for PCa detection. On one hand, this would justify the choice to exclude DCE from dominant sequences for PI-RADSv2 score assessment, which is still a topic of discussion [34–36]; on the other hand, this would be food for thought regarding the complex debate of the financial benefits of including time- and computational-demanding DKI acquisition in prostate mpMRI acquisition protocol [14]. Regarding the comparison of the 3D and 2D advanced models, high diagnostic performances were shown by both advanced models, although the sensitivity was slightly lower and the specificity higher for the model built using 2D ROI, even though the resulting AUCs were similar and above 0.99, thereby suggesting great accuracy for the quantitative parameters extracted from VOI. This confirmed the hypothesis that tridimensional regions of interest allow for a more complete description of the lesion [37] and increased the number of points included in the statistical feature computation, thereby leading to results that were, in principle, more reliable and less vulnerable to sampling errors [38].

Our study presents several limitations. First of all, even if the lesions selected as PI-RADS 4–5 were confirmed during biopsy, uncertainty in histological radiological correlations may still remain when determining HT VOIs performed on the basis of radiological images. Such uncertainties could be ruled out using MR-guided biopsy techniques, which could adopt the advantages of new technologies, such as 3D printing, and could be used to develop personalized mold from diagnostic images to obtain histopathological slices exactly corresponding to the acquired slice in mpMRI, as an example [39]. In addition, due to the small sample size (< 100 cases), we could not evaluate the prediction accuracy for a nonbinary classification task (i.e., the additional inclusion of PI-RADS 3 lesions), neither could we test the reproducibility of the proposed method in a separate validation group of patients.

4. Materials and Methods

4.1. Patient Cohort

The study was approved by the Institutional Review Board (9/19). All mpMRI data acquired from March 2017 to August 2018 from a single center were retrospectively checked. A total of 65 patients were selected according to the following inclusion criteria: PI-RADS 4–5 at mpMRI, PSA > 4 ng/mL, age older than 18 years at the time of the study, and available results of biopsy. Exclusion criteria included inadequate MR images and unbiopsied lesions.

4.2. MR Imaging

mpMRI examinations were performed on a 3T Biograph mMR (Siemens Healthcare, Erlangen, Germany) with a body surface coil. The imaging protocols included a T2W (Repetition Time [TR] = 4010 ms, Echo Time [TE] = 112 ms, in plane field of view [FOV] = 200 × 200 mm^2, number of slices = 26, resolution = 0.6 × 0.6 mm2, slice thickness = 3 mm), DWI (TR = 7000 ms, TE = 86 ms, in plane FOV = 260 × 220 mm^2, number of slices = 26, resolution = 2 × 2 mm^2, slice thickness = 3 mm, b values = 0, 250, 500 (4 averages), 1000, 1500 (6 averages), 2000, 2500 (8 averages) s/mm^2), 6 gradient echo Volumetric Interpolated Breath-hold Examination (VIBE) sequences at variable flip angles (FAs) for T1 mapping (TR = 5.58 ms, TE = 1.83 ms, FAs = (2°, 5°, 8°, 12°, 15°, 20°), in plane FOV = 243 × 260 × 80 mm^3, slice gap 20%, resolution = 1.4 ×1.4 × 3.0 mm^3), and a dynamic scan with 60 consecutives phases with a VIBE sequence (TR = 5.58 ms, TE = 1.83 ms, FA = 20°, FOV = 243 × 260 × 80 mm^3, resolution = 1.4 × 1.4 × 3.0 mm^3, temporal resolution = 9 s/phase). Intravenous contrast injections started at the end of the first phase of dynamic scan at a dose of 0.1 mmol/kg of body weight and at the highest rate compatible with the patient's age and compliance (up to 5 mL/s)

4.3. PI-RADS

The PI-RADS assignment was performed by two radiologists experienced in urogenital imaging. They inspected, in consensus, T2W, DWI, ADC maps, and DCE images in order to identify prostatic lesions in accordance to PI-RADS v2 guidelines [40]. Of the PI-RADS 4 and PI-RADS 5 lesions, 100% were confirmed to be cancer on biopsy.

4.4. ADC and DKI Maps Calculation

ADC maps were computed using the in-line software of the Biograph scanner, selecting b-values from 0 to 1500. DKI maps, i.e., D and K, were computed using a voxel-wise fitting procedure implemented in Matlab (The MathWorks Inc., Natick, MA, USA).

4.5. Pharmacokinetic Map Calculation

Pharmacokinetic maps were obtained with the commercial software Tissue 4D (Siemens Healthcare, Erlangen, Germany). After an automated step of motion correction of the VIBE sequences at variable FAs with the dynamic VIBE sequence, the Toft model [41] was chosen for pharmacokinetic parameter calculations. The arterial input function (AIF) used for the analysis was set to "intermediate", on the basis of population-based AIFs built in Tissue 4D. Finally, 3D maps of K^{trans}, K_{ep}, v_e, and iAUC were obtained [23].

4.6. Image Preprocessing

Before feature extraction, some preprocessing steps were performed for each subject, i.e., the image acquired at b = 0 was non-rigidly coregistered to the T2W image in order to correct for spatial distortion typical of DWI acquisition. The registration was performed using the Elastix software (v. 4.9.0 [42]), and the resulting transform was used to warp the volumes acquired at the other b-values and the corresponding ADC, D, and K maps. In addition, K^{trans}, K_{ep}, v_e, and iAUC maps were resampled to match the resolution of the T2W image.

4.7. VOI/ROI Segmentation

3D VOI segmentations were manually obtained. Two experienced radiologists were asked to consensually draw the 3D VOI in the biopsied lesions with PI-RADS 4–5 and in HT on T2W images, while also looking at the b = 1000 coregistered volume. During the segmentation procedure, the radiologists were blinded to both the histological results and all clinical information relative to the retrospective prostate MR images. The segmentation was done using in-house developed software for region labeling. The 2D ROIs were automatically obtained in Matlab from 3D VOIs, with the 2D section with the longest major axis chosen for each.

4.8. Feature Extraction

The first order features were extracted from T2W, ADC, D, K, K^{trans}, K_{ep}, v_e, and iAUC for the 3D VOIs and 2D ROIs. First, each image was normalized, limiting its dynamics within the segmentation to $\mu \pm 3\sigma$ [43], then 13 first order features were extracted from the intensity histogram computed on 256 bins, namely, energy, entropy, kurtosis, maximum (Max), mean, mean absolute deviation (Mad), median, minimum (Min), root mean square (Rms), skewness, standard deviation (Std), uniformity, and variance.

In addition, second order features were also computed for the T2W and ADC images. Gray Level Co-occurrence Matrix (GLCM) [44], which was computed by 3D analysis of the tumor region with 26-voxel connectivity, was chosen, simultaneously taking into account the neighboring properties of the voxels in all 3D directions [45] after image quantization on 32 grey levels. The obtained features included energy, contrast, entropy, homogeneity, correlation, sum average, variance, dissimilarity, and auto correlation.

4.9. Multivariable Analysis

Three classification tasks were analyzed: PI-RADS 4–5 vs. HT on 3D VOI in the adv3D, which was computed using first order features from T2W, ADC, D, K, K^{trans}, K_{ep}, v_e, and iAUC, PI-RADS 4–5 vs. HT on 2D ROI in the adv2D, and PI-RADS 4–5 vs. HT on 3D VOI in the std3D, which was computed using the first and second order features from T2W and ADC.

The multivariable predictive models were obtained following the method described by Vallières et al. [45], using an imbalance-adjusted bootstrap resampling (IABR) on 1000 samples at each step.

First, from the large initial set of features, a reduced feature set of 25 features was computed through a stepwise forward feature selection scheme for each classification task. The first feature was chosen as the one that maximized Spearman's rank correlation regarding the outcome. Then, the features were added one at a time to maximize a linear combination of Spearman's rank correlation (between the feature and the outcome) and the Maximal Information Coefficient (between the feature and the features that were yet to be included in the reduced set) [46].

Then, from the reduced feature set, logistic regression models of order i from 1 to 10 that would best predict the outcome under investigation were obtained using another stepwise forward feature selection. This procedure involved adding features that maximized the 0.632 + bootstrap area under the receiver operating characteristic curve (AUC) [47] to the ith model one by one.

Finally, for each classification task, the prediction model was obtained by choosing the order that maximized the AUC and computing the final model logistic regression coefficients for the aforementioned combination of features using IABR.

5. Conclusions

In this work, we proposed a radiomic approach to differentiate between PI-RADS 4–5 lesions and HT using different prediction models. The proposed comparisons, including one between models constructed from standard mpMR acquisition protocol (including ADC and T2W) and advanced acquisition protocol (with the addition of DCE and DKI) and another between models derived from features extracted from 3D VOIs or 2D ROIs, provided interesting insights into these sensitive discussion topics amongst the scientific community. This work paved the way toward further studies of these topics, potentially evaluating nonbinary outcomes, tumor aggressiveness, and reproducibility of the computed features in wider cohorts of patients. More extensive work could enable the scientific community to more confidently suggest guidelines regarding the choice of the most confident, but not redundant, acquisition protocol, and of the most appropriate postprocessing pipeline to accurately detect and characterize PCa.

Author Contributions: S.M. and C.C. conceived the study; C.C., L.B., A.R., G.D.C., and M.P. enrolled the patients and acquired data; S.M., V.B., and L.B. performed the data analysis; S.M. and V.B. wrote the original draft; C.C., M.S., and A.R. reviewed and edited the manuscript. All authors read and agreed to the published version of the manuscript.

Funding: This work was supported by "Ricerca Corrente" Grant from Italian Ministry of Health (IRCCS SDN).

Conflicts of Interest: The authors declare no conflict of interest.

References

1. Bray, F.; Ferlay, J.; Soerjomataram, I.; Siegel, R.L.; Torre, L.A.; Jemal, A. Global cancer statistics 2018: GLOBOCAN estimates of incidence and mortality worldwide for 36 cancers in 185 countries. *CA Cancer J. Clin.* **2018**, *68*, 394–424. [CrossRef] [PubMed]
2. Hegde, J.V.; Mulkern, R.V.; Panych, L.P.; Fennessy, F.M.; Fedorov, A.; Maier, S.E.; Tempany, C.M.C. Multiparametric MRI of prostate cancer: An update on state-of-the-art techniques and their performance in detecting and localizing prostate cancer. *J. Magn. Reson. Imaging* **2013**, *37*, 1035–1054. [CrossRef] [PubMed]
3. De Rooij, M.; Hamoen, E.H.J.; Fütterer, J.J.; Barentsz, J.O.; Rovers, M.M. Accuracy of multiparametric MRI for prostate cancer detection: A meta-analysis. *Am. J. Roentgenol.* **2014**, *202*, 343–351. [CrossRef] [PubMed]
4. Fütterer, J.J.; Briganti, A.; De Visschere, P.; Emberton, M.; Giannarini, G.; Kirkham, A.; Taneja, S.S.; Thoeny, H.; Villeirs, G.; Villers, A. Can clinically significant prostate cancer be detected with multiparametric magnetic resonance imaging? A systematic review of the literature. *Eur. Urol.* **2015**, *68*, 1045–1053. [CrossRef]
5. Weinreb, J.C.; Barentsz, J.O.; Choyke, P.L.; Cornud, F.; Haider, M.A.; Macura, K.J.; Margolis, D.; Schnall, M.D.; Shtern, F.; Tempany, C.M.; et al. PI-RADS prostate imaging—Reporting and data system: 2015, version 2. *Eur. Urol.* **2016**, *69*, 16–40. [CrossRef]
6. Zhao, C.; Gao, G.; Fang, D.; Li, F.; Yang, X.; Wang, H.; He, Q.; Wang, X. The efficiency of multiparametric magnetic resonance imaging (mpMRI) using PI-RADS Version 2 in the diagnosis of clinically significant prostate cancer. *Clin. Imaging* **2016**, *40*, 885–888. [CrossRef]
7. Chung, A.G.; Shafiee, M.J.; Kumar, D.; Khalvati, F.; Haider, M.A.; Wong, A. Discovery radiomics for multi-parametric MRI prostate cancer detection. *arXiv* **2015**, arXiv:1509.00111.
8. Xu, M.; Fang, M.; Zou, J.; Yang, S.; Yu, D.; Zhong, L.; Hu, C.; Zang, Y.; Dong, D.; Tian, J.; et al. Using biparametric MRI radiomics signature to differentiate between benign and malignant prostate lesions. *Eur. J. Radiol.* **2019**, *114*, 38–44. [CrossRef]
9. Schoots, I.G. MRI in early prostate cancer detection: How to manage indeterminate or equivocal PI-RADS 3 lesions? *Transl. Androl. Urol.* **2018**, *7*, 70–82. [CrossRef]
10. Sun, Y.; Reynolds, H.M.; Parameswaran, B.; Wraith, D.; Finnegan, M.E.; Williams, S.; Haworth, A. Multiparametric MRI and radiomics in prostate cancer: A review. *Australas. Phys. Eng. Sci. Med.* **2019**, *42*, 3–25. [CrossRef]
11. Rosenkrantz, A.B.; Sigmund, E.E.; Johnson, G.; Babb, J.S.; Mussi, T.C.; Melamed, J.; Taneja, S.S.; Lee, V.S.; Jensen, J.H. Prostate cancer: Feasibility and preliminary experience of a diffusional kurtosis model for detection and assessment of aggressiveness of peripheral zone cancer. *Radiology* **2012**, *264*, 126–135. [CrossRef] [PubMed]
12. Suo, S.; Chen, X.; Wu, L.; Zhang, X.; Yao, Q.; Fan, Y.; Wang, H.; Xu, J. Non-Gaussian water diffusion kurtosis imaging of prostate cancer. *Magn. Reson. Imaging* **2014**, *32*, 421–427. [CrossRef] [PubMed]

13. Tamura, C.; Shinmoto, H.; Soga, S.; Okamura, T.; Sato, H.; Okuaki, T.; Pang, Y.; Kosuda, S.; Kaji, T. Diffusion kurtosis imaging study of prostate cancer: Preliminary findings. *J. Magn. Reson. Imaging* **2014**, *40*, 723–729. [CrossRef] [PubMed]
14. Brancato, V.; Cavaliere, C.; Salvatore, M.; Monti, S. Non-Gaussian models of diffusion weighted imaging for detection and characterization of prostate cancer: A systematic review and meta-analysis. *Sci. Rep.* **2019**, *9*, 16837. [CrossRef] [PubMed]
15. Kumar, V.; Gu, Y.; Basu, S.; Berglund, A.; Eschrich, S.A.; Schabath, M.B.; Forster, K.; Aerts, H.J.W.L.; Dekker, A.; Fenstermacher, D.; et al. Radiomics: The process and the challenges. *Magn. Reson. Imaging* **2012**, *30*, 1234–1248. [CrossRef]
16. Lambin, P.; Rios-Velazquez, E.; Leijenaar, R.; Carvalho, S.; Van Stiphout, R.G.P.M.; Granton, P.; Zegers, C.M.L.; Gillies, R.; Boellard, R.; Dekker, A.; et al. Radiomics: Extracting more information from medical images using advanced feature analysis. *Eur. J. Cancer* **2012**, *48*, 441–446. [CrossRef]
17. Gillies, R.J.; Kinahan, P.E.; Hricak, H. Radiomics: Images are more than pictures, they are data. *Radiology* **2016**, *278*, 563–577. [CrossRef]
18. Aerts, H.J.W.L.; Velazquez, E.R.; Leijenaar, R.T.H.; Parmar, C.; Grossmann, P.; Cavalho, S.; Bussink, J.; Monshouwer, R.; Haibe-Kains, B.; Rietveld, D.; et al. Decoding tumour phenotype by noninvasive imaging using a quantitative radiomics approach. *Nat. Commun.* **2014**, *5*, 4006. [CrossRef]
19. Incoronato, M.; Aiello, M.; Infante, T.; Cavaliere, C.; Grimaldi, A.M.; Mirabelli, P.; Monti, S.; Salvatore, M. Radiogenomic analysis of oncological data: A technical survey. *Int. J. Mol. Sci.* **2017**, *18*, 805. [CrossRef]
20. Diehn, M.; Nardini, C.; Wang, D.S.; McGovern, S.; Jayaraman, M.; Liang, Y.; Aldape, K.; Cha, S.; Kuo, M.D. Identification of noninvasive imaging surrogates for brain tumor gene-expression modules. *Proc. Natl. Acad. Sci. USA* **2008**, *105*, 5213–5218. [CrossRef]
21. Segal, E.; Sirlin, C.B.; Ooi, C.; Adler, A.S.; Gollub, J.; Chen, X.; Chan, B.K.; Matcuk, G.R.; Barry, C.T.; Chang, H.Y.; et al. Decoding global gene expression programs in liver cancer by noninvasive imaging. *Nat. Biotechnol.* **2007**, *25*, 675–680. [CrossRef] [PubMed]
22. Li, H.; Zhu, Y.; Burnside, E.S.; Huang, E.; Drukker, K.; Hoadley, K.A.; Fan, C.; Conzen, S.D.; Zuley, M.; Net, J.M.; et al. Quantitative MRI radiomics in the prediction of molecular classifications of breast cancer subtypes in the TCGA/TCIA data set. *npj Breast Cancer* **2016**, *2*, 16012. [CrossRef] [PubMed]
23. Monti, S.; Aiello, M.; Incoronato, M.; Grimaldi, A.M.; Moscarino, M.; Mirabelli, P.; Ferbo, U.; Cavaliere, C.; Salvatore, M. DCE-MRI pharmacokinetic-based phenotyping of invasive ductal carcinoma: A radiomic study for prediction of histological outcomes. *Contrast Media Mol. Imaging* **2018**, *2018*, 5076269. [CrossRef] [PubMed]
24. Yip, S.S.F.; Aerts, H.J.W.L. Applications and limitations of radiomics. *Phys. Med. Biol.* **2016**, *61*, R150–R166. [CrossRef] [PubMed]
25. Chaddad, A.; Kucharczyk, M.J.; Niazi, T. Multimodal radiomic features for the predicting gleason score of prostate cancer. *Cancers* **2018**, *10*, 249. [CrossRef] [PubMed]
26. Chaddad, A.; Niazi, T.; Probst, S.; Bladou, F.; Anidjar, M.; Bahoric, B. Predicting Gleason score of prostate cancer patients using radiomic analysis. *Front. Oncol.* **2018**, *8*, 630. [CrossRef]
27. Chen, T.; Li, M.; Gu, Y.; Zhang, Y.; Yang, S.; Wei, C.; Wu, J.; Li, X.; Zhao, W.; Shen, J. Prostate cancer differentiation and aggressiveness: Assessment with a radiomic-based model vs. PI-RADS v2. *J. Magn. Reson. Imaging* **2019**, *49*, 875–884. [CrossRef]
28. Hermie, I.; Van Besien, J.; De Visschere, P.; Lumen, N.; Decaestecker, K. Which clinical and radiological characteristics can predict clinically significant prostate cancer in PI-RADS 3 lesions? A retrospective study in a high-volume academic center. *Eur. J. Radiol.* **2019**, *114*, 92–98. [CrossRef]
29. Wang, J.; Wu, C.J.; Bao, M.L.; Zhang, J.; Wang, X.N.; Zhang, Y.D. Machine learning-based analysis of MR radiomics can help to improve the diagnostic performance of PI-RADS v2 in clinically relevant prostate cancer. *Eur. Radiol.* **2017**, *27*, 4082–4090. [CrossRef]
30. Hectors, S.J.; Cherny, M.; Yadav, K.K.; Beksaç, A.T.; Thulasidass, H.; Lewis, S.; Davicioni, E.; Wang, P.; Tewari, A.K.; Taouli, B. Radiomics features measured with multiparametric magnetic resonance imaging predict prostate cancer aggressiveness. *J. Urol.* **2019**, *202*, 498–505. [CrossRef]
31. Toivonen, J.; Perez, I.M.; Movahedi, P.; Merisaari, H.; Pesola, M.; Taimen, P.; Boström, P.J.; Pohjankukka, J.; Kiviniemi, A.; Pahikkala, T.; et al. Radiomics and machine learning of multisequence multiparametric

prostate MRI: Towards improved non-invasive prostate cancer characterization. *PLoS ONE* **2019**, *14*, e0217702. [CrossRef] [PubMed]
32. Franiel, T.; Hamm, B.; Hricak, H. Dynamic contrast-enhanced magnetic resonance imaging and pharmacokinetic models in prostate cancer. *Eur. Radiol.* **2011**, *21*, 616–626. [CrossRef] [PubMed]
33. Dercle, L.; Ammari, S.; Bateson, M.; Durand, P.B.; Haspinger, E.; Massard, C.; Jaudet, C.; Varga, A.; Deutsch, E.; Soria, J.C.; et al. Limits of radiomic-based entropy as a surrogate of tumor heterogeneity: ROI-area, acquisition protocol and tissue site exert substantial influence. *Sci. Rep.* **2017**, *7*, 7952. [CrossRef] [PubMed]
34. Greer, M.D.; Brown, A.M.; Shih, J.H.; Summers, R.M.; Marko, J.; Law, Y.M.; Sankineni, S.; George, A.K.; Merino, M.J.; Pinto, P.A.; et al. Accuracy and agreement of PIRADSv2 for prostate cancer mpMRI: A multireader study. *J. Magn. Reson. Imaging* **2017**, *45*, 579–585. [CrossRef] [PubMed]
35. Greer, M.D.; Shih, J.H.; Lay, N.; Barrett, T.; Kayat Bittencourt, L.; Borofsky, S.; Kabakus, I.M.; Law, Y.M.; Marko, J.; Shebel, H.; et al. Validation of the dominant sequence paradigm and role of dynamic contrast-enhanced imaging in PI-RADS version 2. *Radiology* **2017**, *285*, 859–869. [CrossRef] [PubMed]
36. Taghipour, M.; Ziaei, A.; Alessandrino, F.; Hassanzadeh, E.; Harisinghani, M.; Vangel, M.; Tempany, C.M.; Fennessy, F.M. Investigating the role of DCE-MRI, over T2 and DWI, in accurate PI-RADS v2 assessment of clinically significant peripheral zone prostate lesions as defined at radical prostatectomy. *Abdom. Radiol.* **2019**, *44*, 1520–1527. [CrossRef]
37. Parmar, C.; Velazquez, E.R.; Leijenaar, R.; Jermoumi, M.; Carvalho, S.; Mak, R.H.; Mitra, S.; Shankar, B.U.; Kikinis, R.; Haibe-Kains, B.; et al. Robust radiomics feature quantification using semiautomatic volumetric segmentation. *PLoS ONE* **2014**, *9*, e102107. [CrossRef]
38. O'Connor, J.P.B.; Rose, C.J.; Waterton, J.C.; Carano, R.A.D.; Parker, G.J.M.; Jackson, A. Imaging intratumor heterogeneity: Role in therapy response, resistance, and clinical outcome. *Clin. Cancer Res.* **2015**, *21*, 249–257. [CrossRef]
39. Baldi, D.; Aiello, M.; Duggento, A.; Salvatore, M.; Cavaliere, C. MR imaging-histology correlation by tailored 3d-printed slicer in oncological assessment. *Contrast Media Mol. Imaging* **2019**, *2019*, 1071453. [CrossRef]
40. Vargas, H.A.; Hötker, A.M.; Goldman, D.A.; Moskowitz, C.S.; Gondo, T.; Matsumoto, K.; Ehdaie, B.; Woo, S.; Fine, S.W.; Reuter, V.E.; et al. Updated prostate imaging reporting and data system (PIRADS v2) recommendations for the detection of clinically significant prostate cancer using multiparametric MRI: Critical evaluation using whole-mount pathology as standard of reference. *Eur. Radiol.* **2016**, *26*, 1606–1612. [CrossRef]
41. Tofts, P.S.; Parker, G.J.M. DCE-MRI: Acquisition and analysis techniques. In *Clinical Perfusion MRI: Techniques and Applications*; Cambridge University Press: Cambridge, UK, 2013; pp. 58–74.
42. Klein, S.; Staring, M.; Murphy, K.; Viergever, M.A.; Pluim, J.P.W. Elastix: A toolbox for intensity-based medical image registration. *IEEE Trans. Med. Imaging* **2010**. [CrossRef]
43. Collewet, G.; Strzelecki, M.; Mariette, F. Influence of MRI acquisition protocols and image intensity normalization methods on texture classification. *Magn. Reson. Imaging* **2004**, *22*, 81–91. [CrossRef] [PubMed]
44. Haralick, R.M.; Dinstein, I.; Shanmugam, K. Textural features for image classification. *IEEE Trans. Syst. Man Cybern.* **1973**, *3*, 610–621. [CrossRef]
45. Vallières, M.; Freeman, C.R.; Skamene, S.R.; El Naqa, I. A radiomics model from joint FDG-PET and MRI texture features for the prediction of lung metastases in soft-tissue sarcomas of the extremities. *Phys. Med. Biol.* **2015**, *60*, 5471–5496. [CrossRef] [PubMed]
46. Reshef, D.N.; Reshef, Y.A.; Finucane, H.K.; Grossman, S.R.; McVean, G.; Turnbaugh, P.J.; Lander, E.S.; Mitzenmacher, M.; Sabeti, P.C. Detecting novel associations in large data sets. *Science* **2011**, *334*, 1518–1524. [CrossRef] [PubMed]
47. Sahiner, B.; Chan, H.P.; Hadjiiski, L. Classifier performance prediction for computer-aided diagnosis using a limited dataset. *Med. Phys.* **2008**, *35*, 1559–1570. [CrossRef]

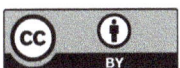

© 2020 by the authors. Licensee MDPI, Basel, Switzerland. This article is an open access article distributed under the terms and conditions of the Creative Commons Attribution (CC BY) license (http://creativecommons.org/licenses/by/4.0/).

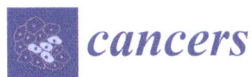

Article

Role of Baseline and Post-Therapy 18F-FDG PET in the Prognostic Stratification of Metastatic Castration-Resistant Prostate Cancer (mCRPC) Patients Treated with Radium-223

Matteo Bauckneht [1,*], Selene Capitanio [1], Maria Isabella Donegani [2], Elisa Zanardi [3,4], Alberto Miceli [2], Roberto Murialdo [5], Stefano Raffa [2], Laura Tomasello [3], Martina Vitti [2], Alessia Cavo [6], Fabio Catalano [7], Manlio Mencoboni [6], Marcello Ceppi [8], Cecilia Marini [2,9], Giuseppe Fornarini [7], Francesco Boccardo [3,4], Gianmario Sambuceti [1,2] and Silvia Morbelli [1,2]

1. Nuclear Medicine Unit, IRCCS Ospedale Policlinico San Martino, 16132 Genoa, Italy; selene.capitanio@hsanmartino.it (S.C.); sambuceti@unige.it (G.S.); silviadaniela.morbelli@hsanmartino.it (S.M.)
2. Department of Health Sciences (DISSAL), University of Genova, 16132 Genoa, Italy; isabella.donegani@gmail.com (M.I.D.); albertomiceli23@gmail.com (A.M.); stefanoraffa@live.com (S.R.); vitti.martina@hotmail.it (M.V.); cecilia.marini@unige.it (C.M.)
3. Academic Unit of Medical Oncology, IRCCS Ospedale Policlinico San Martino, 16132 Genoa, Italy; elisa.zanardi@unige.it (E.Z.); laura.tomasello@hsanmartino.it (L.T.); fboccardo@unige.it (F.B.)
4. Department of Internal Medicine and Medical Specialties (DIMI), University of Genoa, 16132 Genoa, Italy
5. Internal Medicine Unit, IRCCS Ospedale Policlinico San Martino, 16132 Genoa, Italy; roberto.murialdo@hsanmartino.it
6. Oncology Unit, Villa Scassi Hospital, 16149, Genova, Italy; alessia.cavo@asl3.liguria.it (A.C.); manlio.mencoboni@asl3.liguria.it (M.M.)
7. Medical Oncology Unit, IRCCS Ospedale Policlinico San Martino, 16132 Genoa, Italy; catalan.fab@gmail.com (F.C.); giuseppe.fornarini@hsanmartino.it (G.F.)
8. Clinical Epidemiology Unit, IRCCS Ospedale Policlinico San Martino, 16132 Genoa, Italy; marcello.ceppi@hsanmartino.it
9. CNR Institute of Molecular Bioimaging and Physiology (IBFM), 20090 Segrate (MI), Italy
* Correspondence: matteo.bauckneht@hsanmartino.it; Tel.: +39-0105553038; Fax: +39-0105556911

Received: 26 November 2019; Accepted: 17 December 2019; Published: 20 December 2019

Abstract: Radium-223 dichloride (Ra223) represents the unique bone-directed treatment option that shows an improvement in overall survival (OS) in metastatic castrate resistant prostate cancer (mCRPC). However, there is an urgent need for the identification of reliable biomarkers to non-invasively determine its efficacy (possibly improving patients' selection or identifying responders' after therapy completion). 18F-Fluorodeoxyglucose (FDG)-avidity is low in naïve prostate cancer, but it is enhanced in advanced and chemotherapy-refractory mCRPC, providing prognostic insights. Moreover, this tool showed high potential for the evaluation of response in cancer patients with bone involvement. For these reasons, FDG Positron Emission Tomography (FDG-PET) might represent an effective tool that is able to provide prognostic stratification (improving patients selection) at baseline and assessing the treatment response to Ra223. We conducted a retrospective analysis of 28 mCRPC patients that were treated with Ra223 and submitted to bone scan and FDG-PET/CT for prognostic purposes at baseline and within two months after therapy completion. The following parameters were measured: number of bone lesions at bone scan, SUVmax of the hottest bone lesion, metabolic tumor volume (MTV), and total lesion glycolysis (TLG). In patients who underwent post-therapy 18F-Fluorodeoxyglucose Positron Emission Tomography/Computed Tomography (FDG-PET/CT), (20/28), PET Response Criteria in Solid Tumors (PERCIST), and European Organization for Research and Treatment of Cancer (EORTC) criteria were applied to evaluate the metabolic treatment response. The difference between end of therapy and baseline values was also calculated for Metabolic Tumor Volume (MTV),

TLG, prostate-specific antigen (PSA), alkaline phosphatase (AP), and lactate dehydrogenase (LDH) (termed deltaMTV, deltaTLG, deltaPSA, deltaAP and deltaLDH, respectively). Predictive power of baseline and post-therapy PET- and biochemical-derived parameters on OS were assessed by Kaplan–Meier, univariate and multivariate analyses. At baseline, PSA, LDH, and MTV significantly predicted OS. However, MTV (but not PSA nor LDH) was able to identify a subgroup of patients with worse prognosis, even after adjusting for the number of lesions at bone scan (which, in turn, was not an independent predictor of OS). After therapy, PERCIST criteria were able to capture the response to Ra223 by demonstrating longer OS in patients with partial metabolic response. Moreover, the biochemical parameters were outperformed by PERCIST in the post-treatment setting, as their variation after therapy was not informative on long term OS. The present study supports the role of FDG-PET as a tool for patient's selection and response assessment in mCRPC patients undergoing Ra223 administration.

Keywords: Radium-223; positron emission tomography; FDG; castrate resistant prostate cancer

1. Introduction

Radium-223 dichloride (Ra223) is a radionuclide that selectively binds to areas of increased bone turnover in bone metastases. The short range of energy delivery that is typical of its apha-emission makes Ra223 an effective therapeutic approach for symptomatic patients with bone metastatic castration-resistant prostate cancer (mCRPC) [1].

Besides documenting its effect on pain palliation, the pivotal phase 3 Alpharadin in Symptomatic Prostate Cancer Patients (ALSYMPCA) trial demonstrated the prognostic benefit that is induced by this radio-metabolic approach that prolonged overall survival (OS) and delayed time to the first symptomatic skeletal event with respect to the placebo arm [1]. However, in the last few years, some retrospective studies suggested that the OS benefit in real-life patients might be lower than that reported in the ALSYMPCA study [2–5]. These evidences might be explained either by the suboptimal sequence of Ra223 use in the castrate-resistant phase or as the result of a suboptimal selection of patients with poorer prognostic clinical characteristics. A similar consideration also applies to the monitoring of therapy effectiveness: a number of limitations hamper the direct evaluation of bone lesion evolution asking for a combined approach while using clinical, biochemical (e.g. prostate-specific antigen (PSA), serum alkaline phosphatase (AP)), and imaging assessments [6]. However, this approach is also hampered by the so-called flare effect: the early and transient rise in the PSA levels or tracer uptake at bone scan, followed by a later decline that is commonly observed in prostate cancer patients treated with chemotherapy, luteinizing hormone-releasing hormone, and even Ra223 [7]. Indeed, the role of imaging for capturing response to Ra223 is still unclear and data regarding the most accurate modality for evaluating treated patients are lacking.

In this framework, while 18F-Fluorodeoxyglucose Positron Emission Tomography/Computed Tomography (FDG-PET/CT) is not indicated in naïve prostate cancer, as they have low FDG-avidity, mCRPC patients, and, even more, chemotherapy-refractory mCRPC are characterized by higher FDG uptake. For this reason, FDG has been proposed as a tool that is able to aggressively identify disease in mCRPC [8–11], and more in general molecular imaging with PET has high potential for the evaluation of response in cancer patients with bone involvement [12]. Based on these considerations, FDG-PET/CT might represent an effective tool for measuring disease burden and aggressiveness at baseline and for assessing the treatment response to Ra223 in mCRPC.

In the present retrospective, single center study, we aimed to evaluate the potential role of FDG-PET/CT in patient's selection and evaluation of response in a cohort of mCRPC treated with Ra223. To this aim, FDG-avid metabolic tumor burden at baseline and post-therapy of patients that were treated with Ra223 was computed and its relationship with biochemical parameters as well as progression-free (PFS) and overall survival (OS) was assessed.

2. Patients and Methods

2.1. Study Protocol

We conducted a retrospective review of mCRPC patients treated with Ra223 and submitted to FDG-PET/CT at baseline and within two months after therapy between September 2016 and November 2018 in our institution. All of the patients with an available baseline FDG-PET/CT scan were included (regardless of the availability of a post-therapy scan). By contrast, patients with an available post-therapy were only included when a baseline scan was available in the 30 days preceding Ra223 administration. Patients were candidate to FDG-PET/CT, in agreement with the evidence reported in national guidelines of the Italian Association of Medical Oncology (AOIM) on the emerging role of FDG-PET/CT in patients with mCRPC or in patients with poorly differentiated prostate cancer (Gleason score ≥ 8) [13,14]. According to our standard procedure, all of the patients signed a written informed consent form, which encompassed the use of anonymized data for retrospective research purposes, before each PET/CT scan.

All of the patients obviously had to fulfill all of the inclusion criteria for Ra223 treatment and they were treated with standard Ra223 regimen encompassing six administrations every four weeks (55 KBq/kg, intravenously). According to the established selection criteria for Ra223 patient's selection [13], in the previous four weeks preceding the first administration, each patient underwent contrast enhanced CT (ceCT) and bone scan, in order to select mCRPC patients with symptomatic bone metastases in the absence of visceral metastases (with the exception for lymph nodes with maximum diameter < 3 cm). Similarly, a bone marrow reserve fulfilling the hematologic criteria necessary for administering Ra223 and Eastern Cooperative Oncology Group (ECOG) performance status of 0–1 (life expectancy greater than six months) were verified [13]. Clinical and biochemical variables at baseline, in course and at the end of therapy, also had to be available at the time of our study. These variables included: ECOG performance status, PSA, AP, and lactate dehydrogenase (LDH). During treatment, the patients were maintained under androgen deprivation therapy.

2.2. Imaging Procedures

Bone scan and FDG-PET/CT were performed according to European Association of Nuclear Medicine (EANM) Guidelines [15,16], as detailed in the Supplementary Materials. Briefly, bone scan was acquired 3 h after the injection of 740 MBq of 99mTc-methilen diphosphonate. A dual-head gamma camera (Millennium; GE Healthcare, Boston, USA) that was equipped with a parallel-hole, low-energy, high-resolution collimator on a 10% energy window centered on the 99mTc photopeak was used to acquire planar whole-body acquisitions, and, if needed, Single Photon Emission Computed Tomography (SPECT) images. FDG-PET/CT was performed while using a 16-slices PET/CT hybrid system (Hirez-Biograph 16, Siemens Medical Solutions, Munich, Germany). After blood glucose levels measurement (to ensure blood glucose levels <160 mg/dL), fasting patients underwent the intravenous injection of 300–400 MBq of FDG. The patients were asked to drink 500 mL of water 1h prior to image acquisition and empty the bladder just before the acquisition start. Imaging started 60 ± 15 minutes after tracer administration. The acquired PET data were reconstructed into a 128 × 128 matrix using an iterative reconstruction algorithm (three iterative steps, eight subsets). Raw images were scatter-corrected and processed while using a three-dimensional (3D) Gaussian filter, while CT was used for attenuation correction. Image quality control documented a spatial resolution of 4.0 mm full width at half-maximum.

2.3. Image Analysis

The bone scan images were qualitatively evaluated, and number of lesions present at baseline and after therapy was recorded. The following semiquantitative parameters were computed on both baseline and post-therapy FDG-PET/CT scans: maximum standard uptake value (SUVmax) of the hottest bone lesion, Metabolic Tumor Volume (MTV) and Total Lesion Glycolysis (TLG). MTV was estimated from the volumes of interest SUV isocontours that were automatically drawn by setting a relative threshold of 40% of the SUVmax [17]. TLG was calculated as SUVmean × MTV. All of the semiquantitative variables were estimated at baseline and after therapy to calculate their difference (termed deltaMTV and deltaTLG, respectively). However, deltaSUVmax was not calculated, as the hottest bone lesion at post-therapy FDG-PET/CT might not correspond to the hottest lesion at baseline. The metabolic response to Ra223 was also evaluated by two independent readers (MB, SM) while using PET Response Criteria in Solid Tumors (PERCIST) and European Organization for Research and Treatment of Cancer (EORTC) criteria [18,19], see also Supplementary Materials for details on PERCIST and EORTC criteria). The PET readers were blinded to ceCT and bone scan results. DeltaPSA, deltaAP, and deltaLDH were also calculated as the difference between post-therapy and baseline levels.

2.4. Statistical Analysis

PFS and OS curves were computed according to Kaplan–Meier with the Log Rank test determining statistical significance. This analysis was performed by dividing the population into tertiles for all tested variables, with the only exception of bone scan lesions whose number was divided in ≤ 6, 6–20, and > 20, as performed in a sub-analysis of the ALSYMPCA study [1]. A binary classification of response to therapy was applied to PERCIST scores due to the small numbers involved, as previously described [20]. In particular, patients showing partial metabolic response (PMR) were considered as "responders", while stable metabolic disease (SMD) and progressive metabolic disease (PMD) were classified as "non-responders". A set of univariate and multivariate Cox proportional hazard models were fitted to the data to assess the predictive value of baseline parameters: in univariate analyses, OS and PFS were modeled as a function of each tested variable. Subsequently, all of the tested variables were tentatively included in a multivariate Cox's model by means of a step-down (backward) procedure, based on the likelihood ratio test: variables with a p value < 0.1 were removed from the model. Proportionality assumptions were assessed, as previously described [21]. Analyses were conducted with IBM-SPSS release 23 (IBM, Armonk, USA).

3. Results

The interrogation of our database identified 28 mCRPC patients who met the inclusion criteria and they were submitted to baseline FDG-PET/CT. Within this cohort, six patients died before treatment completion, while two refused the post-therapy FDG-PET/CT, but were still alive at the time of database interrogation. Accordingly, functional imaging at both time points was available in 20 subjects. The median interval between the two PET/CT scan was 213 days. Table 1 summarizes the overall patient's characteristics. Once completed the treatment protocol, the 20 remaining patients were monitored for twelve months after the post-therapy PET/CT. During this one-year follow-up, further 10/20 (50%) patients died. Figure S1 reports OS in the whole study cohort (since treatment start).

3.1. Prognostic Role of Baseline Parameters

As shown in Figure 1, Kaplan–Meyer analysis revealed that the biochemical parameters PSA, AP, and LDH, as well as the FDG imaging ones MTV and TLG provided a risk stratification power. In fact, the death rate was highest in mCRPC patients' candidates to Ra223 clustered within the highest tertile for each of them ($p < 0.01$, respectively). By contrast, the whole body bone scan was devoid of this prognostic penetrance, since mortality rate was remarkably similar among patients with low, intermediate, or high number of detectable bone lesions [1]. Univariate analysis that reported a significant association between overall survival and PSA, LDH, and MTV confirmed this observation ($p < 0.01$ each, respectively), as shown in Table 2 (see also Table S1 for the univariate analysis including the same variables as categorial). Multivariate Cox Regression analysis reported that each of these variables was characterized an additive predictive capability (Table 2, see also Table S1 for the multivariate analysis, including the same variables as categorial). By contrast, no baseline clinical or imaging variable was able to predict the PFS.

Table 1. Patients characteristics.

	Baseline (n = 28)	End of Therapy (n = 20)	p
Age	76.71 ± 7.1	-	-
Gleason score at diagnosis	-	-	-
5	1 (3.6%)	-	-
6	6 (21.4%)	-	-
7	9 (32.1%)	-	-
8	9 (32.1%)	-	-
9	2 (7.2%)	-	-
10	1 (3.6%)	-	-
Time evolution of prostate cancer (months)	90.59 ± 156.3	-	-
Time gap from diagnosis to mCRPC (months)	40.22 ± 54.7	-	-
Number of previous systemic therapies for mCRPC	-	-	-
1	8 (28.6%)	-	-
2	6 (21.4%)	-	-
3	7 (25%)	-	-
4	6 (21.4%)	-	-
5	1 (3.6%)	-	-
ECOG score	-	-	-
0	5 (17%)	3 (15%)	p = ns
1	23 (82%)	17 (85%)	p = ns
Number of Ra223 administered doses	-	5.3 ± 1.1	-
Pain response	-	6 (30%)	-
Lab tests	-	-	-
Hemoglobin (g/dL)	12.34 ± 1.6	10.87 ± 1.1	$p < 0.05$
White Blood Cells (x10^9/L)	6.6 ± 2.2	5.5 ± 1.9	$p < 0.05$
Platelets (x10^9/L)	236 ± 72.9	214.7 ± 84.3	p = ns
PSA (ng/mL)	119.25 ± 171.5	347.80 ± 468.1	$p < 0.01$
AP (UI/L)	213.3 ± 295.4	133.46 ± 159.1	$p < 0.05$
LDH (UI/L)	265.23 ± 112.1	317.36 ± 241.9	$p < 0.05$
Bone scintigraphy parameters	-	-	-
1–6 lesions	7 (25%)	9 (45%)	p = ns
6-20 lesions	9 (32%)	3 (15%)	p = ns
> 20 lesions	9 (32%)	4 (20%)	p = ns
Superscan	3 (10%)	4 (20%)	p = ns
Extraosseus involvement	-	-	-
Lymph nodes	4 (14.3%)	6 (30%)	-
Prostate	2 (7%)	2 (1%)	-
FDG PET/CT parameters	-	-	-
SUVmax of the hottest bone lesion	7.25 ± 3.4	8.04 ± 4.3	ns
MTV (cm3)	352.71 ± 384.3	468.01 ± 489.9	$p < 0.01$
TLG	1358.92 ± 1560.9	1877.69 ± 2179.13	$p < 0.01$

Of note, focusing the survival analysis on the 12 patients showing >20 bone lesions at bone scan, neither PSA, AP, nor LDH serum levels significantly predicted OS, while MTV was able to stratify three different prognostic classes ($p < 0.01$, Figure 2). Again, the multivariate analysis confirmed these data (Cox Regression, backward stepwise, LR; $p < 0.0001$).

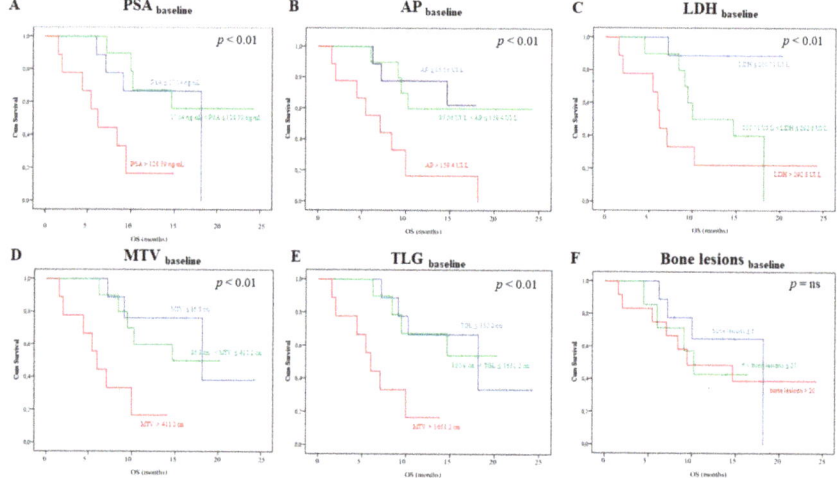

Figure 1. Kaplan–Meyer analysis including baseline biochemical and imaging variables. Each panel show the overall survival (OS) curves depending on baseline prostate-specific antigen (PSA), alkaline phosphatase (AP), lactate dehydrogenase (LDH), metabolic tumor volume (MTV), total lesion glycolysis (TLG), and bone lesions, respectively. In each case, but Panel F, patients were divided in three tertiles (first tertile: blue; second tertile: green; third tertile: orange). Following a subgroup analysis proposed in the ALSYMPCA study, in Panel F, patients were divided in three subgroups according to the number bone lesions at bone scan in < 6 (blue), 6–19 (green), and > 20 (orange) bone metastases, respectively.

Table 2. The prognostic role of baseline parameters: uni- and multivariate analyses.

	df	\multicolumn{4}{c}{Univariate Analysis}			\multicolumn{4}{c}{Multivariate Analysis}
	df	p	H.R.	\multicolumn{2}{c}{95% CI}	p	H.R.	\multicolumn{2}{c}{95% CI}
PSA	1	0.001	1.007	1.003 - 1.010	0.004	1.007	1.002 - 1.011
AP	1	0.020	1.001	0.000 - 0.001	0.443	*		
LDH	1	0.001	1.009	1.004 - 1.015	0.010	1.009	1.002 - 1.016
Number of bone lesions	1	0.960	1.009	−0.002 - 0.019	0.300	*		
SUVmax	1	0.976	1.001	−0.055 - 0.057	0.204	*		
MTV	1	0.001	1.002	1.001 - 1.003	0.044	1.002	1.000 - 1.003
TLG	1	0.134	5×10^{-005}	0.339 - 0.733	0.411	*		

* = excluded from the final model.

3.2. FDG PET/CT in the Response Evaluation Following Ra223

Table 1 sumamrizes the overall clinical characteristics of the 20 patients who underwent FDG-PET/CT post therapy evaluation. Ra223 administration caused a measurable response in most of the tested variables. In particular, hematopoietic response was confirmed by a decrease in hemoglobin levels and in white blood cells count, while the decrease in platelet number did not reach the statistical significance. AP showed a significant decrease. Nevertheless, the suggested reduction in osteoblastic activity was devoid of any significant risk prediction power, as reported in Supplementary Materials Figure S2, Panel B. The tumor burden indexes showed an opposite response that roughly approached 25% for LDH and almost 300% for PSA. Again, this response was not able to stratify patient's outcome (Figure S2, Panels A and C), which confirmed a relevant interference of the so-called "flair effect" after radiometabolic treatment of bone lesions.

A completely different consideration applied to imaging indexes of treatment effectiveness. PERCIST scores significantly predicted OS (Figure 3, $p < 0.05$), while this prognostic penetrance did not reach statistical significance for EORTC, deltaMTV, and deltaTLG evaluations.

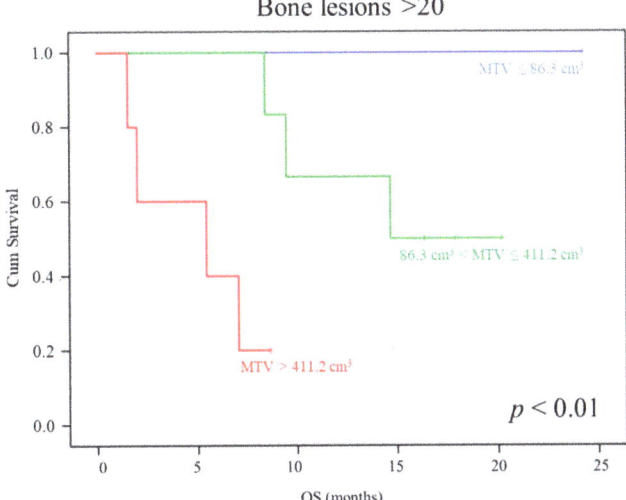

Figure 2. MTV prognostic power in patients showing >20 lesions at bone scan. OS curves depending on baseline MTV (first tertile: blue; second tertile: green; third tertile: orange) in the subgroup of patients showing > 20 bone lesions at bone scan.

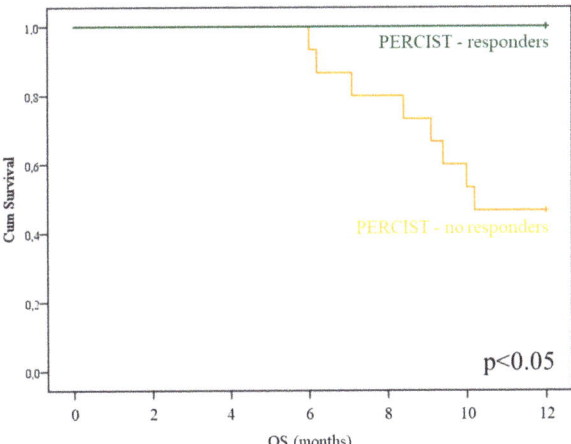

Figure 3. PET Response Criteria in Solid Tumors (PERCIST) prognostic power in Radium-223 treated patients. OS curves depending on PERCIST score (PMR: blue; SMD+PMD: green) in the subgroup of patients submitted to post-therapy 18F-Fluorodeoxyglucose Positron Emission Tomography/Computed Tomography (FDG-PET/CT).

Multivariate Cox analysis, including deltaPSA, deltaAP, deltaLDH, and PERCIST score, confirmed the additive value of PERCIST score with respect to all of the remaining variables ($p = 0.012$). In agreement with this finding, the imaging index virtually preserved its capability to predict the response to treatment in patients with the highest increase in PSA after Ra223 administration, as suggested by the almost significant p value ($p = 0.1$ in each subgroup, see also Figure 4) and the emblematic example reported in Figure 5.

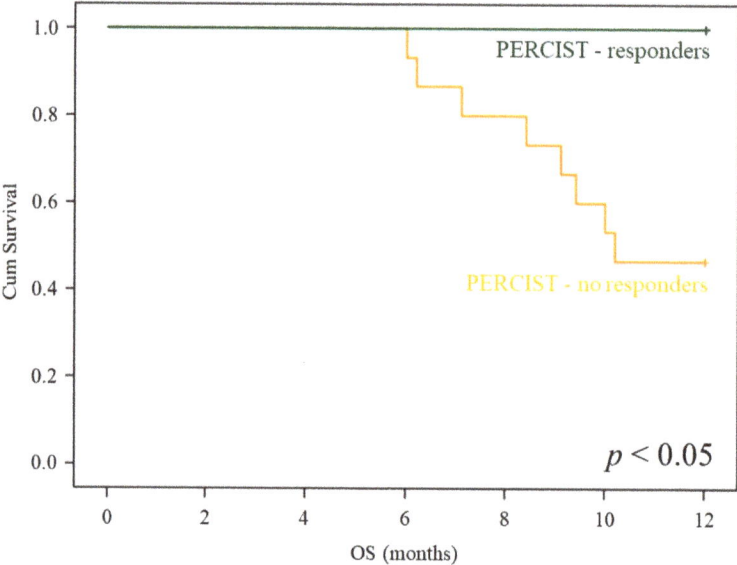

Figure 4. PERCIST prognostic stratification in deltaPSA classes. OS curves depending on PERCIST score (PMR: blue; SMD+PMD: green) in the subgroups of patients submitted to post-therapy FDG-PET/CT classified on the basis of the deltaPSA class.

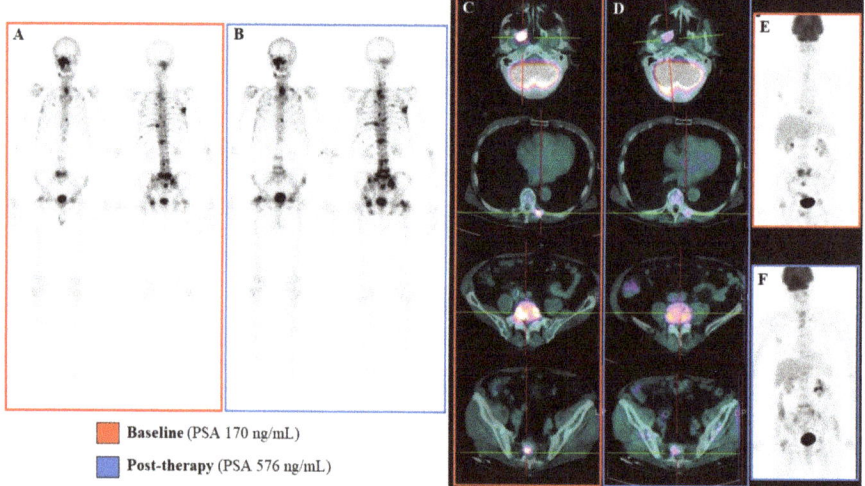

Figure 5. Emblematic example of mismatch between metabolic and biochemical/bone scan response. In this emblematic case a mismatch between metabolic data and biochemical/bone scan results was observed. At baseline the bone scan revealed the presence of several osteoblastic bone lesions (Panel **A**) that were mainly FDG-avid (Panels **C** and **E**). The post-therapy evaluation, performed six weeks after Ra223 protocol completion, showed the persistence of osteoblastic bone lesions that were occasionally more extended and diphosphonate-avid (Panel **B**). This finding was paralleled by increased serum PSA levels (576 vs 170 ng/mL at baseline). However, the post-therapy FDG PET/CT showed a significant reduction in bone lesions FDG uptake, leading to a Partial Metabolic Response according to PERCIST criteria (Panels **D** and **F**).

4. Discussion

The present results support the role of both baseline and post-therapy FDG-PET/CT in mCRPC patients treated with Ra223. In fact, MTV evaluation of baseline metabolically active skeletal disease burden was able to predict OS with an additive independent value, as documented by multivariate Cox regression analysis. By contrast, the number of lesions, as assessed by bone scan, was characterized by a largely less evident prognostic penetrance. Similarly, biochemical biomarkers PSA, AP, and LDH confirmed their predictive value when assessed before Ra223 treatment. However, their response to therapy was virtually devoid of any prognostic penetrance. By contrast, PET-based evaluations and, in particular, PERCIST criteria, were able to predict the response to Ra223 by demonstrating a lower mortality rate in patients with partial metabolic response.

4.1. Patient's Selection for Ra223

Patients' selection is a crucial point when discussing the role of Ra223 in mCRPC patients. In 2018, the European Medicines Agency (EMA) issued a specific note on the indications for treatment with Ra223 in a review of an ongoing phase 3 trial by the EMA's Pharmacovigilance Risk Assessment Committee, basically moving Ra223 to a third-line of treatment of mCRPC patients (EMA/500948/2018; https://www.ema.europa.eu/en/documents/press-release/ema-restricts-use-prostate-cancer-medicine-xofigo_en.pdf). The observation of increased the risk of fractures, in the absence of statistically significant survival benefit in patients with <6 bone lesions enrolled in the ERA-223 study, receiving Ra223 in combination with abiraterone acetate plus prednisone/prednisolone, motivated this action [22]. In fact, patients with lower skeletal disease burden might have a larger proportion of Ra223 homing to healthy bone, as compared to patients with extensive bone metastases. Indeed, sites of bony metastases are known to have a higher bone turnover and the sequestration of administered Ra223 (the so-called "sink-effect"), which might limit Ra223 deposition in the non-diseased skeleton [23,24]. However, besides the mere number of bone lesions, a huge variability in Ra223-avid bone disease can be observed. Preclinical prostate cancer models showed that the short range of alpha particles results in a lower tumor control-rate of large metastatic deposits as compared to near eradication of small lesions [25]. These data suggest the inadequacy of the mere bone lesion number count in the identification of the right candidate to Ra223.

Previous studies showed that the quantification of skeletal tumor burden by means of bone scintigraphy or 18F-NaF PET/CT might predict patients' OS and reflect the risk of hematological toxicity related to Ra223 administration [26,27]. The present study is in keeping with these evidences as also FDG-PET/CT-derived tumor volume and not the mere number of bone lesions predicted patients' prognosis. However, the present findings further extend this evidence by demonstrating the specific weight of metabolic active tumor burden.

Indeed, the higher predictive value of 18F-FDG PET/CT with respect to bone scan might be due to its capability to capture bone marrow involvement, which is obviously underestimated by the simple osteoblastic bone disease detected by bone scan (and even by 18F-NaF-PET/CT) [28]. On the other hand, the detection of FDG-avid de-differentiated and non-osteoblastic bone disease [10,29,30] might mirror greater tumour aggressiveness, also possibly predicting the lower Ra223 accumulation and the consequent low-response rate. Moreover, as the added prognostic value of the extent of metabolic active disease was preserved in patients showing >20 bone lesions at bone scan, FDG-PET/CT might play a role in the selection of patients with larger tumour burden. This finding is of potential clinical relevance, since high-volume bone disease predicts higher degrees of haematological toxicity and the selection of this group of patients for Ra223 should be even more thoughtful [26,31]. Finally, if confirmed in larger studies, the highlighted FDG-PET/CT capability rule out high-risk candidates to Ra223 might be relevant for the cost/effectiveness of Ra223 administration, thus reducing the risk of ineffective treatments in patients with worst prognosis and higher risk of hematological toxicity.

4.2. Post-Therapy Assessment

In the ALSYMPCA trial, Ra223 showed a modest effect on serum PSA levels, which reached a ≥30% reduction in just 16% of treated patients, despite improving OS [1]. Moreover, a minor correlation between OS and PSA changes at week 12 was observed [32] and, especially during the first three months of treatment, possible flare phenomena have been described [33–35]. AP and LDH kinetics under Ra223 administration has been proposed as an alternative approach to the PSA monitoring [1,36]. However, post-hoc analyses from the ALSYMPCA trial showed that these biomarkers did not meet the needed statistical surrogacy requirement for OS [32]. Therefore, the low predictive value of these biochemical biomarkers raises the urgent need for the identification of novel biomarkers, even if the dynamic monitoring of AP and LDH serum levels is still recommended during Ra223 administration.

Even though imaging was not routinely performed in the ALSYMPCA trial, imaging with bone-targeted radiopharmaceuticals has been proposed as a tool for monitoring treatment response when clinically indicated [1]. However, bon flare phenomenon resulting in false-positive tracer uptake, even in responsive cases, has been described [23,37,38], which complicates the evaluation of response at a single patient level. Recently, the 2 + 2 rule has been proposed for overcoming this limitation of osteotropic radiotracers [26,34,39]. However, its reliability in the clinical setting still needs to be validated. On the other hand, ceCT scan can be used in case of suspicious disease progression. However, in prostate cancer metastatic lymph nodes can be normal sized resulting false-negative at anatomic imaging [40,41], profoundly underpowering the accuracy of this tool in the evaluation of response to Ra223. In this scenario, 18F-Fluorocholine or 68Ga-PSMA PET/CT have been recently proposed as promising tools for monitoring the response to Ra223 treatment [31,42–45].

To the best of our knowledge, a case report of mCRPC [46], a small case series [47], and a phase IIa metastatic breast cancer study represent the sole available reports on FDG-PET/CT used for the evaluation of Ra223 response [48]. In the present study, the application of PERCIST criteria to FDG-PET/CT images overpowered bone scan and biochemical parameters in the evaluation of response to Ra223 treatment. Moreover, a trend in the post-treatment prognostic assessment was maintained when the PERCIST classes were analyzed in patients experiencing an increase in PSA levels. This latter finding suggests the potential role for FDG-PET/CT in the identification of the PSA-flare phenomenon. The observed discordance in the bone imaging patterns between bone scan and FDG-PET/CT after Ra223 administration might be related to bone marrow metastases, which cannot be detected by bone scintigraphy. Importantly, these discordances have been observed, not only in case of disease progression, but also in metabolic responders, although the magnitude of this discordance seems to be larger in cases of progression. On one side, this finding fits with the acknowledged limited efficacy of Ra223 in bone marrow metastases, as consistent with its mode of action [34,49–51]. On the other hand, it highlights a need for optimal clinical management of Ra223-treated patients who present with marrow metastases at baseline.

4.3. Limitations

The present study has some drawbacks. First, the relatively small population. However, its monocentric nature represents one of its strengths. Accordingly, all of the enrolled patients were submitted to FDG-PET/CT while using the same PET/CT scanner avoiding the possible influence of inter-scanner variability on PET results. Second, in the multivariate analyses, we did not consider other potential prognostic factors in the cohort able to influence OS and, consequently, the impact of the different response criteria investigated. Finally, bone scan images were qualitatively evaluated, while the application of semi-quantification tools [26,52] might have provided the estimation of the "osteoblastic tumor volume", improving the comparison between bone scan and metabolic parameters that were obtained by FDG-PET/CT.

5. Conclusions

FDG-PET/CT can represent a widely available method for directly measuring active de-differentiated tumor burden in mCRPC patients' candidates to Ra223, providing prognostic information overpowering biochemical and other imaging parameters. After treatment, it can assess tumor load reduction particularly in patients showing increased PSA, helping in the differential diagnosis between progression and pseudoprogression (related to the PSA flare phenomenon).

Supplementary Materials: The following are available online at http://www.mdpi.com/2072-6694/12/1/31/s1: Supplementary Materials, Table S1: prognostic role of baseline parameters as categorical variables: uni- and multivariate analyses. Figure S1: OS in the whole study cohort. Figure S2: Reduction in osteoblastic activity.

Author Contributions: Study concept and design M.B., S.M., G.S., S.C.; recruitment and collection data: M.I.D., E.Z., A.M., S.R., L.T., R.M., M.V., A.C., F.C., M.M., G.F., C.M.; quality control of data and algorithm: M.B.; data analysis, statistical analysis and interpretation: M.B., M.C., G.S.; manuscript preparation: M.B., S.C., S.M., G.S.; editing, review, supervision, approval final version of the manuscript, all authors. All authors have read and agreed to the published version of the manuscript.

Funding: M.B. and S.M. were supported by grants from Italian Ministry of Health—5 × 1000 funds 2016.

Conflicts of Interest: SM received speaker honoraria from General Electric and Eli-Lilly. The other authors declare they have no conflict of interest.

References

1. Parker, C.; Nilsson, S.; Heinrich, D.; Helle, S.I.; O'Sullivan, J.M.; Fosså, S.D.; Chodacki, A.; Wiechno, P.; Logue, J.; Seke, M.; et al. ALSYMPCA Investigators. Alpha emitter radium-223 and survival in metastatic prostate cancer. *N. Engl. J. Med.* **2013**, *369*, 213–223. [CrossRef] [PubMed]
2. Parikh, S.; Murray, L.; Kenning, L.; Bottomley, D.; Din, O.; Dixit, S.; Ferguson, C.; Handforth, C.; Joseph, L.; Mokhtar, D.; et al. Real-world outcomes and factors predicting survival and completion of radium 223 in metastatic castrate-resistant prostate cancer. *Clin. Oncol.* **2018**, *30*, 548–555. [CrossRef] [PubMed]
3. Wong, W.W.; Anderson, E.M.; Mohammadi, H.; Daniels, T.B.; Schild, S.E.; Keole, S.R.; Choo, C.R.; Tzou, K.S.; Bryce, A.H.; Ho, T.H.; et al. Factors associated with survival following radium-223 treatment for metastatic castration-resistant prostate cancer. *Clin. Genitourin. Cancer* **2017**, *15*, e969–e975. [CrossRef] [PubMed]
4. Frantellizzi, V.; Farcomeni, A.; Follacchio, G.A.; Pacilio, M.; Pellegrini, R.; Pani, R.; De Vincentis, G. A 3-variable prognostic score (3-PS) for overall survival prediction in metastatic castration-resistant prostate cancer treated with 223Radium-dichloride. *Ann. Nucl. Med.* **2018**, *32*, 142–148. [CrossRef]
5. Saad, F.; Carles, J.; Gillessen, S.; Heidenreich, A.; Heinrich, D.; Gratt, J.; Lévy, J.; Miller, K.; Nilsson, S.; Petrenciuc, O.; et al. Radium-223 International Early Access Program Investigators. Radium-223 and concomitant therapies in patients with metastatic castration-resistant prostate cancer: An international, early access, open-label, single-arm phase 3b trial. *Lancet Oncol.* **2016**, *17*, 1306–1316. [CrossRef]
6. Clamp, A.; Danson, S.; Nguyen, H.; Cole, D.; Clemons, M. Assessment of therapeutic response in patients with metastatic bone disease. *Lancet Oncol.* **2004**, *5*, 607–616. [CrossRef]
7. Castello, A.; Macapinlac, H.A.; Lopci, E.; Santos, E.B. Prostate-specific antigen flare induced by 223RaCl2 in patients with metastatic castration-resistant prostate cancer. *Eur. J. Nucl. Med. Mol. Imaging* **2018**, *45*, 2256–2263. [CrossRef]
8. Oyama, N.; Akino, H.; Suzuki, Y.; Kanamaru, H.; Miwa, Y.; Tsuka, H.; Sadato, N.; Yonekura, Y.; Okada, K. Prognostic value of 2-deoxy-2-[F-18]fluoro-D-glucose positron emission tomography imaging for patients with prostate cancer. *Mol. Imaging Biol.* **2002**, *4*, 99–104. [CrossRef]
9. Meirelles, G.S.; Schöder, H.; Ravizzini, G.C.; Gönen, M.; Fox, J.J.; Humm, J.; Morris, M.J.; Scher, H.I.; Larson, S.M. Prognostic value of baseline [18F] fluorodeoxyglucose positron emission tomography and 99mTc-MDP bone scan in progressing metastatic prostate cancer. *Clin. Cancer Res.* **2010**, *16*, 6093–6096. [CrossRef]
10. Jadvar, H.; Desai, B.; Ji, L.; Conti, P.S.; Dorff, T.B.; Groshen, S.G.; Pinski, J.K.; Quinn, D.I. Baseline 18F FDG PET/CT parameters as imaging biomarkers of overall survival in castrate-resistant metastatic prostate cancer. *J. Nucl. Med.* **2013**, *54*, 1195–1201. [CrossRef]

11. Vargas, H.A.; Wassberg, C.; Fox, J.J.; Wibmer, A.; Goldman, D.A.; Kuk, D.; Gonen, M.; Larson, S.M.; Morris, M.J.; Scher, H.I.; et al. Bone metastases in castration-resistant prostate cancer: Associations between morphologic CT patterns, Glycolytic activity, and androgen receptor expression on PET and overall survival. *Radiology* **2014**, *271*, 220–229. [CrossRef] [PubMed]
12. Capitanio, S.; Bongioanni, F.; Piccardo, A.; Campus, C.; Gonella, R.; Tixi, L.; Naseri, M.; Pennone, M.; Altrinetti, V.; Buschiazzo, A.; et al. Comparisons between glucose analogue 2-deoxy-2-((18)F)fluoro-D-glucose and (18)F-sodium fluoride positron emission tomography/computed tomography in breast cancer patients with bone lesions. *World J. Radiol.* **2016**, *8*, 200–209. [CrossRef] [PubMed]
13. AIOM 2019 Prostate Cancer Guidelines. Available online: https://www.aiom.it/linee-guida-aiom-carcinoma-della-prostata-2019/14 (accessed on 23 November 2019).
14. Jadvar, H. Prostate cancer: PET with 18F-FDG, 18F- or 11C-acetate, and 18F- or 11C-choline. *J. Nucl. Med.* **2011**, *52*, 81–89. [CrossRef]
15. Boellaard, R.; Delgado-Bolton, R.; Oyen, W.J.; Giammarile, F.; Tatsch, K.; Eschner, W.; Verzijlbergen, F.J.; Barrington, S.F.; Pike, L.C.; Weber, W.A.; et al. European Association of Nuclear Medicine (EANM). FDG PET/CT: EANM procedure guidelines for tumour imaging: Version 2.0. *Eur. J. Nucl. Med. Mol. Imaging* **2015**, *42*, 328–354. [CrossRef] [PubMed]
16. Van den Wyngaert, T.; Strobel, K.; Kampen, W.U.; Kuwert, T.; van der Bruggen, W.; Mohan, H.K.; Gnanasegaran, G.; Delgado-Bolton, R.; Weber, W.A.; Beheshti, M.; et al. The EANM practice guidelines for bone scintigraphy. *Eur. J. Nucl. Med. Mol. Imaging* **2016**, *43*, 1723–1738. [CrossRef] [PubMed]
17. Kruse, V.; Mees, G.; Maes, A.; D'Asseler, Y.; Borms, M.; Cocquyt, V.; Van De Wiele, C. Reproducibility of FDG PET based metabolic tumor volume measurements and of their FDG distribution within. *Q. J. Nucl. Med. Mol. Imaging* **2015**, *59*, 462–468. [PubMed]
18. Young, H.; Baum, R.; Cremerius, U.; Herholz, K.; Hoekstra, O.; Lammertsma, A.A.; Pruim, J.; Price, P. Measurement of clinical and subclinical tumour response using [18F]-fluorodeoxyglucose and positron emission tomography: Review and 1999 EORTC recommendations. European Organization for Research and Treatment of Cancer (EORTC) PET Study Group. *Eur. J. Cancer* **1999**, *35*, 1773–1782. [CrossRef]
19. Wahl, R.L.; Jacene, H.; Kasamon, Y.; Lodge, M.A. From RECIST to PERCIST: Evolving Considerations for PET response criteria in solid tumors. *J. Nucl. Med.* **2009**, *50*, 122S–150S. [CrossRef]
20. Rossi, G.; Bauckneht, M.; Genova, C.; Rijavec, E.; Biello, F.; Mennella, S.; Dal Bello, M.G.; Cittadini, G.; Bruzzi, P.; Piva, R.; et al. Comparison between 18F-FDG-PET- and CT-based criteria in non-small cell lung cancer (NSCLC) patients treated with Nivolumab. *J. Nucl. Med.* **2019**. [CrossRef]
21. Grambsch, P.M.; Therneau, T.M. Proportional hazards tests and diagnostics based on weighted residuals. *Biometrika* **1994**, *81*, 515–526. [CrossRef]
22. Smith, M.; Parker, C.; Saad, F.; Miller, K.; Tombal, B.; Ng, Q.S.; Boegemann, M.; Matveev, V.; Piulats, J.M.; Zucca, L.E.; et al. Addition of radium-223 to abiraterone acetate and prednisone or prednisolone in patients with castration-resistant prostate cancer and bone metastases (ERA 223): A randomised, double-blind, placebo-controlled, phase 3 trial. *Lancet Oncol.* **2019**, *20*, 408–419. [CrossRef]
23. Nilsson, S.; Larsen, R.H.; Fosså, S.D.; Balteskard, L.; Borch, K.W.; Westlin, J.E.; Salberg, G.; Bruland, O.S. First clinical experience with alpha-emitting radium-223 in the treatment of skeletal metastases. *Clin. Cancer Res.* **2005**, *11*, 4451–4459. [CrossRef] [PubMed]
24. Beauregard, J.M.; Hofman, M.S.; Kong, G.; Hicks, R.J. The tumour sink effect on the biodistribution of 68Ga-DOTA-octreotate: Implications for peptide receptor radionuclide therapy. *Eur. J. Nucl. Med. Mol. Imaging* **2012**, *39*, 50–56. [CrossRef] [PubMed]
25. Dondossola, E.; Casarin, S.; Paindelli, C.; De-Juan-Pardo, E.M.; Hutmacher, D.W.; Logothetis, C.J.; Friedl, P. Radium 223-Mediated Zonal Cytotoxicity of Prostate Cancer in Bone. *J. Natl. Cancer Inst.* **2019**, *111*, 1042–1050. [CrossRef]
26. Føsbol, M.O.; Petersen, P.M.; Kjaer, A.; Mortensen, J. 223Ra Therapy of Advanced Metastatic Castration-Resistant Prostate Cancer: Quantitative Assessment of Skeletal Tumor Burden for Prognostication of Clinical Outcome and Hematologic Toxicity. *J. Nucl. Med.* **2018**, *59*, 596–602. [CrossRef]
27. Etchebehere, E.C.; Araujo, J.C.; Fox, P.S.; Swanston, N.M.; Macapinlac, H.A.; Rohren, E.M. Prognostic factors in patients treated with 223ra: The role of skeletal tumor burden on baseline 18F-fluoride PET/CT in predicting overall survival. *J. Nucl. Med.* **2015**, *56*, 1177–1184. [CrossRef]

28. Raynor, W.Y.; Al-Zaghal, A.; Zadeh, M.Z.; Seraj, S.M.; Alavi, A. Metastatic Seeding Attacks Bone Marrow, Not Bone: Rectifying Ongoing Misconceptions. *PET Clin.* **2019**, *14*, 135–144. [CrossRef]
29. Jadvar, H. Is There Use for FDG-PET in Prostate Cancer? *Semin. Nucl. Med.* **2016**, *46*, 502–506. [CrossRef]
30. Fox, J.J.; Gavane, S.C.; Blanc-Autran, E.; Nehmeh, S.; Gönen, M.; Beattie, B.; Vargas, H.A.; Schöder, H.; Humm, J.L.; Fine, S.W.; et al. Positron Emission Tomography/Computed Tomography-Based Assessments of Androgen Receptor Expression and Glycolytic Activity as a Prognostic Biomarker for Metastatic Castration-Resistant Prostate Cancer. *JAMA Oncol.* **2018**, *4*, 217–224. [CrossRef]
31. Etchebehere, E.C.; Araujo, J.C.; Milton, D.R.; Erwin, W.D.; Wendt, R.E., 3rd; Swanston, N.M.; Fox, P.; Macapinlac, H.A.; Rohren, E.M. Skeletal tumor burden on baseline 18F-fluoride PET/CT predicts bone marrow failure after 223Ra therapy. *Clin. Nucl. Med.* **2016**, *41*, 268–273. [CrossRef]
32. Sartor, O.; Coleman, R.E.; Nilsson, S.; Heinrich, D.; Helle, S.I.; O'Sullivan, J.M.; Vogelzang, N.J.; Bruland, Ø.; Kobina, S.; Wilhelm, S.; et al. An exploratory analysis of alkaline phosphatase, lactate dehydrogenase, and prostate-specific antigen dynamics in the phase 3 ALSYMPCA trial with radium-223. *Ann. Oncol.* **2017**, *28*, 1090–1097. [CrossRef] [PubMed]
33. Gillessen, S.; Omlin, A.; Attard, G.; de Bono, J.S.; Efstathiou, E.; Fizazi, K.; Halabi, S.; Nelson, P.S.; Sartor, O.; Smith, M.R.; et al. Management of patients with advanced prostate cancer: Recommendations of the St Gallen Advanced Prostate Cancer Consensus Conference (APCCC) 2015. *Ann. Oncol.* **2015**, *26*, 1589–1604. [CrossRef] [PubMed]
34. Scher, H.I.; Morris, M.J.; Stadler, W.M.; Higano, C.; Basch, E.; Fizazi, K.; Antonarakis, E.S.; Beer, T.M.; Carducci, M.A.; Chi, K.N.; et al. Trial design and objectives for castration-resistant prostate cancer: Updated recommendations from the prostate cancer clinical trials working group 3. *J. Clin. Oncol.* **2016**, *34*, 1402–1418. [CrossRef] [PubMed]
35. Poeppel, T.D.; Handkiewicz-Junak, D.; Andreeff, M.; Becherer, A.; Bockisch, A.; Fricke, E.; Geworski, L.; Heinzel, A.; Krause, B.J.; Krause, T.; et al. EANM guideline for radionuclide therapy with radium-223 of metastatic castration-resistant prostate cancer. *Eur. J. Nucl. Med. Mol. Imaging* **2018**, *45*, 824–845. [CrossRef] [PubMed]
36. Heinrich, D.; Gillessen, S.; Heidenreich, A.; Keizman, D.; O'Sullivan, J.M.; Carles, J.; Wirth, M.; Miller, K.; Procopio, G.; Gratt, J.; et al. Changes in alkaline phosphatase (ALP) dynamics and overall survival (OS) in metastatic castration-resistant prostate cancer (mCRPC) patients treated with radium-223 in an international early access program (EAP). *Ann. Oncol.* **2016**, *27*, 751P. [CrossRef]
37. Keizman, D.; Fosboel, M.O.; Reichegger, H.; Peer, A.; Rosenbaum, E.; Desax, M.C.; Neiman, V.; Petersen, P.M.; Mueller, J.; Cathomas, R.; et al. Imaging response during therapy with radium-223 for castration-resistant prostate cancer with bone metastases-analysis of an international multicenter database. *Prostate Cancer Prostatic Dis.* **2017**, *20*, 289–293. [CrossRef]
38. McNamara, M.A.; George, D.J. Pain, PSA flare, and bone scan response in a patient with metastatic castration-resistant prostate cancer treated with radium-223, a case report. *BMC Cancer* **2015**, *15*, 371. [CrossRef]
39. Yoneyama, S.; Miyoshi, Y.; Tsutsumi, S.; Kawahara, T.; Hattori, Y.; Yokomizo, Y.; Hayashi, N.; Yao, M.; Uemura, H. Value of bone scan index for predicting overall survival among patients treated with radium-223 for bone metastatic castration-resistant prostate cancer. *J. Clin. Oncol.* **2018**, *36*, 216. [CrossRef]
40. O'Sullivan, G.J.; Carty, F.L.; Cronin, C.G. Imaging of bone metastasis: An update. *World J. Radiol.* **2015**, *7*, 202–211. [CrossRef]
41. Perez-Lopez, R.; Mateo, J.; Mossop, H.; Blackledge, M.D.; Collins, D.J.; Rata, M.; Morgan, V.A.; Macdonald, A.; Sandhu, S.; Lorente, D.; et al. Diffusion-weighted imaging as a treatment response biomarker for evaluating bone metastases in prostate cancer: A pilot study. *Radiology* **2017**, *283*, 168–177. [CrossRef]
42. Etchebehere, E.; Brito, A.E.; Rezaee, A.; Langsteger, W.; Beheshti, M. Therapy assessment of bone metastatic disease in the era of 223radium. *Eur. J. Nucl. Med. Mol. Imaging* **2017**, *44*, 84–96. [CrossRef] [PubMed]
43. Evangelista, L.; Zorz, A. Re: Response Assessment of 223Ra Treatment: Should a Fluorocholine PET/CT Be Performed? *Clin. Nucl. Med.* **2018**, *43*, 867–868. [PubMed]
44. Thomas, L.; Balmus, C.; Ahmadzadehfar, H.; Essler, M.; Strunk, H.; Bundschuh, R.A. Assessment of Bone Metastases in Patients with Prostate Cancer-A Comparison between 99mTc-Bone-Scintigraphy and [68Ga]Ga-PSMA PET/CT. *Pharmaceuticals* **2017**, *10*, 68. [CrossRef] [PubMed]

45. Uprimny, C.; Kroiss, A.; Nilica, B.; Buxbaum, S.; Decristoforo, C.; Horninger, W.; Virgolini, I.J. (68)Ga-PSMA ligand PET versus (18)F-NaF PET: Evaluation of response to (223)Ra therapy in a prostate cancer patient. *Eur. J. Nucl. Med. Mol. Imaging* **2015**, *42*, 362–363. [CrossRef]
46. Maruyama, K.; Utsunomia, K.; Nakamoto, T.; Kawakita, S.; Murota, T.; Tanigawa, N. Utility of F-18 FDG PET/CT for Detection of Bone Marrow Metastases in Prostate Cancer Patients Treated with Radium-223. *Asia Ocean. J. Nucl. Med. Biol.* **2018**, *6*, 61–67.
47. Iizuka, J. Evaluating radium-223 response in metastatic castration-resistant prostate cancer with imaging. *Asia Pac. J. Clin. Oncol.* **2018**, *14*, 16–23. [CrossRef]
48. Coleman, R.; Aksnes, A.K.; Naume, B.; Garcia, C.; Jerusalem, G.; Piccart, M.; Vobecky, N.; Thuresson, M.; Flamen, P. A phase IIa, nonrandomized study of radium-223 dichloride in advanced breast cancer patients with bone-dominant disease. *Breast Cancer Res. Treat.* **2014**, *145*, 411–418. [CrossRef]
49. Suominen, M.I.; Fagerlund, K.M.; Rissanen, J.P.; Konkol, Y.M.; Morko, J.P.; Peng, Z.; Alhoniemi, E.J.; Laine, S.K.; Corey, E.; Mumberg, D.; et al. Radium-223 inhibits osseous prostate cancer growth by dual targeting of cancer cells and bone microenvironment in mouse models. *Clin. Cancer Res.* **2017**, *23*, 4335–4346. [CrossRef]
50. Suominen, M.I.; Rissanen, J.P.; Käkönen, R.; Fagerlund, K.M.; Alhoniemi, E.; Mumberg, D.; Ziegelbauer, K.; Halleen, J.M.; Käkönen, S.M.; Scholz, A. Survival benefit with radium-223 dichloride in a mouse model of breast cancer bone metastasis. *J. Natl. Cancer Inst.* **2013**, *105*, 908–916. [CrossRef]
51. Lange, P.H.; Vessella, R.L. Mechanisms, hypotheses and questions regarding prostate cancer micrometastases to bone. *Cancer Metastasis Rev.* **1998**, *17*, 331–336. [CrossRef]
52. Fiz, F.; Dittman, H.; Campi, C.; Morbelli, S.; Marini, C.; Brignone, M.; Bauckneht, M.; Piva, R.; Massone, A.M.; Piana, M.; et al. Assessment of Skeletal Tumor Load in Metastasized Castration-Resistant Prostate Cancer Patients: A Review of Available Methods and an Overview on Future Perspectives. *Bioengineering (Basel)* **2018**, *5*, 58. [CrossRef] [PubMed]

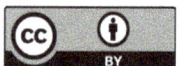

© 2019 by the authors. Licensee MDPI, Basel, Switzerland. This article is an open access article distributed under the terms and conditions of the Creative Commons Attribution (CC BY) license (http://creativecommons.org/licenses/by/4.0/).

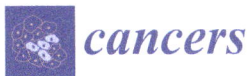

Article

The Role of 18F-FDG PET/CT in Staging and Prognostication of Mantle Cell Lymphoma: An Italian Multicentric Study

Domenico Albano [1], Riccardo Laudicella [2], Paola Ferro [3], Michela Allocca [4], Elisabetta Abenavoli [4], Ambra Buschiazzo [5], Alessia Castellino [6], Agostino Chiaravalloti [7,8], Annarosa Cuccaro [9], Lea Cuppari [10], Rexhep Durmo [1], Laura Evangelista [11], Viviana Frantellizzi [12], Sofya Kovalchuk [13], Flavia Linguanti [4], Giulia Santo [14], Matteo Bauckneht [15,*] and Salvatore Annunziata [16] on behalf of Young Italian Association of Nuclear Medicine (AIMN) Working Group

1. Nuclear Medicine, University of Brescia, Spedali Civili Brescia, 25123 Brescia, Italy; doalba87@libero.it (D.A.); rexhep.durmo@gmail.com (R.D.)
2. Nuclear Medicine Unit, Department of Biomedical and Dental Sciences and Morpho-Functional Imaging, University of Messina, 98125 Messina, Italy; riclaudi@hotmail.it
3. Nuclear Medicine Department, IRCCS San Raffaele Hospital, 20132 Milan, Italy; paola.paolina01@gmail.com
4. Nuclear Medicine Unit, Department of Experimental and Clinical Biomedical Sciences, University of Florence, 50134 Florence, Italy; michimedn2@gmail.com (M.A.); elisabettabenavoli@gmail.com (E.A.); flavialinguanti@hotmail.it (F.L.)
5. Nuclear Medicine Department, S. Croce e Carle Hospital Cuneo, 12100 Cuneo, Italy; ambra.buschiazzo@gmail.com
6. Hematology Division, S. Croce e Carle Hospital Cuneo, 12100 Cuneo, Italy; castellino.al@ospedale.cuneo.it
7. Department of Biomedicine and Prevention, University Tor Vergata, 00133 Rome, Italy; agostino.chiaravalloti@gmail.com
8. IRCCS Neuromed, 86077 Pozzilli, Italy
9. Istituto di Ematologia, Fondazione Policlinico Universitario A. Gemelli IRCCS, Università Cattolica del Sacro Cuore, 00168 Rome, Italy; annarosa.cuccaro@gmail.com
10. Nuclear Medicine and Molecular Imaging Unit, Veneto Institute of Oncology IOV-IRCCS, 35128 Padua, Italy; lea.cuppari@aulss2.veneto.it
11. Nuclear Medicine Unit, Department of Medicine – DIMED, University of Padua, 35121 Padua, Italy; laura.evangelista@unipd.it
12. Department of Molecular Medicine, Sapienza University of Rome, 00185 Rome, Italy; viviana.frantellizzi@uniroma1.it
13. Hematology Unit, Department of Experimental and Clinical Biomedical Sciences, University of Florence, 50134 Florence, Italy; sofya.kovalchuk@unifi.it
14. Nuclear Medicine Unit, Department of Interdisciplinary Medicine, University of Bari Aldo Moro, 70124 Bari, Italy; giuliasanto92@gmail.com
15. Nuclear Medicine, IRCCS Policlinico San Martino, 16132 Genova, Italy
16. Institute of Nuclear Medicine, Fondazione Policlinico Universitario A. Gemelli IRCCS, Università Cattolica del Sacro Cuore, 00168 Rome, Italy; salvatoreannunziata@live.it
* Correspondence: matteo.bauckneht@hsanmartino.it or matteo.bauckneht@gmail.com; Tel.: +39-010-555-3038

Received: 6 October 2019; Accepted: 19 November 2019; Published: 21 November 2019

Abstract: Mantle cell lymphoma (MCL) is an aggressive lymphoma subtype with poor prognosis in which 18F-FDG-PET/CT role in treatment response evaluation and prediction of outcome is still unclear. The aim of this multicentric study was to investigate the role of 18F-FDG-PET/CT in staging MCL and the prognostic role of Deauville criteria (DC) in terms of progression-free survival (PFS) and overall survival (OS). We retrospectively enrolled 229 patients who underwent baseline and end-of-treatment (eot) 18F-FDG-PET/CT after first-line therapy. EotPET/CT scans were visually interpreted according to DC. The sensitivity, specificity, positive predictive value, negative predictive value and accuracy of PET/CT for evaluation of bone marrow (BM) were 27%, 100%, 100%, 48% and

57%, respectively. The sensitivity, specificity, positive predictive value, negative predictive value and accuracy of PET/CT for evaluation of the gastrointestinal (GI) tract were 60%, 99%, 93%, 90% and 91%, respectively. At a median follow-up of 40 months, relapse occurred in 104 cases and death in 49. EotPET/CT results using DC significantly correlated with PFS, not with OS. Instead, considering OS, only MIPI score was significantly correlated. In conclusion, we demonstrated that MCL is an FDG-avid lymphoma and 18F-FDG-PET/CT is a useful tool for staging purpose, showing good specificity for BM and GI evaluation, but suboptimal sensitivity. EotPET/CT result was the only independent significant prognostic factor that correlated with PFS.

Keywords: mantle cell lymphoma; 18F-FDG PET/CT; prognosis; Deauville criteria

1. Introduction

Mantle cell lymphoma (MCL) accounts for 3% to 6% of all non-Hodgkin lymphoma and it is an aggressive lymphoma subtype with a high recurrence and mortality rate [1]. In the era of personalized and precision medicine, strong prognostic tools are needed in all lymphoma subtypes, such as MCL, to accurately predict possible further relapse of disease or death and to improve their treatment management. For this end-point, both clinical and imaging parameters are nowadays available, such as clinical scores and fluorine-18-fluorodeoxyglucose positron emission tomography/computed tomography (18F-FDG-PET/CT) derived parameters. MCL International Prognostic Index (MIPI) is the first prognostic index suited for MCL patients and may serve as an important tool to facilitate risk-adapted treatment decisions in patients with advanced stage MCL [2]. At the same time, FDG-PET/CT at the end of first-line therapy is recognized as a powerful prognostic tool in many lymphoma subtypes. The Deauville score criteria (DC) and subsequent Lugano criteria were proposed in this setting and nowadays they are commonly accepted as a tool to evaluate response to treatment and prognosis in both interim and end-of-therapy setting in some lymphoma subtypes as in Hodgkin lymphoma (HL) and large B-cell lymphoma (DLBCL) [3,4]. For other less common lymphoma subtypes such as MCL, there is no clear scientific evidence of the role of these criteria in treatment evaluation and prognostication, although theoretically they can be considered valid. A recent editorial by Bailly et al. [5] underlined the lack of scientific evidences of a proven role of these criteria in MCL. Moreover, 18F-FDG-PET/CT at baseline has been recently evaluated to complete the staging of disease at diagnosis, with possible implication of different prognostic risk in the follow-up. The aim of this study was to evaluate the role of 18F-FDG-PET/CT in patients with MCL as follows: assessing its power in staging MCL; evaluating DC as a predictive tool in response to therapy and as a prognostic tool in terms of progression-free survival (PFS) and overall survival (OS); testing the combination of clinical and imaging parameters in order to identify different risk classes able to predict the outcomes.

2. Results

2.1. Tumor Characteristics

Among 229 patients with histological proven MCL, there was a prevalence of male ($n = 172$) compared to female ($n = 57$); the average age was 65.1 years (range: 29–88). Patients were staged according to the Ann Arbor system as follows: stage I ($n = 4$), stage II ($n = 9$), stage III ($n = 32$) and stage IV ($n = 184$). B-symptoms, bulky disease and splenomegaly were described in 65, 40 and 101 patients, respectively. LDH level resulted high in 93 cases, β2-microglobulin in 65 and MIPI score was greater than 6 in 130 patients. Proliferative index Ki-67 was available in 183 patients, being low in 65 (36%) and high in 118 (64%) subjects. Baseline features of the patients are summarized in Table 1.

Table 1. Baseline features of our population.

Variables		Patients n (%)	Average (Range)
Age (years)			65.1 (29–88)
Sex			
	male	172 (75%)	
	female	57 (25%)	
Tumor stage at diagnosis (Ann Arbor)			
	I	4 (2%)	
	II	9 (4%)	
	III	32 (14%)	
	IV	184 (80%)	
Blastoid variant		26 (11%)	
B symptoms		65 (28%)	
LDH			
	≤245 U/L	121 (57%)	
	>245 U/L	93 (43%)	
β2-microglobulin			
	≤2.8 mg/L	108 (62%)	
	>2.8 mg/L	65 (38%)	
MIPI score			
	low-intermediate (≤6)	99 (43%)	
	high-intermediate (>6)	130 (57%)	
Bulky disease		40 (17%)	
Splenomegaly		101 (44%)	
Ki-67 score			
	≤15%	65 (36%)	
	>15%	118 (64%)	

LDH: lactate dehydrogenase; MIPI: mantle cell lymphoma international prognostic index.

2.2. 18F-FDG PET/CT Evaluation for Initial Staging

All patients had abnormal 18F-FDG PET/CT showing the presence of at least one lesion with increased FDG uptake consistent with MCL. 18F-FDG PET/CT scans detected nodal disease in 216 (94%) patients. Splenic involvement was detected by PET/CT in 100 (44%) patients.

Considering bone marrow (BM) biopsy as reference, BM disease was reported in 136 (59%) patients, while 18F-FDG PET/CT showed a focal uptake, compatible with BM involvement, in 37 (16%) subjects. Sensitivity (SE), specificity (SP), positive predictive value (PPV), negative predictive value (NPV) and accuracy (AC) of 18F-FDG-PET/CT in evaluating BM were 27% (20–35%), 100% (96–100%), 100%, 48% (46–51%) and 57% (50–63%); negative likelihood ratio was 0.73. No false positive findings for BM involvement were registered at PET/CT; however, 99 false negative findings were registered (Table 2). Agreement between the two techniques was low (Cohen's k = 0.23).

Table 2. Agreement between 18F-FDG PET/CT and BM biopsy and GI endoscopy findings.

PET/CT Findings	BM Biopsy		GI Endoscopy	
	Positive	Negative	Positive	Negative
Positive	37 (16%)	0 (0%)	28 (12%)	2 (1%)
Negative	99 (43%)	93 (41%)	19 (8%)	180 (79%)
Total	136 (59%)	93 (41%)	47 (21%)	182 (79%)

BM: bone marrow; GI: gastrointestinal.

18F-FDG PET/CT resulted positive for gastrointestinal (GI) tract involvement in 30 (13%) cases: among them, in 13 showing gastric uptake, 1 in gastro-duodenal junction uptake, 2 in the duodenum, 12 in the colon, 1 in sigma and 1 in the cecum. Considering GI endoscopy as standard of reference, 47 patients had a GI involvement of MCL. SE, SP, PPV, NPV and AC of 18F-FDG-PET/CT were 60% (44–74%), 99% (96–100%), 93% (78–98%), 90% (87–93%), 91% (86–94%) respectively; positive and negative likelihood ratios were 54.21 and 0.41, respectively (Table 2). Agreement between the two techniques was quite good (Cohen's k = 0.67).

2.3. Role of 18F-FDG PET/CT in Predicting Survival

Application of Deauville Criteria

According to DC, 186 (81%) patients were categorized as eotPET negative (score 1–3) (Figure 1) and 43 (19%) as a positive scan (score 4–5) (Figure 2). At a median follow-up of 40 months, relapse and/or progression of lymphoma was found in 104 patients with a mean time of 31.2 months (range: 3–145) from the diagnosis, and death was found in 49 cases with a mean time of 33.9 months (range 3–145). Considering patients with relapse/progression of disease, a negative eotPET/CT scans applying DC were registered in 74 cases, whilst a positive scan in 30 (in particular, Deauville score 4 in thirteen cases and Deauville score 5 in seventeen). Instead, among patients who died during the course of the disease, eotPET/CT applying DC was positive in 20 (in particular, score 4 in seven cases and score 5 in thirteen) and negative in 27 (in particular, score 1 in 17 subjects, score 2 in nine and score 3 in one). Patients with eot positive PET/CT underwent subsequent second-line chemotherapy regimen according to institutional protocol.

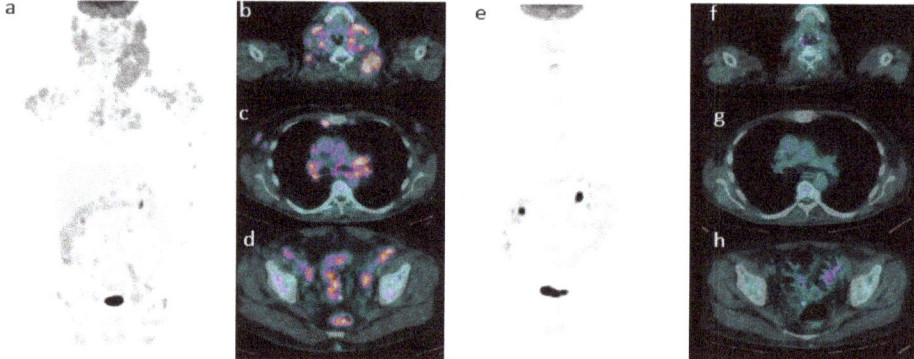

Figure 1. Emblematic example of complete metabolic response. A representative case of a 56-year-old male with stage III MCL. (**a**) Baseline maximum intensity projection (MIP), showing diffuse hypermetabolic disease in (**b**) laterocervical, (**c**) mediastinal and (**d**) iliac nodes. (**e**) PET/CT after chemotherapy showing a complete metabolic response (Deauville score 1) with no 18F-FDG uptake (**f–h**) with the disappearance of previous lesions.

The median PFS and OS were 28 months (range 3–145 months) and 34 months (range 3–145 months) respectively; with estimated 2-year PFS and OS rates of 73% and 84%, and 3-year PFS and OS rates of 56% and 75%, respectively.

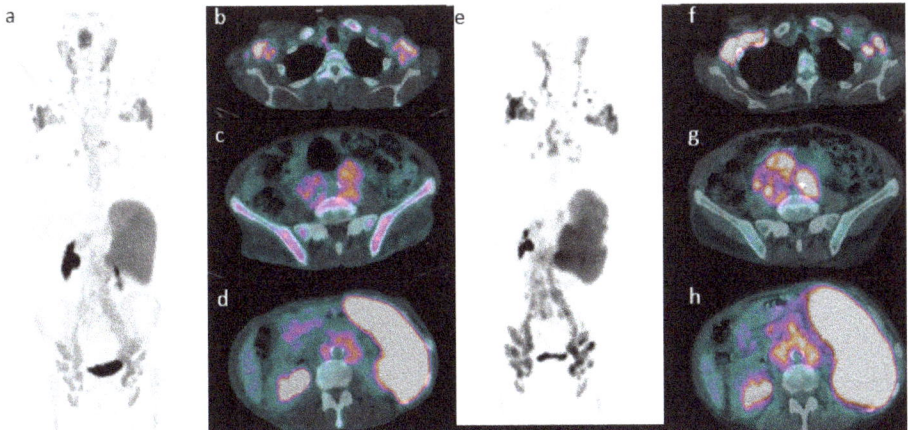

Figure 2. Emblematic example of progressive disease. A representative case of a 65-year-old male with stage III MCL. (**a**) Baseline maximum intensity projection (MIP, showing diffuse hypermetabolic disease in (**b**) laterocervical, axillary, (**c**) iliac and (**d**) inguinal nodes and in spleen. (**e**) PET/CT after chemotherapy showing a metabolic progression of disease (Deauville score 5) with the appearance of new lesions (**f–h**).

At univariate analysis, DC and MIPI score were the only parameters significantly related to PFS (Figure 3); other clinical/pathological features (sex, age, splenomegaly, bulky disease, stage, blastoid variant, β2-microglobulin and LDH level) were not associated with the outcome. PFS was significantly shorter in patients with eotPET/CT DC positive compared to negative (12 vs. 32 months, $p < 0.001$). At multivariate analysis, only metabolic feature (Deauville score) was confirmed to be an independent prognostic factor for PFS ($p < 0.001$). Combining DC (≤3 and >3) and MIPI score (≤6 and >6), PFS was significantly longer in eotPET negative patients independently from MIPI score ($p < 0.001$) (Figure 4). Median PFS was 82 months in patients with low-intermediate MIPI score (≤6) and a negative eotPET/CT (DC ≤ 3); 62 months in patients with high MIPI score (>6) and a negative eotPET/CT; 25 months in patients with low-intermediate MIPI score and a positive eotPET/CT (DC 4 or 5), and 12 months in patients with high MIPI score and a positive eotPET/CT.

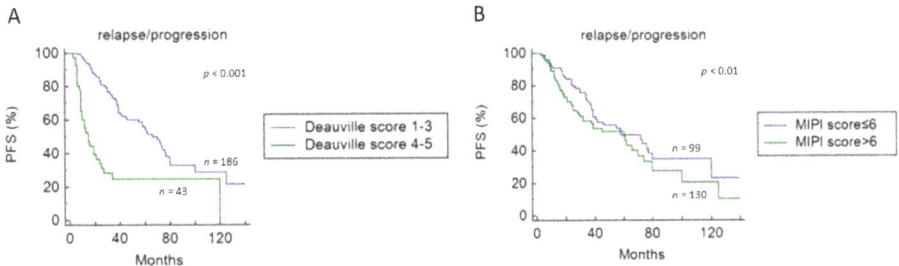

Figure 3. Progression-free survival (PFS) curves according to end-of-treatment PET/CT results using (**A**) Deauville criteria and (**B**) MIPI score.

Instead, considering OS, only MIPI score resulted as significantly correlated (Figure 5), both at univariate and multivariate analysis ($p = 0.017$) (Table 3). EotPET/CT according to DC did not predict OS (31 vs. 37.5 months, $p = 0.814$) (Figure 5).

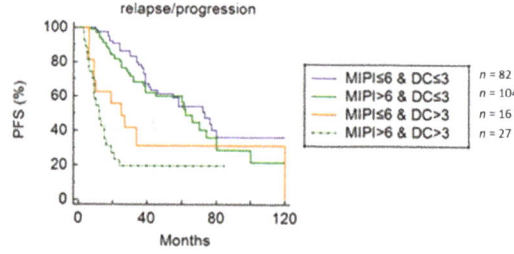

Figure 4. Progression-free survival curve combining MIPI score and Deauville score groups.

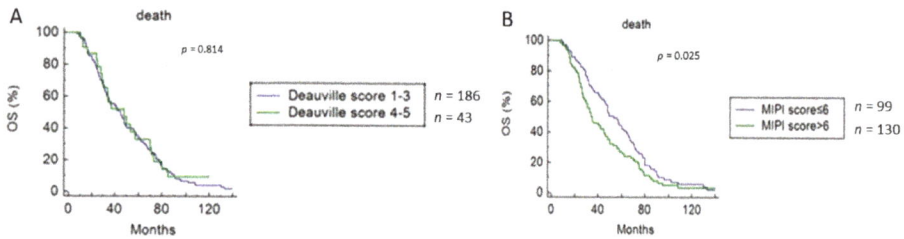

Figure 5. Overall survival (OS) curves according to end-of-treatment PET/CT results using (**A**) Deauville criteria and (**B**) MIPI score.

Table 3. Univariate and multivariate analyses for PFS and OS.

Variables	Univariate Analysis		Multivariate Analysis	
	p-Value	HR (95% CI)	*p*-Value	HR (95% CI)
	PFS			
Sex	0.451	0.845 (0.548–1.306)		
Age	0.153	1.530 (0.838–3.097)		
MIPI score	0.009	0.713 (0.482–1.056)	0.174	1.219 (0.915–1.623)
LDH level	0.163	0.742 (0.488–1.128)		
B2 microglobulin	0.458	0.831 (0.511–1.353)		
Ki-67 score	0.066	0.653 (0.415–1.028)		
Bulky disease	0.153	1.722 (0.992–2.987)		
Splenomegaly	0.087	0.703 (0.472–01049)		
Stage acc Ann Arbor	0.855	0.957 (0.589–1.531)		
Blastoid variant	0.185	0.598 (0.282–1.270)		
Deauville score	<0.001	0.137 (0.073–0.259)	<0.001	4.059 (2.573–6.403)
Treatment regimen	0.655	0.857 (0.519–1.243)		
	OS			
Sex	0.211	1.759 (0.577–6.033)		
Age	0.375	1.270 (0.722–2.369)		
MIPI score	0.025	0.711 (0.527–0.959)	0.017	1.204 (1.032–1.403)
LDH level	0.709	0.942 (0.690–1.287)		
B2 microglobulin	0.524	1.128 (0.778–1.635)		
Ki67 score	0.195	1.250 (0.891–1.754)		
Bulky disease	0.390	0.828 (0.539–1.272)		
Splenomegaly	0.287	0.846 (0.622–1.150)		
Stage acc Ann Arbor	0.393	0.859 (0.606–1.217)		
Blastoid variant	0.075	0.618 (0.363–1.051)		
Deauville score	0.814	1.055 (0.671–1.660)		
Treatment regimen	0.598	1.001 (0.571–1.460)		

PFS: progression-free survival; OS: overall survival; HR: hazard ratio; CI: confidence interval; N: number.

Treatment regimen (R-CHOP regimen vs. other chemotherapy regimen) did not influence outcome survival considering both PFS and OS.

3. Discussion

MCL is an aggressive B-cell non-Hodgkin lymphoma with a fast-growing course, high-risk of relapse and need for early treatment. Patients affected by MCL typically present with advanced-stage disease and extranodal involvement with a predilection for BM and GI tract, where routine conventional techniques such as CT have a suboptimal accuracy [6]. A correct and an early identification of initial and extranodal disease may be crucial because it could potentially affect patient's management and therapeutic choice. 18F-FDG PET/CT has shown a high accuracy in the detection of nodal involvement [7–9], but a low sensitivity in BM and GI tract, being inadequate to replace BM biopsy and GI endoscopy in disease staging [10–12]. In the present study, we demonstrated a very low sensitivity of PET/CT in the evaluation of BM involvement (27%), but with a specificity equal to 100%. No case of false-positive findings on BM at PET/CT were recorded, but there were 99 cases of false-negative PET. Thus, the need for BM biopsy seems to be mandatory in case of negative BM PET/CT. Previous studies [10–12] reported a very low pretreatment PET scan accuracy to detect BM involvement, very low with sensitivity ranging from 12% to 51%. A comparison between our paper and others is not easy due to the different population number and features evaluated. Recently, Morgan et al. [13] projected a voxel-based analysis of the iliac bones for classifying BM disease in MCL founding a good sensitivity and specificity (100% and 87.5%, respectively); this method seems to be very promising but less practical and reproducible and it has been validated only on a small sample of patients. The potential role of 18F-FDG PET/CT in evaluating lymphoma BM involvement remains a challenge; this is a non-invasive technique well studied in HL and DLBCL, but with controversial and limited evidence [14,15]. Several studies have proven that 18F-FDG PET/CT can be an accurate method for the evaluation of BM involvement in patients affected by DLBCL considering focal highly 18F-FDG-avid lesions as reference standard; on the other hand the absence of a focal uptake does not exclude the presence of BM involvement. Our results confirmed similar evidences also in MCL, suggesting to avoid a BM biopsy in case of positive PET/CT scan.

Also, for the GI tract, our results showed that 18F-FDG PET/CT revealed a good specificity but a low sensitivity (60%), being in agreement with other published papers [9,12,16]. It was already demonstrated that an increased 18F-FDG bowel uptake may be common, especially in diabetic patients [17,18], thus reducing the diagnostic accuracy of the evaluation of this district.

Another crucial topic to consider in MCL is the prognostication; nowadays, neither clinical nor imaging prognostic markers are available in MCL setting. MIPI score [2] was an attempt created to better classify patients with MCL and predict prognosis, but its validation has shown conflicting results [19,20]. Other histopathological features, such as blastoid variant and Ki-67 score, have been investigated without shared evidence [21]. Instead, the prognostic value of 18F-FDG-PET/CT in MCL remains under debate [16,22–25]. In 2009, a five-point scale system called Deauville criteria (DC) was introduced to analyze 18F-FDG PET/CT results after treatment in lymphoma [26]; this scale used the mediastinum and liver activity as the reference standard, and has been recommended for reporting both interim and end-of-treatment PET for FDG-avid lymphoma (both HL and NHL, especially DLBCL) [3,4,27]. In our paper, we tried to validate this score also in MCL, obtaining some strong results; patients with a negative end-of-treatment PET/CT (DC1-3) had significantly longer PFS than patients with a positive PET/CT (DC4,5). Similar results in small cohort of patients were reported by other authors [20,22,28]. However, this evidence was not confirmed for OS, where DC seems to not influence the outcome survival. This could be explained to the fact that eotPET/CT results were used to guide subsequent management and further treatments, as second-line chemotherapy regimen.

The treatment of MCL is a challenge and often stays unsatisfactory; complete responses to the standard chemotherapy regimens are not common. Czuczman et al. [29] in a multicenter open-label single-arm phase II study showed that the complete metabolic response at PET/CT was a predictor of outcome survival. In addition to qualitative 18F-FDG PET/CT analysis using DC, also semiquantitative PET/CT parameters have been studied as prognostic factors, like SUVmax, with controversial results. Karam et al. [30] and Bodet-Milin et al. [16], in patients affected by MCL, suggested SUVmax thresholds of 5 and 6, respectively, to stratify patients into high-risk versus low-risk groups and to predict OS and disease-free survival. On the other hand, no prognostic impact of SUVmax was demonstrated by other groups [10,12,24]. Recently in the LyMa-PET Project [23], it was demonstrated that SUVmax was the only independent prognostic factor for PFS and OS; moreover, authors suggested a scoring system combining MIPI and SUVmax (using a cutoff of 10.3) to help the outcome prediction. In our study, eotPET/CT results using DC were superior than the MIPI score in PFS, while for OS only the MIPI score resulted as an independent prognostic factor.

Instead, no clinical or histological variables, like blastoid variant and B2 microglobulin, showed significant association with outcome survival in our analysis; this is partially in contradiction with literature [1] and related probably to heterogeneity of population studied.

Also, Ki-67 score seems not to be related to PET/CT features and outcome survival despite that in other lymphoma subtypes significant correlation was demonstrated [31,32].

The present study has some limitations. First, this is a retrospective multicentric study, so heterogeneous features in our population in terms of clinical baseline parameters and treatment schemes could be found. Despite this, so far and to best of our knowledge, the present study is the first large series of MCL patients aimed to assess the diagnostic and prognostic role of 18F-FDG PET/CT. Second, although this study showed the independent prognostic value for PFS of end-of-treatment PET/CT, the role of semi-quantitative PET/CT parameters, in terms of SUVs, should be further analyzed. Third, more complex statistical analysis, like a deep learning approach, might have improved data analysis.

4. Materials and Methods

4.1. Patients

Between January 2007 and December 2018 in nine Italian Nuclear Medicine Centers, 229 patients with newly diagnosed, histologically proven MCL were retrospectively enrolled. The histopathological diagnosis was based on the World Health Organization criteria [33]. The inclusion criteria were as follows: patients with a histological confirmation of MCL; age ≥18 years; availability of BM biopsy and GI endoscopy at time of diagnosis; availability of baseline and end of treatment 18F-FDG PET/CT results in all patients; and availability of clinical/radiologic follow-up data for at least 12 months. Patients with concomitant malignancies were excluded. We further reviewed the follow medical records of these patients: epidemiological features (age at diagnosis, sex), clinical data (tumor stage, MIPI score, bulky disease, splenomegaly, B symptoms, lactate-dehydrogenase (LDH) level, β2-microglobulin level), histopathological data (Ki-67 score, blastoid variant), metabolic features by 18F-FDG PET/CT, treatment modalities and follow-up data. LDH level, β2-microglobulin and MIPI score were dichotomized using cutoff values of 245 U/L, 2.8 mg/L and 6 respectively. Tumor stage according to Ann Arbor classification was divided in early (I and II) and advanced (III and IV) disease. The bulky disease was defined when the maximum width was equal or greater than one-third of the internal transverse diameter of the thorax or at an alternative site as any mass measuring 10 cm or more by any imaging study. Proliferative activity, expressed by Ki-67 score, was available in 183 patients; average Ki-67 was 25% (range 1–95%). The Ki-67 expression level was arbitrarily dichotomized using a cut-off of 15% as suggested by other authors [24,34].

All patients were treated according to the institution's standard protocol with chemotherapy regimen related to the stage of disease, age and institutional internal protocol. Eighty-two patients were treated according to R-CHOP (Rituximab, Cyclophoshpamide, Hydroxydaunomycin, Oncovin, Prednisone) regimen, sixty-eight with R-DHAP (dexamethasone, cytarabine, cisplatin), thirty-nine with R-Bendamustina, twenty-four with BCVPP (Carmustine, Cyclophosphamide, Vinblastine, Procarbazine, and Prednisone), twelve with MBVD (Myocet+BVD). In one case, chemotherapy was followed by the involved field radiotherapy. Four patients (2%) underwent only radiotherapy due to the early stage of disease (stage I).

4.2. 18F-FDG PET/CT Imaging and Interpretation

All patients underwent baseline 18F-FDG PET/CT and a subsequent PET/CT at completion of first-line therapy (eotPET/CT). PET/CT studies were performed following EANM guidelines [35]. Baseline PET/CT was performed within 14 days before the first cycle of chemotherapy and end-of-treatment PET/CT was done at least three weeks after the completion of chemotherapy or 12 weeks after completion of radiotherapy.

18F-FDG-PET/CT was performed after at least 6 h of fasting and with glucose level lower than 150 mg/dL. An activity of 3.5–4.5 MBq/Kg of 18F-FDG was administered intravenously and scans were acquired about 60 min after injection, usually from the skull basis to the mid-thigh. Owing to the multicenter nature of the study, the exams were acquired on different PET/CT scanners: Discovery STE or 690 (GE Healthcare Technologies, Milwaukee, Wisconsin, USA), Discovery IQ (GE Healthcare Technologies), Discovery LS (GE Healthcare Technologies), Gemini TFEGXL (Philips Medical Systems, Cleveland, OH, USA) and Biograph 16 (Siemens Healthcare, Erlangen, Germany). Standard parameters used were: CT: 80 mA, 120 Kv without contrast; 2.5–4 min per bed-PET-step of 15 cm; the reconstruction was performed in a 128×128 matrix and with a 60 cm field-of-view.

Patients were instructed to void before imaging acquisition, no oral or intravenous contrast agents were administrated and no bowel preparation was used for any patient; written consent was obtained before studies. The PET images were visually analyzed and readers had knowledge of clinical history. PET/CT scans were interpreted visually by two nuclear medicine physicians (DA, SA) with experience in this field and the discordance was resolved by a consensus between the two imaging readers.

For the interpretation of images, each focal tracer uptake deviating from physiological distribution and background and uptake higher than liver activity was considered as suggestive for lymphoma.

In the evaluation of BM involvement, PET/CT findings were considered positive in the presence of isolated/multiple focal uptakes in the BM that could not be explained by benign findings on the underlying CT scan or patient's medical history (like fractures, spondylodiscitis, etc.). In the evaluation of GI involvement, PET/CT findings were considered positive in the presence of isolated/multiple intense focal uptakes in the GI tract. Accuracy of 18F-FDG PET/T results was evaluated considering further evaluations: lesions with 18F-FDG PET/CT uptakes were considered as true-positives if further analyses confirmed the malignant nature, and false-positive if further evaluations showed no malignant lesions. Lesions without 18F-FDG PET/CT uptakes were considered as true negative if further analyses confirmed the absence of neoplastic lesions and false-negative if further evaluations showed malignant ones. Eot 18F-FDG PET/CT was interpreted by visual analysis using the Deauville 5-point scale [4]. According to Deauville Criteria (DC), 18F-FDG PET was interpreted as follows: 1 = no uptake above background, 2 = uptake equal to or lower than mediastinum, 3 = uptake higher than mediastinum and lower than liver, 4 = uptake moderately increased compared to the liver and 5 = uptake markedly increased compared to the liver. Eot 18F-FDG PET/CT scans were considered negative for scores 1 to 3 and positive for scores 4 to 5.

4.3. Statistical Analysis

Our statistical analysis was carried out using MedCalc Software version 17.1 for Windows (Ostend, Belgium). Categorical variables were described as the calculation of simple and relative frequencies, while the numeric variables were described as average, minimum and maximum. We calculated SE, SP, PPV, NPV and AC based on Bayes's law, with 95% confidence intervals, considering final diagnosis as a reference.

The PFS was calculated from the date of diagnosis of MCL to the date of first relapse, progression of disease or the last follow-up date. The OS was calculated from the date of diagnosis of MCL to the date of death from any cause or the last follow-up date.

Survival curves were plotted according to the Kaplan–Meier method and differences between several groups were investigated by using a two-tailed log rank test. Cox regression was used to evaluate the hazard ratio (HR) and its confidence interval (CI). A p-value of <0.05 was considered statistically significant and the adjusted significant p-value after Bonferroni's correction was 0.038.

5. Conclusions

In conclusion, in this study, we demonstrated that MCL is an FDG-avid lymphoma and that 18F-FDG PET/CT is a useful tool for staging purpose, which should be considered in the diagnostic flow-chart of this patients in concert with other modalities.

PET/CT showed good specificity for BM and GI evaluation but suboptimal sensitivity. Moreover, eotPET post-therapy PET/CT results, evaluated according to Deauville criteria, can be considered powerful prognostic information in order to stratify the progressive patients.

Author Contributions: Study concept and design, D.A., S.A., R.L., M.B.; recruitment and collection data, D.A., S.A., M.B., R.D., A.B., A.C. (Alessia Castellino), L.C., P.F., V.F., A.C. (Agostino Chiaravalloti), F.L., E.A., M.A., G.S., A.C. (Annarosa Cuccaro), S.K.; quality control of data and algorithm, L.E., M.B., R.L.; data analysis, statistical analysis and interpretation, D.A., S.A.; manuscript preparation, D.A., S.A., R.L., M.B.; editing, review, supervision, approval final version of the manuscript, all authors.

Funding: This research received no external funding.

Conflicts of Interest: The authors declare they have no conflict of interest.

References

1. Vose, J.M. Mantle cell lymphoma: 2017 update on diagnosis, risk-stratification, and clinical management. *Am. J. Hematol.* **2017**, *92*, 806–813. [CrossRef] [PubMed]
2. Hoster, E.; Dreyling, M.; Klapper, W.; Gisselbrecht, C.; van Hoof, A.; Kluin-Nelemans, H.C.; Pfreundschuh, M.; Reiser, M.; Metzner, B.; Einsele, H.; et al. A new prognostic index (MIPI) for patients with advanced-stage mantle cell lymphoma. *Blood* **2008**, *111*, 558–565. [CrossRef] [PubMed]
3. Barrington, S.F.; Mikhaeel, N.G.; Kostakoglu, L.; Meignan, M.; Hutchings, M.; Müeller, S.P.; Schwartz, L.H.; Zucca, E.; Fisher, R.I.; Trotman, J.; et al. Role of imaging in the staging and response assessment of lymphoma: Consensus of the International Conference on Malignant Lymphomas Imaging Working Group. *J. Clin. Oncol.* **2014**, *32*, 3048–3058. [CrossRef] [PubMed]
4. Cheson, B.D.; Fisher, R.I.; Barrington, S.F.; Cavalli, F.; Schwartz, L.H.; Zucca, E.; Lister, T.A. Recommendations for initial evaluation, staging, and response assessment of Hodgkin and non-Hodgkin lymphoma: The Lugano classification. *J. Clin. Oncol.* **2014**, *32*, 3059–3068. [CrossRef] [PubMed]
5. Bailly, C.; Carlier, T.; Touzeau, C.; Arlicot, N.; Kraeber-Bodéré, F.; Le Gouill, S.; Bodet-Milin, C. Interest of FDG-PET in the Management of Mantle Cell Lymphoma. *Front Med (Lausanne)* **2019**, *6*, 70. [CrossRef]
6. Maddocks, K. Update on Mantle cell lymphoma. *Blood* **2018**, *132*, 1647–1656. [CrossRef]
7. Gill, S.; Wolf, M.; Prince, H.M.; Januszewicz, H.; Ritchie, D.; Hicks, R.J.; Seymour, J.F. 18F Fluorodeoxyglucose positron emission tomography scanning for staging, response assessment, and disease surveillance in patients with Mantle cell lymphoma. *Clin. Lymphoma Myeloma* **2008**, *8*, 158–165. [CrossRef]
8. Alavi, A.; Shrikanthan, S.; Aydin, A.; Talanow, R.; Schuster, S. Fluorodeoxyglucose-positron-emission tomography findings in Mantle cell lymphoma. *Clin. Lymphoma Myeloma Leuk.* **2011**, *11*, 261–266. [CrossRef]
9. Albano, D.; Ferro, P.; Bosio, G.; Fallanca, F.; Re, A.; Tucci, A.; Ferreri, A.J.M.; Angelillo, P.; Gianolli, L.; Giubbini, R.; et al. Diagnostic and Clinical Impact of Staging 18F-FDG PET/CT in Mantle-Cell Lymphoma: A Two-Center Experience. *Clin. Lymphoma Myeloma Leuk.* **2019**, *19*, e457–e464. [CrossRef]
10. Brepoels, L.; Stroobants, S.; De Wever, W.; Dierickx, D.; Vandenberghe, P.; Thomas, J.; Mortelmans, L.; Verhoef, G.; De Wolf-Peeters, C. Positron emission tomography in mantle cell lymphoma. *Leuk. Lymphoma* **2008**, *49*, 1693–1701. [CrossRef]

11. Cohen, J.B.; Hall, N.C.; Ruppert, A.S.; Jones, J.A.; Porcu, P.; Baiocchi, R.; Christian, B.A.; Penza, S.; Benson, D.M.; Flynn, J.; et al. Association of pre-transplantation positron emission tomography/computed tomography and outcome in mantle cell lymphoma. *Bone Marrow Transplant.* **2013**, *48*, 1212–1217. [CrossRef] [PubMed]
12. Hosein, P.J.; Pastorini, V.H.; Paes, F.M.; Eber, D.; Chapman, J.R.; Serafini, A.N.; Alizadeh, A.A.; Lossos, I.S. Utility of positron emission tomography scans in mantle cell lymphoma. *Am. J. Hematol.* **2011**, *86*, 841–845. [CrossRef] [PubMed]
13. Morgan, R.; Perry, M.; Kwak, J.; Jensen, A.; Kamdar, M. Positron emission tomography-based analysis can accurately predict bone marrow involvement with Mantle Cell Lymphoma. *Clin. Lymphoma Myeloma Leuk.* **2018**, *18*, 731–736. [CrossRef] [PubMed]
14. Adams, H.J.A.; Kwee, T.C.; de Keizer, B.; Fijnheer, R.; de Klerk, J.M.; Littooij, A.S.; Nievelstein, R.A. Systematic review and meta-analysis on the diagnostic performance of FDG-PET/CT in detecting bone marrow involvement in newly diagnosed Hodgkin lymphoma: Is bone marrow biopsy still necessary? *Ann. Oncol.* **2014**, *25*, 921–927. [CrossRef]
15. Adams, H.J.A.; Kwee, T.C.; de Keizer, B.; Fijnheer, R.; de Klerk, J.M.; Nievelstein, R.A. FDG PET/CT for the detection of bone marrow involvement in diffuse large B cell lymphoma: Systematic review and meta-analysis. *Eur. J. Nucl. Med. Mol. Imaging* **2014**, *41*, 565–574. [CrossRef]
16. Bodet-Milin, C.; Touzeau, C.; Leux, C.; Sahin, M.; Moreau, A.; Maisonneuve, H.; Morineau, N.; Jardel, H.; Moreau, P.; Gallazini-Crépin, C.; et al. Prognostic impact of 18F-fluorodeoxyglucose positron emission tomography in untreated mantle cell lymphoma: A retrospective study from GOELAMS group. *Eur. J. Nucl. Med. Mol. Imaging* **2010**, *37*, 1633–1642. [CrossRef]
17. Gontier, E.; Fourme, E.; Wartski, M.; Blondet, C.; Bonardel, G.; Le Stanc, E.; Mantzarides, M.; Foehrenbach, H.; Pecking, A.P.; Alberini, J.L. High and typical 18F-FDG bowel uptake in patients treated with metformin. *Eur. J. Nucl. Med. Mol. Imaging* **2008**, *35*, 95–99. [CrossRef]
18. Bybel, B.; Greenberg, I.D.; Paterson, J.; Ducharme, J.; Leslie, W.D. Increased F-18 FDG intestinal uptake in diabetic patients on metformin: A matched case-control analysis. *Clin. Nucl. Med.* **2011**, *36*, 452–456. [CrossRef]
19. Shah, J.J.; Fayad, L.; Romaguera, J. Mantle Cell International Prognostic Index (MIPI) not prognostic after R-hyper-CVAD. *Blood* **2008**, *112*, 2583. [CrossRef]
20. Mato, A.R.; Svodoba, J.; Feldman, T.; Zielonka, T.; Agress, H.; Panush, D.; Miller, M.; Toth, P.; Lizotte, P.M.; Nasta, S.; et al. Post-treatment (not interim) positron emission tomography-computed tomography scan status is highly predictive of outcome in mantle cell lymphoma patients treated with R-HyperCVAD. *Cancer* **2012**, *118*, 3565–3570. [CrossRef]
21. Tiemann, M.; Schrader, C.; Klapper, W.; Dreyling, M.H.; Campo, E.; Norton, A.; Berger, F.; Kluin, P.; Ott, G.; Pileri, S.; et al. Histopathology, cell proliferation indices and clinical outcome in 304 patients with mantle cell lymphoma (MCL): A clinicopathological study from the European MCL Network. *Br. J. Haematol.* **2005**, *131*, 29–38. [CrossRef] [PubMed]
22. Lamonica, D.; Graf, D.A.; Munteanu, M.C.; Czuczman, M.S. 18F-FDG PET for Measurement of Response and Prediction of Outcome to Relapsed or Refractory Mantle Cell Lymphoma Therapy with Bendamustine-Rituximab. *J. Nucl. Med.* **2017**, *58*, 62–68. [CrossRef] [PubMed]
23. Bailly, C.; Carlier, T.; Barriolo-Rieding, A.; Casasnovas, O.; Gyan, E.; Meignan, M.; Moreau, A.; Burroni, B.; Djaileb, L.; Gressin, R.; et al. Prognostic value of FDG-PET in patients with mantle cell lymphoma: Results from the LyMa-PET Project. *Haematologica* **2019**. [CrossRef] [PubMed]
24. Albano, D.; Bosio, G.; Bianchetti, N.; Pagani, C.; Re, A.; Tucci, A.; Giubbini, R.; Bertagna, F. Prognostic role of baseline 18F-FDG PET/CT metabolic parameters in mantle cell lymphoma. *Ann. Nucl. Med.* **2019**, *33*, 449–458. [CrossRef]
25. Kedmi, M.; Avivi, I.; Ribakovsky, E.; Benyamini, N.; Davidson, T.; Goshen, E.; Tadmor, T.; Nagler, A.; Avigdor, A. Is there a role for therapy response assessment with 2-[fluorine-18] fluoro-2-deoxy-D-glucose-positron emission tomography/computed tomography in mantle cell lymphoma? *Leuk. Lymphoma* **2014**, *55*, 2484–2489. [CrossRef]
26. Meignan, M.; Gallamini, A.; Haioun, C.; Polliack, A. Report on the Second International Workshop on interim positron emission tomography in lymphoma held in Menton, France, 8–9 April 2010. *Leuk Lymphoma.* **2010**, *51*, 2171–2180. [CrossRef]

27. Fallanca, F.; Alongi, P.; Incerti, E.; Ginaolli, L.; Picchio, M.; Kayani, I.; Bomanji, J. Diagnostic accuracy of FDG PET/CT for clinical evaluation at the end of treatment of HL and NHL: A comparison of the Deauville Criteria (DC) and the International Harmonization Project Criteria (IHPC). *Eur. J. Nucl. Med. Mol. Imaging* **2016**, *43*, 1837–1840. [CrossRef]
28. Klener, P.; Fronkova, E.; Belada, D.; Forsterova, K.; Pytlik, R.; Kalinova, M.; Simkovic, M.; Salek, D.; Mocikova, H.; Prochazka, V.; et al. Alternating R-CHOP and R-cytarabine is a safe and effective regimen for transplant-ineligible patients with a newly diagnosed mantle cell lymphoma. *Hematol. Oncol.* **2018**, *36*, 110–115. [CrossRef]
29. Czuczman, M.S.; Goy, A.; Lamonica, D.; Graf, D.A.; Munteanu, M.C.; van der Jagt, R.H. Phase II study of bendamustine combined with rituximab in relapsed/refractory mantle cell lymphoma: Efficacy, tolerability, and safety findings. *Ann. Hematol.* **2015**, *94*, 2025–2032. [CrossRef]
30. Karam, M.; Ata, A.; Irish, K.; Feustel, P.J.; Mottaghy, F.M.; Stroobants, S.G.; Verhoef, G.E.; Chundru, S.; Douglas-Nikitin, V.; Wong, C.O.; et al. FDG positron emission tomography/computed tomography scan may identify mantle cell lymphoma patients with unusually favorable outcome. *Nucl. Med. Comm.* **2009**, *30*, 770–778. [CrossRef]
31. Novelli, A.; Briones, J.; Flotats, A.; Sierra, J. PET/CT Assessment of Follicular Lymphoma and High Grade B Cell Lymphoma-Good Correlation with Clinical and Histological Features at Diagnosis. *Adv. Clin. Exp. Med.* **2015**, *24*, 325–330. [CrossRef] [PubMed]
32. Meyer, H.J.; Wienke, A.; Surov, A. Correlations Between Imaging Biomarkers and Proliferation Index Ki-67 in Lymphomas: A Systematic Review and Meta-Analysis. *Clin. Lymphoma Myeloma Leuk.* **2019**, *19*, 266–272. [CrossRef] [PubMed]
33. Jaffe, E.S.; Harris, N.L.; Stein, H.; Vardinam, J.W. *Tumours of Haematopoietic and Lymphoid Tissues: World Health Organization Classification of Tumours, Pathology, and Genetics*; IARC Press: Lyon, France, 2001; Volume 3.
34. Albano, D.; Bosio, G.; Camoni, L.; Farina, M.; Re, A.; Tucci, A.; Giubbini, R.; Bertagna, F. Prognostic role of baseline ^{18}F-FDG PET/CT parameters in MALT lymphoma. *Hematol. Oncol.* **2019**, *37*, 39–46.
35. Boellaard, R.; Delgado-Bolton, R.; Oyen, W.J.; Giammarile, F.; Tatsch, K.; Eschner, W.; Verzijlbergen, F.J.; Barrington, S.F.; Pike, L.C.; Weber, W.A.; et al. FDG PET/CT: EANM procedure guidelines for tumour imaging: Version 2.0. *Eur. J. Nucl. Med. Mol. Imaging* **2015**, *42*, 328–354. [CrossRef]

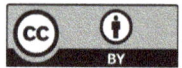

© 2019 by the authors. Licensee MDPI, Basel, Switzerland. This article is an open access article distributed under the terms and conditions of the Creative Commons Attribution (CC BY) license (http://creativecommons.org/licenses/by/4.0/).

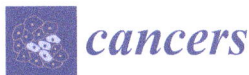

Article

Consensus Procedures in Oncological Imaging: The Case of Prostate Cancer

Stefano Fanti [1], Wim Oyen [2,3] and Elisabetta Lalumera [4,*]

[1] Department of Experimental, Diagnostic and Specialty Medicine—DIMES, University of Bologna, and Nuclear Medicine Division, Policlinico S.Orsola, 40138 Bologna, Italy; stefano.fanti@aosp.bo.it
[2] Department of Radiology and Nuclear Medicine, Rijnstate Hospital, 6815 Arnhem, The Netherlands; wjg.oyen@gmail.com
[3] Department of Biomedical Sciences, Humanitas University and Department of Nuclear Medicine, Humanitas Clinical and Research Center, 20126 Milan, Italy
[4] Psychology Department, Milano-Bicocca University, 20126 Milan, Italy
* Correspondence: elisabetta.lalumera@unimib.it

Received: 27 September 2019; Accepted: 12 November 2019; Published: 14 November 2019

Abstract: Recently, there has been increasing interest in methodological aspects of advanced imaging, including the role of guidelines, recommendations, and experts' consensus, the practice of self-referral, and the risk of diagnostic procedure overuse. In a recent Delphi study of the European Association for Nuclear Medicine (EANM), panelists were asked to give their opinion on 47 scientific questions about imaging in prostate cancer. Nine additional questions exploring the experts' attitudes and opinions relating to the procedure of consensus building itself were also included. The purpose was to provide insights into the mechanism of recommendation choice and consensus building as seen from the experts' point of view. Results: Regarding the factors likely to influence the willingness to refer a patient for imaging, the most voted were incorporation into guidelines and data from scientific literature, while personal experience and personal relationship were chosen by a small minority. Regarding the recommendations more relevant to prescribe an imaging procedure, it resulted the incorporation into guidelines promoted by scientific societies (59% of votes); these guidelines also resulted the more trusted. With respect to patients' preferences considered when prescribing an imaging procedure, the most voted was accuracy, resulted more important than easy access and time to access to the procedure. The majority of the experts expressed the opinion that there is a scarce use of imaging procedures in prostate cancer. With respect to the most relevant factor to build consensus, it resulted the transparency of the process (52% of votes), followed by multidisciplinarity of contributors. The main obstacle to incorporation of modern imaging procedures into guidelines resulted the lack of primary literature on clinical impact. Conclusions: Firstly, the panelists portray themselves as having Evidence-Based Medicine oriented and scientifically inclined attitudes and preferences. Secondly, guidelines and recommendations from scientific societies, especially clinical ones, are positively taken into account as factors influencing decisions, but panelists tend to consider their own appraisal of the scientific literature as more relevant. Thirdly, in respect of overuse, panelists do not think that advanced diagnostic procedures are overutilized in the specific case of Prostate Cancer, but rather they are underutilized.

Keywords: nuclear medicine; guidelines; prostate cancer; overutilization; epistemology; consensus

1. Introduction

Production of clinical practice guidelines (hereinafter "guidelines") and consensus statements is of paramount importance for the medical community. This is because the availability of an increasing number of therapeutic and diagnostic options for many diseases requires careful choices, and evidence-based data such as meta-analyses are not always sufficient to drive appropriate use of medical options [1,2]. This is arguably more relevant in the field of advanced medical imaging, where the evaluation of a new diagnostic technique is often not obtainable from evidence cased on randomized controlled trials (RCT), for both conceptual and practical reasons [3].

Even though conspicuous efforts have been made recently to improve and standardize guidelines [4,5], they are still far from being a perfect tool, as philosophers of medicine and methodologists have outlined. They are inevitably outdated in respect of the development of new technologies, they are seldom followed in clinical practice, and they intrinsically need further clinical judgment in order to be appropriately applied to the individual patient's case [6–9]. Moreover, it has recently been pointed out that scarce adherence to guidelines and recommendations favors self-referral and excessive compliance with patients' requests, factors that may cause overuse of diagnostic procedures [10,11]. In addition to these problematic aspects, guidelines are likely to be affected by bias as they are promoted by professional organizations which may tend to select experts from among their members [12,13].

Literature on the functioning of guideline development groups and their attitudes (the view from inside) is relatively scarce [14–16]. Here we take Prostate Cancer (PC) as a case study and illustrate and discuss how experts themselves involved in a consensus conference judge the procedures of consensus building, referral, and compliance with guidelines.

Available diagnostic options at various stages of the disease require careful consideration. A number of imaging methods to study PC have been suggested. These include methods which have been available for decades, for example, computed tomography (CT), bone scintigraphy (BS), and trans rectal ultrasound (TRU), as well as methods which have been introduced more recently, such as whole-body magnetic resonance imaging (MRI), multiparametric MRI, and positron emission tomography (PET). However, there is significant disagreement about the usefulness of such approaches [17–19].

In light of this, the European Association for Nuclear Medicine (EANM), representing nuclear medicine specialists who have been at the forefront of advances in molecular imaging techniques for PC, launched EANM Focus 1 to develop consensus statements in PC. EANM Focus 1 was held in February 2018 and resulted in a consensus on molecular imaging for diagnosis and treatment of prostate cancer. The findings were published in Lancet Oncology in December 2018 [20].

The organizers of EANM focus 1 were also interested in knowing the experts' attitudes and opinions relating to the procedure of consensus building itself as well as guidelines and their problematic aspects. For this reason, the final questionnaire included nine questions specifically focusing on these issues. This article reports and discusses the results of the aforementioned survey. Our goal is to provide insights into the mechanism of recommendation choice and consensus building as seen from the experts' point of view. We are aware that experts' declared attitudes and opinions may not be identical to the actual reasons motivating their decisions in practice. Nevertheless, we believe that their perception of their own role may be of interest in understanding the epistemology of consensus procedures, especially in the relatively new field of imaging epistemology. Moreover, we submit that experts' reflection and self-appraisal on methodological and ethical issues may enhance their commitment to their scientific role.

2. Materials and Methods

EANM Focus 1 was based on a clinical questionnaire proposed and then agreed among the panelists. A modified Delphi process was used to generate consensus on the topics identified. Overall, the questionnaire contained 47 questions, and a 70% cut-off was adopted to determine consensus [21–25]. Three Delphi rounds were conducted, and consensus was achieved in 36 out of 47 clinical questions (77%), as detailed in [20].

In order to address the specific problem of bias from affiliation to a scientific society, a multidisciplinary expert panel was established (hereinafter "the panelists"). The panel consisted of

24 people with representation from all fields involved to ensure a similar number of oncologists (5), urologists (5), radiation oncologists (2), radiologists (4), and nuclear medicine specialists (7). All the panelists were selected on the basis of their international reputation. Furthermore, one pathologist, one molecular biologist, and one radio pharmacist were involved, as well as two patient advocates. The full list of panelists is enclosed in Appendix A.

During the first Delphi round, in addition to the 47 clinical questions, panelists were given nine additional questions specifically designed to evaluate the role of guidelines in respect of clinical practice and the overall approach to consensus building. Questions 48 to 55 are grouped by topic, and their results are shown below. An informal discussion of the findings, without statistical analysis, then follows.

3. Results and Discussion

3.1. Factors to Refer PC Patients for Imaging

Question number 48 was, "Which factors are likely to influence your willingness to refer a patient for an imaging procedure, assuming that availability is not limited?", and panelists were asked to choose all that apply. Results are reported in Table 1.

Table 1. Consensus outcomes for question number 48.

Which Factors are Likely to Influence your Willingness to Refer a Patient for an Imaging Procedure, Assuming that Availability is not Limited?	
Incorporation into guidelines	76.2%
Data from scientific literature	90.5%
Study on cost-effectiveness	52.4%
Patients preferences	42.8%
Personal relationship with imaging professionals	19.0%
Personal experience	23.8%
Out of pocket cost to patient	19.0%
Abstain	4.3%
Unqualified to answer	4.3%

Before moving to further consideration, it is necessary to clarify some possible implications deriving from this question (number 48), as well as from the next (number 49). Some of the answers, and in particular "personal relationship" and "personal experience", may raise an ethical issue. If a "personal relationship" between a medical professional and the imaging professional has the ability to influence the outcome of the patient care, then we could have a major ethical violation. However, this was not the meaning of the answers and rather referred to professional trust that is developed when you personally know the imaging specialist and you are used to personally contacting him in case of any doubtful findings. Wording may seem somewhat vague, and therefore it is important to emphasize that all questions were reviewed and approved by all panelists, before being submitted, and no ethical concern was raised. The main reason to offer those possible answers was related to awareness that doctors may prescribe imaging exams not recommended by guidelines, for nonscientific reasons [26], and we were aimed at evaluating such possibility.

The panelists considered all the possible factors as potential influencers, but some of them were chosen by a small minority. In particular, the personal relationship with imaging professionals was regarded as a possible influencer by less than 20% of the panel. This indicates strong independence from a factor that may have either positive or negative implications.

Indeed, the personal relationship does not have much scientific value. It may be speculated that long-lasting collaboration may result in a fruitful professional relationship. Nonetheless, this factor seems less reliable than others. Surprisingly, the out of pocket cost of the examination for the patient gained the same low percentage of votes, while being a more relevant factor for appropriateness. It could be speculated that the experts regarded as minor the expense of an imaging procedure as compared with the overall costs of treatment. Further considerations regarding patient preference are detailed in question number 51 (see below).

A relatively low number of votes was also scored by the influence of the prescriber's personal experience, confirming that all the factors relating to nonscientific data were regarded as less relevant. Indeed, the first three answers are clearly related to objective scientific facts and gained a clear preference among the experts, while the two answers relating to individual personal perception did not obtain many votes. Factors relating to patient perspective scored somewhere in between. These results are in line with a scientifically oriented approach of the panelists, who clearly preferred rational, evidence-based factors to less measurable issues.

Question number 49 was as question 48, but in this case, panelists were asked to choose one answer only: results are reported in Table 2.

Table 2. Consensus outcomes for question number 49.

Which is the most Relevant Factor Influencing Referral to Imaging? Choose One	
Incorporation into guidelines	23.8%
Data from scientific literature	81.9%
Study on cost-effectiveness	9.5%
Patients preferences	4.7%
Personal relationship with imaging professionals	4.7%
Personal experience	0.0%
Out of pocket cost to patient	0.0%
Abstain	4.3%
Unqualified to answer	4.3%

When it comes to identifying the most relevant factor among the many proposed, there was a clear winner in data from scientific literature. Please note the sum of percentages is greater than 100% because several panelists, despite the question explicitly asking them not to, chose more than one answer. A formal consensus was reached regarding the most relevant factor (data from scientific literature), with almost 82% of the panelists voting for it. This consensus is in line with the principles of EBM (Evidence-based medicine) which consider scientific articles published in peer-reviewed journals as the most valuable source of evidence to decide whether to use a certain imaging procedure or not.

The panelists also considered incorporation into guidelines as a relevant factor, but to a minor extent. It should be mentioned that data from the literature is the prerequisite for proper incorporation into guidelines. Therefore, this factor implies the existence of the previous and most selected factor. The impression is that experts tend to prefer their own evaluation of original articles over guidelines, given that guidelines are only updated several months later.

There is much debate about the problems of timing required to have a new imaging method incorporated into PC guidelines. Previously, before the development of an EBM culture, conventional imaging methods such as CT and BS were incorporated without any formal evaluation of the positive effects on patient outcome. In the 1970's, these methods were simply introduced and rapidly considered mandatory without a specifically designed clinical trial being undertaken. Thirty years later, rapid developments in the field of imaging still pose issues for guideline development. Indeed, new methods such as MRI and PET are available and have been adopted in clinical practice before evidence-generating clinical trials have been performed, resulting in a significant increase in their use. With the growth of medical imaging, the concern that not all examinations are necessary has increased, and it is argued that up to 40% of diagnostic imaging studies may be inappropriate[17-18]. Furthermore, as mentioned, there are intrinsic problems in building EBM literature for diagnostic imaging[11] and this fact has led to significant disagreement in the field of PC imaging. At the Advanced Prostate Cancer Consensus Conference held in St. Gallen there was no consensus on most questions relating to advanced PC imaging [27]. The problem of reliability in the sources of recommendations was further investigated in the next question.

3.2. Source of Recommendations

Question number 50 was, "Which recommendations are more relevant for you when prescribing an imaging procedure?": results are reported in Table 3.

Table 3. EANM (European Association for Nuclear Medicine) consensus outcomes for question number 50.

Which Recommendations are more Relevant for you when Prescribing an Imaging Procedure?	
Guidelines published by Evidence-Based Medicine/Health Technology Assessment authorities	13.6%
Guidelines promoted by scientific societies (imaging)	19.2%
Guidelines promoted by scientific societies (clinical)	59.0%
Local healthcare recommendation	0.0%
Proceeding of consensus multidisciplinary congresses	13.6%
None of the above	9.9%
Abstain	0.0%
Unqualified to answer	4.3%

There could be several reasons why a minority of the panelists chose the option of EBM/Health Technology Assessment-promoted guidelines. Firstly, in the area of prostate cancer, there is a complete lack of such guidelines, and the panel was surely aware of that even if the question did not focus on PC. A more general reason might be the resistance of clinicians to guidelines developed outside their professional control. See also question no. 54.

It is interesting to note that experts regard published studies as the most reliable evidence to influence their willingness to refer a patient for imaging (see question no. 49). On the other hand, EBM guidelines resulting directly from scientific data review are perceived as less reliable than scientific society guidelines.

It is noteworthy that not a single panelist considers local healthcare recommendations as relevant. Once again, this result could relate to the composition of the panel, which is made up of clinicians selected on the basis of their international reputation. This means they may not be keen to adhere to local rules that often tend to limit access to expensive and innovative imaging methods.

3.3. Patients' Preferences

Question number 51 was "Which part of patients' preference are you considering when prescribing an imaging procedure?", and panelists were asked to choose all that apply: results are reported in Table 4.

The suggested answers to this question were slightly tricky because only the first four are genuinely related to patient preference and the fifth (accuracy of the procedure) relates to a scientific point of view. Indeed, it was this answer that received the largest majority of preferences (almost 82%), with the others being selected, but not to such a great extent. It is clear that this finding is related to the paternalistic approach of doctors to patients. When a final decision has to be taken, all patient preferences are duly taken into account, but the most relevant factor remains purely scientific evidence. In other words, the doctor is deciding in favor of the best diagnostic option, the value of which is more important than other factors.

Table 4. EANM consensus outcomes for question number 51.

Which Part of Patients' Preference are you Considering when Prescribing an Imaging Procedure?	
Easy access to the procedure (distance and availability)	54.5%
Time to access to the procedure (waiting list)	45.4%
Cost of the procedure (irrespective whether or not it is covered by healthcare system or insurance)	22.7%
Out of pocket cost to patient	22.7%
Accuracy of the procedure (best available option)	81.8%
None of the above	9.9%
Abstain	0.0%
Unqualified to answer	4.3%

3.4. Degree of Use of Imaging Procedures (See Below)

Question number 52 was, "Which is your overall opinion about the use of imaging procedures in PC?": results are reported in Table 5.

Table 5. EANM consensus outcomes for question number 52.

Which is your Overall Opinion about the Use of Imaging Procedures in PC?	
Overall there is excessive use of imaging procedures in PC	25.0%
There is excessive use of modern imaging procedures in PC	20.0%
Overall there is scarce use of imaging procedures in PC	10.0%
There is scarce use of modern imaging procedures in PC	60.0%
Use of imaging procedures in PC is optimal	10.0%
Abstain	8.7%
Unqualified to answer	4.3%

Question 53 was, "Which is your overall opinion about the use of imaging procedures in PC for BCR/APC (Biochemical Recurrence/Advanced Prostate Cancer)?": results are reported in Table 6.

Table 6. EANM consensus outcomes for question number 53.

Which is your Overall Opinion about the Use of Imaging Procedures in PC for Biochemical Recurrence (BCR)/Advanced Prostate Cancer(APC)?	
Overall there is excessive use of imaging procedures in PC for BCR/APC	10.5%
There is excessive use of modern imaging procedures in PC for BCR/APC	15.8%
Overall there is scarce use of imaging procedures in PC for BCR/APC	5.2%
There is scarce use of modern imaging procedures in PC for BCR/APC	52.6%
Use of imaging procedures in PC is quite optimal for BCR/APC	15.8%
Abstain	9.0%
Unqualified to answer	4.5%

3.5. Trustworthiness of Recommendations

Question 54 was, "Which recommendations do you consider more trustworthy regarding imaging usage?". Results are reported in Table 7.

Table 7. EANM consensus outcomes for question number 54.

Which Recommendations do you Consider more Trustworthy Regarding Imaging Usage?	
Guidelines promoted by clinical scientific societies (European Association of Urology, or similar)	52.4%
Guidelines promoted by imaging scientific societies (European Association for Nuclear Medicine or similar)	19.2%
Guidelines promoted by EBM/HTA authorities	4.7%
Proceeding of consensus multidisciplinary congresses	14.3%
Equally all of the above	14.3%
Abstain	4.5%

This question is closely linked to question number 50, but with the emphasis placed on trustworthiness of recommendations. Once again there is a clear preference for guidelines promoted by clinical scientific societies. This point deserves further consideration. It seems that overall results are mainly influenced by the actual scenario of existing recommendations in the field. As already mentioned, guidelines promoted by clinical scientific societies are more common and more usual.

3.6. Building Consensus

Question number 55 was, "Which factor do you consider most relevant to build consensus on imaging procedures?". Results are reported in Table 8.

The issue of consensus building is complex and controversial, with a number of factors involved and significant consequences for any healthcare system. Despite the fact that only one question in this questionnaire specifically covered the issue, some comments are necessary. The panelists clearly considered transparency of the process as the most relevant factor, thus favoring an EBM-oriented procedure. This is undoubtedly in line with current scientific opinion but contradicts the answers to question nos. 50 and 54, where EBM guidelines gained limited preferences. In other words, EBM methodology is widely recognized as the best option when making a recommendation, but there is resistance to guidelines promoted by EBM/HTA authorities. This fact is easily recognizable in the current practice of preparation of EAU guidelines, which are the most widely used in the treatment of PC.

Table 8. EANM consensus outcomes for question number 55.

Which Factor do you Consider most Relevant to Build Consensus on Imaging Procedures?	
Transparency of the process (evidence based medicine oriented)	52.4%
Participation of expert panelists (imaging specialist)	9.5%
Participation of multidisciplinary expert panelists (clinical specialist)	19.0%
Contribution of all stakeholders (specialists, patients, healthcare)	28.6%
Cost-effectiveness analysis	4.7%
Translational and primary literature data	9.5%
Abstain	0.0%
Unqualified to answer	4.5%

3.7. Incorporation of Imaging into Guidelines

Question 56 was, "Which factor do you consider the most relevant obstacle for the lack of incorporation of modern imaging procedures into guidelines and clinical practice?". Results are reported in Table 9.

Table 9. EANM consensus outcomes for question number 56.

Which Factor do you Consider the most Relevant Obstacle for the Lack of Incorporation of Modern Imaging Procedures into Guidelines and Clinical Practice?	
Lack of primary literature on accuracy (Multicentric Prospective Trials)	9.5%
Lack of primary literature on clinical impact (Multicentric Prospective Trials)	66.6%
Lack of secondary literature (systematic reviews and meta-analyses)	4.7%
Lack of cost-effectiveness analyses	0.0%
Difficulties of access to modern imaging methods	19.0%
Difficulties in communications with imaging specialists	0.0%
Abstain	0.0%
Unqualified to answer	4.5%

This question is based on recognition that modern imaging procedures, such as MRI and PET, have gained widespread use in some countries despite a lack of incorporation into guidelines. Lack of primary literature on the clinical impact of modern imaging procedures is identified as the most relevant factor.

4. Conclusions

We cautiously assume that the panelists' answers to the meta-questions show what they consider to be the right attitudes and preferences to have rather than the attitudes and preferences they actually have. The general picture that emerges is that experts, in their role as panelists, are adequately conscious of their role, that is, of which factors should be taken into account in deciding on imaging procedures within an EBM framework.

The results reported so far can be summarized as follows.

Firstly, the panelists show themselves to have EBM-oriented and scientifically inclined attitudes and preferences (questions 49, 55, and 56).

Secondly, guidelines and recommendations from scientific societies, especially clinical ones, are positively taken into account as factors influencing decisions, but panelists tend to consider their own appraisal of the scientific literature as more relevant and reliable. This is in line with a widespread need to rethink guidelines.

Thirdly, in relation to overutilization, panelists do not think that advanced diagnostic procedures are overutilized in the specific case of PC, but rather they are underutilized. Moreover, in line with the EBM-inclined attitude, they do not consider patient preferences as factors that should influence their decision whether to prescribe a test or not. This result suggests that the issue of overutilization of diagnostic procedures should be considered on a case-by-case basis. Furthermore, additional research should be done to compare the inclinations of medical specialists with those of general practitioners and patients with regard to this topic.

Fourthly, various problems specific to the field have also emerged. These include the relative scarcity of primary literature on the clinical effectiveness of some imaging tests and the predominance of the clinical importance of the procedure over its intrinsic diagnostic accuracy in evaluation and recommendation.

As a final and general suggestion, we submit that questions such as the ones we have posed and analyzed may, in general, enhance the experts' self-appraisal of their role when actively participating in Delphi and consensus procedures, may act as a reminder of good scientific practices, and, therefore, may contribute to better performance on their part.

Author Contributions: Conceptualization, S.F. and W.O.; methodology, S.F.; writing—original draft preparation, S.F. and E.L.; writing—review and editing, S.F. and E.L.

Funding: This research was funded by EANM.

Acknowledgments: The authors wish to thank Silvia Minozzi for Delphi supervision and data analysis; Susanne Koebe, Andreas Felser, and Henrik Silber (EANM) for project management. We would also like to thank all the panelists for their contribution.

Conflicts of Interest: The authors declare no conflict of interest.

Appendix A. —Expert Panel

Name of Expert	Institute	Field of Expertise
Gerald Antoch	University Hospital Düsseldorf, Germany	Radiology
Ian Banks	ECCO & European Men's Health Forum	Patient Advocate
Alberto Briganti	San Raffaele University Hospital, Milan, Italy	Urology
Ignasi Carriò	Hospital de la Santa Creu i Sant Pau, Barcelona, Spain	Nuclear Medicine
Arturo Chiti	Instituto Clinico Humanitas, Milan, Italy	Nuclear Medicine
Noel Clarke	The Christie Hospital	Urological Oncology
Johann De Bono	The Institute of Cancer Research, London, United Kingdom	Medical Oncology
Matthias Eiber	Klinikum rechts der Isar, TUM, München, Germany	Nuclear Medicine
Karim Fizazi	Institut Gustave Roussy, Paris, France	Medical Oncology
Silke Gillessen	Kantonsspital St. Gallen, Switzerland	Medical Oncology
Sam Gledhill	Movember Foundation	Patient Advocate
Uwe Haberkorn	University Hospital Heidelberg, Germany	Nuclear Medicine
Ken Herrmann	Universitätsklinikum Essen, Germany	Nuclear Medicine
Rodney Hicks	Peter Mac Callum Cancer Institute, Melbourne, Australia	Nuclear Medicine
Frédéric Lecouvet	Clinique Universitaires Saint-Luc UCL, Brussels, Belgium	Radiology
Rodolfo Montironi	Ospedali Riuniti Ancona, Italy	Pathology
Joe O'Sullivan	Queen's University Belfast, United Kingdom	Radiation Oncology
Piet Ost	Ghent University Hospital, Belgium	Radiation Oncology
Anwar Padhani	Mount Vernon Cancer Centre, London, United Kingdom	Radiology
Jack Schalken	Radboud UMC, Netherland	Molecular Biology
Howard Scher	Memorial Sloan Kettering Cancer Center, New York, USA	Medical Oncology
Bertrand Tombal	Cliniques Universitaires Saint-Luc; Belgium	Urology
Jeroen van Moorselaar	VU Medisch Centrum, Netherland	Urology
Hendrik Van Poppel	KU Leuven	Urology
Herbert Alberto Vargas	Memorial Sloan Kettering Cancer Center, New York, USA	Radiology
Jochen Walz	Institute Paoli-Calmettes, Marseille, France	Urology
Wolfgang Weber	Memorial Sloan Kettering Cancer Center, New York, USA	Nuclear Medicine
Hans-Jürgen Wester	Technische Universität München, Germany	Radiochemistry

References

1. Woolf, S.H.; Grol, R.; Hutchinson, A.; Eccles, M.; Grimshaw, J. Potential benefits, limitations, and harms of clinical guidelines. *BMJ* **1999**, *318*, 527–530. [CrossRef] [PubMed]

2. Qaseem, A.; Forland, F.; Macbeth, F.; Ollenschläger, G.; Phillips, S.; van der Wees, P. Guidelines International Network: Toward international standards for clinical practice guidelines. *Ann. Intern. Med.* **2012**, *156*, 525–531. [CrossRef] [PubMed]
3. Lalumera, E.; Fanti, S. Randomized Controlled Trials for Diagnostic Imaging: Conceptual and Pratical Problems. *Topoi* **2017**, 1–6. [CrossRef]
4. Brouwers, M.C.; Kho, M.E.; Browman, G.P.; Burgers, J.S.; Cluzeau, F.; Feder, G.; Littlejohns, P. AGREE II: Advancing guideline development, reporting and evaluation in health care. *Cmaj* **2010**, *182*, E839–E842. [CrossRef]
5. Eccles, M.P.; Grimshaw, J.M.; Shekelle, P.; Schünemann, H.J.; Woolf, S. Developing clinical practice guidelines: Target audiences, identifying topics for guidelines, guideline group composition and functioning and conflicts of interest. *Implement. Sci.* **2012**, *7*, 60. [CrossRef]
6. Upshur, R.E. Do clinical guidelines still make sense? No. *Ann. Fam. Med.* **2014**, *12*, 202–203. [CrossRef]
7. Cartwright, N. A philosopher's view of the long road from RCTs to effectiveness. *Lancet* **2011**, *377*, 1400–1401. [CrossRef]
8. Cartwright, N. What evidence should guidelines take note of? *J. Evaluat. Clin. Pract.* **2018**, *24*, 1139–1144. [CrossRef]
9. Cabana, M.D.; Rand, C.S.; Powe, N.R.; Wu, A.W.; Wilson, M.H.; Abboud, P.A.C.; Rubin, H.R. Why don't physicians follow clinical practice guidelines? A framework for improvement. *Jama* **1999**, *282*, 1458–1465. [CrossRef]
10. Hendee, W.R.; Becker, G.J.; Borgstede, J.P.; Bosma, J.; Casarella, W.J.; Erickson, B.A.; Wallner, P.E. Addressing overutilization in medical imaging. *Radiology* **2010**, *257*, 240–245. [CrossRef]
11. Hofmann, B. Too much of a good thing is wonderful? A conceptual analysis of excessive examinations and diagnostic futility in diagnostic radiology. *Med. Health Care Philos.* **2010**, *13*, 139–148. [CrossRef] [PubMed]
12. Grilli, R.; Magrini, N.; Penna, A.; Mura, G.; Liberati, A. Practice guidelines developed by specialty societies: The need for a critical appraisal. *Lancet* **2000**, *355*, 103–106. [CrossRef]
13. Shekelle, P.G. Clinical practice guidelines: what's next? *Jama* **2018**, *320*, 757–758. [CrossRef] [PubMed]
14. Atkins, L.; Smith, J.A.; Kelly, M.P.; Michie, S. The process of developing evidence-based guidance in medicine and public health: A qualitative study of views from the inside. *Implement. Sci.* **2013**, *8*, 101. [CrossRef] [PubMed]
15. Sundberg, L.R.; Garvare, R.; Nyström, M.E. Reaching beyond the review of research evidence: A qualitative study of decision making during the development of clinical practice guidelines for disease prevention in healthcare. *BMC Health Serv. Res.* **2017**, *17*, 344.
16. Raine, R.; Sanderson, C.; Hutchings, A.; Carter, S.; Larkin, K.; Black, N. An experimental study of determinants of group judgments in clinical guideline development. *Lancet* **2004**, *364*, 429–437. [CrossRef]
17. American Urological Association—Clinically Localized Prostate Cancer: AUA/ASTRO/SUO Guideline. Available online: http://www.auanet.org/guidelines/clinically-localized-prostate-cancer-new-(aua/astro/suo-guideline-2017) (accessed on 5 September 2019).
18. Cornford, P.; Bellmunt, J.; Bolla, M.; Briers, E.; De Santis, M.; Gross, T.; Henry, A.M.; Joniau, S.; Lam, T.B.; Mason, M.D.; et al. EAU-ESTRO-SIOG Guidelines on Prostate Cancer. Part II: Treatment of Relapsing, Metastatic, and Castration-Resistant Prostate Cancer. *Eur. Urol.* **2017**, *71*, 630–642. [CrossRef]
19. Mottet, N.; Bellmunt, J.; Bolla, M.; Briers, E.; Cumberbatch, M.G.; De Santis, M.; Fossati, N.; Gross, T.; Henry, A.M.; Joniau, S.; et al. EAU-ESTRO-SIOG Guidelines on Prostate Cancer. Part I: Screening, Diagnosis, and Local Treatment with Curative Intent. *Eur. Urol.* **2017**, *71*, 618–629. [CrossRef]
20. Fanti, S.; Minozzi, S.; Antoch, G.; Banks, I.; Briganti, A.; Carrio, I.; Fizazi, K. Consensus on molecular imaging and theranostics in prostate cancer. *Lancet Oncol.* **2018**, *19*, e696–e708. [CrossRef]
21. Delphi Method/RAND. Available online: https://www.rand.org/topics/delphi-method.html (accessed on 22 September 2019).
22. Landis, J.R.; Koch, G.G. The measurement of observer agreement for categorical data. *Biometrics* **1977**, *33*, 159–174. [CrossRef]
23. Bruinsma, S.M.; Roobol, M.J.; Carroll, P.R.; Klotz, L.; Pickles, T.; Moore, C.M.; Gnanapragasam, V.J.; Villers, A.; Rannikko, A.; Valdagni, R.; et al. Expert consensus document: Semantics in active surveillance for men with localized prostate cancer—Results of a modified Delphi consensus procedure. *Nat. Rev. Urol.* **2017**, *14*, 312–322. [CrossRef] [PubMed]

24. Zafar, S.Y.; Currow, D.C.; Cherny, N.; Strasser, F.; Fowler, R.; Abernethy, A.P. Consensus-based standards for best supportive care in clinical trials in advanced cancer. *Lancet Oncol.* **2012**, *13*, e77–e82. [CrossRef]
25. Hasson, F.; Keeney, S.; McKenna, H. Research guidelines for the Delphi survey technique. *J. Adv. Nurs.* **2000**, *32*, 1008–1015. [PubMed]
26. Simos, D.; Hutton, B.; Graham, I.D.; Arnaout, A.; Caudrelier, J.M.; Clemons, M. Imaging for metastatic disease in patients with newly diagnosed breast cancer: Are doctor's perceptions in keeping with the guidelines? *J. Eval. Clin. Pract.* **2015**, *21*, 67–73. [CrossRef] [PubMed]
27. Gillessen, S.; Attard, G.; Beer, T.M.; Beltran, H.; Bossi, A.; Bristow, R.; Carver, B.; Castellano, D.; Chung, B.H.; Clarke, N.; et al. Management of Patients with Advanced Prostate Cancer: The Report of the Advanced Prostate Cancer Consensus Conference APCCC 2017. *Eur. Urol.* **2018**, *73*, 178–211. [CrossRef] [PubMed]

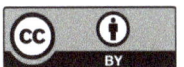

© 2019 by the authors. Licensee MDPI, Basel, Switzerland. This article is an open access article distributed under the terms and conditions of the Creative Commons Attribution (CC BY) license (http://creativecommons.org/licenses/by/4.0/).

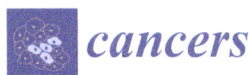

Article

Hybrid ^{18}F-FDG-PET/MRI Measurement of Standardized Uptake Value Coupled with Yin Yang 1 Signature in Metastatic Breast Cancer. A Preliminary Study

Concetta Schiano [1,*], Monica Franzese [1], Katia Pane [1], Nunzia Garbino [1], Andrea Soricelli [1,2], Marco Salvatore [1,†], Filomena de Nigris [3,†] and Claudio Napoli [1,4,†]

1. IRCCS SDN, 80134 Naples, Italy
2. Department of Motor Sciences and Healthiness, University of Naples Parthenope, 80134 Naples, Italy
3. Department of Precision Medicine, University of Campania "Luigi Vanvitelli", 80138 Naples, Italy
4. Department of Advanced Medical and Surgical Sciences, University of Campania "Luigi Vanvitelli", 80138 Naples, Italy
* Correspondence: tina.schiano@gmail.com or cshiano@sdn-napoli.it; Tel.: +39-081-2408260; Fax: +39-081-668841
† Contributed equally to the design of the study.

Received: 5 July 2019; Accepted: 23 September 2019; Published: 26 September 2019

Abstract: Purpose: Detection of breast cancer (BC) metastasis at the early stage is important for the assessment of BC progression status. Image analysis represents a valuable tool for the management of oncological patients. Our preliminary study combined imaging parameters from hybrid ^{18}F-FDG-PET/MRI and the expression level of the transcriptional factor Yin Yang 1 (YY1) for the detection of early metastases. Methods: The study enrolled suspected $n = 217$ BC patients that underwent ^{18}F-FDG-PET/MRI scans. The analysis retrospectively included $n = 55$ subjects. $n = 40$ were BC patients and $n = 15$ imaging-negative female individuals were healthy subjects (HS). Standard radiomics parameters were extracted from PET/MRI image. RNA was obtained from peripheral blood mononuclear cells and YY1 expression level was evaluated by real time reverse transcription polymerase chain reactions (qRT-PCR). An enzyme-linked immuosorbent assay (ELISA) was used to determine the amount of YY1 serum protein. Statistical comparison between subgroups was evaluated by Mann-Whitney U and Spearman's tests. Results: Radiomics showed a significant positive correlation between Greg-level co-occurrence matrix (GLCM) and standardized uptake value maximum (SUVmax) ($r = 0.8$ and $r = 0.8$ respectively) in BC patients. YY1 level was significant overexpressed in estrogen receptor (ER)-positive/progesteron receptor-positive/human epidermal growth factor receptor2-negative (ER+/PR+/HER2-) subtype of BC patients with synchronous metastasis (SM) at primary diagnosis compared to metachronous metastasis (MM) and HS ($p < 0.001$) and correlating significantly with ^{18}F-FDG-uptake parameter (SUVmax) ($r = 0.48$). Conclusions: The combination of functional ^{18}F-FDG-PET/MRI parameters and molecular determination of YY1 could represent a novel integrated approach to predict synchronous metastatic disease with more accuracy than ^{18}F-FDG-PET/MRI alone.

Keywords: breast; imaging; marker; radiomics; Yin Yang 1

1. Introduction

PET and MRI scans are useful instruments to diagnose the presence of metastatic disease providing both morphological and metabolic information [1–3]. However, an exclusive use of imaging technique, has some limitations, such as high cost, sensitivity and specificity [4]. We are confident that the combination of non-invasive methods with the parameters derived from image analysis will be of great interest for clinical practice.

A growing amount of data has established that polycomb oncoprotein Yin Yang 1 (YY1) has a prognostic impact in malignancy [5–7]. YY1 is frequently overexpressed in a wide range of solid and non-solid tumors, regulating a broad class of genes involved in control of both cell cycle and apoptosis. In vitro and in vivo studies have reported the expression of YY1 has been associated with development of a malignant phenotype in some human cancers, tumor progression, metastasis formation, and correlating with poor prognosis and drug/immune resistance [8–17]. However, conflicting results have been shown when YY1 was evaluated during the progression and metastasis of breast cancer (BC). The role of YY1 in metastatic BC has recently been verified by meta-analysis showing that YY1 exhibited significantly high mRNA levels in basal-like BCs versus normal tissues [18]. In contrast, Lieberthal et al. reported an increased expression of YY1 in invasive BC cells [19]. Furthermore, recently, YY1 was reported as anti-oncogene in invasive human BC cells [20]. Specifically, three potential binding sites for YY1 were found on a lincRNA involved in occurrence and progression of human cancers [20]. Moreover, about 70%–80% of diagnosed BCs are estrogen receptor positive and treated with endocrine therapy. However, this treatment is ineffective for patients with metastatic disease [21].

This study represents the first assessment of YY1 mRNA and protein expression levels in peripheral blood from BC patients, which have been correlated with imaging parameters from hybrid ^{18}F-FDG-PET/MRI in order to improve the early detection of metastatic disease.

2. Materials and Methods

2.1. Study Cohort

The study was approved by the institutional ethics committee (IRCCS Fondazione SDN) in accordance with the ethical standard of the Declaration of Helsinki. A written informed consent was obtained from all subjects enrolled (healthy subjects (HS) and BC patients). All clinical-pathological characteristics are reported in Table 1. Exclusion criteria included age <18 years, pregnancy, different cancer detection, and general contraindications for contrast agent injection. All eligible patients had ^{18}F-FDG-PET/MRI scans between 2014 and 2018. Our retrospective study enrolled consecutive suspected $n = 217$ oncological patients that underwent ^{18}F-FDG-PET/MRI scans. Individuals with negative imaging were considered HS ($n = 15$) (Figure 1) [22].

Table 1. Patient clinical-pathological characteristics.

	Number or Values
Total Cohort	52
Healthy Subjects "Control group"	15
Breast cancer group "Synchronous metastasis" (SM)	11
Breast cancer group "Metachronous metastasis" (MM)	26
Mean age (years)	57
Range (min–max)	32–88
TNM	13
T0	1
T1	2
T2	7
T3	3
NA	24

Table 1. *Cont.*

	Number or Values
Tumor Grade	10
G2	8
G3	2
NA	27
Ki 67 Status [a]	12
Low	4
High	8
NA	25
ER Status	15
Negative	3
Positive	12
NA	22
PR Status	15
Negative	3
Positive	12
NA	22
Her2 Status [b]	13
Negative	9
Positive	3
NA	24

[a] Ki67 ≥ 20% was considered High. [b] one Her2 Status was equivocal. NA = Not available.

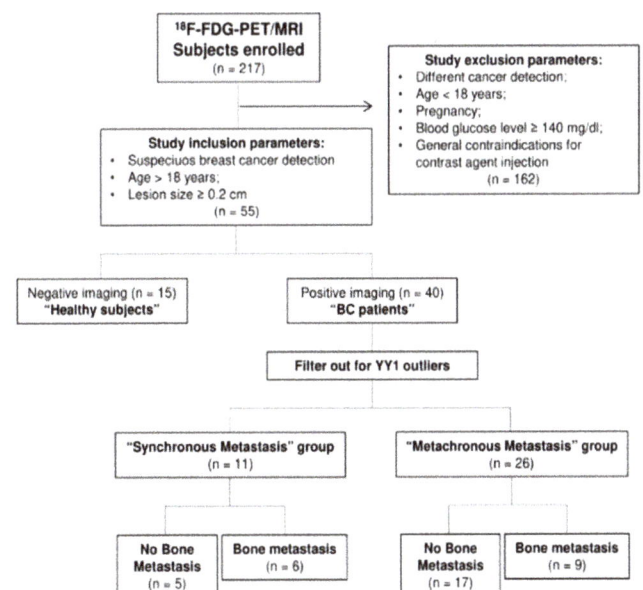

Figure 1. Eligible patients included in the study. Subject flow chart describing inclusion and exclusion criteria for the selection of the patients.

2.2. Sample Collection

Peripheral blood mononuclear cells (PBMCs) and serum aliquots were isolated as previously described [23]. Briefly, PBMCs were isolated by density gradient centrifugation on Histopaque-10771

(Sigma-Aldrich). After centrifugation, white blood cells were recovered and washed twice with phosphate-buffered saline (PBS) pH7.4 (Gibco; Life Technologies/Gibco, Italy). White cells and serum aliquots were frozen at −80 °C at the IRCCS SDN Biobank [24].

2.3. RNA Extraction and Real-Time Quantitative Reverse Transcription Polymerase Chain Reaction (qRT-PCR) Assay

Total RNAs were extracted using Trizol solution (Life Technologies/Gibco, Italy), according to the manufacturer's instructions. The specificity of oligonucleotide pair used was verified with the Basic Local Alignment Search Tool (BLAST), NCBI program and through in-silico polymerase chain reaction (PCR) analysis by UCSC (Genome Browser website) [23]. Primers were designed by Primer 3 software (http://bioinfo.ut.ee/primer3-0.4.0/) and synthesized by Life Technologies [23]. Quantitative real-time PCR was performed according to the supplier protocols (BioRad). Melt curve analysis was performed to verify a single product species. Selective primer sequences used for YY1 (NM_003403) were 5'-CAAAACTAAAACGACACCAAC-3' (Forward) and 5'-TGAAGTCCAGTGAAAAGCGT-3' (Reverse). Ribosomal protein S18 (RPS18; NM_022551) was used as housekeeping gene [23]. All reactions were carried out at least in triplicate for every cDNA template and qRT-PCR data were analyzed by Ct (threshold cycle) approach. The expression levels of the target gene normalized with the internal housekeeping gene were presented as delta-Ct (ΔCt), calculation [23]. The relative expression was estimated among groups considered.

2.4. YY1 Enzyme-Linked Immunosorbent Assay (ELISA) Test

Prior analysis, serum samples were stored at -80 °C. All samples were thawed only once prior to use. For the detection and quantification of our antigen of interest, enzyme-linked immunosorbent assay (ELISA) was used, according to the manufacturer's instructions with signals detection at 450 nm (Biocompare, Italy Cat. number ABIN4973888). Kit detection range was 0.156–10 ng/mL with sensitivity <0.059 ng/mL.

2.5. Hybrid ^{18}F-FDG-PET/MRI Technique

All patients were acquired on both a PET/CT device and on a 3T hybrid PET/MRI system (mMR Biograph; Siemens, Erlangen, Germany, with system sensitivity of 13.2 cps/kBq, transverse resolution of 4.4 mm and axial resolution of 4.5 mm) equipped with a dedicated breast coil, according to previously described acquisition protocols [25,26]. After fasting for 8 hours, patients were administered about 401 ± 32 MBq (mean ± standard deviation) of ^{18}F-FDG was administered to the patients, through an antecubital catheter. ^{18}F-FDG-PET/MRI images were performed concurrently after an uptake period of more than 60 minutes. The protocol was optimized for accurate detection and staging as previously described [25,27], briefly: an axial T2 turbo spin echo sequence; axial and coronal T2 turbo inversion recovery; diffusion weighted imaging (DWI), considered the most specific technique for the breast study. To investigate both morphological and dynamic breast parameters, all patients were injected with gadolinium diethylene triamine pentacetate (GD-DTPA; Magnevist) at 0.1 mmol/kg body weight, The dynamic study provides six axial spoiled gradient echo (SPGRE) 3D VIBE sequence before, during and after injection of contrast agent with variable flip-angle thus making a fat suppression. The attenuation correction is given by the segmentation (DIXON) in tissue classes, obtaining both water and fat maps. PET data are related only to these specific elements. Considering the PET data, the process of image reconstruction is done through an iterative algorithm called OSEM composed by three iterations on a matrix 172 × 172. Its main feature is the noise reduction in regions of low absorption. Image noise control is obtained by dividing data into 21 subsets analyzed cyclically.

2.6. Image Analysis

This study enrolled consecutive n. 217 subjects, of whom n. 15 HS and n. 202 oncological patients that underwent PET/MRI scans (Figure 1). After screening criteria, n. 52 female subjects were retrospectively available for analysis; in detail, 37 were BC patients and 15 HS (Figure 1). BC primary lesions were classified according to the American Joint Committee on Cancer Disease (AJCC) [28]. BC histology was confirmed by immunohistochemistry (IHC) analysis only for few patients diagnosed. Quantitative analysis was performed using PMOD (Version 3.8; PMOD Technologies, Switzerland), which consists of a complete set of tools, able to extrapolate quantitative parameters from the image. After importing all the ^{18}F-FDG-PET/MRI examinations into the PMOD software, the breast lesion automatic segmentation was done on the PET image. A reference cut-off of 41% of the standardized uptake value maximum (SUVmax) and volume of interest (VOI) were reported also on MRI images. Axial T2, DWI, apparent diffusion coefficient (ADC) and post administration 3D VIBE sequence were analyzed. One representative patient case was shown in Figure 2. For all subjects, we considered the following parameters: VOI, SUVmax and standardized uptake value minimum (SUVmin), average, standard deviation (SD), number of pixels and hot average (mean of pixels that presents higher values) of SUV body-weighted (SUVbw) and of SUV lean body mass (SUVlbm). SUVbw was expressed like c(t)/(Injected dose/body weight), where c(t) is tissue radioactivity concentration at time t. While SUVlbm referred to the value of standardized lean body mass absorption. Some texture indices referred to the histogram pixel within a VOI, and others based on to the gray-level co-occurrence matrix (GLCM). This latter matrix is defined as the distribution of co-occurring pixel values (grayscale values, or colors) at a given offset. In this stud, texture indices were: GLCM contrast (measure of the contrast intensity between pixels and its close over the entire image); Statistic Energy (the sum of the squared elements in the GLCM); GLCM sum variance (heterogeneity measure on close pixels).

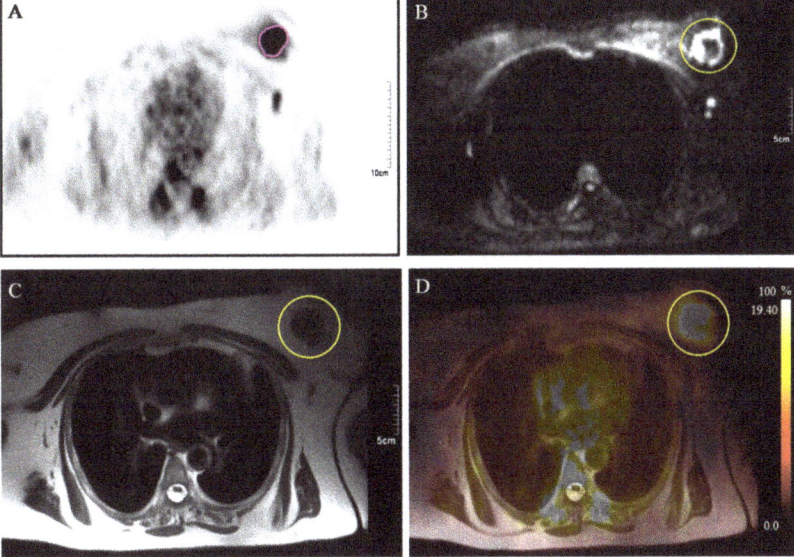

Figure 2. ^{18}F-FDG-PET/MRI scan Images of a 57-year-old patient with a breast heteroplasia with lymph node and bone metastases. The yellow circle indicates the lesion located on the left breast: (**A**) PET image showing uptake after 60 minutes of a segmented lesion (pink depicted); (**B**) Lesion revealed on T2 weighted image acquired on the axial plane; (**C**) hyperintensity of the lesion on diffusion-weighted magnetic resonance imaging; (**D**) ^{18}F-FDG-PET/MRI fusion image.

2.7. Statistical Analysis

Statistical analyses were performed using R environment (http://www.R-project.org). The distribution of biomedical imaging data (PET and MRI) was tested by Shapiro–Wilk test normality. The correlation between the statistical and textural parameters mostly used for breast lesions was evaluated using (Spearman's correlation test). In addition, the Wilcoxon–Mann–Whitney test was used to establish the statistical significance of molecular signature between the different BC groups and HS. To compare different hormone receptor subtypes, Kruskal–Wallis test was performed. For all tests a p value was considered for statistical significance when $p \leq 0.05$ and most significant when $p \leq 0.01$. Spearman's correlation was calculated to compare values of SUV max and YY1 levels.

3. Results

3.1. Study Population and Imaging Features

The mean age of all subject enrolled was 50 ± 4.6 years in HS compared to 53 ± 2.8 years in BC patients.

Moreover, within the metastatic BC cancer patients, we had patients with primary metastases (synchronous disease) and patients who developed metastases during follow-up (metachronous disease),.Thus, the cohort was divided in three groups: (*i*) "Healthy Subjects" (HS) ($n = 15$); (*ii*) "Synchronous Metastasis" (SM), which includes BC patients with one or multiple metastases at primary diagnosis ($n = 11$); and (*iii*) "Metachronous Metastasis" (MM), including BC patients who developed metastasis at follow up ($n = 26$). The metastasis were localized in bone ($n = 9$) and in different site, such as liver, uterus, lung, thyroid, and axillar and thoracic lymph nodes ($n = 17$).

Several features were extrapolated in order to investigate the sensitivity, specificity, and accuracy of ^{18}F-FDG-PET/MRI technique. By integration of high sensitivity of PET with the high spatial and temporal resolution of MRI we obtained information and characterized on the tumor malignancy (Figure 2) and detect small metastasis present in the body (Tumor Volume ≥ 1.2 cm^3 and GLCM_contrast_T2 ≥ 0.002). All features were related to the media pixel histogram within a VOI and to the GLCM, as highlighted by PET and MRI images as reported in Tables 2 and 3.

Table 2. Descriptive statistics of features extracted from PET images.

Synchronous Metastasis Group					
Features	Mean ± SD	Median	Min	Max	Range
Volume	9.54 ± 7.06	8.73	1.91	23.30	21.39
SUV_max	5.16 ± 4.19	3.78	1.33	13.24	11.91
n_voxels	721.86 ± 1247.68	247.00	54.00	3516.00	3462.00
Statistic_Energy	1.01 ± 0.01	0.01	0.01	0.01	0.00
GLCM_contrast	0.04 ± 0.03	0.03	0.00	0.09	0.09
Metachronous Metastasis Group					
Features	Mean ± SD	Median	Min	Max	Range
Volume	27.76 ± 40.35	7.21	2.86	122.19	119.33
SUV_max	5.26 ± 4.88	2.54	1.19	15.14	13.95
n_voxels	945.78 ± 1617.10	142.00	81.00	4998.00	4917.00
Statistic_Energy	1.01 ± 0.01	0.01	0.01	0.01	0.01
GLCM_contrast	0.03 ± 0.03	0.02	0.00	0.10	0.09

Table 3. Descriptive statistics of features extracted from MRI images.

	Synchronous Metastasis Group				
Features	Mean ± SD	Median	Min	Max	Range
Volume	9.33 ± 6.40	8.73	1.56	23.30	21.75
T2_mean	8.72 ± 8.22	6.58	0.16	24.81	24.65
GLCM_contrast_T2	1.87 ± 2.45	0.03	0.00	7.39	7.39
GLCM_entropy_T2	1.87 ± 1.72	0.39	0.06	5.47	5.41
B_value	5.75 ± 4.71	4.42	0.02	14.54	14.52
ADC_mean	5.94 ± 5.06	5.29	0.82	16.23	15.40
GLCM_contrast_ADC	1.01 ± 0.02	0.02	0.00	0.07	0.06
GLCM_entropy_ADC	1.34 ± 0.06	0.37	0.25	0.40	0.15
	Metachronous Metastasis Group				
Features	Mean ± SD	Median	Min	Max	Range
Volume	17.15 ± 22.04	5.02	2.86	54.53	51.67
T2_mean	5.16 ± 5.71	2.09	1.18	15.74	14.56
GLCM_contrast_T2	1.01 ± 0.03	0.01	0.00	0.09	0.08
GLCM_entropy_T2	1.35 ± 0.03	0.36	0.31	0.41	0.10
B_value	4.07 ± 4.14	1.88	1.44	11.58	10.14
ADC_mean	2.97 ± 2.94	1.53	0.45	8.50	8.04
GLCM_contrast_ADC	1.07 ± 0.15	0.01	0.00	0.41	0.40
GLCM_entropy_ADC	0.32 ± 0.13	0.37	0.04	0.38	0.34

3.2. YY1 Molecular Expression in Breast Cancer (BC) Patient

In order to analyze the expression level of YY1, from all patients PBMCs were recovered and total RNAs were extracted. Gene YY1 expression was evaluated in BC patients compared to control samples by real time RT-PCR. Same amount of YY1 has been shown in the MM group compared HS group. Conversely, in the SM group showed a 20-fold increase of YY1 mRNA compared with the HS group and 19-fold increase compared with the MM group ($p \leq 0.01$) using the non-parametric Wilcoxon test (Figure 3A). Moreover, the expression levels of YY1 (mRNA) were compared between MM and SM groups also considering the bone and no bone metastasis, respectively (Figure 3B). In contrast, YY1 protein level, dosed with ELISA assay, showed a significant increase in BC patients (MM and SM respectively, $p < 0.01; p < 0.01$). Differently from the expression trend, protein level of YY1 marker was higher into MM compared with HS group, although we did not know the underlying mechanism (Figure 4A,B).

Up-regulation of YY1 has been shown in estrogen receptor-positive (ER+) BCs [29] however, the regulatory mechanisms are still unknown. In our preliminary analysis, we also found YY1 overexpression in ER+ compared to ER- tumors, taking into account a total of $n = 15$ patients (see Table 1). Interestingly, we observed that YY1 mRNA specifically increased in (ER)-positive/- progesteron receptor-positive (PR+)/-human epidermal growth factor receptor2-negative (HER2-) (ER+/PR+/HER2-) compared to the "triple negative" (ER-/PR-/HER2-) and "triple positive" (ER+/PR+/HER2+) BC subtypes ($p = 0.27$, Kruskal-Wallis test) (Figure 5). Therefore, these data needs to be further elucidated, taking into account larger cohort including also different HER2+ and HER2- combinations such as ER-/PR-/HER2+, not diagnosed in our cases.

3.3. Correlation Between YY1 and FDG-PET/MRI in BC Patients

In order to select ^{18}F-FDG-PET/MRI parameters to correlate with YY1, first we evaluated the association between all imaging features by Spearman correlation test [30]. As shown in Figure 6, a significant positive correlation was observed between textural parameters: GLCM_contrast, SUVmin and SUVmax ($r = 0.8; r = 0.8$ respectively) (Table 2, Table 3 and Supplementary Materials Table S1) [30]. Subsequently, the Spearman test significantly correlated YY1 mRNA level (-ΔCt values) and

^{18}F-FDG-uptake (SUVmax) ($r = 0.48$) in SM patients with invasive BC cancer (Figure 7A,B). As reported in Figure 7B, pink color indicates that there was a negative correlation between YY1 expression reported as ΔCt values and ^{18}F-FDG-uptake. However, considering that small ΔCt values correspond to high gene expression, our preliminary results showed that YY1 mRNA expression and SUVmax reported the same trend (Figure 7B). Instead, no correlation was observed between YY1 protein and ^{18}F-FDG-PET/MRI parameters (data not shown). Overall, our study is the first attempts to evaluate the potential of combining imaging differences between SM and MM breast patient subgroups and YY1 gene expression, for a better diagnostic analysis of tumor metastasis (see Discussion).

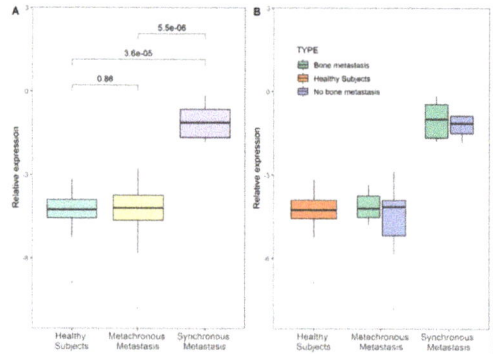

Figure 3. YY1 mRNA level and metastatic breast cancer. Expression level of YY1 in BC patients clustered into "Healthy Subjects" (HS), "Metachronous Metastasis" (MM) and "Synchronous Metastasis" (SM) group. (**A**) YY1 mRNA level in PBMCs from BC patients ($n = 11$ SM and $n = 26$ MM) and HS patients ($n = 15$). Data are reported as (-ΔCt). Each group was compared. (**B**) BC patients for SM and MM group were classified in two categories: no bone metastasis ($n = $ SM and $n = $ MM, respectively) and bone metastasis ($n = 5$ SM and $n = 17$ MM, respectively); the distribution did not show statistically significant difference between two categories included in each group. Statistical analysis was performed by the Wilcoxon test, and p value < 0.05 was considered significant.

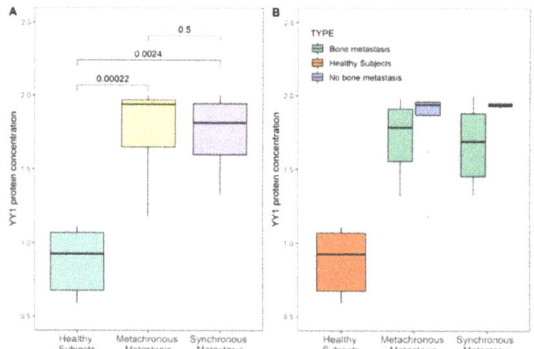

Figure 4. YY1 protein level and metastatic breast cancer. Serum protein level of YY1 in BC patients grouped as "Healthy Subjects" (HS), "Metachronous Metastasis" (MM) and "Synchronous Metastasis" (SM) group. (**A**) Comparison of YY1 protein level between BC patients ($n = 11$ SM and $n = 26$ MM) and HS patients ($n = 15$). Protein concentration is reported as ng/mL. Enzyme-linked immunosorbent assay (ELISA) YY1 protein level in BC patient sera indicated a media concentration of 1.8 ± 0.3 ng/ml in MM and 1.7 ± 0.3 ng/ml in SM patients compared to 0.8 ± 0.3 ng/ml in HS ($p < 0.01$; $p < 0.01$). (**B**) Comparison of YY1 protein level in SM and MM patients subgrouped as: no bone metastasis ($n = 5$ SM and $n = 17$ MM, respectively) and bone metastasis ($n = 5$ SM and $n = 17$ MM, respectively); Statistical significance was determined by Wilcoxon test, p value < 0.05 was considered significant.

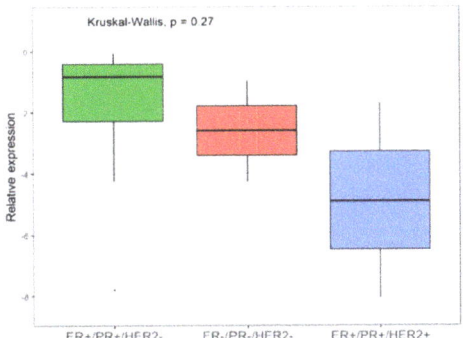

Figure 5. YY1 levels and receptor status in metastatic breast cancer. Comparison of YY1 mRNA level between estrogen receptor -positive/progesteron receptor-positive/human epidermal growth factor receptor2-negative (ER+/PR+/HER2-) compared to the "triple positive" (ER+/PR+/HER2+) and "triple negative" (ER-/PR-/HER2-) BC receptor status. Relative expression is reported as (-ΔCt). Statistical significance was determined by Kruskal-Wallis test, p value <0.05 was considered significant.

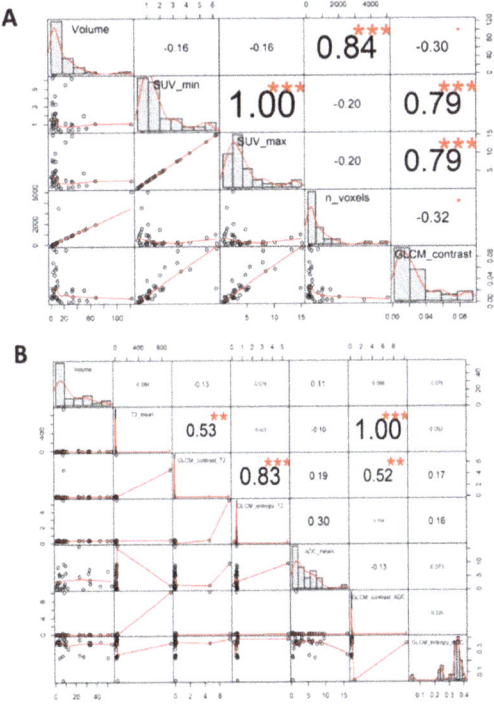

Figure 6. Correlation matrix for radiomics features of PET and MRI images. Correlation charts represent the correlation matrix between the statistical and textural parameters extracted from PET images (**A**) and MRI images (**B**) mostly used for breast lesions. The distribution of each variable is shown on the diagonal. On the bottom of the diagonal: the bivariate scatter plots with a fitted line are displayed. On the top of the diagonal: the value of the correlation plus the significance level as stars. Each significance level is associated to a symbol: p values 0.001; 0.01; 0.05; with symbols "***"; "**"; "*" respectively.

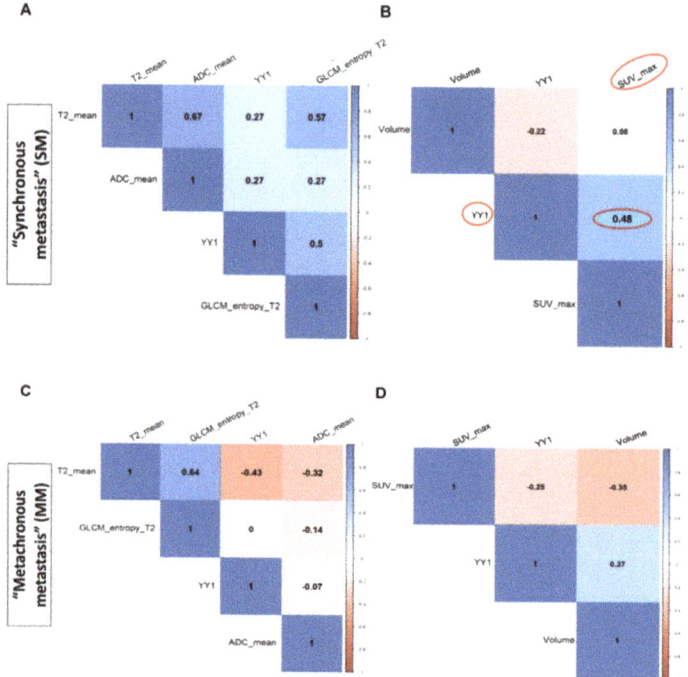

Figure 7. Radiomic features and YY1 molecular analysis. Correlation plot illustrates the Spearman test coefficient between YY1 expression level and PET/RMI parameters across "Synchronous Metatstasis" (SM) (**A**,**B**) and "Metachronous Metatstasis" (MM) BC patients (**C**,**D**). Color scale bar shows the positive correlation in blue and the negative correlation in pink; color intensity represents the strength of the correlation coefficient. Data indicated a statistical significant correlation between YY1mRNA and SUVmax in patients with SM ρ = 0.48. In the Supplementary Materials Table S1 are reported all analyzed findings for each patient at primary diagnosis.

4. Discussion and Conclusions

This preliminary study evaluated the feasibility of using diagnostic imaging and blood circulating level of YY1 as prospective tool to assess the presence of metastasis and tumor grade at diagnosis. The combination of imaging parameters and molecular biomarkers to improve the sensitive and specificity of primary tumor and metastatic lesions diagnosis it is of great interest for both better clinical decision-making and treatment management. To date, an accurate diagnosis of BC patients is difficult due to the tumor heterogeneity of clinical presentation and the co-presence of almost undetectable micro-metastasis. Moreover, based on the expression of hormone receptors in tumor tissues, approximately 70%–80% of BC is ER+ [31–34].

The multifunctional factor YY1 is overexpressed in many types of cancer, including BC [14,35–40] with potential clinical significance [6–10], although Lieberthal et al. reported that a decreased YY1 expression might contribute to the invasive phenotype of metastatic BC cells [19]. However, other authors also previously reported that the YY1 protein level is lower in BC tissue than in the normal breast tissues [29,41,42]. Clearly, more intensive studies are needed to clarify the role of YY1 and its molecular mechanism in BC. Our preliminary data indicated that YY1 transcript in PBMCs of BC subjects showed a significant increase in patients with metastasis at primary diagnosis than the "Healthy Subjects" group. We indicated this group as "Synchronous Metastasis". Interestingly, YY1 was particularly higher in patients BC with bone metastasis although not statistically significant.

In our analysis, we included SM patients with specific BC receptor status; indeed our cohort included about 80% of ER+ tumors, which reflects the recurrence of the majority of breast cancer. As well-known, hormone receptor status is crucial for medical decision-making since strongly related to hormone therapy response. Preliminary data indicated that YY1 might play an important role in ER+ compared to ER- tumors in according to other receptors. Prompted by Lieberthal et al. results on BC model cell lines [19] we evaluated YY1 mRNA level in PBMCs from patients stratified as ER/PR-positive tumors with respect to triple negative (ER-/PR-/HER2-) and triple positive receptor status (ER+/PR+/HER2+). In particular, we observed that YY1 mRNA specifically increased in hormone receptor positive BCs (ER+/PR+/HER2-) compared to the "triple positive" (ER+/PR+/HER2+) and "triple negative" (ER-/PR-/HER2-) subtypes although not statistically significant.

^{18}F-FDG-PET is the gold standard for in vivo evaluation of tumor glucose metabolism and ^{18}F-FDG uptake. In particular, post-contrast MR images were highly correlated to the molecular subtypes of BC, such as normal-like, luminal A and B, HER2-enriched, and basal-like [43]. Additionally, several radiomics features, such as GLCM textural features and SUVs are currently used to classify BC tumor grade [44–46]. In particular, SUVmax is common feature of ^{18}F-FDG-PET that potentially reflects the tumor biology, prognosis and response to treatment [44–46]. Here, we reported for the first time, a correlation of ^{18}F-FDG-PET parameters with YY1 molecular marker. We showed that SUVmax were statistically correlated with blood circulating YY1 mRNAs in a small number of BC patients ($r = 0.48$), suggesting that at higher tumor uptake correspond to high blood level of YY1 (mRNAs). In summary, our study attempts to include another layer of information, which is imaging "phenotype" to tumor metastasis diagnosis. However, imaging phenotype differences between the BC synchronous (SM) and metachronous metastasis (MM) groups, have been so far poorly investigated [47–49]. We assessed if the addition of imaging layer could contribute to better discriminate SM and MM BC subgroups in combination with YY1 gene expression.

Our results, showed a quite weak correlation between imaging and molecular features, although other information could be useful for further consideration. For instance, we found a positive correlation between YY1 expression (mRNA) and SUVmax for SM rather than MM subgroups. SUVmax is routinely used imaging diagnostic parameter [50]. In BC studies, it usually indicates the degree of tumor metabolism and hence can predict its behavior and prognosis [51].

In spite of our observations, the pathogenic role, the release mechanism and cell origin of circulating YY1 in blood remain unknown.

Furthermore, the present study has some limitations, which probably affected also our correlation analysis. It was a retrospective study performed at a single institution with a relatively small number of patients, and recurrence was documented in very few subjects. Moreover, we were unable to analyze overall survival because there were no disease-related deaths among the study population. In detail, in our study, the ROI segmentation was performed automatically. Maybe a manual segmentation could provide more accurate data. Furthermore, the knowledge of the tumor status for each patient would allow a potential correlation between YY1 with the invasiveness of BC. Surely, a larger number of subjects with the same characteristics could improve data sensitivity and specificity. In addition, the data could not be validated internally. Finally, an external validation of our findings would allow us to generalize the results and discriminate YY1 trend in all BC subtypes.

Nevertheless, although there are all the previous limitations and further multicenter studies are needed to confirm our results, all the preliminary data reported above are promising and suggest that a combined approach between different technologies for the clinical diagnosis of BC can provide more differentiated information related to the detection of metastases for treatment decision.

Supplementary Materials: The following are available online at http://www.mdpi.com/2072-6694/11/10/1444/s1: Table S1: Findings evaluated for each BC patient at primary diagnosis.

Author Contributions: Data curation, M.F., K.P. and F.d.N.; Formal analysis, A.S. and M.S.; Methodology, C.S.; Resources, C.N.; Software, M.F., K.P. and N.G.; Supervision, A.S., M.S. and C.N.; Validation, M.F., K.P. and F.d.N.; Writing—original draft, C.S.; Writing—review and editing, F.d.N. and C.N.

Funding: This work was supported by "Ricerca Finalizzata 2011-12 Grant" (project code RF-2011-02349443) and "Ricerca Corrente 2017" (project code RRC-2017) from the Italian Ministry of Health (MS and CN).

Acknowledgments: We thank Teresa Infante, for collaborating to initial sets of YY1 experiments.

Conflicts of Interest: The authors declare that they have no conflict of interest.

Ethical Approval

The study was approved by the institutional ethics committee (IRCCS Fondazione SDN) in accordance with the ethical standard of the Declaration of Helsinki.

Abbreviations

ADC	Apparent Diffusion Coefficient
BC	Breast cancer
DWI	Diffusion Weighted Imaging
ELISA	Enzyme-Linked Immunosorbent Assay
ER	Estrogen Receptor
^{18}F-FDG-PET/MRI	Fluorine-18-fluorodeoxyglucose Positron Emission Tomography/ Magnetic Risonance Imaging
GLCM	Gray Level Co-occurrence Matrix
HER2	Human Epidermal Growth Factor Receptor 2
HS	Healthy subjects
IHC	Immunohistochemistry
MM	Metachronous Metastasis
PBMCs	Peripheral blood mononuclear cells
PET/CT	Positron Emission Tomography/ Computed Tomography
PR	Progesteron Receptor
RT-PCR	Reverse Transcription Polymerase Chain Reaction
SM	Synchronous Metastasis
SUV	Standardized Uptake Value
VOI	Volume of interest
YY1	YY1 Transcription Factor

References

1. Schiano, C.; Soricelli, A.; De Nigris, F.; Napoli, C. New challenges in integrated diagnosis by imaging and osteo-immunology in bone lesions. *Expert Rev. Clin. Immunol.* **2018**, *15*, 289–301. [CrossRef] [PubMed]
2. Werner, M.K.; Schmidt, H.; Schwenzer, N.F. MR/PET: A New Challenge in Hybrid Imaging. *Am. J. Roentgenol.* **2012**, *199*, 272–277. [CrossRef] [PubMed]
3. Schlemmer, H.P.; Pichler, B.J.; Krieg, R.; Heiss, W.D. An integrated MR/PET system: prospective applications. *Abdom. Imaging* **2009**, *34*, 668–674. [CrossRef] [PubMed]
4. Alcantara, D.; Leal, M.P.; Garcia-Bocanegra, I.; Garcia-Martin, M.L.; García-Bocanegra, I.; García-Martín, M.L. Molecular imaging of breast cancer: present and future directions. *Front. Chem.* **2014**, *2*, 112. [CrossRef] [PubMed]
5. Nicholson, S.; Whitehouse, H.; Naidoo, K.; Byers, R. Yin Yang 1 in human cancer. *Crit. Rev. Oncog.* **2011**, *16*, 245–260. [CrossRef] [PubMed]
6. Zaravinos, A.; Spandidos, D.A. Yin Yang 1 expression in human tumors. *Cell Cycle* **2010**, *9*, 512–522. [CrossRef] [PubMed]
7. Zhang, Q.; Stovall, D.B.; Inoue, K.; Sui, G. The oncogenic role of Yin Yang 1. *Crit. Rev. Oncog.* **2011**, *16*, 163–197. [CrossRef]
8. Castellano, G.; Torrisi, E.; Ligresti, G.; Malaponte, G.; McCubrey, J.A.; Nicoletti, F.; Travali, S.; Canevari, S.; Libra, M. Yin Yang 1 overexpression in diffuse large B-cell lymphoma is associated with B-cell transformation and tumor progression. *Cell Cycle* **2010**, *9*, 557–563. [CrossRef]
9. Baritaki, S.; Huerta-Yepez, S.; Sakai, T.; Spandidos, D.A.; Bonavida, B. Chemotherapeutic drugs sensitize cancer cells to TRAIL-mediated apoptosis: up-regulation of DR5 and inhibition of Yin Yang 1. *Mol. Cancer Ther.* **2007**, *6*, 1387–1399. [CrossRef]

10. De Nigris, F.; Zanella, L.; Cacciatore, F.; De Chiara, A.; Fazioli, F.; Chiappetta, G.; Apice, G.; Infante, T.; Monaco, M.; Rossiello, R.; et al. YY1 overexpression is associated with poor prognosis and metastasis-free survival in patients suffering osteosarcoma. *BMC Cancer* **2011**, *11*, 472. [CrossRef]
11. Seligson, D.; Horvath, S.; Huerta-Yepez, S.; Hanna, S.; Garban, H.; Roberts, A.; Shi, T.; Liu, X.; Chia, D.; Goodglick, L.; et al. Expression of transcription factor Yin Yang 1 in prostate cancer. *Int. J. Oncol.* **2005**, *27*, 131–141. [CrossRef]
12. De Nigris, F.; Rossiello, R.; Schiano, C.; Arra, C.; Williams-Ignarro, S.; Barbieri, A.; Lanza, A.; Balestrieri, A.; Giuliano, M.T.; Ignarro, L.J.; et al. Deletion of Yin Yang 1 protein in osteosarcoma cells on cell invasion and CXCR4/angiogenesis and metastasis. *Cancer Res.* **2008**, *68*, 1797–1808. [CrossRef]
13. De Nigris, F.; Botti, C.; de Chiara, A.; Rossiello, R.; Apice, G.; Fazioli, F.; Fiorito, C.; Sica, V.; Napoli, C. Expression of transcription factor Yin Yang 1 in human osteosarcomas. *Eur. J. Cancer* **2006**, *42*, 2420–2424. [CrossRef]
14. Chinnappan, D.; Ratnasari, A.; Andry, C.; King, T.C.; Xiao, D.; Weber, H.C. Transcription factor YY1 expression in human gastrointestinal cancer cells. *Int. J. Oncol.* **2009**, *34*, 1417–1423. [PubMed]
15. Allouche, A.; Nolens, G.; Tancredi, A.; Delacroix, L.; Mardaga, J.; Fridman, V.; Winkler, R.; Boniver, J.; Delvenne, P.; Begon, D.Y. The combined immunodetection of AP-2alpha and YY1 transcription factors is associated with ERBB2 gene overexpression in primary breast tumors. *Breast Cancer Res.* **2008**, *10*, R9. [CrossRef]
16. Begon, D.Y.; Delacroix, L.; Vernimmen, D.; Jackers, P.; Winkler, R. Yin Yang 1 Cooperates with Activator Protein 2 to Stimulate ERBB2 Gene Expression in Mammary Cancer Cells. *J. Biol. Chem.* **2005**, *280*, 24428–24434. [CrossRef] [PubMed]
17. Wu, F.; Lee, A.S. YY1 as a regulator of replication-dependent hamster histone H3.2 promoter and an interactive partner of AP-2. *J. Biol. Chem.* **2001**, *276*, 28–34. [CrossRef]
18. Thomassen, M.; Tan, Q.; Kruse, T.A. Gene expression meta-analysis identifies metastatic pathways and transcription factors in breast cancer. *BMC Cancer* **2008**, *8*, 394. [CrossRef]
19. Lieberthal, J.G.; Kaminsky, M.; Parkhurst, C.N.; Tanese, N. The role of YY1 in reduced HP1alpha gene expression in invasive human breast cancer cells. *Breast Cancer Res.* **2009**, *11*, 42. [CrossRef]
20. Shen, X.; Zhong, J.; Yu, P.; Zhao, Q.; Huang, T. YY1-regulated LINC00152 promotes triple negative breast cancer progression by affecting on stability of PTEN protein. *Biochem. Biophys. Res. Commun.* **2019**, *509*, 448–454. [CrossRef]
21. Hoefnagel, L.D.; Moelans, C.B.; Meijer, S.L.; van Slooten, H.J.; Wesseling, P.; Wesseling, J.; Westenend, P.J.; Bart, J.; Seldenrijk, C.A.; Nagtegaal, I.D.; et al. Prognostic value of estrogen receptor alpha and progesterone receptor conversion in distant breast cancer metastases. *Cancer* **2012**, *118*, 4929–4935. [CrossRef]
22. American Joint Committee on Cancer. *Breast Cancer Staging*, 7th ed.; American Joint Committee on Cancer: Chicago, IL, USA, 2009.
23. Rienzo, M.; Schiano, C.; Casamassimi, A.; Grimaldi, V.; Infante, T.; Napoli, C. Identification of valid reference housekeeping genes for gene expression analysis in tumor neovascularization studies. *Clin. Transl. Oncol.* **2013**, *15*, 211–218. [CrossRef]
24. Mirabelli, P.; Incoronato, M.; Coppola, L.; Infante, T.; Parente, C.A.; Nicolai, E.; Soricelli, A.; Salvatore, M. SDN Biobank: Bioresource of Human Samples Associated with Functional and/or Morphological Bioimaging Results for the Study of Oncological, Cardiological, Neurological, and Metabolic Diseases. *Open J. Bioresour.* **2017**, *4*, 356. [CrossRef]
25. Daye, D.; Signore, A.; Iannace, C.; Vangel, M.; Luongo, A.; Filomena, P.; Mansi, L.; Salvatore, M.; Fuin, N.; Catana, C.; et al. Staging performance of whole-body DWI, PET/CT and PET/MRI in invasive ductal carcinoma of the breast. *Int. J. Oncol.* **2017**, *51*, 281–288.
26. Pace, L.; Nicolai, E.; Luongo, A.; Aiello, M.; Catalano, O.A.; Soricelli, A.; Salvatore, M. Comparison of whole-body PET/CT and PET/MRI in breast cancer patients: Lesion detection and quantitation of ^{18}F-deoxyglucose uptake in lesions and in normal organ tissues. *Eur. J. Radiol.* **2014**, *83*, 289–296. [CrossRef]
27. Catalano, O.A.; Nicolai, E.; Rosen, B.R.; Luongo, A.; Catalano, M.; Iannace, C.; Guimarães, A.; Vangel, M.G.; Mahmood, U.; Soricelli, A.; et al. Comparison of CE-FDG-PET/CT with CE-FDG-PET/MR in the evaluation of osseous metastases in breast cancer patients. *Br. J. Cancer* **2015**, *112*, 1452–1460. [CrossRef]

28. Ehinger, A.; Malmström, P.; Bendahl, P.O.; Elston, C.W.; Falck, A.K.; Forsare, C.; Grabau, D.; Rydén, L.; Stål, O.; Fernö, M.; et al. Histological grade provides significant prognostic information in addition to breast cancer subtypes defined according to St Gallen 2013. *Acta Oncol.* **2017**, *56*, 68–74. [CrossRef]
29. Lee, M.H.; Lahusen, T.; Wang, R.H.; Xiao, C.; Xu, X.; Hwang, Y.S.; He, W.W.; Shi, Y.; Deng, C.X. Yin Yang 1 positively regulates BRCA1 and inhibits mammary cancer formation. *Oncogene* **2012**, *31*, 116–127. [CrossRef]
30. Groheux, D.; Giacchetti, S.; Moretti, J.L.; Porcher, R.; Espié, M.; Lehmann-Che, J.; de Roquancourt, A.; Hamy, A.S.; Cuvier, C.; Vercellino, L.; et al. Correlation of high ^{18}F-FDG uptake to clinical, pathological and biological prognostic factors in breast cancer. *Eur. J. Nucl. Med. Mol. Imaging* **2011**, *38*, 426–435. [CrossRef]
31. Wang, M.Y.; Huang, H.Y.; Kuo, Y.L.; Lo, C.; Sun, H.Y.; Lyu, Y.J.; Chen, B.R.; Li, J.N.; Chen, P.S. TARBP2-Enhanced Resistance during Tamoxifen Treatment in Breast Cancer. *Cancers* **2019**, *11*, 210. [CrossRef]
32. Bray, F.; Ferlay, J.; Soerjomataram, I.; Siegel, R.L.; Torre, L.A.; Jemal, A. Global cancer statistics 2018: GLOBOCAN estimates of incidence and mortality worldwide for 36 cancers in 185 countries. *CA Cancer J. Clin.* **2018**, *68*, 394–424. [CrossRef]
33. Perou, C.M.; Sørlie, T.; Eisen, M.B.; Van De Rijn, M.; Jeffrey, S.S.; Rees, C.A.; Pollack, J.R.; Ross, D.T.; Johnsen, H.; Akslen, L.A.; et al. Molecular portraits of human breast tumours. *Nature* **2000**, *406*, 747–752. [CrossRef]
34. Howlader, N.; Altekruse, S.F.; Li, C.I.; Chen, V.W.; Clarke, C.A.; Ries, L.A.G.; Cronin, K.A. US Incidence of Breast Cancer Subtypes Defined by Joint Hormone Receptor and HER2 Status. *J. Natl. Cancer Inst.* **2014**, *106*. [CrossRef]
35. Wan, M.; Huang, W.; Kute, T.E.; Miller, L.D.; Zhang, Q.; Hatcher, H.; Wang, J.; Stovall, D.B.; Russell, G.B.; Cao, P.D.; et al. Yin Yang 1 plays an essential role in breast cancer and negatively regulates p27. *Am. J. Pathol.* **2012**, *180*, 2120–2133. [CrossRef]
36. Wang, A.M.; Huang, T.T.; Hsu, K.W.; Huang, K.H.; Fang, W.L.; Yang, M.H.; Lo, S.S.; Chi, C.W.; Lin, J.J.; Yeh, T.S. Yin Yang 1 is a target of microRNA-34 family and contributes to gastric carcinogenesis. *Oncotarget* **2014**, *5*, 5002–5016. [CrossRef]
37. Kang, W.; Tong, J.H.; Chan, A.W.; Zhao, J.; Dong, Y.; Wang, S.; Yang, W.; Mc Sin, F.; Ng, S.S.; Yu, J.; et al. Yin Yang 1 contributes to gastric carcinogenesis and its nuclear expression correlates with shorter survival in patients with early stage gastric adenocarcinoma. *J. Transl. Med.* **2014**, *12*, 80. [CrossRef]
38. Bonavida, B.; Kaufhold, S. Prognostic significance of YY1 protein expression and mRNA levels by bioinformatics analysis in human cancers: A therapeutic target. *Pharmacol. Ther.* **2015**, *150*, 149–168. [CrossRef]
39. Shi, J.; Hao, A.; Zhang, Q.; Sui, G. The role of YY1 in oncogenesis and its potential as a drug target in cancer therapies. *Curr. Cancer Drug Targets* **2015**, *15*, 145–157. [CrossRef]
40. Yang, W.; Feng, B.; Meng, Y.; Wang, J.; Geng, B.; Cui, Q.; Zhang, H.; Yang, Y.; Yang, J. FAM3C-YY1 axis is essential for TGFβ-promoted proliferation and migration of human breast cancer MDA-MB-231 cells via the activation of HSF1. *J. Cell. Mol. Med.* **2019**, *23*, 3464–3475. [CrossRef]
41. Zhang, Z.; Zhu, Y.; Wang, Z.; Zhang, T.; Wu, P.; Huang, J. Yin-yang effect of tumor infiltrating B cells in breast cancer: From mechanism to immunotherapy. *Cancer Lett.* **2017**, *393*, 1–7. [CrossRef]
42. Powe, D.G.; Akhtar, G.; Habashy, H.O.; Abdel-Fatah, T.M.; Rakha, E.A.; Green, A.R.; O Ellis, I. Investigating AP-2 and YY1 protein expression as a cause of high HER2 gene transcription in breast cancers with discordant HER2 gene amplification. *Breast Cancer Res.* **2009**, *11*, R90. [CrossRef]
43. Li, H.; Zhu, Y.; Burnside, E.S.; Huang, E.; Drukker, K.; Hoadley, K.A.; Fan, C.; Conzen, S.D.; Zuley, M.; Net, J.M.; et al. Quantitative MRI radiomics in the prediction of molecular classifications of breast cancer subtypes in the TCGA/TCIA data set. *NPJ Breast Cancer* **2016**, *2*, 16012. [CrossRef]
44. Grueneisen, J.; Sawicki, L.M.; Wetter, A.; Kirchner, J.; Kinner, S.; Aktas, B.; Forsting, M.; Ruhlmann, V.; Umutlu, L. Evaluation of PET and MR datasets in integrated ^{18}F-FDG PET/MRI: A comparison of different MR sequences for whole-body restaging of breast cancer patients. *Eur. J. Radiol.* **2017**, *89*, 14–19. [CrossRef]
45. Rahim, M.K.; Kim, S.E.; So, H.; Kim, H.J.; Cheon, G.J.; Lee, E.S.; Kang, K.W.; Lee, D.S. Recent Trends in PET Image Interpretations Using Volumetric and Texture-based Quantification Methods in Nuclear Oncology. *Nucl. Med. Mol. Imaging* **2014**, *48*, 1–15. [CrossRef]
46. Chang, C.C.; Cho, S.F.; Chen, Y.W.; Tu, H.P.; Lin, C.Y.; Chang, C.S. SUV on Dual-Phase FDG PET/CT Correlates With the Ki-67 Proliferation Index in Patients With Newly Diagnosed Non-Hodgkin Lymphoma. *Clin. Nucl. Med.* **2012**, *37*, e189–e195. [CrossRef]

47. Güth, U.; Magaton, I.; Huang, D.J.; Fisher, R.; Schötzau, A.; Vetter, M. Primary and secondary distant metastatic breast cancer: Two sides of the same coin. *Breast* **2014**, *23*, 26–32. [CrossRef]
48. Gerratana, L.; Fanotto, V.; Bonotto, M.; Bolzonello, S.; Minisini, A.M.; Fasola, G.; Puglisi, F. Pattern of metastasis and outcome in patients with breast cancer. *Clin. Exp. Metastasis* **2015**, *32*, 125–133. [CrossRef]
49. Kast, K.; Link, T.; Friedrich, K.; Petzold, A.; Niedostatek, A.; Schoffer, O.; Werner, C.; Klug, S.J.; Werner, A.; Gatzweiler, A.; et al. Impact of breast cancer subtypes and patterns of metastasis on outcome. *Breast Cancer Res. Treat.* **2015**, *150*, 621–629. [CrossRef]
50. Bailly, C.; Bodet-Milin, C.; Bourgeois, M.; Gouard, S.; Ansquer, C.; Barbaud, M.; Sébille, J.C.; Chérel, M.; Kraeber-Bodéré, F.; Carlier, T. Exploring Tumor Heterogeneity Using PET Imaging: The Big Picture. *Cancers* **2019**, *11*, 1282. [CrossRef]
51. Jain, A.; Dubey, I.; Chauhan, M.; Kumar, R.; Agarwal, S.; Kishore, B.; Vishnoi, M.; Paliwal, D.; John, A.; Kumar, N.; et al. Tumor characteristics and metabolic quantification in carcinoma breast: An institutional experience. *Indian J. Cancer* **2017**, *54*, 333. [CrossRef]

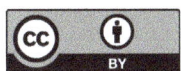 © 2019 by the authors. Licensee MDPI, Basel, Switzerland. This article is an open access article distributed under the terms and conditions of the Creative Commons Attribution (CC BY) license (http://creativecommons.org/licenses/by/4.0/).

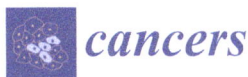

Article

Prognostic Significance of CT-Attenuation of Tumor-Adjacent Breast Adipose Tissue in Breast Cancer Patients with Surgical Resection

Jeong Won Lee [1], Sung Yong Kim [2], Hyun Ju Lee [3], Sun Wook Han [2], Jong Eun Lee [2] and Sang Mi Lee [4,*]

[1] Department of Nuclear Medicine, International St. Mary's Hospital, Catholic Kwandong University College of Medicine, 25 Simgok-ro 100 beon-gil, Seo-gu, Incheon 22711, Korea
[2] Department of Surgery, Soonchunhyang University Cheonan Hospital, 31 Suncheonhyang 6-gil, Dongnam-gu, Cheonan, Chungcheongnam-do 31151, Korea
[3] Department of Pathology, Soonchunhyang University Cheonan Hospital, 31 Suncheonhyang 6-gil, Dongnam-gu, Cheonan, Chungcheongnam-do 31151, Korea
[4] Department of Nuclear Medicine, Soonchunhyang University Cheonan Hospital, 31 Suncheonhyang 6-gil, Dongnam-gu, Cheonan, Chungcheongnam-do 31151, Korea
* Correspondence: c91300@schmc.ac.kr; Tel.: +82-41-570-3540; Fax: +82-41-572-4655

Received: 28 June 2019; Accepted: 6 August 2019; Published: 8 August 2019

Abstract: The purpose of this study was to evaluate the prognostic significance of computed tomography (CT)-attenuation of tumor-adjacent breast adipose tissue for predicting recurrence-free survival (RFS) in patients with breast cancer. We retrospectively enrolled 287 breast cancer patients who underwent pretreatment ^{18}F-fluorodeoxyglucose (FDG) positron emission tomography (PET)/CT. From non-contrast-enhanced CT images of PET/CT, CT-attenuation values of tumor-adjacent breast adipose tissue (TAT HU) and contralateral breast adipose tissue (CAT HU) were measured. Difference (HU difference) and percent difference (HU difference %) in CT-attenuation values between TAT HU and CAT HU were calculated. The relationships of these breast adipose tissue parameters with tumor factors and RFS were assessed. TAT HU was significantly higher than CAT HU ($p < 0.001$). TAT HU, HU difference, and HU difference % showed significant correlations with T stage and estrogen receptor and progesterone receptor status ($p < 0.05$), whereas CAT HU had no significant relationships with tumor factors ($p > 0.05$). Patients with high TAT HU, HU difference, and HU difference % had significantly worse RFS than those with low values ($p < 0.001$). In multivariate analysis, TAT HU and HU difference % were significantly associated with RFS after adjusting for clinico-pathologic factors ($p < 0.05$). CT-attenuation of tumor-adjacent breast adipose tissue was significantly associated with RFS in patients with breast cancer. The findings seem to support the close contact between breast cancer cells and tumor-adjacent adipocytes observed with imaging studies.

Keywords: breast cancer; Hounsfield unit; computed tomography; prognosis; adipose tissue

1. Introduction

Adipose tissue is one of the major components of the human body, found all around the body [1]. In non-lactating human breast tissue, up to 56% of the total breast volume consists of adipose tissue [2]. Although adipose tissue is mainly composed of adipocytes, it is also comprised of various other kinds of cell types including immune cells, endothelial cells, pre-adipocytes, and fibroblasts [1,3]. For a long time, adipose tissue was considered to function as a simple storage organ of excessive energy; however, evidence showed that adipose tissue also function as an endocrine organ secreting hundreds of cell signaling proteins, called adipokines [4]. Previous studies published over the last decade have continuously demonstrated that adipose tissue could play a role in cancer growth, progression, and metastasis by secreting multiple kinds of adipokines, inducing inflammatory micro-environment, remodeling the extracellular matrix, and providing energy to tumor cells [1,3,5]. Furthermore, adipocytes in the close vicinity of cancer cells can have crosstalk with cancer cells, which increases the potential of tumor progression and metastasis [1,3,6]. Because of the close localization between mammary epithelium and breast adipose tissue, breast cancer is considered as one of the most representative malignancies that is in close contact with adipose tissue, along with gastric, colon, and ovary cancers [1,3]. In previous cell-culture and histopathological studies of breast cancer, it has already been proven that breast cancer cells have active interaction with peritumoral adipose tissue, which further enhances aggressiveness and invasiveness of breast cancer cells [1,3,7–9].

In recent clinical studies with imaging examinations, the clinical implication of adipose tissue features on diagnostic images has been investigated in various diseases [10–12]. In addition to the amount of adipose tissue, the qualitative characteristics of adipose tissue has also been studied using imaging modalities such as computed tomography (CT) and positron emission tomography (PET) [10,12–15]. One of the most commonly used imaging features representing qualitative changes in adipose tissue is CT-attenuation of adipose tissue measured on non-contrast-enhanced CT images [10,12–14]. In recent clinical studies with diverse kinds of malignancies, increased CT-attenuation on unenhanced CT images has shown a significant association with worse clinical outcomes, suggesting that increased CT-attenuation might reflect a microenvironment of adipose tissue which promotes cancer cell progression [12–14]. Considering the close localization between breast cancer and breast adipose tissue, the qualitative characteristics of peritumoral breast adipose tissue might have a significant association with the characteristics and clinical outcomes of breast cancer [1]. However, few studies have evaluated the clinical significance of the peritumoral adipose tissue environment using imaging studies [16].

In breast cancer, previous studies have shown the clinical significance of ^{18}F-fluorodeoxyglucose (FDG) PET/CT for staging, differentiating molecular subtypes, and predicting clinical outcomes; therefore, currently, FDG PET/CT is widely used in patients with breast cancer [17–20]. In the present study, we used unenhanced CT images of pretreatment ^{18}F-fluorodeoxyglucose (FDG) PET/CT for measuring CT-attenuation of tumor-adjacent breast adipose tissue and investigated whether it has a significant association with recurrence-free survival (RFS) in patients with breast cancer who underwent curative surgical resection.

2. Results

2.1. Patient Characteristics

Baseline characteristics of the 287 patients enrolled in the present study are shown in Table 1. Of the enrolled patients, 33 (11.5%) were histopathologically confirmed as having triple negative breast cancer. Neoadjuvant chemotherapy was performed in 32 patients (11.1%), and, after curative surgical resection, 282 patients (98.3%) received adjuvant treatments. The median interval between FDG PET/CT and initial treatment was 5.0 days (range, 2–14 days). On PET/CT image analysis of primary breast cancer, 89 patients (31.0%) had a metabolic tumor volume (MTV) of 0.0 cm^3, because maximum standardized uptake values (SUVs) of the primary breast cancer were less than 2.50. The median follow-up duration of the patients was 55.1 months with a range of 6.1–88.9 months, and during the follow-up period, cancer recurrence was found in 30 patients (10.5%).

Table 1. Baseline characteristics of patients (n = 287).

Characteristics		Number (%)	Median (Range)
Age (years)			52 (30–85)
Body mass index			23.8 (16.4–35.2)
Menopausal status	Premenopausal	108 (37.6%)	
	Postmenopausal	179 (62.4%)	
Histopathology	Intraductal carcinoma	252 (87.8%)	
	Intralobular carcinoma	35 (12.2%)	
T stage	T1	136 (47.4%)	
	T2	128 (44.6%)	
	T3	23 (8.0%)	
N stage	N0	190 (66.2%)	
	N1	58 (20.2%)	
	N2	21 (7.3%)	
	N3	18 (6.3%)	
Tumor size (cm)			2.0 (0.4–8.0)
Histologic grade	Grade 1	67 (23.4%)	
	Grade 2	143 (49.7%)	
	Grade 3	77 (26.9%)	
Estrogen receptor statue	Positive	213 (74.2%)	
	Negative	74 (25.8%)	
Progesterone receptor status	Positive	177 (61.7%)	
	Negative	110 (38.3%)	
HER2 status	Positive	142 (49.5%)	
	Negative	145 (50.5%)	
Ki67 expression status	Positive	177 (61.7%)	
	Negative	110 (38.3%)	
Maximum SUV of primary tumor			4.06 (1.10–35.59)
MTV of primary tumor (cm^3)			1.14 (0.0–235.30)
TAT HU			−87.69 (−104.88–−63.36)
CAT HU			−97.54 (−116.85–−70.74)
HU difference			8.66 (−2.67–35.84)
HU difference %			8.94 (−3.15–30.67)
Neoadjuvant chemotherapy	Yes	32 (11.1%)	
	No	255 (88.9%)	
Adjuvant treatment	CTx + RTx + HTx	139 (48.4%)	
	RTx + HTx	82 (28.6%)	
	CTx + HTx	17 (5.9%)	
	CTx + RTx	3 (1.0%)	
	HTx	24 (8.4%)	
	CTx	16 (5.6%)	
	RTx	1 (0.3%)	
	No	5 (1.7%)	

HER2, human epidermal growth factor receptor 2; SUV, standardized uptake value; MTV, metabolic tumor volume; TAT HU, CT-attenuation of tumor-adjacent breast adipose tissue; CAT HU, CT-attenuation of contralateral breast adipose tissue; HU difference, difference of CT-attenuation; HU difference %, percent difference of CT-attenuation; CTx, chemotherapy; RTx, radiotherapy; HTx, hormonal therapy.

2.2. Breast Adipose Tissue Measurement

On the assessment of reproducibility of breast adipose tissue measurement, substantial agreement was shown between the two reviewers for CT-attenuation values, expressed in Hounsfield unit (HU), of tumor-adjacent breast adipose tissue (TAT HU) (concordance correlation coefficient: 0.953; 95% confidence interval: 0.934–0.968) and CT-attenuation values of contralateral breast adipose tissue (CAT HU) (concordance correlation coefficient: 0.951; 95% confidence interval: 0.924–0.972).

Among the enrolled patients, TAT HU was higher than CAT HU in 269 patients (93.7%), showing significant difference between TAT HU and CAT HU ($p < 0.001$). Body mass index (BMI) showed significant negative correlation with both TAT HU ($r = -0.136$, $p = 0.001$) and CAT HU ($r = -0.274$, $p < 0.001$) but showed weaker correlation with TAT HU and no significant correlation with the difference in CT-attenuation values between tumor-adjacent and contralateral breast adipose tissues (HU difference) ($p = 0.231$) and percent difference of CT-attenuation values between tumor-adjacent and contralateral breast adipose tissues (HU difference %) ($p = 0.425$).

In correlation analysis between breast adipose tissue parameters and tumor stage, increased CT-attenuation of peritumoral breast adipose tissue was related with advanced stage (Table 2). For T stage, significant differences of TAT HU, HU difference, and HU difference % were shown on Kruskal—Wallis test ($p < 0.001$ for all; Figure 1). On post-hoc analysis, each T stage group showed significant difference of TAT HU from each other, and HU difference and HU difference % in T2 and T3 stage groups were significantly higher than those in the T1 stage group ($p < 0.05$). For N stage, patients with regional lymph node metastasis had significantly higher HU difference and HU difference % than those with no lymph node metastasis ($p < 0.001$ for all). In contrast, there were no significant differences of CAT HU according to T stage and N stage ($p > 0.05$).

Table 2. Relationship between breast cancer adipose tissue parameters and clinico-histological factors.

Clinico-Histological Factors		TAT HU	CAT HU	HU Difference	HU Difference %
T stage	T1	−88.95 ± 6.53	−96.95 ± 6.61	7.99 ± 6.06	8.08 ± 6.02
	T2	−86.33 ± 5.72	−97.15 ± 7.22	10.82 ± 6.69	10.87 ± 6.23
	T3	−82.67 ± 5.68	−95.43 ± 7.39	12.76 ± 6.18	13.14 ± 5.66
	p-value	<0.001 *	0.505 *	<0.001 *	<0.001 *
N stage	N0	−87.64 ± 6.26	−96.95 ± 6.82	8.63 ± 6.43	8.76 ± 6.27
	N1-3	−86.56 ± 6.56	−98.06 ± 7.97	11.61 ± 6.34	11.63 ± 5.92
	p-value	0.176	0.203	<0.001	<0.001
Histologic grade	Grade 1	−87.62 ± 7.21	−96.28 ± 7.61	8.65 ± 7.11	8.76 ± 6.75
	Grade 2	−87.65 ± 6.23	−96.87 ± 6.71	9.23 ± 6.42	9.32 ± 6.21
	Grade 3	−86.27 ± 5.85	−97.58 ± 6.84	11.21 ± 6.09	11.29 ± 5.83
	p-value	0.288 *	0.391 *	0.013 *	0.013 *
ER status	Positive	−88.03 ± 6.26	−96.76 ± 6.91	8.73 ± 6.34	8.81 ± 6.09
	Negative	−85.11 ± 6.25	−97.36 ± 7.07	12.25 ± 6.46	12.36 ± 6.15
	p-value	<0.001	0.528	<0.001	<0.001
PR status	Positive	−87.94 ± 6.47	−96.60 ± 6.76	8.16 ± 5.73	8.34 ± 5.69
	Negative	−86.22 ± 6.09	−97.23 ± 7.06	12.01 ± 7.08	11.97 ± 6.58
	p-value	0.026	0.318	<0.001	<0.001
HER2 status	Positive	−87.54 ± 5.71	−97.56 ± 6.34	10.02 ± 6.79	10.03 ± 6.49
	Negative	−87.02 ± 6.97	−96.29 ± 7.45	9.27 ± 6.29	9.43 ± 6.10
	p-value	0.488	0.122	0.336	0.426
Ki67 expression status	Positive	−86.72 ± 6.10	−96.88 ± 6.83	10.16 ± 6.76	10.25 ± 6.42
	Negative	−88.01 ± 7.01	−96.72 ± 7.37	8.72 ± 6.25	8.82 ± 6.17
	p-value	0.115	0.856	0.083	0.076
Recurrence	No recur	−87.74 ± 6.27	−96.90 ± 6.74	9.16 ± 6.37	9.25 ± 6.17
	Recur	−83.35 ± 6.00	−97.10 ± 8.62	13.75 ± 6.71	13.85 ± 5.91
	p-value	<0.001	0.882	<0.001	<0.001

* Performed using Kruskal—Wallis test.; ER, estrogen receptor; PR, progesterone receptor; HER2, human epidermal growth factor receptor 2; TAT HU, CT-attenuation of tumor-adjacent breast adipose tissue; CAT HU, CT-attenuation of contralateral breast adipose tissue; HU difference, difference of CT-attenuation; HU difference %, percent difference of CT-attenuation.

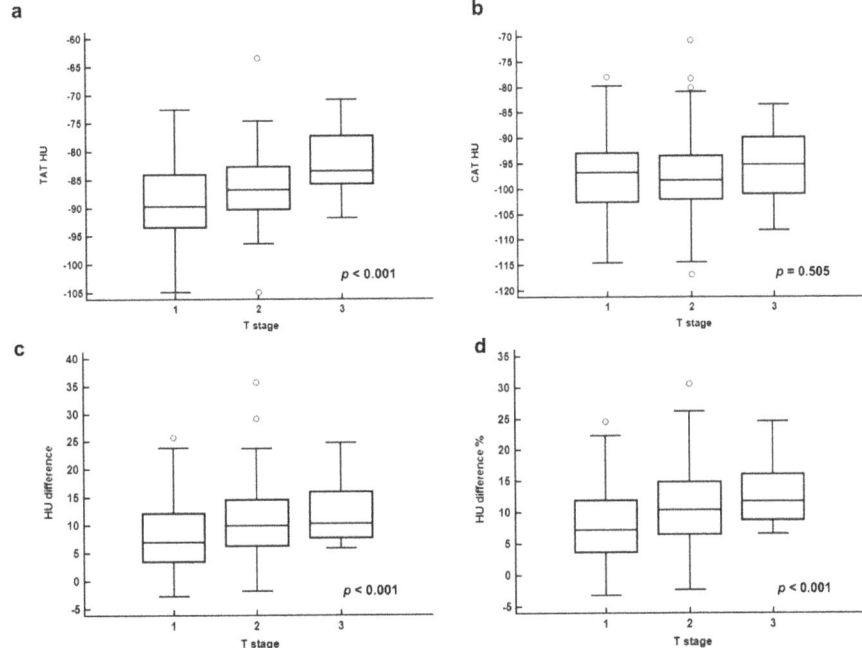

Figure 1. CT-attenuation of tumor-adjacent breast adipose tissue (TAT HU) (**a**), CT-attenuation of contralateral breast adipose tissue (CAT HU) (**b**), difference of CT-attenuation (HU difference) (**c**), and percent difference of CT-attenuation (HU difference %) (**d**), according to T stage.

In correlation analysis with histopathological results, increased CT-attenuation of peritumoral breast adipose tissue was related with aggressive features of breast cancer (Table 2). Patients with negative estrogen receptor (ER) and progesterone receptor (PR) showed higher values of TAT HU, HU difference, and HU difference % than those with positive ER and PR, respectively ($p < 0.05$). Moreover, significant differences of HU difference and HU difference % were observed according to the histologic grade of the primary tumor, showing significantly higher HU difference and HU difference % in patients with histologic grade 3 tumors than in those with grade 1 and grade 2 tumors on post-hoc analysis ($p < 0.05$). In contrast, human epidermal growth factor receptor 2 (HER2) status and Ki67 expression status had no significant correlation with any breast adipose tissue parameters ($p > 0.05$).

In correlation analysis with FDG PET/CT parameters of primary breast cancer lesions, TAT HU, HU difference, and HU difference % showed significant but weak positive correlations with maximum SUV ($r = 0.125$, $p = 0.034$ for TAT HU, $r = 0.266$, $p < 0.001$ for HU difference, and $r = 0.265$, $p < 0.001$ for HU difference %) and MTV of primary tumor ($r = 0.135$, $p = 0.023$ for TAT HU, $r = 0.248$, $p < 0.001$ for HU difference, and $r = 0.241$, $p < 0.001$ for HU difference %).

In comparison, the breast adipose tissue parameters of patients with recurrence showed significantly higher values of TAT HU, HU difference, and HU difference % than those with no recurrence ($p < 0.001$; Figure 2). In contrast, there is no significant difference in CAT HU between those two groups ($p = 0.882$; Figure 2)

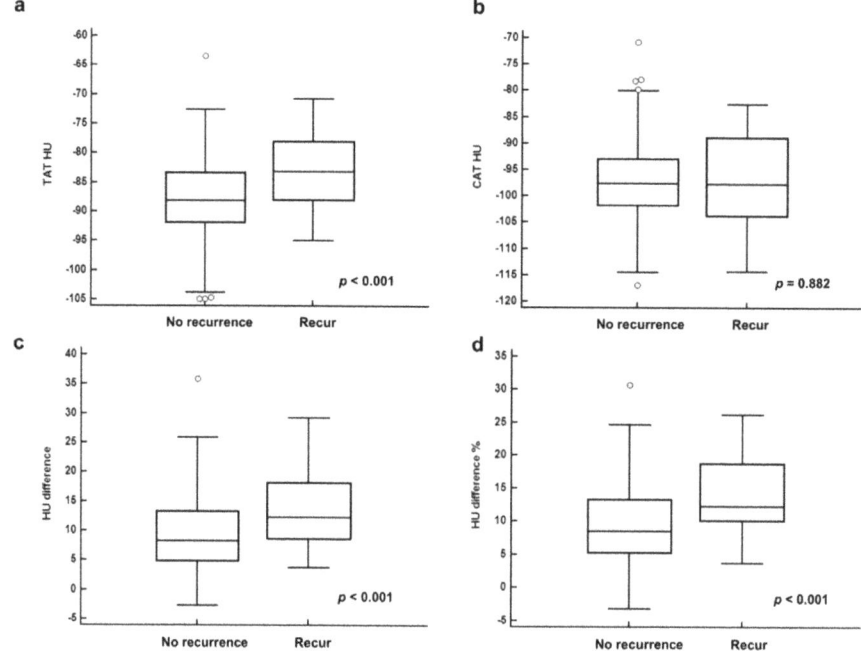

Figure 2. CT-attenuation of tumor-adjacent breast adipose tissue (TAT HU) (**a**), CT-attenuation of contralateral breast adipose tissue (CAT HU) (**b**), difference of CT-attenuation (HU difference) (**c**), and percent difference of CT-attenuation (HU difference %) (**d**) between patients with no recurrence and recurrence.

2.3. Survival Analysis

The prognostic values of breast adipose tissue parameters for predicting RFS were evaluated using univariate Cox regression analysis along with clinico-histological factors and PET/CT parameters of the primary breast cancer. In univariate analysis, TAT HU, HU difference, and HU difference % were significantly associated with RFS ($p < 0.001$ for all; Table 3), while CAT HU showed no statistical significance ($p = 0.786$). Among clinico-histological factors and PET/CT parameters, T stage, N stage, histologic grade, ER status, PR status, Ki67 index, triple negative tumor, and maximum SUV and MTV of primary tumor showed significance in predicting RFS ($p < 0.05$; Table 3).

TAT HU, HU difference, and HU difference % were included in the multivariate analysis for RFS with the addition of eight different covariates in three different models (Table 4). TAT HU and HU difference % remained as significant positive predictors for RFS in all three models after adjustment for age, T stage, N stage, ER status, PR status, Ki67 index, maximum SUV, and MTV ($p < 0.05$). On the other hand, HU difference showed significant association with RFS in models with adjustment for age, T stage, N stage, ER status, PR status, and Ki67 index ($p < 0.05$) but failed to show statistical significance after correcting for maximum SUV and MTV ($p = 0.054$).

Table 3. Univariate analysis for recurrence-free survival.

Variables		p-Value	Hazard Ratio (95% CI)
Age (1-year increase)		0.562	1.01 (0.98–1.04)
BMI (1 kg/m² increase)		0.283	0.93 (0.82–1.06)
Menopausal status (pre vs. post)		0.799	0.91 (0.44–1.89)
T stage	T1 stage	-	1.00
	T2 stage	0.001	11.24 (2.62–48.25)
	T3 stage	<0.001	37.90 (8.17–175.80)
N stage (N0 vs. N1-3)		0.004	2.92 (1.42–6.09)
Histologic grade	Grade 1	-	1.00
	Grade 2	0.873	1.10 (0.34–3.58)
	Grade 3	0.008	4.42 (1.48–13.16)
ER status (positive vs. negative)		<0.001	3.41 (1.66–7.00)
PR status (positive vs. negative)		<0.001	5.22 (2.32–11.74)
HER2 status (positive vs. negative)		0.254	0.65 (0.31–1.36)
Ki67 index (negative vs. positive)		0.005	7.79 (1.85–32.83)
Triple negative tumor (no vs. yes)		0.011	3.00 (1.28–7.03)
Maximum SUV (1.0 increase)		<0.001	1.08 (1.03–1.13)
MTV (1.0 cm³ increase)		<0.001	1.03 (1.02–1.04)
TAT HU (1.0 HU increase)		<0.001	1.10 (1.05–1.16)
CAT HU (1.0 HU increase)		0.786	0.99 (0.94–1.05)
HU difference (1.0 HU increase)		<0.001	1.10 (1.05–1.16)
HU difference % (1.0% increase)		<0.001	1.12 (1.06–1.18)

BMI, body mass index; ER, estrogen receptor; PR, progesterone receptor; HER2, human epidermal growth factor receptor 2; SUV, standardized uptake value; MTV, metabolic tumor volume; TAT HU, CT-attenuation of tumor-adjacent breast adipose tissue; CAT HU, CT-attenuation of contralateral breast adipose tissue; HU difference, difference of CT-attenuation; HU difference %, percent difference of CT-attenuation; HU, Hounsfield units; CI, confidence interval.

Table 4. Multivariate models for recurrence-free survival.

Models		TAT HU (1.0 HU Increase)	HU Difference (1.0 HU Increase)	HU Difference % (1.0% Increase)
Model 1 *	p-value	0.012	0.001	0.001
	Hazard ratio	1.08	1.07	1.09
	(95% CI)	(1.02–1.15)	(1.02–1.19)	(1.02–1.15)
Model 2 †	p-value	0.018	0.044	0.033
	Hazard ratio	1.08	1.06	1.07
	(95% CI)	(1.01–1.16)	(1.00–1.12)	(1.01–1.14)
Model 3 ‡	p-value	0.014	0.054	0.038
	Hazard ratio	1.09	1.05	1.07
	(95% CI)	(1.02–1.16)	(1.00–1.11)	(1.00–1.13)

* Adjusted for age, T stage and N stage; † Adjusted for age, T stage, N stage, estrogen receptor status, progesterone receptor status, and Ki67 index; ‡ Adjusted for age, T stage, N stage, estrogen receptor status, progesterone receptor status, Ki67 index, maximum standardized uptake value, and metabolic tumor volume; CI, confidence interval; TAT HU, CT-attenuation of tumor-adjacent breast adipose tissue; HU difference, difference of CT-attenuation; HU difference %, percent difference of CT-attenuation; HU, Hounsfield units.

For Kaplan—Meier analysis, TAT HU, HU difference, and HU difference % were categorized into two groups according to the optimal cut-off values (−82.50 for TAT HU, 8.50 for HU difference, and 10.00 for HU difference %) determined by receiver operating characteristic (ROC) curve analysis. Kaplan—Meier analysis of enrolled patients stratified by TAT HU, HU difference, and HU difference % showed significantly worse RFS in patients with high values than in those with low values ($p < 0.001$ for all; Figure 3). Patients with high values of TAT HU (75.7% vs. 93.1%), HU difference (82.7% vs. 96.3%), and HU difference % (80.0% vs. 96.8%) showed lower 5-year RFS rates than those with low values.

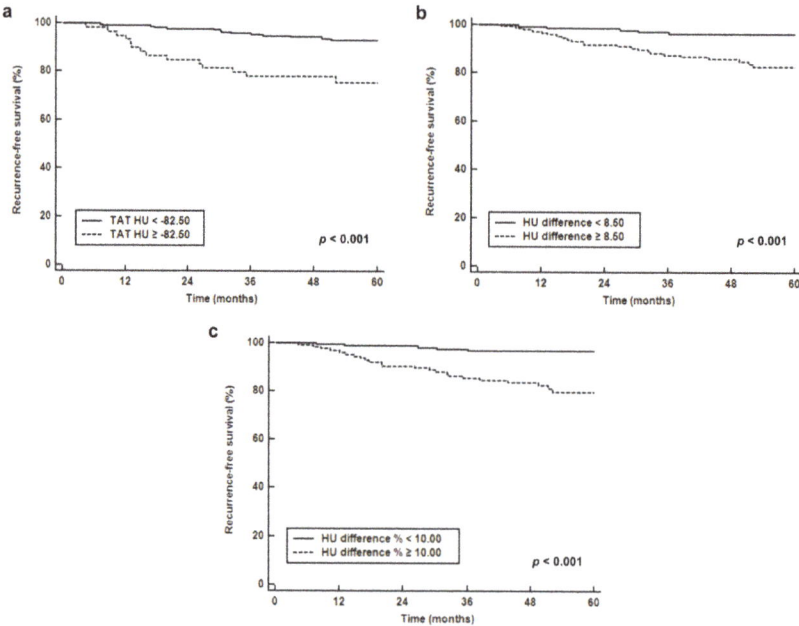

Figure 3. Survival curves. Recurrence-free survival stratified by CT-attenuation of tumor-adjacent breast adipose tissue (TAT HU) (**a**), difference of CT-attenuation (HU difference) (**b**), and percent difference of CT-attenuation (HU difference %) (**c**).

While comparing recurrence rates based on the combination of T stage and TAT HU (Table 5), patients with high TAT HU showed a higher recurrence rate than those with low TAT HU, irrespective of T stage (5.3% vs. 0.9% for T1 stage; 34.1% vs. 12.7% for T2–T3 stage).

Table 5. Recurrence rates according to the combination of T stage and TAT HU.

TAT HU		T Stage	
		T1 Stage	T2–T3 Stage
TAT HU	<−82.50 HU	1/117 (0.9%)	14/110 (12.7%)
	≥−82.50 HU	1/19 (5.3%)	14/41 (34.1%)
	p-value	0.260	0.003

TAT HU, CT-attenuation of tumor-adjacent breast adipose tissue; HU, Hounsfield units.

3. Discussion

In the present study, CT-attenuation of tumor-adjacent breast adipose tissue and difference of CT-attenuation between tumor-adjacent and contralateral breast adipose tissues showed significant association with T stage, tumor characteristics, and RFS in patients with breast cancer. In previous studies with histopathological analysis of resected breast cancer tissue, profound modifications of phenotype and biological features were found in the adipocytes that were present at the invasive front of the breast cancer cells [8,9]. The adipocytes in the vicinity of the breast cancer cells showed decreased cell size and less lipid content when compared to the adipocytes that are located far away from the breast cancer cells [8,9]. These alterations of adipocytes were reproduced in adipocytes which were co-cultivated with cancer cells, showing less differentiated features of adipocytes with decreased expression of adipocyte markers such as adiponectin and resistin and increased expression of matrix metalloproteinase 11, osteopontin, and pro-inflammatory cytokines including tumor necrosis factor-alpha and interleukin-6 [1,8,9,21]. These modified adipocytes are now called cancer-associated adipocytes [1,8,22]. The cancer-associated adipocytes are known to have an active bidirectional crosstalk with cancer cells, inducing fibrotic change in adipose tissue, stimulating tumor progression and metastasis by secreting multiple cytokines and adipokines, and releasing lipid content within the cell to provide source of energy to cancer cells [1,3,21–23]. Previous studies with breast cancer have also demonstrated that expressions of cancer-associated adipocytes-related protein are different according to the subtypes of breast cancer and the interactions between tumor cells and adipocytes can contribute to growth, proliferation, and epithelial-mesenchymal transition of breast cancer cells [23–26].

In a previous study that evaluated the correlation between CT-attenuation of adipose tissue and histopathological results of adipose tissue collected at necropsy in non-human primates, increased CT-attenuation of adipose tissue was significantly associated with smaller adipocytes and increased extracellular matrix fibrosis, which corresponded to the findings in the peritumoral adipose tissue affected by cancer cells [8,10,14]. Therefore, CT-attenuation of adipose tissue has been used as an imaging parameter for the qualitative alterations of adipose tissue in patients with malignant diseases [13,14]. In our study, we measured CT-attenuation in both tumor-adjacent and contralateral breast adipose tissue and tried to find out whether CT-attenuation of tumor-adjacent breast adipose tissue had different features compared to that of the contralateral side. The results of our study demonstrated that increased CT-attenuation was observed in tumor-adjacent breast adipose tissue compared to the contralateral side. Moreover, TAT HU, HU difference, and HU difference % had a significant correlation with the T stage, hormone receptor status, and FDG PET/CT parameters of the primary tumor, while CAT HU showed no significant association with them. These results suggested that qualitative changes had occurred in the peritumoral adipose tissue, which has a positive relationship with tumor aggressiveness.

Given that cancer-associated adipocytes conversely affect the growth and metastasis of cancer cells, it could be hypothesized that CT-attenuation of adipose tissue in patients with malignant diseases has significant prognostic significance for predicting clinical outcomes [5,7,13–15]. In previous studies, CT-attenuations of subcutaneous and visceral adipose tissue measured in the abdomen at the level of the lumbar spine were found to be significant predictors for disease progression-free survival and overall survival [12–15,27]. Previous studies consistently showed that increased CT-attenuation of adipose tissue was significantly associated with worse survival not only in malignant diseases that have close localization with adipose tissue such as pancreatic and prostate cancers, but also in malignant diseases that are remote from abdominal adipose tissue such as head and neck cancer and extremity sarcoma [12–14,27]. In a broad way, breast adipose tissue might be considered as a part of subcutaneous adipose tissue, but it permanently interacts with surrounding mammary epithelial cells consequently having distinctive characteristics from subcutaneous adipose tissue in other body compartments [7]. Considering that even the subcutaneous adipose tissue in remote location had association with cancer progression [13], it is no surprise that tumor-adjacent breast adipose tissue had significant association with cancer recurrence. The results of our study demonstrated that TAT HU and HU difference % were independently associated with RFS event after adjusting for age, tumor stage, ER and PR status, ki67 index, maximum SUV, and MTV, suggesting that perceiving the qualitative characteristics of peritumoral breast adipose tissue, as well as primary tumor features, might be of importance for predicting breast cancer recurrence after surgical resection. Furthermore, the combination of T stage and TAT HU can further improve the stratification of recurrence risk, suggesting that imaging features of tumor-adjacent breast adipose tissue might provide additional prognostic value to tumor stage. Recently, adipocytes have been considered as a new attractive treatment target for breast cancer [7,28,29]. The results of the present study might provide a clue for selecting candidates for future therapy that targets adipocytes in breast cancer patients.

Since the changes in the normal tissue surrounding breast cancer have drawn the attention of researchers, several recent studies have evaluated the clinical implication of imaging findings of tumor-adjacent breast parenchyma on magnetic resonance imaging (MRI) [30,31]. However, in the literature, only a single study has investigated the clinical significance of tumor-adjacent breast adipose tissue on imaging studies [16]. A previous study by Obeid et al. [16] retrospectively enrolled 63 patients with early breast cancer and investigated the association between imaging features of peritumoral breast adipose tissue on MRI images and axillary lymph nodal status. Similar to our study, they defined the peritumoral region as the area which is within a 1-cm spherical extension from the tumor contour. They generated peritumoral adipose volume using voxel intensity filtering and measured five imaging features of peritumoral tissue: mean voxel intensity, standard deviation of voxel intensity, total volume, fat-specific volume, and the fat ratio. Their study demonstrated that significant association was only shown between the fat ratio of peritumoral tissue and the ratio of positive-to-total axillary lymph nodes. On the other hand, the peritumoral fat ratio showed no significant correlation with other histopathologic features such as tumor grade, lymphovascular invasion, extracapsular extension, and tumor size, and the axillary lymph node status also showed no significant correlation with other imaging features of peritumoral tissue including mean voxel intensity. Because different imaging modalities were used in both studies, a direct comparison between our study and the previous studies would be limited. Although both CT and MRI are accurate and effective imaging modalities for adipose tissue measurement, each has different advantages and disadvantages [32,33]. CT is the most well-established method for adipose tissue measurement, and HU is consistent between images on difference scans, while CT scanning has the risk of exposure to high doses of ionizing radiation [32,33]. In contrast, adipose tissue measurements on MRI are expressed in arbitrary units that are difficult to compare between studies and are less reproducible than CT images [32,33]. Therefore, further studies using both CT and MRI in the same patients would be needed to compare the adipose tissue parameters of both modalities. Furthermore, CT-attenuation of only the breast adipose tissue was measured in our study, whereas voxel intensity of whole peritumoral breast tissue, including breast parenchyma and adipose tissue, was measured in the aforementioned study, which could cause differences in the results between the studies [16]. Nonetheless, our study also revealed no significant relationship between N stage and TAT HU, suggesting that the qualitative characteristics of tumor-adjacent breast tissue might have limited value for predicting axillary lymph node metastasis.

Recently, a dual-energy CT system has been introduced to improve tissue differentiation [34]. Using dual-energy CT, virtual non-contrast CT images can be synthesized, which could replace a precontrast CT scan, thereby reducing radiation exposure [34]. In previous studies, CT-attenuation values of various organs in virtual non-contrast CT images have shown close agreement with those in true unenhanced CT images [35,36]. Therefore, future studies are needed to clarify whether CT-attenuation of breast adipose tissue measured on virtual non-contrast CT images of dual-energy CT also has prognostic significance in breast cancer patients, which may form an imaging protocol for evaluating both tumor factors and tumor-adjacent breast tissue factors using a single CT scan.

There are several limitations to our study. Because the study was retrospectively performed in a single center and only the patients who had sufficient breast adipose tissue for the image analysis were included, selection bias is inevitable, which may limit the general application of the results of the present study. Furthermore, having a small number of patients who experienced recurrence could affect the results of survival analysis. Because of the retrospective nature of the study, we cannot compare the histopathological features of tumor-adjacent adipose tissue according to the CT-attenuation. Further studies with histopathological evaluation are needed to elucidate the mechanisms of our results. Lastly, as the present study is the first study to measure the tumor-adjacent breast adipose tissue, there is no established method of calculating CT-attenuation of breast adipose tissue [12,13]. A more sophisticated method, which could properly measure CT-attenuation of tumor-adjacent breast adipose tissue even in patients with a small amount of adipose tissue, would be helpful to confirm the association between breast adipose tissue parameters and clinical outcomes.

4. Materials and Methods

4.1. Study Population

This study was approved by the Institutional Review Board of Soonchunhyang University (Ethic code: SCHCA 2019-05-023, Date: 20 March 2019), and the requirement to obtain informed consent was waived by the board due to its retrospective nature. All procedures in this study were in accordance with the Declaration of Helsinki. Electronic medical records of 393 female patients who had biopsy proven invasive breast cancer and underwent pretreatment FDG PET/CT between February 2012 and December 2016 in our medical center were retrospectively reviewed. Among them, patients (1) who were diagnosed with distant metastasis on staging examinations, (2) who were diagnosed with ductal carcinoma in situ, (3) who had any kind of treatment before FDG PET/CT, (4) who had bilateral breast cancers, (5) who had a previous history of breast surgery, (6) who had a previous history of another malignancy, and (7) who were lost to follow-up within two years after the initial treatment without event were excluded from the study, and 355 patients met the initial eligibility criteria of the study. Of the 355 patients, 68 were excluded from the study during PET/CT image analysis due to insufficient breast adipose tissue for analysis ($n = 55$) and diffuse infiltration of breast cancer lesion ($n = 13$). Therefore, the remaining 287 female patients finally comprised the subjects of the study.

All enrolled patients underwent pretreatment staging examinations which consisted of blood tests, breast ultrasonography, breast MRI, bone scintigraphy, and FDG PET/CT. The BMI for each patient was calculated using the height and weight measured at the time of staging work-up. With the results of staging examinations, clinical TNM stage according to the 7th Edition of the American Joint Committee on Cancer staging system was determined for each patient. ER, PR, HER2, and Ki67 expression status were obtained from histopathological records. ER and PR positive tumors were defined as tumors with 10% or more positively stained cells using immunohistochemistry. A HER2 positive tumor was defined as a tumor with a 3+ score on immunohistochemistry or a tumor with gene amplification on fluorescence in situ hybridization. A tumor with 14% or more Ki67 expression using immunohistochemistry was defined as a Ki67 positive tumor. After staging examinations, all enrolled patients underwent curative surgical resection of breast cancer with or without neoadjuvant chemotherapy and/or adjuvant treatment. All patients were regularly followed up at intervals of 3–6 months with blood test and imaging studies. The duration of follow-up was calculated from the date of the initial treatment to the last date of clinical follow-up at our medical center or to the occurrence of cancer recurrence.

4.2. Image Analysis

All patients underwent FDG PET/CT scanning from the skull base to the proximal thigh in a supine position using a Biograph mCT 128 scanner (Siemens Healthcare, Knoxville, TN, USA) after at least six hours fasting. One hour after intravenous injection of approximately 4.07 MBq/kg of FDG, a non-contrast-enhanced attenuation correction CT scan was performed at 100 mA and 120 kV$_p$ with a slice thickness of 5 mm followed by a PET scan at 1.5 min per bed position. PET images were reconstructed using point-spread-function modeling and time-of-flight reconstruction (2 iterations and 21 subsets) with attenuation correction.

Two expert readers independently reviewed FDG PET/CT images of all patients without knowing clinico-pathological and follow-up results. A United States Food and Drug Administration-approved medical image viewer (OsiriX MD 10.0.3, Pixmeo, Geneva, Switzerland) was used for image analyses. For breast adipose tissue measurement, non-contrast-enhanced CT images of FDG PET/CT were used. A total of four parameters (TAT HU, CAT HU, HU difference, and HU difference %) were measured from breast adipose tissue. We used a 1-cm distance from the tumor margin for defining tumor-adjacent breast adipose tissue. A spheroid-shaped volume-of-interest (VOI) that includes the entire breast cancer lesion and surrounding breast tissue within a 1-cm distance to the tumor margin was manually drawn (Figure 4). Afterwards, another spheroid-shaped VOI of the same size was drawn over the contralateral breast tissue in the same quadrant of the breast tissue (Figure 4). A CT-attenuation range of −200 and −50 HU was used to define breast adipose tissue within VOIs. The mean CT-attenuation value of the area within the CT-attenuation range of breast adipose tissue was measured for each VOI and defined as TAT HU and CAT HU. Using TAT HU and CAT HU, HU difference and HU difference % were calculated as follows: (HU difference) = (TAT HU) − (CAT HU) while (HU difference %) = ((CAT HU) − (TAT HU))/(CAT HU) × 100. Using FDG PET images, we measured two metabolic parameters of primary breast cancer lesion, maximum SUV and MTV. A spheroid-shaped VOI was drawn over the primary cancer lesion on fused PET/CT images including the whole tumor lesion. The maximum SUV of the primary breast cancer lesion was measured. A total volume of voxels that had SUV of 2.50 or greater within VOI was measured and defined as MTV of primary cancer lesion.

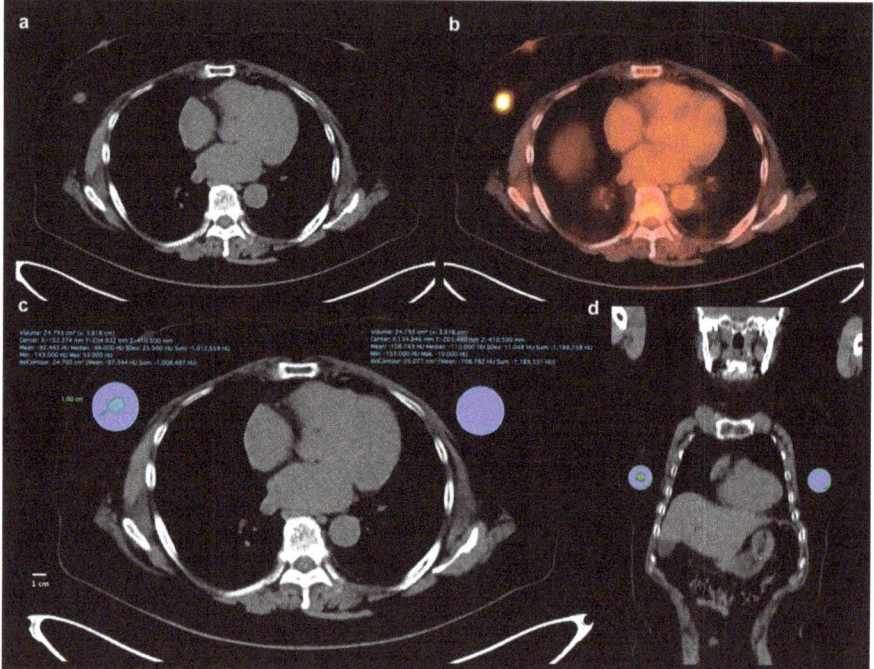

Figure 4. Measurement example of CT-attenuation of tumor-adjacent breast adipose tissue and contralateral breast adipose tissue. A 62-year-old woman underwent FDG PET/CT for staging work-up of right breast cancer, histopathologically confirmed as invasive ductal carcinoma. A mass lesion with intensely increased FDG uptake is observed in outer aspect of right breast, (**a**,**b**), showing maximum SUV of 8.44. A spheroid-shaped volume-of-interest that includes peritumoral breast tissue within a 1-cm distance from the tumor margin was manually drawn over the ipsilateral breast tissue, (**c**,**d**). Another spheroid-shaped volume-of-interest of the same size was drawn over the contralateral breast tissue in the same quadrant of the breast, (c,d). Within the volume-of-interests drawn in bilateral breast tissues, the area of breast adipose tissue defined as an area with CT-attenuation range between −200 and −50 HU was automatically delineated. Mean CT-attenuation value of breast adipose tissue was measured for each VOI (c): −92.463 HU for tumor-adjacent breast adipose tissue and −108.743 for contralateral breast adipose tissue.

4.3. Statistical Analysis

To assess the reproducibility of measurement of TAT HU and CAT HU between the two readers, concordance correlation coefficients for TAT HU and CAT HU were calculated. Paired *t* test was performed to assess the difference between TAT HU and CAT HU. A Student's *t* test and Kruskal—Wallis test were performed to compare the differences in four breast adipose tissue parameters between groups. After performing the normality test, Spearman rank correlation coefficients were calculated for the breast adipose tissue parameters with regard to BMI and maximum SUV and MTV of the primary breast cancer lesion. The primary endpoint of the present study was RFS. Univariate and multivariate survival analyses using the Cox proportional hazards regression model were performed to assess the association between variables and RFS. Of the four breast adipose tissue parameters, those with a *p*-value of less than 0.10 in univariate analysis were included in multivariate analysis. In the multivariate analysis of breast adipose tissue parameters, three different models with eight different covariates (age, T stage, N stage, ER status, PR status, Ki67 index, maximum SUV, and MTV) were constructed. The significances of the association between breast adipose tissue parameters and RFS were evaluated after adjusting for these eight covariates. For breast adipose tissue parameters that showed statistical significance in univariate survival analysis, the optimal cut-off values were determined using ROC curve analysis, and survival curves for RFS according to the cut-off values were estimated using the Kaplan—Meier method. All statistical analyses were performed using MedCalc Statistical Software version 19.0.3 (MedCalc Software bvba, Ostend, Belgium). A *p*-value of <0.05 was considered statistically significant.

5. Conclusions

TAT HU and HU difference % were independent predictors for RFS in patients with breast cancer, suggesting that qualitative alterations of tumor-adjacent breast adipose tissue may have significant association with tumor recurrence. TAT HU and HU difference % had a significant relationship with T stage and hormone receptor status of breast cancer, and patients with increased CT-attenuation of peritumoral adipose tissue had worse survival. Although further studies are warranted to confirm the results, the results of our study seem to support the close interaction between breast cancer cells and tumor-adjacent adipocytes observed with imaging studies.

Author Contributions: Conceptualization, J.W.L., S.M.L.; methodology, J.W.L., S.Y.K., S.M.L.; formal analysis, J.W.L., S.Y.K., H.J.L., S.M.L.; data curation, H.J.L, S.W.H., J.E.L., S.M.L.; writing—original draft preparation, J.W.L.; writing—review & editing, S.Y.K., H.J.L., S.W.H., J.E.L., S.M.L.; visualization, J.W.L.; supervision, S.W.H, S.M.L.; funding acquisition, J.W.L., S.M.L.

Funding: This work was supported by Soonchunhyang University Research Fund and the National Research Foundation of Korea (NRF) grant funded by the Korean government (Ministry of Science and ICT) (grant number: NRF-2017R1C1B5075905 and NRF-2018R1C1B5040061).

Conflicts of Interest: The authors declare no conflict of interest.

References

1. Duong, M.N.; Geneste, A.; Fallone, F.; Li, X.; Dumontet, C.; Muller, C. The fat and the bad: Mature adipocytes, key actors in tumor progression and resistance. *Oncotarget* **2017**, *8*, 57622–57641. [CrossRef] [PubMed]
2. Vandeweyer, E.; Hertens, D. Quantification of glands and fat in breast tissue: An experimental determination. *Ann. Anat.* **2002**, *184*, 181–184. [CrossRef]
3. Guaita-Esteruelas, S.; Guma, J.; Masana, L.; Borras, J. The peritumoural adipose tissue microenvironment and cancer. The roles of fatty acid binding protein 4 and fatty acid binding protein 5. *Mol. Cell. Endocrinol.* **2018**, *462*, 107–118. [CrossRef] [PubMed]
4. Lehr, S.; Hartwig, S.; Sell, H. Adipokines: A treasure trove for the discovery of biomarkers for metabolic disorders. *Proteom. Clin. Appl.* **2012**, *6*, 91–101. [CrossRef] [PubMed]
5. Divella, R.; De Luca, R.; Abbate, I.; Naglieri, E.; Daniele, A. Obesity and cancer: The role of adipose tissue and adipo-cytokines-induced chronic inflammation. *J. Cancer* **2016**, *7*, 2346–2359. [CrossRef]
6. Engin, A.B.; Engin, A.; Gonul, I.I. The effect of adipocyte-macrophage cross-talk in obesity-related breast cancer. *J. Mol. Endocrinol.* **2019**. [CrossRef] [PubMed]
7. Choi, J.; Cha, Y.J.; Koo, J.S. Adipocyte biology in breast cancer: From silent bystander to active facilitator. *Prog. Lipid. Res.* **2018**, *69*, 11–20. [CrossRef] [PubMed]

8. Dirat, B.; Bochet, L.; Dabek, M.; Daviaud, D.; Dauvillier, S.; Majed, B.; Wang, Y.Y.; Meulle, A.; Salles, B.; Le Gonidec, S.; et al. Cancer-associated adipocytes exhibit an activated phenotype and contribute to breast cancer invasion. *Cancer Res.* **2011**, *71*, 2455–2465. [CrossRef] [PubMed]
9. Fletcher, S.J.; Sacca, P.A.; Pistone-Creydt, M.; Colo, F.A.; Serra, M.F.; Santino, F.E.; Sasso, C.V.; Lopez-Fontana, C.M.; Caron, R.W.; Calvo, J.C.; et al. Human breast adipose tissue: Characterization of factors that change during tumor progression in human breast cancer. *J. Exp. Clin. Cancer Res.* **2017**, *36*, 26. [CrossRef] [PubMed]
10. Murphy, R.A.; Register, T.C.; Shively, C.A.; Carr, J.J.; Ge, Y.; Heilbrun, M.E.; Cummings, S.R.; Koster, A.; Nevitt, M.C.; Satterfield, S.; et al. Adipose tissue density, a novel biomarker predicting mortality risk in older adults. *J. Gerontol. A Biol. Sci. Med. Sci.* **2014**, *69*, 109–117. [CrossRef] [PubMed]
11. Lee, J.W.; Lee, H.S.; Na, J.O.; Lee, S.M. Effect of adipose tissue volume on prognosis in patients with non-small cell lung cancer. *Clin. Imaging* **2018**, *50*, 308–313. [CrossRef] [PubMed]
12. Lee, J.W.; Lee, S.M.; Chung, Y.A. Prognostic value of CT attenuation and FDG uptake of adipose tissue in patients with pancreatic adenocarcinoma. *Clin. Radiol.* **2018**, *73*, 1056.e1–1056.e10. [CrossRef] [PubMed]
13. Lee, J.W.; Ban, M.J.; Park, J.H.; Lee, S.M. Visceral adipose tissue volume and CT-attenuation as prognostic factors in patients with head and neck cancer. *Head Neck* **2019**, *41*, 1605–1614. [CrossRef] [PubMed]
14. Veld, J.; Vossen, J.A.; De Amorim Bernstein, K.; Halpern, E.F.; Torriani, M.; Bredella, M.A. Adipose tissue and muscle attenuation as novel biomarkers predicting mortality in patients with extremity sarcomas. *Eur. Radiol.* **2016**, *26*, 4649–4655. [CrossRef]
15. Yoo, I.D.; Lee, S.M.; Lee, J.W.; Baek, M.J.; Ahn, T.S. Usefulness of metabolic activity of adipose tissue in FDG PET/CT of colorectal cancer. *Abdom. Radiol. (NY)* **2018**, *43*, 2052–2059. [CrossRef]
16. Obeid, J.P.; Stoyanova, R.; Kwon, D.; Patel, M.; Padgett, K.; Slingerland, J.; Takita, C.; Alperin, N.; Yepes, M.; Zeidan, Y.H. Multiparametric evaluation of preoperative MRI in early stage breast cancer: Prognostic impact of peri-tumoral fat. *Clin. Transl. Oncol.* **2017**, *19*, 211–218. [CrossRef]
17. Caresia Aroztegui, A.P.; Garcia Vicente, A.M.; Alvarez Ruiz, S.; Delgado Bolton, R.C.; Orcajo Rincon, J.; Garcia Garzon, J.R.; de Arocha Torres, M.; Garcia-Velloso, M.J. 18F-FDG PET/CT in breast cancer: Evidence-based recommendations in initial staging. *Tumour Biol.* **2017**, *39*. [CrossRef]
18. Lee, S.S.; Bae, S.K.; Park, Y.S.; Park, J.S.; Kim, T.H.; Yoon, H.K.; Ahn, H.J.; Lee, S.M. Correlation of molecular subtypes of invasive ductal carcinoma of breast with glucose metabolism in FDG PET/CT: Based on the Recommendations of the St. Gallen Consensus Meeting 2013. *Nucl. Med. Mol. Imaging* **2017**, *51*, 79–85. [CrossRef]
19. Kitajima, K.; Yamano, T.; Miyoshi, Y.; Enoki, T.; Yamakado, K. Prognostic value of FDG-PET/CT prior to breast cancer treatment—Comparison with MRS and DWI. *J. Nucl. Med.* **2019**, *60* (Suppl. 1), 603.
20. Onner, H.; Canaz, F.; Dincer, M.; Isiksoy, S.; Sivrikoz, I.A.; Entok, E.; Erkasap, S. Which of the fluorine-18 fluorodeoxyglucose positron emission tomography/computerized tomography parameters are better associated with prognostic factors in breast cancer? *Medicine (Baltimore)* **2019**, *98*, e15925. [CrossRef]
21. Ribeiro, R.J.; Monteiro, C.P.; Cunha, V.F.; Azevedo, A.S.; Oliveira, M.J.; Monteiro, R.; Fraga, A.M.; Principe, P.; Lobato, C.; Lobo, F.; et al. Tumor cell-educated periprostatic adipose tissue acquires an aggressive cancer-promoting secretory profile. *Cell. Physiol. Biochem.* **2012**, *29*, 233–240. [CrossRef] [PubMed]
22. Dirat, B.; Bochet, L.; Escourrou, G.; Valet, P.; Muller, C. Unraveling the obesity and breast cancer links: A role for cancer-associated adipocytes? *Endocr. Dev.* **2010**, *19*, 45–52. [CrossRef] [PubMed]
23. Bochet, L.; Lehuede, C.; Dauvillier, S.; Wang, Y.Y.; Dirat, B.; Laurent, V.; Dray, C.; Guiet, R.; Maridonneau-Parini, I.; Le Gonidec, S.; et al. Adipocyte-derived fibroblasts promote tumor progression and contribute to the desmoplastic reaction in breast cancer. *Cancer Res.* **2013**, *73*, 5657–5668. [CrossRef] [PubMed]
24. Jung, Y.Y.; Lee, Y.K.; Koo, J.S. Expression of cancer-associated fibroblast-related proteins in adipose stroma of breast cancer. *Tumour Biol.* **2015**, *36*, 8685–8695. [CrossRef] [PubMed]
25. Ando, S.; Barone, I.; Giordano, C.; Bonofiglio, D.; Catalano, S. The Multifaceted mechanism of leptin signaling within tumor microenvironment in driving breast cancer growth and progression. *Front. Oncol.* **2014**, *4*, 340. [CrossRef] [PubMed]
26. Huang, C.K.; Chang, P.H.; Kuo, W.H.; Chen, C.L.; Jeng, Y.M.; Chang, K.J.; Shew, J.Y.; Hu, C.M.; Lee, W.H. Adipocytes promote malignant growth of breast tumours with monocarboxylate transporter 2 expression via beta-hydroxybutyrate. *Nat. Commun.* **2017**, *8*, 14706. [CrossRef] [PubMed]

27. McDonald, A.M.; Fiveash, J.B.; Kirkland, R.S.; Cardan, R.A.; Jacob, R.; Kim, R.Y.; Dobelbower, M.C.; Yang, E.S. Subcutaneous adipose tissue characteristics and the risk of biochemical recurrence in men with high-risk prostate cancer. *Urol. Oncol.* **2017**, *35*, 663.e615–663.e621. [CrossRef]
28. Li, Q.; Xia, J.; Yao, Y.; Gong, D.W.; Shi, H.; Zhou, Q. Sulforaphane inhibits mammary adipogenesis by targeting adipose mesenchymal stem cells. *Breast Cancer Res. Treat.* **2013**, *141*, 317–324. [CrossRef]
29. Bochet, L.; Meulle, A.; Imbert, S.; Salles, B.; Valet, P.; Muller, C. Cancer-associated adipocytes promotes breast tumor radioresistance. *Biochem. Biophys. Res. Commun.* **2011**, *411*, 102–106. [CrossRef]
30. Nabavizadeh, N.; Klifa, C.; Newitt, D.; Lu, Y.; Chen, Y.Y.; Hsu, H.; Fisher, C.; Tokayasu, T.; Olshen, A.B.; Spellman, P.; et al. Topographic enhancement mapping of the cancer-associated breast stroma using breast MRI. *Integr. Biol. (Camb.)* **2011**, *3*, 490–496. [CrossRef]
31. Wu, J.; Li, B.; Sun, X.; Cao, G.; Rubin, D.L.; Napel, S.; Ikeda, D.M.; Kurian, A.W.; Li, R. Heterogeneous enhancement patterns of tumor-adjacent parenchyma at MR imaging are associated with dysregulated signaling pathways and poor survival in breast cancer. *Radiology* **2017**, *285*, 401–413. [CrossRef] [PubMed]
32. Kullberg, J.; Brandberg, J.; Angelhed, J.E.; Frimmel, H.; Bergelin, E.; Strid, L.; Ahlstrom, H.; Johansson, L.; Lonn, L. Whole-body adipose tissue analysis: Comparison of MRI, CT and dual energy X-ray absorptiometry. *Br. J. Radiol.* **2009**, *82*, 123–130. [CrossRef] [PubMed]
33. Pescatori, L.C.; Savarino, E.; Mauri, G.; Silvestri, E.; Cariati, M.; Sardanelli, F.; Sconfienza, L.M. Quantification of visceral adipose tissue by computed tomography and magnetic resonance imaging: Reproducibility and accuracy. *Radiol. Bras.* **2019**, *52*, 1–6. [CrossRef] [PubMed]
34. Goo, H.W.; Goo, J.M. Dual-energy CT: New horizon in medical imaging. *Korean J. Radiol.* **2017**, *18*, 555–569. [CrossRef] [PubMed]
35. Toepker, M.; Moritz, T.; Krauss, B.; Weber, M.; Euller, G.; Mang, T.; Wolf, F.; Herold, C.J.; Ringl, H. Virtual non-contrast in second-generation, dual-energy computed tomography: Reliability of attenuation values. *Eur. J. Radiol.* **2012**, *81*, e398–e405. [CrossRef]
36. Jamali, S.; Michoux, N.; Coche, E.; Dragean, C.A. Virtual unenhanced phase with spectral dual-energy CT: Is it an alternative to conventional true unenhanced phase for abdominal tissues? *Diagn. Interv. Imaging* **2019**. [CrossRef]

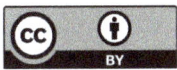

© 2019 by the authors. Licensee MDPI, Basel, Switzerland. This article is an open access article distributed under the terms and conditions of the Creative Commons Attribution (CC BY) license (http://creativecommons.org/licenses/by/4.0/).

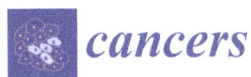

Article

In Vivo Assessment of VCAM-1 Expression by SPECT/CT Imaging in Mice Models of Human Triple Negative Breast Cancer

Christopher Montemagno [1], Laurent Dumas [1,2], Pierre Cavaillès [3], Mitra Ahmadi [1], Sandrine Bacot [1], Marlène Debiossat [1], Audrey Soubies [1], Loic Djaïleb [1], Julien Leenhardt [1], Nicolas De Leiris [1], Maeva Dufies [4], Gilles Pagès [4,5], Sophie Hernot [6], Nick Devoogdt [6], Pascale Perret [1], Laurent Riou [1], Daniel Fagret [1], Catherine Ghezzi [1,†] and Alexis Broisat [1,*,†]

1. Laboratory of Bioclinical Radiopharmaceutics, Universite Grenoble Alpes, Inserm, CHU Grenoble Alpes, LRB, 38000 Grenoble, France
2. Advanced Accelator Applications, 01630 Saint-Genis-Pouilly, France
3. Natural Barriers and Infectiosity, Universite Grenoble Alpes, CNRS, CHU Grenoble Alpes, TIMC-IMAG, 38000 Grenoble, France
4. Biomedical Department, Centre Scientifique de Monaco, 980000 Monaco, Monaco
5. Institute for Research on Cancer and Aging of Nice, Universite Cote d'Azur, CNRS UMR 7284, INSERM U1081, Centre Antoine Lacassagne, 061489 Nice, France
6. Laboratory of In Vivo Cellular and Molecular Imaging, ICMI-BEFY, Vrije Universiteit Brussel, Laarbeeklan 103, B-1090 Brussels, Belgium
* Correspondence: alexis.broisat@inserm.fr; Tel.: +33-47663-7102
† Contributed equally to this work.

Received: 5 June 2019; Accepted: 19 July 2019; Published: 23 July 2019

Abstract: Recent progress in breast cancer research has led to the identification of Vascular Cell Adhesion Molecule-1 (VCAM-1) as a key actor of metastatic colonization. VCAM-1 promotes lung-metastases and is associated with clinical early recurrence and poor outcome in triple negative breast cancer (TNBC). Our objective was to perform the in vivo imaging of VCAM-1 in mice models of TNBC. The Cancer Genomic Atlas (TCGA) database was analyzed to evaluate the prognostic role of VCAM-1 in TNBC. MDA-MB-231 (VCAM-1+) and control HCC70 (VCAM-1-) TNBC cells were subcutaneously xenografted in mice and VCAM-1 expression was assessed in vivo by single-photon emission computed tomography (SPECT) imaging using ^{99m}Tc-cAbVCAM1-5. Then, MDA-MB-231 cells were intravenously injected in mice and VCAM-1 expression in lung metastasis was assessed by SPECT imaging after 8 weeks. TCGA analysis showed that VCAM-1 is associated with a poor prognosis in TNBC patients. In subcutaneous tumor models, ^{99m}Tc-cAbVCAM1-5 uptake was 2-fold higher in MDA-MB-231 than in HCC70 ($p < 0.01$), and 4-fold higher than that of the irrelevant control ($p < 0.01$). Moreover, ^{99m}Tc-cAbVCAM1-5 uptake in MDA-MB-231 lung metastases was also higher than that of ^{99m}Tc-Ctl ($p < 0.05$). ^{99m}Tc-cAbVCAM1-5 is therefore a suitable tool to evaluate the role of VCAM-1 as a marker of tumor aggressiveness of TNBC.

Keywords: triple negative breast cancer; VCAM-1; SPECT imaging; sdAbs

1. Introduction

Breast cancer (BC) is the most common female malignancy, accounting for more than 30% of all malignant tumors in women [1]. Breast cancer is a heterogeneous disease consisting of various subtypes with distinct molecular and pathological profiles [2,3]. Triple Negative Breast Cancer (TNBC) subtypes represent 10% to 20% of BC and are characterized by the lack of progesterone receptor, estrogen receptor and human epidermal growth factor receptor 2 expression [4]. TNBC are mostly associated with poor clinical outcome and high rate of metastasis and relapse following treatment [5,6]. Lung, bones, brain and liver are the most common sites of distant metastasis. Despite intense clinical research efforts, only limited advances have been obtained in the management of BC metastases.

Recent studies have led to the identification of new genes and mechanisms that mediate metastatic colonization [7]. Among them, Vascular Cell Adhesion Molecule-1 (VCAM-1) plays a key role in BC progression and metastatic processes [8,9]. VCAM-1 belongs to the immunoglobulin super family group of adhesion molecules. It is a 110 kDa glycoprotein mainly expressed at the endothelial cells surface during inflammation, but also by macrophages and dendritic cells [10]. The ability of VCAM-1 expressed by endothelial cells to bind tumor cells suggest that it could contribute to metastatic spread. Indeed, VCAM-1 expression on endothelial cells plays a key role in angiogenesis, in tumor cell transmigration, and therefore promotes tumor development and dissemination of tumor cells [11].

In the last few years, a growing interest into VCAM-1 expression on tumor cells has emerged. In BC, the overexpression of VCAM-1 on tumor cells correlates with early relapse and poor patient outcome [12,13]. The direct interaction of VCAM-1 with its ligand Very-Late Antigen -4 (VLA-4) expressed on leukocytes allows tumor cell survival in lungs and consequently lung metastasis [14]. Moreover, VCAM-1 is involved in the transition from dormant micro-metastases to overt macro-metastases in bones, a turning point in BC progression [13,15]. Inhibition of the VCAM-1 and VLA-4 interaction impairs bone metastasis progression and lung colonization [13,14,16]. VCAM-1 is also involved into chemoresistance and tumor immune escape [17–19]. Therefore, VCAM-1 is a key player with multiple functionalities in directing the metastatic spread. VCAM-1 expression could be induced by pro-inflammatory cytokines, such as Tumor Necrosis Factor-α (TNF-α), IL-1 or IL-6, major mediators of tumor progression [19].

To assess the role of VCAM-1 in the metastatic phenotype of BC, nuclear imaging may represent a powerful tool. We recently developed a single domain antibody (sdAb)-based radiotracer targeting VCAM-1 called ^{99m}Technetium-cAbVCAM1-5 (^{99m}Tc-cAbVCAM1-5), which is ongoing clinical transfer for detection of inflamed atherosclerosis lesions [20,21]. The aim of the present study was to assess VCAM-1 expression using ^{99m}Tc-cAbVCAM1-5 in subcutaneous and lung metastasis mice models of TNBC.

2. Results

2.1. VCAM-1 Is Overexpressed in TNBC and Associated with Decreased OS

980 breast cancer patients of The Cancer Genomic Atlas (TCGA) were analyzed for VCAM-1 mRNA levels and subsequent overall survival (OS) follow-up (Figure 1). VCAM-1 expression was higher in TNBC ($n = 114$) as compared to non-TNBC patients ($n = 866$) ($p < 0.001$, Figure 1A). High VCAM-1 expression was associated with decreased OS in TNBC but not in non-TNBC patients (respectively $p = 0.035$ and $p = 0.6886$, Figure 1B,C). TNF-α mRNA expression is overexpressed in TNBC as compared to non-TNBC patients ($p < 0.001$, Figure 1A).

2.2. MDA-MB-231 Cells Overexpress VCAM-1 mRNA and Protein

The expression of VCAM-1 was first assessed on two TNBC cell lines. VCAM-1 mRNA levels were undetectable at the basal level or following TNF-α stimulation in HCC70 cells. However, MDA-MB-231 cells expressed VCAM-1 mRNA basal levels. They were induced by a 3.5-fold upon TNF-α stimulation (1.0 ± 0.1 vs. 3.5 ± 1.3, $p < 0.05$, Figure 2A). Consistently, VCAM-1 protein was undetectable in HCC70 cells whereas MDA-MB-231 expressed basal VCAM-1 protein levels and TNF-α induced a 3.5-fold increase of these basal levels (Figure 2B,C, Figure S1).

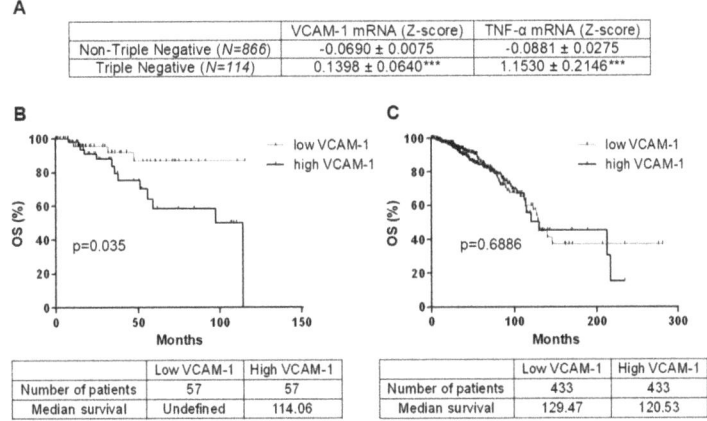

Figure 1. VCAM-1 is overexpressed in Triple-Negative Breast Cancer (TNBC) and associated with a decrease of overall survival. (**A**) Expression of VCAM-1 and TNF-α in TNBC and Non-TNBC were compared in TCGA datasets for breast cancer. Values represent the z scores for $\log_2$-transformed normalized RNA-seq read counts. (**B**,**C**) Kaplan-Meier analysis of OS of TNBC (**B**) and Non-TNBC (**C**) patients. OS (months) were calculated from patient subgroups with VCAM-1 mRNA levels that were less or greater than the median value. Statistical significance (p-value) is indicated. *** $p < 0.001$. Nb: Number.

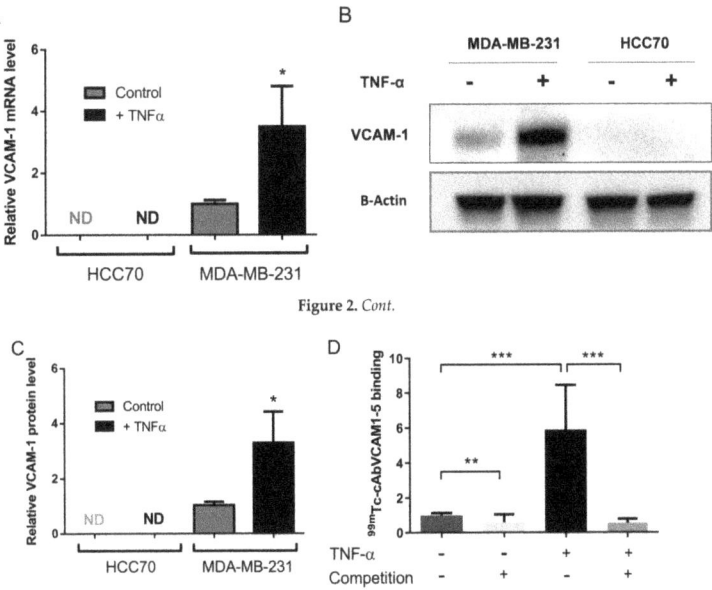

Figure 2. MDA-MB-231 cells overexpress VCAM-1 mRNA and protein upon TNF-α stimulation. MDA-MB-231 and HCC70 cells were treated or not for 18 h with TNF-α (50 ng/mL) and VCAM-1 expression was assessed by RT-qPCR (**A**) and WB (**B**). (**C**) Bands of WB were quantified using ImageJ software. (**D**) ^{99m}Tc-AbVCAM1-5 binding was performed on MDA-MB-231 cells stimulated or not with TNF-α, in the presence or absence of a 100-fold excess of unlabeled cAbVCAM1-5. Unspecific binding was estimated by ^{99m}Tc-AbVCAM1-5 incubation on HCC70 cells. Results are expressed in fold-change vs. untreated and unstimulated MDA-MB-231 $N = 6$ per condition. * $p < 0.05$; ** $p < 0.01$; *** $p < 0.001$; ND, not detected.

2.3. ^{99m}Tc-cAbVCAM1-5 Binds Specifically to VCAM-1 Expressing TNBC Cells

Unlabeled cAbVCAM1-5 bound to VCAM-1-positive MDA-MB-231 but not to VCAM-1-negative HCC70 cells (Figure S2). ^{99m}Tc-cAbVCAM1-5 affinity was evaluated on both mouse and human recombinant protein and found to be in the nanomolar range scale (Kd = 12.5 ± 3.6 nM for mVCAM-1 and 36.3 ± 7.0 nM for hVCAM-1) (Figure S3). To further demonstrate the specificity of the binding on MDA-MB-231 cells, in vitro competition studies were then performed to determine the ability of the radiolabeled ^{99m}Tc-cAbVCAM1-5 to bind specifically to MDA-MB-231 (Figure 2D). ^{99m}Tc-cAbVCAM1-5 binding to TNF-α stimulated cells was 5-fold higher than to unstimulated cells (5.8 ± 2.6 vs. 1.0 ± 0.2, respectively, $p < 0.001$). Moreover, the addition of an excess of unlabeled cAbVCAM1-5 significantly decreased ^{99m}Tc-cAbVCAM1-5 binding on unstimulated and on stimulated MDA-MB-231 cells by 42% ($p < 0.01$) and 90% ($p < 0.001$), respectively. These results demonstrated that ^{99m}Tc-cAbVCAM1-5 binds specifically to VCAM-1 expressing cells.

2.4. SPECT/CT Imaging of VCAM-1 in Subcutaneous Tumor Model

^{99m}Tc-cAbVCAM1-5 potential to perform in vivo imaging of VCAM-1-expressing tumors was then evaluated. Whole-body SPECT/CT images of mice subcutaneously implanted with MDA-MB-231 and HCC70 tumors are presented in Figure 3A and in Figure S4. ^{99m}Tc-cAbVCAM1-5 uptake was readily detectable in MDA-MB-231 tumors, whereas a weak signal was detectable from HCC70 tumor and from MDA-MB-231 or HCC70 tumors using the irrelevant ^{99m}Tc-Ctl (Figure 3A). Quantification of SPECT images confirmed that ^{99m}Tc-cAbVCAM1-5 uptake in MDA-MB-231 tumors (1.7 ± 0.5% ID/cm^3) was significantly higher than in HCC70 tumors (0.9 ± 0.2% ID/cm^3, $p < 0.01$), whereas ^{99m}Tc-Ctl uptake was similar in HCC70 and in MDA-MB-231 tumors (0.6 ± 0.1 vs. 0.6 ± 0.2% ID/cm^3, respectively) (Figure 3B) and significantly lower than ^{99m}Tc-cAbVCAM1-5 tumor uptake in MDA-MB-231 ($p < 0.01$) and HCC70 tumors ($p < 0.05$). The biodistribution of ^{99m}Tc-cAbVCAM1-5 and ^{99m}Tc-Ctl determined ex vivo by gamma-well counting was in accordance with that obtained following SPECT image quantification, thereby demonstrating the accuracy of the method (Figure 3C and Figure S5). Specific ^{99m}Tc-cAbVCAM1-5 uptake in lymphoid organs was observed which was consistent with VCAM-1 expression (Table S1).

2.5. Ex Vivo Assessment of VCAM-1 Expression in Subcutaneous Tumors

Since VCAM-1 is also involved in inflammatory and angiogenic processes, we next determined which part of its expression was attributable to tumor cells (human VCAM-1), or to the inflammatory and endothelial cells (mouse VCAM-1) using RT-qPCR (Figure 4). Consistently with in vitro results, hVCAM-1 mRNA was expressed by MDA-MD-231 but was not detectable in HCC70 tumors. Moreover, hVCAM-1 expression was nearly 4-fold higher than that of mVCAM-1 in MDA-MB-231 xenograft tumors ($p < 0.001$), suggesting that the hVCAM-1 expression by tumor cells was the predominant form present in MDA-MB-231 subcutaneous xenografts. Interestingly, no significant difference was observed in mVCAM-1 mRNA expression between HCC70 and MDA-MB-231 tumors (1.6 ± 1.0 vs. 1.0 ± 0.1). This results strongly suggests that the signal obtained on SPECT/CT images reflects VCAM-1-expressing tumor cells.

2.6. SPECT/CT Imaging of VCAM-1 in an Experimental Metastasis Model

Because VCAM-1 is involved in lung colonization we next investigated the ability of ^{99m}Tc-cAbVCAM1-5 to perform its imaging in an experimental metastasis model. Representative SPECT/CT images are presented in Figure 5A and in Figure S6.

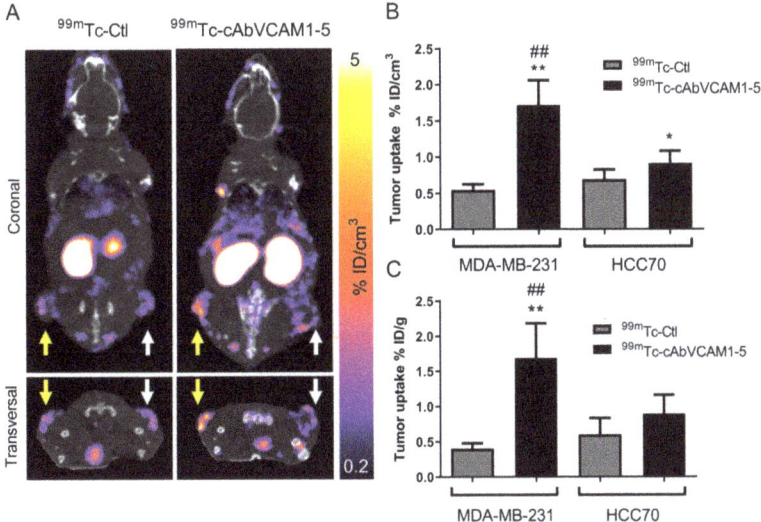

Figure 3. In vivo biodistribution of ^{99m}Tc-cAbVCAM1-5 in mice bearing HCC70 and MDA-MB-231 tumor xenografts. (**A**) Representative coronal and transversal views of fused SPECT/CT images of HCC70 (right hind limb, white arrow) and MDA-MB-231 (left hind limb, yellow arrow) tumor-bearing mice at 1 h after i.v injection of ^{99m}Tc-cAbVCA1M-5 or ^{99m}Tc-Ctl. (**B**) In vivo quantification of ^{99m}Tc-cAbVCAM1-5 and ^{99m}Tc-Ctl tumor uptake from SPECT images. (**C**) Ex vivo quantification of ^{99m}Tc-cAbVCAM1-5 and ^{99m}Tc-Ctl tumor uptake from post-mortem biodistribution studies. Results were expressed as % ID/cm^3 (imaging) and % ID/g (ex vivo) of tumor. Statistics: * $p < 0.05$, ** $p < 0.01$ vs. ^{99m}Tc-Ctl; ## $p < 0.01$ vs. HCC70.

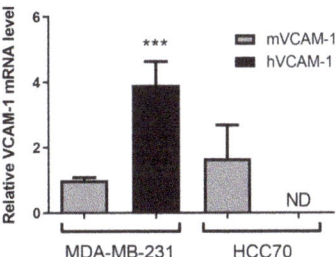

Figure 4. Ex vivo assessment of VCAM-1 expression by RT-qPCR. 50 mg of MDA-MB-231 and HCC70 xenografts were harvested and tested for human and mice VCAM-1 expression by RT-qPCR. *** $p < 0.001$ vs. MDA-MB-231 mVCAM-1.

^{99m}Tc-cAbVCAM1-5 lung uptake was readily observable, whereas a weak signal was obtained with ^{99m}Tc-Ctl (Figure 5A). Quantification of SPECT/CT images confirmed that the lung uptake was 2.5-fold higher with ^{99m}Tc-cAbVCAM1-5 than ^{99m}Tc-Ctl (1.7 ± 0.4 vs. 0.7 ± 0.1% ID/cm^3, $p < 0.05$, Figure 5B). When performing image quantification of pulmonary activity, the volume of interest contains a mixture of tissue and air, thereby leading to an underestimation of the uptake. ^{99m}Tc-cAbVCAM1-5 lung uptake was therefore further evaluated using ex vivo gamma-well counting (Figure 5C) and autoradiography (Figure 6A,B). Using these two technics, ^{99m}Tc-cAbVCAM1-5 uptake was found to represent ~3% ID/g and 4–5 fold-higher value than that obtained with ^{99m}Tc- Ctl ($p < 0.05$ for both technics). ^{99m}Tc-cAbVCAM1-5 uptake was also evaluated in lung-metastasis free mice and found to be 3-fold lower than lung-metastasis bearing mice ($p < 0.05$, Figure S7).

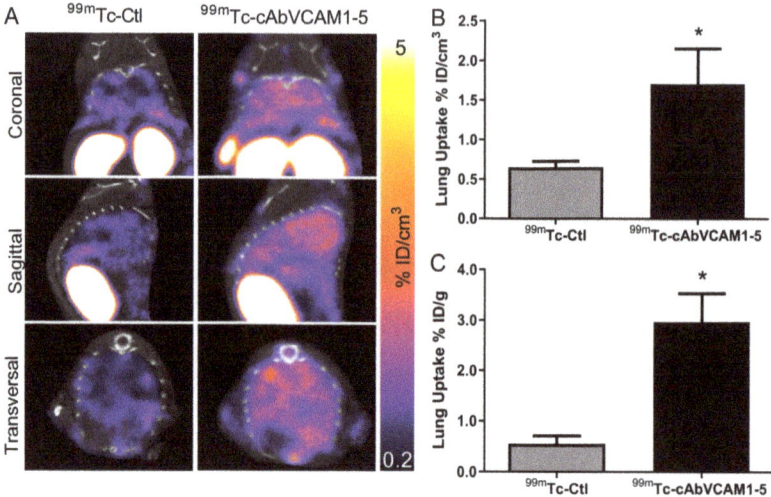

Figure 5. In vivo biodistribution of ^{99m}Tc-cAbVCAM1-5 in a pulmonary experimental metastasis model. (**A**) Representative coronal and transversal views of fused SPECT/CT images of MDA-MB-231 lung metastases at 1 h after i.v. injection of ^{99m}Tc-cAbVCAM1-5 or ^{99m}Tc-Ctl. (**B**) In vivo quantification of ^{99m}Tc-cAbVCAM1-5 and ^{99m}Tc-Ctl lung uptake from SPECT images. (**C**) Ex vivo quantification of ^{99m}Tc-cAbVCAM1-5 and ^{99m}Tc-Ctl lung uptake from post-mortem biodistribution studies. Results were expressed as % ID/cm^3 (imaging) and % ID/g (ex vivo) of tumor. Statistics: * $p < 0.05$ vs. ^{99m}Tc-Ctl.

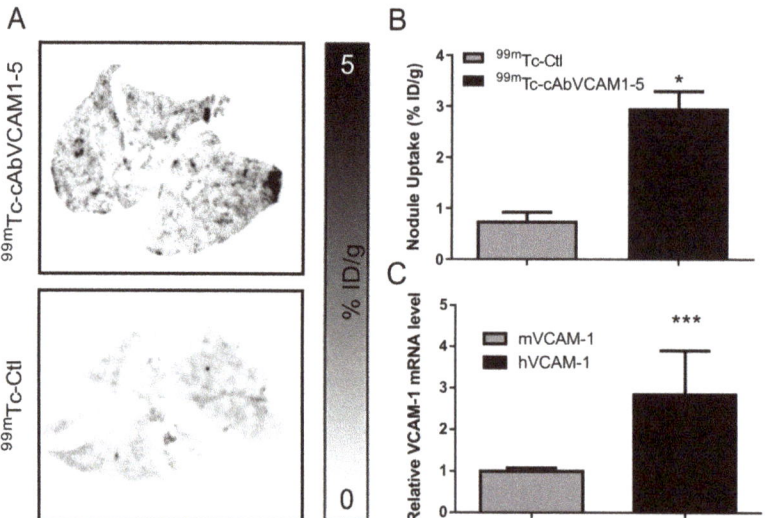

Figure 6. Ex vivo assessment of ^{99m}Tc-cAbVCAM1-5 uptake in metastatic nodules and assessment of VCAM-1 expression by RT-qPCR. (**A**) Autoradiography on 20 µm metastasis-containing lung slices. (**B**) Autoradiographic image quantification of ^{99m}Tc-cAbVCAM1-5 and ^{99m}Tc-Ctl uptake in MDA-MB-231 metastatic nodules. * $p < 0.05$ vs. ^{99m}Tc-Ctl. (**C**) 50 mg of lung containing metastases (MDA-MB-231) were harvested and tested for human and mice VCAM-1 expression by RT-qPCR. *** $p < 0.001$ vs. MDA-MB-231 mVCAM-1.

2.7. Ex Vivo Assessment of VCAM-1 Expression in the Experimental Metastasis Model

As in the subcutaneous xenograft study, VCAM-1 lung expression was assessed by RT-qPCR (Figure 6C). Both mVCAM-1 and hVCAM-1 mRNA were expressed, with the predominant expression of hVCAM-1 in tumors. Indeed, hVCAM-1 was nearly 3-fold more expressed than mVCAM-1 (2.8 ± 1.1 vs. 1.0 ± 0.1, $p < 0.001$). This results strongly suggests that the ^{99m}Tc-cAbVCAM1-5 imaging reflects VCAM-1 tumor cells expression in this model.

3. Discussion

Despite major advances in fundamental knowledge and therapeutic opportunities, BC remains the leading form of malignancy among women [1]. If the 5-year relative survival of BC is almost 100% when the cancer is restricted to the breast, the prognosis of patients with metastatic BC is unfavorable with a 5-year survival rate of 25% [22]. Moreover, among women initially diagnosed without metastasis, 20 to 25% will develop a metastatic disease in the next 5 years [23]. Despite intense clinical research efforts, there is still a strong need for novel molecular target and therapies to improve management of BC metastases [24]. The identification of genes and mechanisms involved in metastatic processes and the development of effective treatments against metastatic BC are outstanding challenges in current experimental and clinical research. In the past few years, growing interest into tumorigenicity and metastatic processes has led to the identification of VCAM-1 as a key actor for tumor growth, metastasis and angiogenesis [25].

In BC, VCAM-1 expression on tumor cells is an important actor for metastatic colonization of lungs and bones [9]. In the lungs VCAM-1 binds to α4β1 integrin expressed on macrophages triggering the activation of the PI3K/Akt survival pathway in cancer cells [14]. In bone, VCAM-1 expressing tumor cells binds to α4β1 integrin-expressing osteoclast progenitors to mediate osteolytic metastasis [13]. Moreover, VCAM-1 expression seems to be correlated to poor outcome in BC [12]. The results provided by the TCGA analysis showed that VCAM-1 is overexpressed in TNBC in comparison to Non-TNBC. Moreover, VCAM-1 expression is associated with a poor prognosis only in TNBC patients. In addition to BC, VCAM-1 increased expression has also been described in other cancer types such as glioblastoma, gastric and ovarian cancer. In these cancers, VCAM-1 expression correlated with the tumor grade [26–28]. Considering the role of VCAM-1 in directing the metastatic spread, VCAM-1 imaging agents could be used to (1) understand the biological role of VCAM-1 in metastatic processes and (2) to evaluate the prognostic value of VCAM-1 expression in clinical practice. Therefore, radiotracers have been developed for VCAM-1 imaging in tumors [29,30].

Our group recently developed ^{99m}Tc-cAbVCAM1-5, a radiotracer targeting VCAM-1 which is ongoing clinical transfer for the detection of inflamed atherosclerotic lesions [20,21,31]. The purpose of the present study was to evaluate this new tool for the pre-clinical nuclear imaging of VCAM-1 in TNBC. Two TNBC cell lines were employed, MDA-MB-231 and HCC70. The MDA-MB-231 cell line is highly metastatic whereas few results were available on HCC70. In vitro experiments demonstrated that MDA-MB-231 expressed hVCAM-1 mRNA and protein, and that expression was increased after TNF-α stimulation which is consistent with previous studies [19]. TNF-α is a key activator of VCAM-1 through NF-κB signaling [32]. A bundle of evidences links TNF-α and NF-κB pathway to tumor survival, growth and invasion [33,34]. The results provided by the TCGA showed higher TNF-α expression in TNBC in comparison to Non-TNBC tumors. These results suggest that the TNF-α/VCAM-1 axis is a relevant target in TNBC. As demonstrated by in vitro competition studies, the ^{99m}Tc-cAbVCAM1-5 tracer specifically binds human VCAM-1. Using this imaging agent, subcutaneous MDA-MB-231 tumors were successfully visualized by SPECT/CT imaging, whereas significantly lower signals were found in HCC70 tumors (which do not express hVCAM-1 mRNA and protein) or using the negative irrelevant control sdAb, thereby indicating that the signal was specific and predominantly attributable to tumor cell expressing VCAM-1 rather than murine endothelial or inflammatory cells. These results were in agreement with the level of murine and human VCAM-1 mRNA determined in tumor biopsies by RT-qPCR. Additional studies are however warranted in order to investigate if, similarly to that has been observed in vitro, in vivo hVCAM-1 expression in MDA-MB-231 tumor cells can be increased by TNF-α or other cytokines present in the microenvironment, leading to increased ^{99m}Tc-cAbVCAM1-5 uptake.

Therefore, ^{99m}Tc-cAbVCAM1-5 is a validated tool to investigate the role of VCAM-1 in metastatic processes. However our results support that using VCAM-1 as a tumor inflammatory marker should be carefully considered due to the potential expression of VCAM-1 by tumor cells themselves.

Because of VCAM-1 is aberrantly expressed in BC cells and mediates lung metastasis, ^{99m}Tc-cAbVCAM1-5 imaging was further studied in an experimental lung metastasis model with MDA-MB-231 cells. According to SPECT/CT quantifications, ^{99m}Tc-cAbVCAM1-5 lung uptake was 3-fold higher than that of ^{99m}Tc-Ctl whereas it was found to be 5-fold higher by ex vivo gamma-well counting. This difference can be attributed to the fact that when performing in vivo lung imaging quantification, the volume of interest contains a mixture of tissue and air, thereby leading to underestimation of the uptake.

Autoradiography further confirmed that ^{99m}Tc-cAbVCAM1-5 uptake was localized in metastatic nodules, and RT-qPCR showed that, in the whole lung, hVCAM-1 expression was found to be 3-fold higher than mVCAM-1 indicating that ^{99m}Tc-cAbVCAM1-5 uptake highlights presence of tumor cells rather than inflammatory processes. This result is consistent with a previous study demonstrating VCAM-1 tumor expression rather than endothelial cells one in lung metastasis of BC patients [14]. ^{99m}Tc-cAbVCAM-1 is therefore a validate tool to study the prognostic value of VCAM-1 in the metastatic disease.

Other VCAM-1-targeting radiotracers have been developed. ^{99m}Tc-cAbVCAM1-5 tumor uptake was comparable to that obtained by Scalici et al. using ^{111}In-tVCAM-4, an indium-111 labeled peptide targeting VCAM-1 [30]. Indeed, in an experimental mouse model of metastatic ovarian cancer, ^{111}In-tVCAM-4 uptake in tumor was of ~2% ID/g at 4 h post-injection. Using a ^{68}Ga-labeled Single Chain Variable Fragment, Zhang et al. obtained a ~5% ID/g tumor uptake in a mouse model of melanoma. Nevertheless, due to the fast blood clearance of sdAbs-based imaging agents, ^{99m}Tc-cAbVCAM1-5 tumor-to-blood ratio (5 at 2 h) favorably compared to that of this imaging agent (2 at 3 h) [29].

4. Materials and Methods

4.1. Patients—Online Data

Normalized RNA sequencing (RNA-Seq) data of The Cancer Genome Atlas (TCGA) were downloaded from cBioportal (Breast Invasive Carcinoma—TCGA Provisional; RNA-Seq V2) [35]. Data were available for 980 BC tumor samples (866 Non-TNBC and 114 TNBC). The results published here are based upon data generated by the TCGA Research Network [36,37].

4.2. Cell Lines and Culture Conditions

MDA-MB-231 cells were cultured with Dulbecco's Modified Eagle's Medium supplemented with 10% fetal bovine serum and 1% penicillin-streptomycin. HCC70 cells were cultured using Roswell Park Memorial Institute-1640 medium, supplemented with 10% fetal bovine serum and 1% penicillin-streptomycin.

4.3. RT-qPCR Assay

HCC70 and MDA-MB-231 cells were stimulated or not with Tumor Necrosis Factor-α (TNF-α, 50 ng/mL, Peprotech®, Rocky Hill, NJ, USA) for 18 h. Cell lysis and extraction of total RNA from cell lines were performed using PureLink™ RNA Mini Kit (ThermoFisher Scientific, Illkirch, France) according to the manufacturer's protocol. Reverse transcription (RT) was performed using an iScript Reverse transcription kit (iScript RT supermix; BioRad, Hercules, CA, USA). The reaction mixtures were incubated at 25 °C for 5 min, 46 °C for 20 min, 95 °C for 1 min and held at 4 °C. For the assessment of VCAM-1 expression in xenograft tumors and in metastatic nodules, 20–50 mg of tissue was ground (PureLink™ RNA Mini Kit; ThermoFisher Scientific), and the same protocol as for the in vitro assay was applied. Quantitative Polymerase Chain Reaction (qPCR) was performed on the resulting cDNA with the Fast SYBR Green Master Mix (ThermoFisher Scientific, Illkirch, France), using a Real Time PCR system (Applied Biosystem StepOne Plus; ThermoFisher Scientific). The primer sequences were as follows: human VCAM-1 (hVCAM-1) Forward, 5′-AGTTGAAGGATGCGGGAGTA-3′, Reverse 5′-ACCCCTTCAT GTTGGCTTTTC-3′; murine VCAM-1 (mVCAM-1) Forward, 5′- GCCACCCTCACCTTAATTGC -3′, Reverse 5′- TCAGAACAACCGAATCCCCA-3′. The expression levels of mRNAs were normalized to the endogenous control actin, and were calculated with the formula $2^{-\Delta\Delta CT}$. The primer sequence for actin was as follows: Forward, 5′-CTCCTGAGCGCAAGTACTCC-3′, Reverse 5′-TGTTTTCT GCGCAAGTTAGG-3′.

4.4. Western Blot Assay

HCC70 and MDA-MB-231 cells were treated or not with TNF-α (50 ng/mL) for 18 h. Total proteins were extracted with RIPA buffer. Proteins were separated by 7.5% denaturing SDS-PAGE and transferred onto a nitrocellulose membrane. The membrane was incubated with the anti-VCAM-1 antibody (1/2000; Rabbit anti-VCAM-1, ab134047 Abcam®, Cambridge, UK). As a loading control, the membrane was probed with an anti-β-actin antibody (1/10,000; Beckton Dickinson). Revelation was assessed using the chemiluminescence ECL kit (BioRad). Bands were quantified by densitometry using ImageJ software.

4.5. Flow Cytometry

MDA-MB-231 and HCC70 cells (200.000) treated or not with TNF-α (50 ng/mL) for 18 h were collected and washed with phosphate buffered saline solution (PBS). Cells were incubated with cAbVCAM1-5 (10 µg/mL) and then with an anti-poly histidine antibody (anti-6x His tag antibody, ab9108 Abcam), followed by a AlexaFluor®488-anti-Rabbit-IgG (Goat anti-Rabbit IgG H&L, AlexaFluor®488, ab150077 Abcam). Binding was measured on a FACS Accuri C6 analyzer (BD Biosciences, San Jose, CA, USA). Background fluorescence was determined by measuring the fluorescent signal from cells stained with the irrelevant control sdAb.

4.6. Saturation Binding Experiments and In Vitro Competition Studies

Saturation binding experiments was determined on 96-well plates coated with mouse or human recombinant VCAM-1 protein (100 ng/well; R&D Systems, Minneapolis, MN, USA). Serial diluations of ^{99m}Tc-cAbVCAM1-5 were incubated for 1 h at room temperature before being washed 5 times with PBS-polysorbate 0.1%. The radioactivity in each well was then determined using a γ-counter (Wizard^2; Perkin Elmer, Courtaboeuf, France) and corrected for unspecific binding. Binding curves were fitted using a non linear regression equation (specific binding: $y = B_{max} \times x/(K_D + x)$, with x being the radioligand concentration, K_D being the dissociation constant, and B_{max} being the maximum number of binding sites, or receptor density) (GraphPad Prism, version 6, software, San Diego, CA, USA), to determine K_D values.

For in vitro competition studies, 12,000 HCC70 and MDA-MB-231 cells were coated in 96-well plates (Stripwell™ Plate, Corning®, Corning, NY, USA) in their respective culture medium. After 24 h, cells were treated with 50 ng/mL of TNF-α for 18 h. Then, cells were rinsed with PBS and fixed with paraformaldehyde (PFA) 4% for 10 min. Following 1 h of saturation with PBS-BSA 1%, cells were incubated with 30 nM of ^{99m}Tc-cAbVCAM1-5 in the absence or presence of a 100-fold excess of unlabeled cAbVCAM1-5 at room temperature for 1 h before being washed 5 times with PBS-Tween 0.05%. Bound activity was determined using a gamma-counter (Wizard^2, Perkin Elmer) and results were corrected from nonspecific binding determined on HCC70 cells.

4.7. Tumor Models

All animal procedures conformed to French government guidelines (Articles R214-87 to R214-126; European directive 2010/63/UE). They were performed in an approved facility (C385161 0005) under permit APAFIS#3690-2016011916045217 v4 and APAFIS#8683-2017012611031820 v3 from the French Ministry of Research. To evaluate ^{99m}Tc-cAbVCAM1-5 biodistribution and tumor uptake, 12 female BALB/c nu/nu mice (5 weeks old) were subcutaneously inoculated into the left flank with MDA-MB-231 (3×10^6) and into the right flank with HCC70 (3×10^6), in a 2:1 PBS/Matrigel® (Corning) mixture. The tumors were allowed to grow for 3 weeks to reach ~150–200 mm^3. For the experimental metastasis model, 9 female C.B17 SCID (Severe Combined ImmunoDeficient) mice (5 weeks old) were intravenously injected with MDA-MB-231 cells (1 M in 150 µL) in PBS. Eight weeks later, SPECT/CT imaging and biodistribution studies were performed.

4.8. SPECT/CT Imaging

For the subcutaneous xenograft study, mice were divided in 2 groups: tumor bearing mice injected with (i) the human/mouse cross-reactive sdAb ^{99m}Tc-cAbVCAM1-5 ($n = 6$) or (ii) with the irrelevant control sdAb, ^{99m}Tc-Ctl ($n = 6$). The previously described BcII10a control sdAb was used in this study (20). SPECT/CT acquisitions were performed 1 hour after intravenous injection of 57.6 ± 9.8 MBq of ^{99m}Tc-cAbVCAM1-5 or ^{99m}Tc-Ctl. The cAbVCAM1-5 and control sdAbs were radiolabeled as previously described using the tricarbonyl method [20]. Whole body SPECT/CT acquisitions were performed using a dedicated system (nanoSPECT-CT; Mediso, Budapest, Hungary). For the experimental metastasis study, mice were injected with 61.9 ± 16.2 MBq of ^{99m}Tc-cAbVCAM1-5 ($n = 5$) or the irrelevant ^{99m}Tc-Ctl ($n = 4$). Biodistributions were also performed on healthy mice ($n = 4$). SPECT/CT acquisition was centered on the thoracic region. CT and SPECT acquisitions were reconstructed and fused using Nucline software (Mediso), and SPECT quantification based on CT was performed using VivoQuant^{TM} (InviCRO, Boston, MA, USA). For the xenograft tumor model, a 50 mm^3 sphere was drawn at the center of the tumor on the basis of the CT image. For the metastasis assay, total quantification of pulmonary tracer uptake based on the CT image was performed. ^{99m}Tc-sdAbs activity was expressed as a percentage of the injected dose per cm^3 (% ID/cm^3).

4.9. Post-Mortem Analysis

Two hours after injection and immediately following SPECT/CT image acquisitions, anesthetized mice were euthanized using CO_2 and tumors (either subcutaneous or the whole lungs with metastasis) were harvested along with other organs. Samples were weighed and their radioactivity determined with a γ-counter (Wizard^2, PerkinElmer, Courtaboeuf, France). Results were corrected for decay, injected dose and organ weight and expressed as % ID/g. Subcutaneous tumors were then immediately frozen in −40 °C isopentane, whereas metastatic lungs were inflated with a 1:1 mixture of PBS/Optimal Cutting Temperature prior being frozen. In order to investigate whether the VCAM-1 expression status determined in vitro on HCC70 and MDA-MB-231 cells was preserved in vivo, RT-qPCR was performed on HCC70 and MDA-MB-231 subcutaneous tumor slices and tissue samples. Moreover, due to the fact that ex vivo counting on lung with metastases reflects a mixture of healthy tissue and tumor uptake, lung autoradiography was performed to precisely evaluate the tumor uptake. To that purpose, 20 µm-thick lung slices, together with reference organs of known activities, were exposed overnight on an autoradiographic film which was then scanned using a phosphoimager (Fujifilm BAS-5000, FUJIFILM, Montigny, France). Slices were then stained with hematoxylin-eosin and regions of interest were delineated on tumor nodules, thereby allowing the quantification of ^{99m}Tc-cAbVCAM1-5 or ^{99m}Tc-Ctl uptake as a percentage of injected dose per gram (% ID/g).

4.10. Statistics

For the in vitro and mice experiments: Data were expressed as mean ± standard deviation and analyzed using an unpaired Mann Whitney test for inter group analysis. Significance of linear correlations was assessed with a Pearson's test. p values < 0.05 were considered significant. Data were analyzed with Prism 7.0 (GraphPad Software).

For patients: The Student's t-test was used to compare continuous variables. Overall survival (OS) was defined as the time between surgery and the date of death from any cause. The Kaplan-Meier method was used to produce survival curves and analyses of censored data were performed using Cox models. Data were analyzed with Prism 7.0 (GraphPad Software).

5. Conclusions

In the two mouse models of TNBC, SPECT imaging of VCAM-1 was successfully performed and the signal originated from the tumor was found to reflect hVCAM-1 expression by cancer cells rather than mVCAM-1 expression by the tumor stroma. ^{99m}Tc-cAbVCAM1-5 can therefore be used as a preclinical tool to evaluate the role of VCAM-1 expression by tumor cells in tumor development and metastasis. In clinical practice, VCAM-1 expression has been reported to be correlated with poorer outcome in TNBC but also in other cancer type such as glioblastoma and ovarian cancer, and VCAM-1 imaging has been proposed as a tool for the assessment of tumor aggressiveness. Further studies will however be necessary to evaluate the prognostic value of ^{99m}Tc-cAbVCAM1-5 tumor imaging in clinical practice.

Supplementary Materials: The following are available online at http://www.mdpi.com/2072-6694/11/7/1039/s1, Figure S1: MDA-MB-231 cells overexpress VCAM-1 protein upon TNF-α. Table S1: Biodistribution of 99mTc-cAbVCAM1-5 in athymic nude mice bearing HCC70 and MDA-MB-231 xenografts. Figure S2: cAbVCAM1-5 binds to MDA-MB-231 but not to HCC70 cells. Figure S3: Affinity of 99mTc-cAbVCAM1-5 for mVCAM-1 and hVCAM-1. Figure S4: Representative Maximum Intensity Projection views of fused SPECT/CT images of HCC70 and MDA-MB-231 tumor-bearing mice 1h after i.v injection of 99mTc-cAbVCAM1-5 or 99mTc-Ctl. Figure S5: Correlation between tumor uptake as determined by SPECT image quantification and by ex vivo biodistribution studies. Figure S6: Representative Maximal Intensity (MIP) of fused SPECT/CT views of MDA-MB-231 lung metastases at 1h after i.v injection of 99mTc-cAbVCAM1-5 of 99mTc-Ctl. One lung-metastases free mouse wal also injected with 99mTc-cAbVCAM1-5. Figure S7: Ex vivo quantification of 99mTc-cAbVCAM1-5 in SCID mice bearing MDA-MB-231 lung metastasis.

Author Contributions: Conceptualization, C.M., A.B., C.G., D.F; methodology, C.M., P.C., A.B., C.G., D.F; formal analysis, C.M., L.D., P.C., M.A., S.B., M.D., A.S., L.D., J.L., N.L., M.D., G.P., S.H., N.D., P.P., L.R., A.B., C.G., D.F; investigation, C.M., L.D., P.C., M.A., S.B., M.D., A.S., L.D., J.L., N.L., M.D., G.P., S.H., N.D., P.P., L.R; resources, C.M., L.D., P.C., M.A., S.B., M.D., A.S., L.D., J.L., N.L., M.D., G.P., A.B., C.G., D.F.; writing—original draft preparation, C.M, A.B., C.G; writing—review and editing, C.M., L.D., P.C., M.A., S.B., M.D., A.S., L.D., J.L., N.L., M.D., G.P., S.H., N.D., P.P., L.R., A.B., C.G., D.F.; visualization, C.M., A.B., C.G., D.F; supervision, A.B, D.F., C.G.; funding acquisition, A.B., C.G., D.F.

Funding: This research received no external funding.

Acknowledgments: This work was partly funded by France Life Imaging, grant "ANR-11-INBS-0006".

Conflicts of Interest: The authors declare no conflict of interest.

References

1. Ferlay, J.; Steliarova-Foucher, E.; Lortet-Tieulent, J.; Rosso, S.; Coebergh, J.W.W.; Comber, H.; Forman, D.; Bray, F. Cancer incidence and mortality patterns in Europe: Estimates for 40 countries in 2012. *Eur. J. Cancer* **2013**, *49*, 1374–1403. [CrossRef] [PubMed]
2. Perou, C.M.; Sorlie, T.B.; Eisen, C.; Van De Rijn, M.; Jeffrey, S.S.; Rees, C.A.; Pollack, J.R.; Ross, D.T.; Johnsen, H.; Akslen, L.A.; et al. Molecular portraits of human breast tumours. *Nature* **2000**, *747–752*. [CrossRef] [PubMed]
3. Sorlie, T.; Tibshirani, R.; Parker, J.; Hastie, T.; Marron, J.S.; Nobel, A.; Deng, S.; Johnsen, H.; Pesich, R.; Geisler, S.; et al. Repeated observation of breast tumor subtypes in independent gene expression data sets. *Proc. Natl. Acad. Sci. USA* **2003**, *100*, 8418–8423. [CrossRef] [PubMed]

4. Reis-Filho, J.S.; Tutt, A.N.J. Triple negative tumours: A critical review: Triple negative tumours. *Histopathology* **2007**, *52*, 108–118. [CrossRef] [PubMed]
5. Dent, R.; Trudeau, M.; Pritchard, K.I.; Hanna, W.M.; Kahn, H.K.; Sawka, C.A.; Lickley, L.A.; Rawlinson, E.; Sun, P.; Narod, S.A. Triple-Negative Breast Cancer: Clinical Features and Patterns of Recurrence. *Clin. Cancer Res.* **2007**, *13*, 4429–4434. [CrossRef] [PubMed]
6. Haffty, B.G.; Yang, Q.; Reiss, M.; Kearney, T.; Higgins, S.A.; Weidhaas, J.; Harris, L.; Hait, W.; Toppmeyer, D. Locoregional Relapse and Distant Metastasis in Conservatively Managed Triple Negative Early-Stage Breast Cancer. *J. Clin. Oncol.* **2006**, *24*, 5652–5657. [CrossRef] [PubMed]
7. Lorusso, G.; Rüegg, C. New insights into the mechanisms of organ-specific breast cancer metastasis. *Semin. Cancer Biol.* **2012**, *22*, 226–233. [CrossRef]
8. Minn, A.J.; Gupta, G.P.; Siegel, P.M.; Bos, P.D.; Shu, W.; Giri, D.D.; Viale, A.; Olshen, A.B.; Gerald, W.L.; Massagué, J. Genes that mediate breast cancer metastasis to lung. *Nature* **2005**, *436*, 518. [CrossRef]
9. Chen, Q.; Massague, J. Molecular Pathways: VCAM-1 as a Potential Therapeutic Target in Metastasis. *Clin. Cancer Res.* **2012**, *18*, 5520–5525. [CrossRef]
10. Cook-Mills, J.M.; Marchese, M.E.; Abdala-Valencia, H. Vascular cell adhesion molecule-1 expression and signaling during disease: Regulation by reactive oxygen species and antioxidants. *Antioxid. Redox Signal.* **2011**, *15*, 1607–1638. [CrossRef]
11. Schlesinger, M.; Bendas, G. Vascular cell adhesion molecule-1 (VCAM-1)-An increasing insight into its role in tumorigenicity and metastasis: VCAM-1 in tumorigenicity. *Int. J. Cancer* **2015**, *136*, 2504–2514. [CrossRef] [PubMed]
12. Maimaiti, Y.; Wang, C.; Mushajiang, M.; Tan, J.; Huang, B.; Zhou, J.; Huang, T. Overexpression of VCAM-1 is correlated with poor survival of patients with breast cancer. *Int. J. Clin. Exp. Pathol.* **2016**, *9*, 7451–7457.
13. Lu, X.; Mu, E.; Wei, Y.; Riethdorf, S.; Yang, Q.; Yuan, M.; Yan, J.; Hua, Y.; Tiede, B.J.; Lu, X.; et al. VCAM-1 Promotes Osteolytic Expansion of Indolent Bone Micrometastasis of Breast Cancer by Engaging α4β1-Positive Osteoclast Progenitors. *Cancer Cell* **2011**, *20*, 701–714. [CrossRef] [PubMed]
14. Chen, Q.; Zhang, X.H.-F.; Massagué, J. Macrophage Binding to Receptor VCAM-1 Transmits Survival Signals in Breast Cancer Cells that Invade the Lungs. *Cancer Cell* **2011**, *20*, 538–549. [CrossRef] [PubMed]
15. Kang, Y. Dissecting Tumor-Stromal Interactions in Breast Cancer Bone Metastasis. *Endocrinol. Metab.* **2016**, *31*, 206. [CrossRef] [PubMed]
16. Cao, H.; Zhang, Z.; Zhao, S.; He, X.; Yu, H.; Yin, Q.; Zhang, Z.; Gu, W.; Chen, L.; Li, Y. Hydrophobic interaction mediating self-assembled nanoparticles of succinobucol suppress lung metastasis of breast cancer by inhibition of VCAM-1 expression. *J. Control. Release* **2015**, *205*, 162–171. [CrossRef] [PubMed]
17. Wu, T.-C. The Role of Vascular Cell Adhesion Molecule-1 in Tumor Immune Evasion. *Cancer Res.* **2007**, *67*, 6003–6006. [CrossRef] [PubMed]
18. Lin, K.-Y.; Lu, D.; Hung, C.-F.; Peng, S.; Huang, L.; Jie, C.; Murillo, F.; Rowley, J.; Tsai, Y.-C.; He, L.; et al. Ectopic Expression of Vascular Cell Adhesion Molecule-1 as a New Mechanism for Tumor Immune Evasion. *Cancer Res.* **2007**, *67*, 1832–1841. [CrossRef]
19. Wang, P.-C.; Weng, C.-C.; Hou, Y.-S.; Jian, S.-F.; Fang, K.-T.; Hou, M.-F.; Cheng, K.-H. Activation of VCAM-1 and Its Associated Molecule CD44 Leads to Increased Malignant Potential of Breast Cancer Cells. *Int. J. Mol. Sci.* **2014**, *15*, 3560–3579. [CrossRef]
20. Broisat, A.; Hernot, S.; Toczek, J.; De Vos, J.; Riou, L.M.; Martin, S.; Ahmadi, M.; Thielens, N.; Wernery, U.; Caveliers, V.; et al. Nanobodies Targeting Mouse/Human VCAM1 for the Nuclear Imaging of Atherosclerotic Lesions. *Circ. Res.* **2012**, *30*, 927–937. [CrossRef]
21. Dumas, L.S.; Briand, F.; Clerc, R.; Brousseau, E.; Montemagno, C.; Ahmadi, M.; Bacot, S.; Soubies, A.; Perret, P.; Riou, L.M.; et al. Evaluation of Antiatherogenic Properties of Ezetimibe Using ^{3}H-Labeled Low-Density-Lipoprotein Cholesterol and ^{99m}Tc-cAbVCAM1–5 SPECT in ApoE$^{-/-}$ Mice Fed the Paigen Diet. *J. Nucl. Med.* **2017**, *58*, 1088–1093. [CrossRef] [PubMed]
22. Mariotto, A.B.; Etzioni, R.; Hurlbert, M.; Penberthy, L.; Mayer, M. Estimation of the Number of Women Living with Metastatic Breast Cancer in the United States. *Cancer Epidemiol. Biomark. Prev.* **2017**, *26*, 809–815. [CrossRef] [PubMed]
23. Group EBCTC. Effects of chemotherapy and hormonal therapy for early breast cancer on recurrence and 15-year survival: An overview of the randomised trials. *Lancet* **2005**, *365*, 1687–1717. [CrossRef]

24. Eckhardt, B.L.; Francis, P.A.; Parker, B.S.; Anderson, R.L. Strategies for the discovery and development of therapies for metastatic breast cancer. *Nat. Rev. Drug Discov.* **2012**, *11*, 479–497. [CrossRef] [PubMed]
25. Sharma, R.; Sharma, R.; Khaket, T.P.; Dutta, C.; Chakraborty, B.; Mukherjee, T.K. Breast cancer metastasis: Putative therapeutic role of vascular cell adhesion molecule-1. *Cell Oncol.* **2017**, *40*, 199–208. [CrossRef] [PubMed]
26. Ding, Y.-B.; Chen, G.-Y.; Xia, J.-G.; Zang, X.-W.; Yang, H.-Y.; Yang, L. Association of VCAM-1 overexpression with oncogenesis, tumor angiogenesis and metastasis of gastric carcinoma. *World J. Gastroenterol.* **2003**, *9*, 1409. [CrossRef] [PubMed]
27. Liu, Y.-S.; Lin, H.-Y.; Lai, S.-W.; Huang, C.-Y.; Huang, B.-R.; Chen, P.-Y.; Wei, K.-C.; Lu, D.-Y. MiR-181b modulates EGFR-dependent VCAM-1 expression and monocyte adhesion in glioblastoma. *Oncogene* **2017**, *36*, 5006–5022. [CrossRef]
28. Huang, J.; Zhang, J.; Li, H.; Lu, Z.; Shan, W.; Mercado-Uribe, I.; Liu, J. VCAM1 expression correlated with tumorigenesis and poor prognosis in high grade serous ovarian cancer. *Am. J. Transl. Res.* **2013**, *5*, 336.
29. Zhang, X.; Liu, C.; Hu, F.; Zhang, Y.; Wang, J.; Gao, Y.; Jiang, Y.; Zhang, Y.; Lan, X. PET Imaging of VCAM-1 Expression and Monitoring Therapy Response in Tumor with a ^{68}Ga-Labeled Single Chain Variable Fragment. *Mol. Pharm.* **2018**, *15*, 609–618. [CrossRef]
30. Scalici, J.M.; Thomas, S.; Harrer, C.; Raines, T.A.; Curran, J.; Atkins, K.A.; Conaway, M.R.; Duska, L.; Kelly, K.A.; Slack-Davis, J.K. Imaging VCAM-1 as an Indicator of Treatment Efficacy in Metastatic Ovarian Cancer. *J. Nucl. Med.* **2013**, *54*, 1883–1889. [CrossRef]
31. Broisat, A.; Toczek, J.; Dumas, L.S.; Ahmadi, M.; Bacot, S.; Perret, P.; Slimani, L.; Barone-Rochette, G.; Soubies, A.; Devoogdt, N.; et al. 99mTc-cAbVCAM1-5 Imaging Is a Sensitive and Reproducible Tool for the Detection of Inflamed Atherosclerotic Lesions in Mice. *J. Nucl. Med.* **2014**, *55*, 1678–1684. [CrossRef] [PubMed]
32. Rajan, S.; Ye, J.; Bai, S.; Huang, F.; Guo, Y.-L. NF-κB, but not p38 MAP Kinase, is required for TNF-α-induced expression of cell adhesion molecules in endothelial cells. *J. Cell. Biochem.* **2008**, *105*, 477–486. [CrossRef] [PubMed]
33. Li, B.; Vincent, A.; Cates, J.; Brantley-Sieders, D.M.; Polk, D.B.; Young, P.P. Low Levels of Tumor Necrosis Factor Increase Tumor Growth by Inducing an Endothelial Phenotype of Monocytes Recruited to the Tumor Site. *Cancer Res.* **2009**, *69*, 338–348. [CrossRef] [PubMed]
34. Cai, X.; Cao, C.; Li, J.; Chen, F.; Zhang, S.; Liu, B.; Zhang, W.; Zhang, X.; Ye, L. Inflammatory factor TNF-alpha promotes the growth of breast cancer via the positive feedback loop of TNFR1/NF-κB (and/or p38)/p-STAT3/HBXIP/TNFR1. *Oncotarget* **2017**, *8*, 58338–58352. [PubMed]
35. The cBioPortal for Cancer Genomics. Available online: https://www.cbioportal.org/study/summary?id=brca_tcga (accessed on 19 July 2019).
36. Cerami, E.; Gao, J.; Dogrusoz, U.; Gross, B.E.; Sumer, S.O.; Aksoy, B.A.; Jacobsen, A.; Byrne, C.J.; Heuer, M.L.; Larsson, E.; et al. The *cBio Cancer* Genomics Portal: An Open Platform for Exploring Multidimensional Cancer Genomics Data: Figure 1. *Cancer Discov.* **2012**, *2*, 401–404. [CrossRef] [PubMed]
37. Gao, J.; Aksoy, B.A.; Dogrusoz, U.; Dresdner, G.; Gross, B.; Sumer, S.O.; Sun, Y.; Jacobsen, A.; Sinha, R.; Larsson, E.; et al. Integrative Analysis of Complex Cancer Genomics and Clinical Profiles Using the cBioPortal. *Sci. Signal.* **2013**, *6*, pl1. [CrossRef]

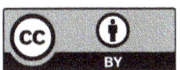

© 2019 by the authors. Licensee MDPI, Basel, Switzerland. This article is an open access article distributed under the terms and conditions of the Creative Commons Attribution (CC BY) license (http://creativecommons.org/licenses/by/4.0/).

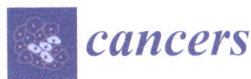

Article

Circulating miRNAs in Untreated Breast Cancer: An Exploratory Multimodality Morpho-Functional Study

Mariarosaria Incoronato [1,*], Anna Maria Grimaldi [1], Peppino Mirabelli [1], Carlo Cavaliere [1], Chiara Anna Parente [1], Monica Franzese [1], Stefania Staibano [2], Gennaro Ilardi [2], Daniela Russo [2], Andrea Soricelli [1,3], Onofrio Antonio Catalano [4,*] and Marco Salvatore [1]

1. IRCCS SDN, 80143 Naples, Italy; agrimaldi@sdn-napoli.it (A.M.G.); pmirabelli@sdn-napoli.it (P.M.); ccavaliere@sdn-napoli.it (C.C.); caparente@sdn-napoli.it (C.A.P.); mfranzese@sdn-napoli.it (M.F.); soricelli@uniparthenope.it (A.S.); direzionescientifica@sdn-napoli.it (M.S.)
2. Department of Advanced Biomedical Sciences, Federico II University, 80131 Naples, Italy; staibano@unina.it (S.S.); gennaro.ilardi@gmail.com (G.I.); danielarusso83@yahoo.it (D.R.)
3. Department of Motor Sciences & Wellness, University of Naples Parthenope, 80133 Naples, Italy
4. Department of Radiology, Athinoula A. Martinos Center for Biomedical Imaging, Massachusetts General Hospital, Harvard Medical School, Charlestown, MA 02129, USA
* Correspondence: mincoronato@sdn-napoli.it (M.I.); onofriocatalano@yahoo.it (O.A.C.)

Received: 24 May 2019; Accepted: 20 June 2019; Published: 22 June 2019

Abstract: The aim of this study was to identify new disease-related circulating miRNAs with high diagnostic accuracy for breast cancer (BC) and to correlate their deregulation with the morpho-functional characteristics of the tumour, as assessed in vivo by positron emission tomography/magnetic resonance (PET/MR) imaging. A total of 77 untreated female BC patients underwent same-day PET/MR and blood collection, and 78 healthy donors were recruited as negative controls. The expression profile of 84 human miRNAs was screened by using miRNA PCR arrays and validated by real-time PCR. The validated miRNAs were correlated with the quantitative imaging parameters extracted from the primary BC samples. Circulating miR-125b-5p and miR-143-3p were upregulated in BC plasma and able to discriminate BC patients from healthy subjects (miR-125-5p area under the receiver operating characteristic ROC curve (AUC) = 0.85 and miR-143-3p AUC = 0.80). Circulating CA15-3, a soluble form of the transmembrane glycoprotein Mucin 1 (MUC-1) that is upregulated in epithelial cancer cells of different origins, was combined with miR-125b-5p and improved the diagnostic accuracy from 70% (CA15-3 alone) to 89% (CA15-3 plus miR-125b-5p). MiR-143-3p showed a strong and significant correlation with the stage of the disease, apparent diffusion coefficient (ADC_{mean}), reverse efflux volume transfer constant (Kep_{mean}) and maximum standardized uptake value (SUV_{max}), and it might represent a biomarker of tumour aggressiveness. Similarly, miR-125b-5p was correlated with stage and grade 2 but inversely correlated with the forward volume transfer constant ($Ktrans_{mean}$) and proliferation index (Ki67), suggesting a potential role as a biomarker of a relatively more favourable prognosis. In situ hybridization (ISH) experiments revealed that miR-143-3p was expressed in endothelial tumour cells, miR-125-5p in cancer-associated fibroblasts, and neither in epithelial tumour cells. Our results suggested that miR-125-5p and miR-143-3p are potential biomarkers for the risk stratification of BC, and Kaplan-Maier plots confirmed this hypothesis. In addition, the combined use of miR-125-b-5p and CA15-3 enhanced the diagnostic accuracy up to 89%. This is the first study that correlates circulating miRNAs with in vivo quantified tumour biology through PET/MR biomarkers. This integration elucidates the link between the plasmatic increase in these two potential circulating biomarkers and the biology of untreated BC. In conclusion, while miR-143-3b and miR-125b-5p provide valuable information for prognosis, a combination of miR-125b-5p with the tumour marker CA15-3 improves sensitivity for BC detection, which warrants consideration by further validation studies.

Keywords: circulating miRNAs; breast cancer; imaging parameters; PET/MRI; biomarkers

1. Introduction

According to GLOBOCAN 2018, a project of the International Agency for Research on Cancer (IARC), approximately 2.1 million women (1.7 million in 2012) were diagnosed with breast cancer (BC) worldwide, and there were approximately 6.9 million women (6.3 million in 2012) who had been diagnosed with BC in the previous five years [1]. BC is also the most common cause of cancer death among women, with 627,000 deaths in 2018. Early diagnosis plays a major role in fighting BC. However, on a worldwide scale, breast imaging techniques such as screening mammography and ultrasound have intrinsic limitations related to economic costs, limited technology availability in underdeveloped countries, the necessity of well-trained radiologists, and an overall unsatisfactory performance regarding the images. Screening mammography performance indexes vary considerably for sensitivity and specificity, influencing the ability of mammography to reach its full potential for decreasing BC mortality [2]; moreover, ultrasound plus mammography can indicate cancers in high-risk women, but the number of false positives are increased [3].

Circulating biomarkers are biomolecules released into the bloodstream by both tumour cells and other types of neighbouring cells [4]. Their quantification and identification are considered an economical, non-invasive diagnostic method that provides information on the presence and/or absence of the disease as well as its evolution. To date, the carcinoembryonic antigen (CEA) [5] and the soluble form of Mucin 1 (MUC-1) protein (CA15-3) [6] are the most commonly used serum biomarkers for the clinical monitoring of BC patients. Although these biomarkers have been recognized from the international healthcare system as molecules used for the management of BC patients, current guidelines suggest that they fail in the early diagnosis of the disease, having a clinical role only during follow-up [7]. Therefore, there is a compelling need to discover potential biomarkers that might be useful for diagnosing BC. The ideal tumour marker should have high specificity, sensitivity and predictive value and be detectable by an accurate, rapid, simple and inexpensive method that might also be used in countries with less access to expensive technology. In recent decades, non-coding RNA molecules (miRNAs) have emerged as a new class of regulatory genes involved in many cellular processes, such as development, differentiation, proliferation, apoptosis and the response to stress. In their mature form, these single-stranded small molecules are 19 to 25 nucleotides in length and are able to silence gene expression at the post-transcriptional level, thus inhibiting protein translation. They act by recognizing a sequence within the 3' and/or 5' untranslated region (UTR) of their mRNA target [8]. miRNAs can exert their action in cancers through both tumour suppression and oncogenic mechanisms [9,10]. Due to their structural characteristics, functions and tissue specificity, miRNAs have been proposed as a new class of biomarkers for the screening of different tumours. Recent discoveries have shown that miRNAs are also present in biological fluids, such as blood [11], urine [12], sputum [13] and saliva [14]; moreover, they were found to be aberrantly expressed in different human cancers and feature unprecedented levels of diagnostic specificity and sensitivity that are associated with tumour burden and malignant progression [15,16]. Additionally, circulating miRNAs are extremely stable against degradation by RNase, easily collected through non-invasive methods (blood sampling), resistant to repeated freeze/thaw cycles and easily identified by nucleic acid amplification techniques (real-time PCR). These factors also make their collection possible in third-world countries and underserved areas. Taken together, these findings highlight the potential usefulness of these molecules as promising biomarkers. To date, many studies have identified different circulating miRNAs as new biomarkers for BC detection; however, the results are discordant [17]. Moreover, they have not been assessed in conjunction with diagnostic imaging, which is used for quantifying the extent of the disease and provides information related to tumour aggressiveness representing an obligatory step for treatment planning. The use of diagnostic imaging to extract quantitative parameters related to the morphology, metabolism and functionality of tumours, as well as to correlate specific imaging parameters with tissue biomarkers, is an emerging research topic [18,19]. The aim of our study was to identify potential new disease-related circulating miRNAs with high diagnostic accuracy for BC and to elucidate the relationship between their circulating deregulation and tumour characteristics, including stage at presentation and the functional quantification of tumour metabolism and perfusion, by using same-day positron emission tomography/magnetic resonance (PET/MR) imaging. Since PET/MR scanners have been approved for use less than 8 years ago, with very few installed worldwide, PET/MR is currently clinically used for BC diagnosis and treatment planning in only an extremely limited number of highly specialized centres that have both the expertise of scanner use and a strong oncologic breast programme. In these centres, PET/MR is used for the whole-body and local staging of newly diagnosed BC cases that are amenable to curative resection, either without or after neoadjuvant treatments, and as problem-solving technology in complicated, more advanced cases. PET/MR is currently not mentioned in the National Comprehensive Cancer Network (NCCN) guidelines or in any other scientific organization/society guidelines despite its higher performances than those of any other non-invasive imaging modality. In fact, the accuracy of PET/MR staging outperformed that of PET/computed tomography (CT) (the most accurate of the routinely clinically approved imaging modalities) on a per patient analysis (98% versus 75%) and was also capable of demonstrating bony metastases not detected by same-day PET/CT in up to 12% of the cases [20,21]. These results have been confirmed by other authors who showed that, in a lesion-per-lesion analysis, PET/MR had higher sensitivity than PET/CT in detecting bony lesions (0.924 and 0.6923, respectively). Moreover, PET/MR also had a better sensitivity than PET/CT in detecting contralateral tumours (1 and 0.25, respectively) and all lesions together (0.89 and 0.77, respectively) [22]. To the best of our knowledge, this is the first study that aimed to correlate the deregulated expression of disease-related circulating miRNAs with the morphological, metabolic and functional parameters of BC lesions (tumour metabolism, cellular density and vascularisation) extracted through a hybrid PET/MR scanner. The plasma samples of BC patients and healthy donors were analysed for miRNA expression, and for each BC patient, PET/MR was used to ascertain the stage of the disease as well as the metabolic, diffusion and perfusion characteristics of the primary cancer. In silico studies and in situ hybridization (ISH) experiments were also performed to better understand miRNA expression in tissue and their cellular localization. Last, we correlated the expression levels of the validated miRNAs with immunohistochemical markers of BC, stage of disease and PET/MR-derived functional and metabolic biomarkers of primary cancer.

2. Results

2.1. Identification and Validation of a Plasma miRNA Signature for Breast Cancer Detection

The study design is illustrated in Figure 1A. The healthy and BC subjects were age-matched (p-value = 0.157), and the clinicopathological characteristics of the study participants are reported in Table 1. By using the miScript miRNA PCR Array, we found that five (miR-125b-5p, miR-143-3p, miR-145-5p, miR-100-5p and miR-23a-3p; Figure 1B–D) out of the 84 miRNAs analysed were significantly (p-value < 0.05) upregulated in the plasma samples of 27 BC patients vs. 14 healthy donors, with a fold change ≥1.5. RT-PCR was conducted to confirm the array results in a study population of 46 healthy donors and 64 naïve BC patients (Supplementary Figure S1). Then, a logistic regression model (Supplementary Table S1A) identified miR-125b-5p and miR-143-3p as the circulating miRNAs able to effectively discriminate affected from unaffected subjects. A logistic stepwise regression model confirmed these results (Supplementary Table S1B). Moreover, the results were corroborated by expanding the case studies to 78 healthy donors and 77 naïve BC patients (Figure 1A, Validation II). In fact, as shown in Figure 2A,B, we confirmed that miR-125b-5p and miR-143-3p were significantly upregulated in the plasma of BC patients with a fold change of 3.3 and 3.2, respectively. These results were confirmed by logistic stepwise regression analysis (Figure 2C).

Table 1. Detailed clinicopathological characteristics of the study participants.

Healthy Control Samples ($n = 78$)	
Age range	28–84 years
Mean ± S.D.	51.05 ± 11.26
Breast Cancer Samples ($n = 77$)	
Age range	28–82 years
Mean ± S.D.	53.68 ± 12.02
Subtype	
Luminal A	16
Luminal B	50
HER2+	7
Triple negative	4
Ki67	
Low (1–20%)	21
High (21–100%)	56
Grade	
G1	1
G2	41
G3	35
Stage	
Stage I	1
Stage II	12
Stage III	42
Stage IV	22

S.D.: standard deviation; HER2+: Human epidermal growth factor receptor positive.

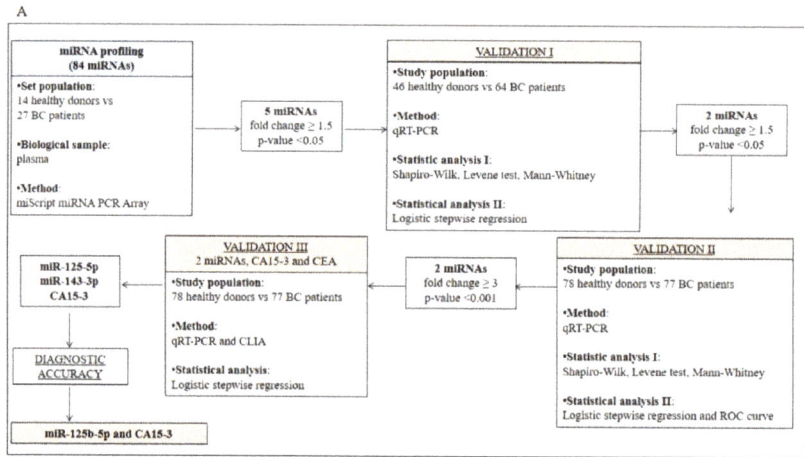

Figure 1. *Cont.*

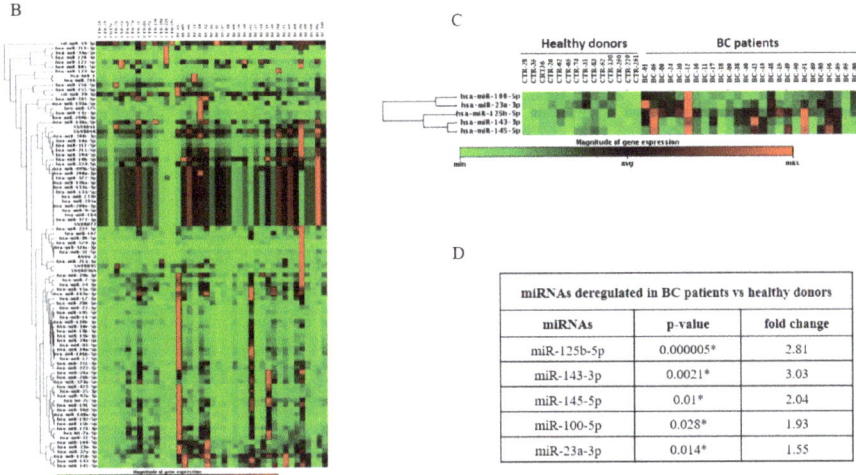

Figure 1. Study design for the identification of circulating miRNAs and protein biomarkers able to discriminate breast cancer (BC) patients from healthy donors (**A**). miRNA expression analysis in a set population of 14 healthy donors (CTR) and 27 BC subjects. Expression analysis of 84 miRNAs by using a 96-well miScript miRNA PCR Array (**B**). * miRNAs significantly upregulated ($p < 0.05$) in BC patients vs. healthy donors (**C,D**).

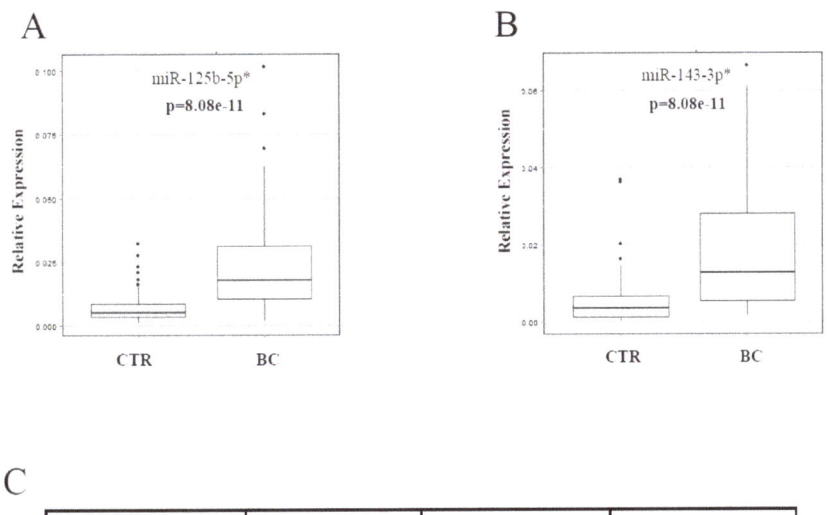

Figure 2. Validation II. Relative expression of miRNAs selected in a study population of 78 healthy donors (CTR) and 77 breast cancer (BC) subjects. Box plot analyses performed to show the relative expression of miR-125b-5p (**A**) and miR-143-3p (**B**) in the plasma samples of healthy donors vs. BC patients. Logistic stepwise regression analysis (**C**). * miRNAs that significantly ($p < 0.05$) estimate the probability of having BC.

2.2. Diagnostic miRNA Signature-Based Model Compared with Established BC Markers

Receiver operating characteristic (ROC) curve analyses showed that miR-125b-5p (area under the ROC curve (AUC) = 0.85) and miR-143-3p (AUC = 0.80) were able to discriminate BC patients from healthy donors (Figure 3A,B). Then, we compared the AUC value of the selected miRNAs with the AUC value of the traditional BC biomarkers CA15-3 and CEA. As reported in Figure 3C,D, the AUC values of CA15-3 (0.70) and CEA (0.68) were lower than those calculated for miR-125b-5p and miR-143-3p. Based on these results, a logistic stepwise regression analysis was performed considering the miR-125b-5p, miR-143-3p, CA15-3 and CEA molecules as independent variables (Figure 1A, Validation III). According to Table 2, miR-125b-5p, miR-143-3p and CA15-3 were significantly correlated with the disease, although the statistical significance of CA15-3 was lower than that of the miRNAs. Based on these findings, the diagnostic accuracy of each biomarker was evaluated. To this end, the cut-off values of miR-125b-5p and miR-143-3p were calculated, and the clinical cut-off values of CA15-3 and CEA were already known (CA15-3 = 35 UI/mL and CEA = 3 UI/mL). Using the "closest to top-left" method, we defined the cut-off value of miR-125b-5p as 0.0090 and that of miR-143-3p as 0.0064, both related to relative expression. Among the analysed molecules, miR-125b-5p showed the highest diagnostic accuracy (Table 3).

Table 2. Validation III. Logistic stepwise regression on the indicated molecules in a cohort of 78 CTR and 77 BC subjects. * Molecules that significantly ($p < 0.05$) estimate the probability of having a tumour.

Circulating Biomarkers	Estimate	Std. Error	p-Value
miR-125b-5p *	9.018	2.401	0.000248
miR-143-3p *	1.017×10^1	2.644	0.000179
CA15-3 *	2.123×10^{-3}	8.984×10^{-4}	0.01941
CEA	4.866×10^{-3}	7.095×10^{-3}	0.4939

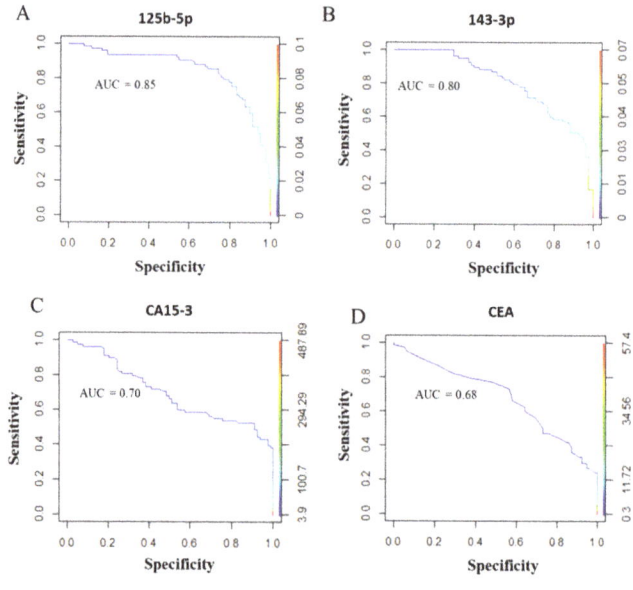

Figure 3. ROC curve analyses and AUC values of miR-125-5p (**A**), miR-143-3p (**B**), CA15-3 (**C**), and CEA (**D**) for discriminating BC patients from healthy controls in 76 BC patients and 78 healthy donors. ROC: Receiver operating characteristic; AUC: area under the ROC curve; CEA: carcinoembryonic antigen.

Table 3. Diagnostic accuracy of the indicated circulating biomarkers.

miR-125b-5p	Disease +	Disease −	Total	Sensitivity	Specificity	Diagnostic Accuracy
Test +	61 (TP)	16 (FP)	77	0.79	0.79	0.79
Test −	16 (FN)	62 (TN)	78	(CI 0.68–0.88)	(CI 0.69–0.88)	(CI 0.72–0.85)
Total	77	78	155			
miR-143-3p	**Disease +**	**Disease −**	**Total**	**Sensitivity**	**Specificity**	**Diagnostic accuracy**
Test +	53 (TP)	20 (FP)	73	0.69	0.74	0.72
Test −	24 (FN)	58 (TN)	82	(CI 0.57–0.79)	(CI 0.63–0.84)	(CI 0.64–0.79)
Total	77	78	155			
CA15-3	**Disease +**	**Disease −**	**Total**	**Sensitivity**	**Specificity**	**Diagnostic accuracy**
Test +	29 (TP)	1 (FP)	30	0.38	0.99	0.68
Test −	47 (FN)	75 (TN)	122	(CI 0.27–0.50)	(CI 0.93–1.00)	(CI 0.60–0.76)
Total	76	76	152			
CEA	**Disease +**	**Disease −**	**Total**	**Sensitivity**	**Specificity**	**Diagnostic accuracy**
Test +	25 (TP)	8 (FP)	73	0.33	0.89	0.61
Test −	51 (FN)	68 (TN)	82	(CI 0.23–0.45)	(CI 0.80–0.95)	(CI 0.53–0.69)
Total	76	76	152			

CI: confidence interval 95%; Disease +: BC patients, Disease −: healthy donors, TP: True Positive TP, FP: False Positive, FN: False Negative and TN: True Negative. CEA: carcinoembryonic antigen and BC: breast cancer.

2.3. Co-Expression Analysis of Circulating miR-125b-5p, miR-143-3p and miR-145-5p and Their Association with Immunohistochemical Markers of BC

Although miR-145-5p was not able to estimate the probability of pathology (Supplementary Table S1), it is transcribed from a putative miR-143/145 cluster on chromosome 5 in humans (5q33). Therefore, co-expression analyses by Spearman's test were performed not only for miR-125b-5p and miR-143-3p but also for miR-145-5p. As reported in Figure 4A, we found that miR-143-3p and miR-145-5p were strongly co-expressed (ρ: 0.93; p-value $< 2 \times 10^{-16}$) in the plasma samples of BC patients, and the expression levels of miR-125b-5p were significantly correlated with those of miR-143-3p (ρ: 0.57; p-value $= 2 \times 10^{-4}$) and miR-145-5p (ρ: 0.56; p-value $= 6 \times 10^{-6}$), although to a limited extent.

The immunohistochemical (IHC) reports of the enrolled BC patients were used to determine the receptor status (oestrogen, progesterone, and human epidermal growth factor receptor 2), cellular differentiation status (grade) and proliferation index (Ki67) of the tumour lesions. No association was found between the expression levels of miR-125-5p, miR-143-3p and miR-145-5p and the hormonal receptor status of the lesions (Estrogen Receptor positive or negative: ER+/−, Progesteron receptor positive or negative: PR +/− and Human epidermal growth factor receptor positive or negative: HER2 +/−; Supplementary Table S2) or with tumour subtypes (all p-values > 0.05). Nevertheless, only miR-125b-5p was significantly associated with the Ki67 proliferation index (Figure 4B, p-value = 0.038) and the differentiation status of tumour cells (Figure 4C, p-value = 0.003). Specifically, we found that in the presence of a low Ki67 index and a low grade, the expression levels of miR-125b-5p were increased, suggesting its inverse correlation with the aggressiveness of the disease.

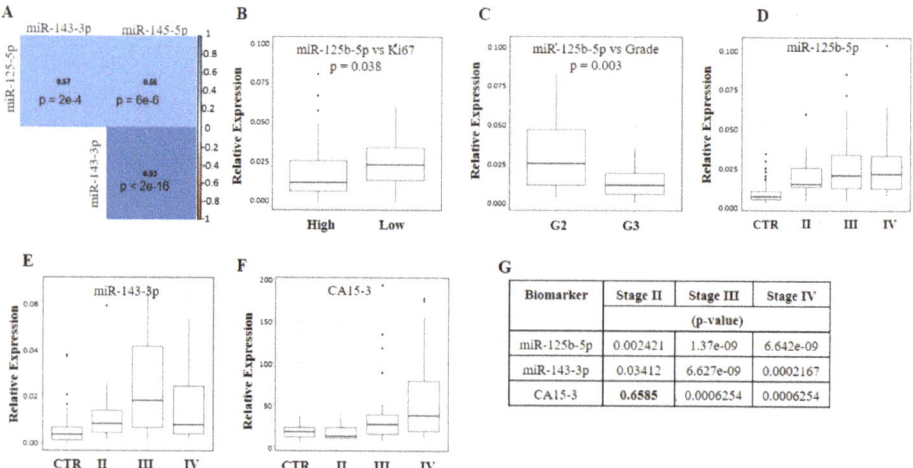

Figure 4. Correlation studies. Co-expression analyses of miR-125b-5p, miR-143-3p and miR-145-5p (**A**). Expression levels of miR-125b-5p vs. Ki67 (low <20%; high ≥20%) (**B**), and grade (**C**). Expression levels of miR-125b-5p (**D**), miR-143-3p (**E**), and CA15-3 (**F**) vs. stage. Statistical significance (**G**). Non-significant results are reported in bold.

2.4. Correlation Analysis of Circulating miR-125b-5p, miR-143-3p and miR-145-5p with Quantitative Imaging Parameters of Tumour Lesions

The BC patients enrolled in this study underwent same-day contrast-enhanced fluorodeoxyglucose (CE-FDG)-PET/MR and blood collection to better correlate circulating miR-125-5p and miR-143-3p with the morphological, metabolic and functional imaging features of BC (Figure 4). No significant correlations were found between the miRNA expression levels and lesion size (Supplementary Table S2). The plasma levels of miR-125b-5p increased significantly at stage II, reaching higher expression levels at stage III and remained unchanged at stage IV compared to stage III (Figure 4D,G). This trend confirmed that the expression levels of miR-125b-5p were variable and depended on the severity of the disease. Additionally, the expression levels of miR-143-3p (Figure 4E,G) became significantly higher in stage III and drastically decreased in stage IV, reaching expression values close to those of healthy donors. This result suggests that at stage IV, this molecule is not required for the maintenance of the pathology. It is known that CA15-3 levels increase in the late stage of the disease, so its relationship with clinical staging was also evaluated. As reported in Figure 4F,G, in our cohort, CA15-3 was not able to diagnose stage II, but its levels increased significantly at stage III, reaching the maximum concentration at stage IV. This was in agreement with the known performance of CA15-3. In addition, no correlations were found between CA15-3 and grade (p-value = 0.761) or subtypes (p-value = 0.450).

Correlation analyses between miR-125b-5p and miR-143-3p levels and PET/MR-based tumour biomarkers were performed by grouping the data according to staging. Only the statistically significant results were reported (Table 4); we found a strong and significant correlation between circulating miR-143-3p and the mean initial area under the concentration curve (iAUC$_{mean}$) and the mean reverse efflux volume transfer constant (Kep$_{mean}$) (for both, ρ: 0.943, p-value = 0.005) in the stage II group. Perfusion parameters such as iAUC and Kep are generally correlated with tumour vascularisation [23,24], suggesting that the plasmatic overexpression of miR-143-3p in BC patients might correlate with angiogenesis. The correlation between iAUC and miR-143-3p persisted at stage III but was lost at stage IV, where its relative expression drastically decreased (see Figure 4B). Notably, there was a strong correlation index between miR-143-3p and the maximum standardized uptake value (SUV$_{max}$) (ρ: 0.829 and p-value = 0.042) at stage II, although the statistical significance was borderline. SUV is a biomarker of tumour metabolism. This result together with those reported above suggest that miR-143-3p could be correlated with tumour aggressiveness. miR-125-5p was significantly inversely correlated with the mean forward volume transfer constant (Ktrans$_{mean}$) and the proliferation index Ki67 at stage IV (Table 4). Ktrans$_{mean}$, like iAUC and Kep, is a perfusion parameter linked to tumour vascularisation [24]. Since the highest plasma concentration of miR-125b-5p was associated with a low Ki67 index (Figure 4B) and grade G2 (Figure 4C) and inversely correlated with Ktrans$_{mean}$ (Table 4), these results suggest that the highest plasma values of miR-125b-5p might predict a better prognosis.

Table 4. Correlation studies among the miRNAs selected and the imaging parameters extracted from tumour lesions. The table reports ρ and *p*-values ($p < 0.05$ was considered statistically significant).

	Stage II				Stage III		Stage IV	
	iAUC$_{mean}$	Ki67	Kep$_{mean}$	SUV$_{max}$	iAUC$_{mean}$	Ki67	Ki67	Ktrans$_{mean}$
miR-125-5p	ns	ns	ns	ns	ns	ns	−0.513 *p*-value 0.029	−0.421 *p*-value 0.040
miR-143-3p	0.943 *p*-value 0.005	ns	0.943 *p*-value 0.005	0.829 *p*-value 0.042	0.938 *p*-value 0.044	ns	ns	ns

ns indicates non-significant results. iAUC$_{mean}$: area under the concentration curve; SUV$_{max}$: maximum standardized uptake value; Kep$_{mean}$: mean reverse efflux volume transfer constant; Ktrans$_{mean}$: mean forward volume transfer constantin.

2.5. In Silico Studies

Large publicly funded projects have generated extensive and freely available multi-assay data resources. To date, The Cancer Genome Atlas (TCGA) represents the largest available resource for multi-assay cancer genomics data that includes ~30000 cases of major primary cancers, including BC (TCGA-BRCA) [25]. To evaluate whether the upregulation of circulating miR-125b-5p, miR-143-3p and miR-145-5p in the plasma samples of BC patients reflected their tumour tissue expression, we performed in silico studies by using the TCGA-BRCA database. We also included miR-145-5p in order to perform co-expression analyses. We found that in BC tissue specimens, the expression of miR-125b-5p, miR-143-3p and miR-145-5p was significantly lower compared to that in normal tissues (Supplementary Figure S2A) and that their downregulation was not correlated with the stage of the disease (Supplementary Figure S2B).

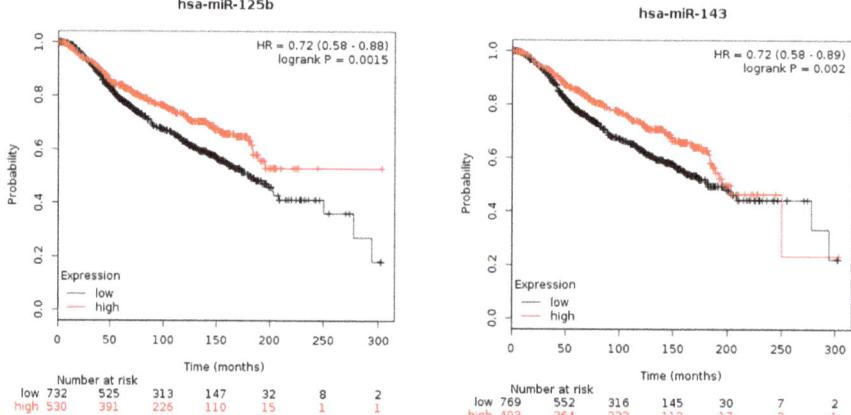

Figure 5. Kaplan-Meier plots, which are based on breast cancer data from the METABRIC database, illustrate the survival probability for patients with low or high miR-125b (upper panel) and miR-143 (lower panel) expression levels in breast cancer. Hazard ratios (HRs) and p-values (log-rank test) were generated.

In addition, we found that the downregulation of miR-143-3p and miR-145-5p in BC tissues (Supplementary Figure S2C) showed a lower correlation index compared to that we found in the plasma samples of BC patients (compare Figure 4A with Supplementary Figure S2C: ρ: 0.93 vs. ρ: 0.28). Taken together, these results showed an opposite expression trend of miR-125-5p, miR-143-3p and miR-145-5p in cancer tissue versus plasma.

Since we were unable to monitor patients during follow-up, a survival analysis was performed for both miR-125b-5p and miR-143-3p by using the miRpower software (http://kmplot.com/analysis/index.php?p=service&cancer=breast_mirna). This software uses publicly available BC data from different databases, including data from large databases such as TCGA and Molecular Taxonomy of Breast Cancer International Consortium (METABRIC). To generate Kaplan-Meier curves, we selected the option to auto select the best cut-off for defining high and low groups. The algorithm computes all possible cut-off values between the lower and upper quartiles and uses the best performing threshold. The hazard ratios (HRs) and p-values (log-rank test) were calculated. By using the TCGA dataset, the Kaplan-Meier plots were not statistically significant for miR-125b-5p or miR-143-3p (data not shown), so the METABRIC dataset was used. As reported in Figure 5, we found that high tissue expression levels of miR-125b-5p were associated with the best prognosis (upper panel), and this result was in agreement with those obtained correlating this miRNA with grade, Ki67 and Ktrans$_{mean}$. The effect of high expression levels of miR-143 on the survival of BC patients varied with age, and higher values contributed to worse prognoses starting at 250 months (lower panel). This result was in part in agreement with those obtained correlating this miRNA with the imaging parameters linked with tumour aggressiveness. It is necessary to point out that the miRpower software did not discriminate miR-143-3p from miR-143-5p, grouping them in miR-143, and miR-125b-5p from miR-125b-3p, grouping them in miR-125b.

2.6. Cellular Origin of miR-125b-5p, miR-143-3p and miR-145-5p in Normal and BC Tissues

To corroborate the obtained results and confirm the in silico data, we performed ISH experiments. We hypothesized that release of miR-125b-5p, miR-143-3p and miR-145-5p into the bloodstream did not originate from tumour cells. As reported in Figure 6, the results confirmed that the expression of miR-143-3p (B) and miR-145-5p (C) was low or absent in epithelial tumour tissue (right) but high in endothelial cells, highlighting their vascular origin, as anticipated by correlation studies among miRNAs with image biomarkers. In addition, in benign breast tissue, miR-143-3p stained in glandular epithelial and endothelial cells (Figure 6B, left), and miR-145-5p was expressed with the strongest staining intensity in myoepithelial cells and endothelial cells (Figure 6C, left panel). Moreover, miR-125b-5p was weakly expressed in normal tissue (Figure 6D, left) and low-to-absent in neoplastic cells (Figure 6D, right). This supported the hypothesis that miR-125b-5p could have a stromal origin. This hypothesis was further confirmed by the result shown in Figure 6E, in which miR-125b-5p expression occurred in cancer-associated fibroblasts. Taken together, these results confirmed that the BC plasma upregulation of miR-125-5p and miR-143-3p could be related to their overexpression in endothelial and fibroblast cells and not in tumour epithelial cells.

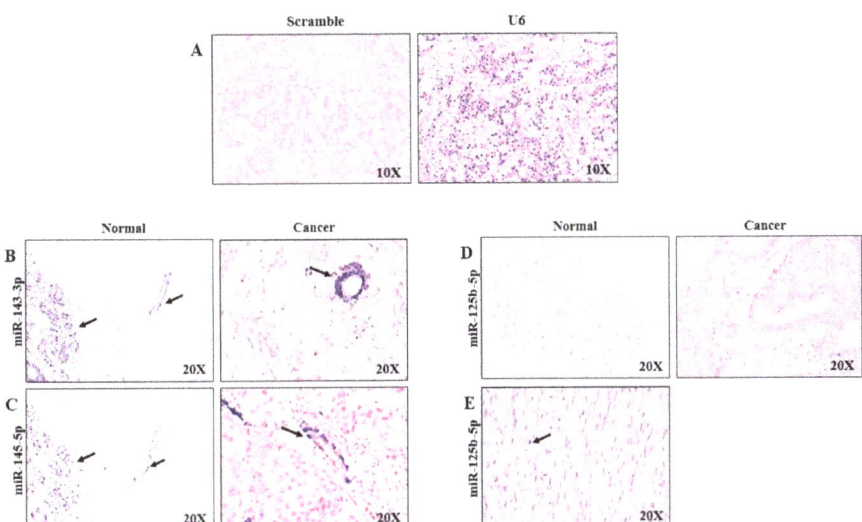

Figure 6. In situ hybridization staining patterns in benign and malignant breast tissues. Scrambled miR negative control probe and U6 positive control probe (**A**). miR-143-3p in normal (left) and BC tissues (right) (**B**). miR-145-5p in normal (left) and BC tissues (right) (**C**). miR-125b-5p in normal (left) and BC tissues (right) (**D**). miR-125b-5p in stromal tumour tissue (**E**). BC: breast cancer.

2.7. Combining Diagnostic test Results to Increase Accuracy

Since the relationship between upregulated circulating miRNA expression and the functional characteristics of tumour lesions was clarified, we next sought to optimize their diagnostic role by evaluating a combined detection of miR-125b-5p and miR-143-3p with CA15-3. As reported in Figure 7A, we found that combining the diagnostic test results of miR-125b-5p and CA15-3 improved the accuracy (AUC = 0.89) compared to the same molecules analysed individually (see Figure 3: miR-125-5p, AUC = 0.85; CA15-3, AUC = 0.68). In contrast, combining miR-143-3p and CA15-3 reduced the diagnostic accuracy (data not shown). Additionally, the combined analysis of miR-125b-5p and miR-143-3p did not improve the accuracy (Figure 7B, AUC = 0.85) in comparison to the same molecules analysed individually (see Figure 3: miR-125-5p, AUC = 0.85; miR-143-3p, AUC = 0.80).

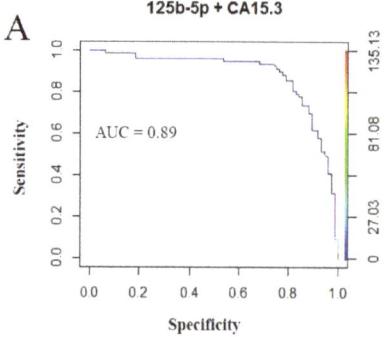 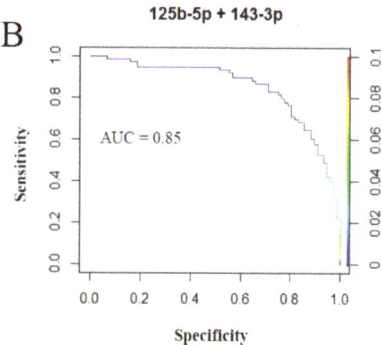

Figure 7. ROC curve analyses and AUC values combining the profiles of miR-125b-5p and CA15-3 (**A**) and miR-125-5p and miR-143-3p (**B**) for discriminating BC patients from healthy patients. ROC: Receiver operating characteristic; AUC: area under the ROC curve; BC: breast cancer.

3. Discussion

The detection of BC is pivotal for proper patient management, especially at an early stage. However, the currently utilized technology, which is heavily based on screening mammography and ultrasound (in specific patient populations), is imperfect, with limited accessibility in underdeveloped/underserved areas and might be economically challenging. Therefore, there is a compelling need to identify new biomarkers that might be diagnostically advantageous. Due to their structural and functional characteristics, microRNAs have been proposed as a new class of biomarkers for cancer screening; in fact, they are stable, deregulated, and found in different biological fluids, including blood that can be easily withdrawn in the field and subsequently processed in centralized laboratories. To date, circulating biomarkers that are able to diagnose BC with high specificity and sensitivity are lacking, so our study aimed to (i) identify new circulating miRNAs for the diagnosis of BC; (ii) to elucidate the relationship between their circulating deregulation and the functional characteristics of tumour lesions for in vivo investigation through PET/MR; and (iii) understand the link between circulating miRNA deregulation and their origin in the primary tumour.

By using the miScript miRNA PCR Array, we found that five miRNAs (miR-125b-5p, miR-143-3p, miR-145-5p, miR-100-5p and miR-23a-3p) were significantly ($p \leq 0.0005$) overexpressed in the plasma samples of BC patients compared to healthy subjects and defined miR-125b-5p and miR-143-3p as the best molecules able to estimate the probability of having the disease. The circulating levels of miR-125b-5p and miR-143-3p are of intense debate in the scientific literature, especially in BC. Matamala et al. [26] found that circulating miR-143 was upregulated in BC patients; on the contrary, some studies showed a downregulation of circulating miR-143 in BC patients [27–30], and others found no significant deregulation of circulating miR-125b and miR-143 in BC patients [30]. These discrepancies could be explained by the usage of serum rather than plasma [31]. Regardless of whether the choice of the biological sample can affect the result, different studies reported the upregulation of miR-125b in the serum samples of BC patients [32–34]. These discrepancies highlight the need to standardize protocols, including sample collection, storage, choice of the starting biological material, and processing. To better understand the biological basis and clinical implications of miR-125b-5p and miR-143-3p, we performed a correlation analysis between the circulating expression of the deregulated disease-related miRNAs and the metabolic and functional characteristics of the primary tumour, also taking into consideration the TNM (Tumour Lymph Nodes Metastasis) classification of malignant tumours stage of the disease. For this purpose, we employed biomarkers extracted from a hybrid clinically approved PET/MR scanner. We decided to use PET/MR since it couples two modalities (FDG-PET and MR) capable of sampling different biological features of cancers in vivo, specifically glucose metabolism through PET and cellular density plus tissue perfusion through MR. The advantages arising from the simultaneous acquisition of PET- and MR-derived biomarkers in investigating BC biology have been shown by some exploratory studies that demonstrated the capability of PET/MR to predict BC subtypes, including those with a better prognosis [19,35]. In this study, we found that the expression of circulating miR-143-3p was strongly and significantly correlated with iAUC$_{mean}$ at stage II (ρ: 0.943, p-value = 0.005) and at stage III (ρ: 0.938, p-value = 0.044) and with Kep$_{mean}$ at stage II (ρ: 0.943, p-value = 0.005). Both iAUC$_{mean}$ and Kep$_{mean}$ are perfusion parameters that provide information on tumour vascularisation, suggesting that miR-143-3p overexpression in the plasma samples of BC patients could be linked to tumour angiogenesis. Our hypothesis was in agreement with the editorial comment of Almeida and Calin [36] that argued the possible critical role of these miRNAs in the neoangiogenesis of lung cancer. To confirm this hypothesis and to further validate our results, we performed ISH experiments on BC and normal breast tissue specimens and found that miR-143-3p had a clear vascular endothelial origin. In addition, we also found that miR-143-3p was correlated with SUV$_{max}$ at stage II (ρ: 0.829, p-value = 0.042). The SUV parameter reflects the metabolic activity of tumours, so we speculate that miR-143-3p could have a role in neoangiogenesis and that its overexpression in the plasma samples of BC patients could be correlated with the aggressiveness of the disease, both in terms of tumour vascularisation and metabolic activity. This hypothesis was in part corroborated by the survival analysis performed *in silico* by using the miRpower software.

Another interesting result correlated the expression levels of miR-125b-5p with IHC biomarkers and imaging parameters. We concluded that miR-125b-5p was inversely associated with the proliferation index Ki67 (p-value = 0.038), grading (p-value = 0.003) and the perfusion imaging parameter Ktrans$_{mean}$ (ρ: −0.421, p-value = 0.040) and that its expression occurred in cancer-associated fibroblasts. These findings suggest that the highest concentration of miR-125b-5p could be correlated with a better prognosis, and the survival analysis confirmed this hypothesis. This is in agreement with the "seed and soil" hypothesis, which postulates that different components of the tumour microenvironment (the soil) may have stimulatory or inhibitory effects on tumour progression (the seed) [37], and with recent studies showing that miR-125b-5p overexpression in BC cell lines could inhibit cell proliferation, migration and invasion [38,39].

One of the limitations of this study is the sample size (n = 77 BC patients). In fact, the heterogeneity and complexity of BC make it challenging to find a unique circulating signature of pathology with high diagnostic accuracy. Each circulating biomarker released in the blood of affected patients exists as a consequence of genetic and/or epigenetic alterations linked to the pathology. Breast carcinoma is divided into different subtypes with different genetic characteristics [40,41], which can affect the release of specific miRNAs in the blood. Moreover, the variety of biomarkers and the difference in concentration in the blood might be influenced by the stage, so the analysis of a cohort not homogeneous for staging could be a limitation, and the BC patients included in this cohort are lacking stage I and grade 1 (one patient for each condition). Therefore, a limitation of our study is the paucity of stage I and II cancers. However, this is unavoidable in studies that recruit clinically justified PET acquisition since, as per the Clinical Practice Guidelines in Oncology (NCCN guidelines), PET is not indicated in the initial work-up of clinical stage I, II, or operable stage III (NCCN Guidelines Version 1.2019, accessed on 22th May 2019).

This staging group heterogeneity might lead to different results in different cohorts. Another limitation was the inability of monitoring patients during follow-up to better understand the prognostic and predictive role of miR-125b-5p and miR-143-3p. Nevertheless, the strengths of this study included the analysis performed on naïve patients as well as the availability of the same-day imaging parameters that provided information related to the morpho-functional characteristics of the primary cancers to correlate circulating miRNAs with in vivo quantified tumour biology. We performed a combined detection of miR-125b-5p and miR-143-3p with CA15-3 to improve the diagnostic accuracy. As suggested by guidelines, CA15-3 is not recommended for BC diagnosis [42,43], and our result (CA15-3$_{AUC}$ = 0.70) was in agreement with those of Liu and colleagues (CA15-3$_{AUC}$ = 0.71 [44]), Zaleski and colleagues (CA15-3$_{AUC}$ = 0.72 [45]) and Zajkowska and colleagues (CA15-3$_{AUC}$ = 0.70 [46]). Nevertheless, the coupled analysis of miR-125b-5p and CA15-3 increased the diagnostic accuracy up to AUC = 0.89. To the best of our knowledge, this is one of the best results published so far and the first study that combines the expression of a circulating miRNA with the expression of an established BC tumour marker. The combined detection of plasma miR-125b-5p and serum CA15-3 improved the diagnostic accuracy of BC detection up to ~90%, suggesting that this signature could be used for the diagnosis of BC. In addition, for stage II, the expression levels of CA15-3 were not correlated with the pathology (p-value = 0.658), whereas those of miR-125b-5p were (p-value = 0.002). The combined analysis of miR-125b-5p and CA 15-3 not only improved diagnostic accuracy in its entirety but also provided additional diagnostic information at less advanced pathological stages, suggesting the use of miRNAs as potential diagnostic circulating biomarkers that warrants consideration by further validation studies.

4. Materials and Methods

4.1. Participants and Study Design

This Health Insurance Portability and Accountability Act–compliant prospective study was approved by the institutional review board. All procedures performed in studies involving human participants were in accordance with the ethical standards of the institutional and/or national research committee and with the principles of the 1964 Declaration of Helsinki and its later amendments or comparable ethical standards. Informed consent was obtained from all individual participants included in the study. For study enrolment, all participants provided written informed consent before undergoing imaging PET/MR and blood collection. Between September 2012 and November 2015 at the IRCCS SDN Institute, 221 female Caucasian patients with BC who underwent a clinically indicated same-day CE-FDG-PET/MR and blood collection were evaluated for inclusion in this study. Plasma haemolysation was evaluated as described by Kirschner MB and colleagues [47]. The inclusion criteria for BC patients were as follows: (i) diagnosis of BC by core biopsy report; (ii) absence of any prior surgical or pharmacological treatment for BC (naïve); (iii) negative previous personal oncological history; (iv) age > 18 years; (v) CE-FDG-PET/MR and blood collection were performed on the same day; and (vi) fasting for at least 8 hours. The exclusion criteria for BC patients were as follows: (i) pregnancy; (ii) blood glucose levels > 140 mg/dL (7.77 mmol/L); (iii) artefacts affecting PET/MR images; (iv) standard contraindications for MR; (v) performance of CE-FDG-PET/MR and blood collection on different days; and (vi) plasma haemolysation. Blood samples of age-matched healthy donors were collected; their inclusion criteria were as follows: (i) >18 years of age; (ii) negative previous personal oncological history; (iii) absence of suspected BC as confirmed by ultrasound and/or mammography during the last 6 months from enrolment; iv) absence of a family history of BC; and (v) fasting for at least 8 hours. The exclusion criteria for healthy donors were the presence of one or more of the criteria reported above, including haemolysed plasma. We recruited 77 BC patients and 78 healthy donors for a total of 155 plasma/serum samples. The clinicopathological characteristics of the enrolled patients are reported in Table 1, and the whole study design is shown in Figure 1A.

This study was approved by the institutional Ethics Committee (Protocol Number: Prot2-11, approved 06/07/2011 by Ethical Committee IRCCS Fondazione SDN). This article does not describe any studies with animals performed by any of the authors

4.2. PET/MR Data Acquisition

PET/MR was performed with a Biograph mMR imager (Siemens Healthiness, Erlangen, Germany). First, a whole-body protocol was used to assess the overall extent of cancer and provide the NM stage. Thereafter, a dedicated breast protocol to provide both metabolic and functional biomarkers of primary cancer and its T stage was acquired. For total body acquisition, we used a 16-channel head-neck coil and three or four 12-channel body coils depending on the patient's height; for breast acquisition, a 4-channel breast coil was employed. Acquisitions were performed according to previously described protocols [19,20,35,48,49]. All patients fasted for at least 8 h before the procedure. They received

401 ± 32 MBq (mean ± standard deviation) of 18F-FDG intravenously. After a 60-min incubation time, PET and MR data were acquired simultaneously. The mean total time for the PET/MR examination was 107.87 ± 18.92 min [19].

4.3. Data Processing and Multiparametric Analysis

The PET data obtained from the PET/MR examinations were processed with comparable reconstruction and correction algorithms. Emission data were corrected for randomness, dead time, scatter, and attenuation.

Lymph node involvement and distant metastases were assessed on the entire dataset of PET/MR sequences for the purpose of NM staging. The primary tumour size and infiltration of neighbouring structures were evaluated on the dedicated breast PET/MR protocol for T staging [50].

The dynamic contrast-enhanced (DCE)-MRI images were processed through commercially available and clinically approved software for estimating tissue perfusion (Tissue 4D, Siemens Healthiness) according to the same established procedures provided by the manufacturer manual and widely used in the published literature. The pharmacokinetic modelling is based on a two-compartment Toft's model that allows for the calculation of the following: the transfer constant between vascular, extravascular, and extracellular space (EES) (Ktrans); volume of EES (Ve); constant reflux between EES and blood plasma (kep); initial area under the concentration curve (iAUC) [51,52]. Ktrans is a parameter related to vessel permeability and tissue blood flow. The volume of the extravascular extracellular space Ve is a marker of cell density, kep is a transfer constant from the extracellular/extravascular space to plasma, and iAUC is related to the blood volume in the tissue of interest [51].

After automatic motion correction and registration of the pre- and post-contrast acquisitions, T1 mapping was automatically obtained from the multiple flip angle pre-contrast part of the DCE-MRI sequence. Arterial input function (AIF) was related to the gadolinium dose injected and automatically modelled by a bi-exponential function using an intermediate population-derived mode provided by the software. On each single slice, a region-of-interest (ROI) was manually plotted around the tumour excluding the neighbouring vessels (internal mammary arteries and heart chambers) to compute the MR perfusion biomarker maps that were stored in the system.

For the subsequent tumour ROI analysis, PET/MR datasets (PET acquisition, dynamic axial T1 weighted post-contrast, dynamic axial T1 weighted subtracted contrast-enhanced images, axial T2 weighted sequences, axial apparent diffusion coefficient (ADC) map, and perfusion maps for Ktrans, Ve, kep and iAUC) were simultaneously evaluated on a clinically approved hybrid imaging workstation (Syngo.via, Siemens Healthiness) allowing the visual and quantitative comparison of the multiparametric data.

The maximum standardized uptake value (SUVmax) was automatically calculated by using an iso-contour automatic volume-of-interest (VOI) method of tissue delineation that selected a fixed threshold fraction (40%) of the peak activity in the tumour.

To obtain Ktrans, Ve, Kep and iAUC, the subtracted dynamic post-contrast T1-weighted series that best visualized the tumour was chosen. ROIs were manually drawn around the tumour on each image of that series, copied and then pasted on the corresponding Ktrans, Ve, Kep and iAUC maps. The values of all the ROIs were averaged. To obtain the ADC values, the ROIs were drawn on each image of the high-b value (800 s/mm^2) diffusion-weighted imaging (DWI), copied and then pasted on the ADC maps. The values of all the ROIs were averaged.

While the ROIs were drawn around the tumours, care was taken to avoid including large feeding vessels and areas of frank necrosis, as seen on T2 weighted and subtracted dynamic post-contrast T1-weighted images.

The maximal diameter of the tumour was measured on every single slice of the reference subtracted dynamic post-contrast T1-weighted images. The measurements were performed by a radiologist and a nuclear medicine physician with more than 5 years of experience. The whole-body and breast PET/MR protocols were derived from the published literature [20,35].

4.4. Plasma Sampling, RNA Extraction and Reverse Transcription

Blood samples were collected immediately before FDG injection. For each patient, a total of 10.5 mL of venous blood was collected in BD Vacutainer® 3 mL ethylenediaminetetraacetic acid (EDTA) tubes (Becton Dikinson, Franklin Lakes, NJ, USA) and 7.5 mL serum separating tubes. Blood was processed within 1 h of harvest. Plasma and serum were obtained from the whole blood samples by centrifugation at 1900× g for 10 min at 4 °C. The supernatant was further centrifuged at 16,000× g for 10 min at 4 °C and stored in aliquots of 0.5 mL at −80 °C until analysis. The samples were stored at −80 °C at the SDN Biobank (IRCCS DSN, Naples, Italy) [53]. The extraction of total RNA from 200 µL of plasma was performed within 1 year of storage at −80 °C using an miRNeasy Serum/Plasma Kit (Qiagen, Hilden, Germany) according to the manufacturer's instructions. Briefly, 3.5 µL of *Caenorhabditis elegans* miR-39 (cel-miR-39, 1.6 × 108 copies/µL) was added as the spike-in control after the denaturing solution. Total RNA (including miRNAs) was eluted in 14 µL of RNase-free water. Reverse transcription was performed using the miScript II RT Kit (Qiagen, Hilden, Germany) according to the manufacturer's instructions. Because extracellular miRNAs are less than 1% of the total RNA recovered [54] their concentration is often under the detection limits of spectrophotometric devices, so we decided to use a fixed volume rather than a fixed miRNA amount for qRT-PCR. To this aim, 1.5 µL of total RNA was added to the HiSpect Buffer (Qiagen, Hilden, Germany), nucleic acid mix and reverse transcriptase in a final volume of 20 µL. Reactions were incubated for 60 min at 37 °C and then for 5 min at 95 °C to inactivate the miScript Reverse Transcriptase mix (Qiagen, Hilden, Germany). At the end of the reactions, the resulting cDNAs were stored undiluted at −20 °C. The cycling conditions for real-time PCR were as follows: 15 min at 95 °C as the initial activation step, followed by 3-step cycling including denaturation (15 s at 94 °C), annealing (30 s at 55 °C) and extension (30 s at 70 °C) for a total of 40 cycles.

4.5. miRNA Microarray and Validation by Real-Time PCR (qRT-PCR)

By using the miScript miRNA PCR Array (Qiagen; MIHS-106Z), the expression profile of 84 human miRNAs (Supplementary Table S3) from the plasma samples of naïve BC patients and healthy donors were screened according to the manufacturer's protocol. The miScript miRNA PCR Array profiles the expression of 84 human miRNAs known to be deregulated in different cancers and are best characterized in miRBase. miRNA profiles were initially checked against a set population of 41 plasma samples (14 plasma samples from healthy donors and 27 from BC patients at diagnosis) on a MyiQ PCR system (Bio-Rad, Hercules, CA, USA). To identify interindividual variability, we did not pool plasma samples from each group (BC patients and healthy donors), but each sample was individually analysed by miRNA PCR arrays. The 96-well array also included $n = 2$ miRNA isolation controls, $n = 6$ "Housekeeping" snRNAs, $n = 2$ miRNA Reverse Transcription Controls (miRTC) and $n = 2$ Positive PCR Controls (PPC). Briefly, 200 µL of RNase-free water was added to each 20 µL of reverse transcription reaction, and 100 µL of diluted cDNA was used to prepare a reaction mix according to the manufacturer's protocol. For data analysis, the Baseline and Threshold settings, which were the same across all PCR runs, were from cycle 2 to cycle 15 for Baseline and 20 for Threshold. By using a data analysis tool (GeneGlobe Data Analysis Center, Qiagen, Hilden, Germany), the threshold cycle (CT) values were exported, and the steps performed by the software were as follows: any CT value ≥ 33 was considered negative; if the RNA sample was of high quality, the cycling programme was correctly run and the threshold was correctly defined, the value of the positive PCR control wells from the CT samples (CTPPC) should be 19 ± 2 or 15 ± 2; if the CT values of the reverse transcription control are less than 7, no inhibition of the reverse transcription reaction is apparent; the ΔCT value for each mature miRNA profiled is calculated using the formula $\Delta CT = CT_{miRNA} - CT_{normalizer}$. The relative expression for each miRNA was calculated as $2^{-\Delta CT}$, and the criteria for the selection of miRNAs differentially expressed between the two populations with a statistical significance were a fold change ≥ 1.5 and a *p*-value < 0.05. Data validations were performed by qRT-PCR screening for only the following molecules: miR-125b-5p, miR-143-3p, miR-145-5p, miR-100-5p and miR-23a-3p. The Qiagen miScript SYBR Green PCR Kit was used for qPCR according to the manufacturer's protocol on the

Bio-Rad MyiQ PCR system. To determine the best standard genes to normalize our data, BestKeeper software was used [55]. By analysing $n = 41$ plasma samples, we found that the best normalizer included in the miScript miRNA PCR Array was the exogenous cel-mir 39. The MiScript Primers Assay was purchased from Qiagen (Qiagen, Hilden, Germany).

4.6. TCGA Data Processing

TCGA Breast Invasive Carcinoma (TCGA-BRCA project, February 2018) transcriptome profiling data (miRNA Expression Quantification) and clinical metadata were extracted from the Genomic Data Commons (GDC) portal (https://portal.gdc.cancer.gov/) for primary tumour ($n = 1096$ files for 1078 BC cases) and normal solid tissue ($n = 104$ files for 104 normal cases) using the open source R software and the TCGAbiolinks R package [56]. For the miRNA datasets, we selected the level-3 miRNA-Seq data, which were produced on Illumina HiSeq 2000 sequencers (Illumina Ventures, San Diego, CA, USA) The miRNA-Seq expression level-3 data contains raw read counts ($n = 1881$ miRNAs). The miRNA raw counts were filtered as follows: we calculated the mean value for duplicated BC cases and filtered out miRNA counts with null expression values on both conditions (tumour/normal) for a total of 1625 filtered counts. We considered only 1625 filtered miRNAs for the normalization step. Filtered raw counts were normalized using the Upper Quartile approach, and the patients with "−Inf" normalized values were removed for a total of 1076 tumours. The normalized counts were used to evaluate miR-125b-5p, miR-143-3p and miR-145-5p expression levels (tumour vs. normal) as log2-transformed relative expression values. We performed a Wilcoxon test to assess the statistical significance between tumour and normal conditions and calculated the adjusted *p*-value for each selected miRNA profile. We also reported miRNA tumour expression profiles based on the American Joint Committee on Cancer (AJCC) TNM staging. We grouped the clinical stages into four categories: (1) stage I; (2) stage II; (3) stage III; and (4) stage IV. We filtered out data with unassessed stage (stage x) or unreported information. Finally, we carried out a Spearman correlation analysis among the selected miRNA profiles and reported the associated *p*-values.

4.7. In Situ Hybridization

ISH was performed on formalin-fixed and paraffin-embedded tissue specimens surgically resected from patients diagnosed with BC. For each case analysed (a total of 22 breast tissues), we selected a block of tissue fixed in formalin and embedded in paraffin representative of the tumour and used it to obtain 4 µm-thick sections mounted on Superfrost Plus slides (Thermo Fisher Scientific, Waltham, MA, USA). The paraffin sections were placed in an oven at 60 °C for 45 min the day before ISH was performed and were stored overnight at 4 °C. Double digoxigenin (DIG)-labelled miRCURY LNA™ microRNA detection probes (Exiqon, Vedbæk, Denmark) were employed in this study. Specifically, we used 60 nM miR-145-5p target probe (Exiqon, Cat #619865-360), 60 nM miR-143-3p target probe (Exiqon, Cat #619872-360), 60 nM miR-125-5p target probe (Exiqon, Cat #611756-360), 40 nM scramble miR negative control probe (Exiqon, Cat #90-001) and 10 nM U6 positive control probe (Exiqon, Cat #90-002). The detection of microRNA by ISH was performed using the Enhanced miRCURY LNA microRNA ISH Optimization Kit (Exiqon, Vedbæk, Denmark) according to the manufacturer's protocol. Briefly, formalin-fixed paraffin-embedded sections were deparaffinized in xylene, rehydrated through solutions of ethanol to phosphate-buffered saline (PBS, pH 7.4) and pre-treated by enzymatic digestion (Proteinase K at 20 µg/mL for 30 min at 37 °C). Hybridization was performed by adding 60 nM LNA detection probes diluted in Exiqon hybridization buffer (Exiqon, Vedbæk, Denmark, Cat #90000) to each slide and incubating for 1 h at 60 °C in a hybridizer oven. After hybridization, the sections were washed under stringent conditions. Stringent washes were performed in pre-heated saline-sodium citrate (SSC) buffers in 5-min washes at 60 °C: once in 5× SSC, twice in 1× SSC and twice in 0.2× SSC. Then, the slides were placed in 0.2× SSC at room temperature and washed in PBS with 0.1% Tween-20. The sections were blocked against the unspecific binding of the detection antibody using a blocking solution according to the manufacturer's recommendations at room temperature for 15 min. The chromogenic detection of the miRNA LNA-ISH probe was performed with anti- anti-digoxygenin -alkaline phosphatase conjugate (1:800 dilution of the conjugate in blocking reagent, Roche Diagnostics GmbH, Mannheim, Germany) and incubated at room temperature for 1 h. Enzymatic development was performed by incubating the slides with 4-nitro-blue tetrazolium (NBT) and 5-bromo-4-chloro-3′-indolyl phosphate (BCIP) substrate (Roche) at 30 °C overnight to allow the formation of dark-blue 4-nitro-blue tetrazolium formazan precipitate. The following day, the sections were washed twice for 5 min in KTBT buffer (50 mM Tris–HCl, 150 mM NaCl, 10 mM KCl) and then shortly twice in water. Counterstaining using ISH nuclear fast red was performed for 1 min at room temperature. The sections were rinsed in tap water for 10 min, dehydrated through an increasing gradient of ethanol solutions and mounted with Eukitt mounting medium (VWR, Herlev, Denmark). A scrambled probe and U6 small nuclear RNA-specific probe were used as controls.

4.8. Measurement of CA 15-3

The CA15-3 serology test was performed in accordance with the manufacturer's protocols and reference intervals. Specifically, this tumour marker was measured in 155 serum samples ($n = 78$ healthy donors and $n = 77$ BC patients) on a Dimension Vista®1500 System (Siemens Healthcare Diagnostics Inc., Tarrytown, NY, USA) that uses the LOCI method (Siemens Healthcare Diagnostics, Eschborn, Germany), a homogeneous sandwich chemiluminescent immunoassay-based LOCI® technology (Siemens Healthcare Diagnostics, Eschborn, Germany). The threshold value provided by the supplying company for CA15-3 was 35 UI/mL. For serum tumour marker determination, when its level exceeded a threshold value, the samples were considered to be positive; otherwise, they were considered to be negative.

4.9. Statistical Analysis

Statistical analyses were performed using the open source R Statistical Software. All p-values were two-sided, and $p < 0.05$ was considered statistically significant. We used Shapiro–Wilk analysis and the Levene test to assess the normality and homoscedasticity of the distribution of the data, respectively. We performed the Mann-Whitney non-parametric test to compare the expression of the selected miRNAs between the two groups (BC and healthy controls). Furthermore, stepwise logistic regression was implemented to assess the association between miRNA expression and the probability of pathology. ROC curves were constructed for each miRNA, CA15-3 and CEA, and AUC values with 95% confidence intervals were calculated to evaluate the predictive power of the selected molecules for detecting BC. We evaluated the diagnostic accuracy of each circulating miRNA, CA15-3 and CEA, and their combination. The non-parametric Spearman's rank-order correlation and Mann-Whitney U test were performed to verify the correlations/associations among the biological markers and imaging parameters. To assess the association between the molecular and imaging parameters, the data were grouped according to positive or negative expression of ER, PR and HER2 receptors, low or high expression of Ki67 (low ≤20% and high >20%), grading, and staging as I, II, III, and IV, according to BC guidelines.

5. Conclusions

Our study highlighted that the addition of PET/MR biomarkers led to a better understanding of the relationships between circulating miRNAs and tumour biology in our BC population. Nevertheless, further studies with larger samples and a more homogeneous distribution of tumour subtypes and staging are needed to confirm our results.

Supplementary Materials: The following are available online at http://www.mdpi.com/2072-6694/11/6/876/s1: Table S1: Statistical analyses, Table S2: Correlation analysis among the indicated miRNAs and hormonal receptor status of the lesions in a cohort of 77 BC patients, Table S3: Array Layout, Figure S1: Validation I: Relative expression of the selected miRNAs in a study population of 46 healthy donors (CTR) and 64 BC subjects, Figure S2: Expression analysis of miR-125b-5p, miR-143-3p and miR-145-5p by using the TCGA database.

Author Contributions: Conception and design: M.I. and O.A.C.; development of methodology: M.I., O.A.C., A.S. and S.S.; acquisition of data: M.I., O.A.C., P.M., C.C., G.I. and D.R.; analysis and interpretation of data: M.I., A.M.G., C.C., C.A.P. and M.F.; writing, review, and/or revision of the manuscript: M.I., A.M.G., O.A.C., C.C. and P.M.; study supervision: M.S.

Funding: This work was supported by the Ministry of Health under contract "Ricerca Corrente RRC-2019-2366651" and in part under contract "5 per mille 2014 5M-2353583".

Acknowledgments: We would like to thank Silvia Varricchio for technical support on the ISH assay.

Conflicts of Interest: The authors declare no conflict of interest.

References

1. Bray, F.; Ferlay, J.; Soerjomataram, I.; Siegel, R.L.; Torre, L.A.; Jemal, A. Global cancer statistics 2018: GLOBOCAN estimates of incidence and mortality worldwide for 36 cancers in 185 countries. *CA A Cancer J. Clin.* **2018**, *68*, 394–424. [CrossRef] [PubMed]
2. Carney, P.A.; Sickles, E.A.; Monsees, B.S.; Bassett, L.W.; Brenner, R.J.; Feig, S.A.; Smith, R.A.; Rosenberg, R.D.; Bogart, T.A.; Browning, S.; et al. Identifying Minimally Acceptable Interpretive Performance Criteria for Screening Mammography. *Radiology* **2010**, *255*, 354–361. [CrossRef] [PubMed]
3. Berg, W.A.; Blume, J.D.; Cormack, J.B.; Mendelson, E.B.; Lehrer, D.; Bohm-Velez, M.; Pisano, E.D.; Jong, R.A.; Evans, W.P.; Morton, M.J.; et al. Combined screening with ultrasound and mammography vs. mammography alone in women at elevated risk of breast cancer. *JAMA J. Am. Med Assoc.* **2008**, *299*, 2151–2163. [CrossRef] [PubMed]
4. Maric, P.; Ozretic, P.; Levanat, S.; Oreskovic, S.; Antunac, K.; Beketic-Oreskovic, L. Tumor Markers in Breast Cancer—Evaluation of their Clinical Usefulness. *Coll. Antropol.* **2011**, *35*, 241–247. [PubMed]
5. Duffy, M.J. Serum tumor markers in breast cancer: Are they of clinical value? *Clin. Chem.* **2006**, *52*, 345–351. [CrossRef]
6. Kufe, D.W. MUC1-C oncoprotein as a target in breast cancer: Activation of signaling pathways and therapeutic approaches. *Oncogene* **2013**, *32*, 1073–1081. [CrossRef] [PubMed]
7. Lin, N.U.; Thomssen, C.; Cardoso, F.; Cameron, D.; Cufer, T.; Fallowfield, L.; Francis, P.A.; Kyriakides, S.; Pagani, O.; Senkus, E.; et al. International guidelines for management of metastatic breast cancer (MBC) from the European School of Oncology (ESO)-MBC Task Force: Surveillance, staging, and evaluation of patients with early-stage and metastatic breast cancer. *Breast* **2013**, *22*, 203–210. [CrossRef]
8. Lytle, J.R.; Yario, T.A.; Steitz, J.A. Target mRNAs are repressed as efficiently by microRNA-binding sites in the 5' UTR as in the 3' UTR. *Proc. Natl. Acad. Sci. USA* **2007**, *104*, 9667–9672. [CrossRef]
9. Esquela-Kerscher, A.; Slack, F.J. Oncomirs—MicroRNAs with a role in cancer. *Nat. Rev. Cancer* **2006**, *6*, 259–269. [CrossRef]
10. Kent, O.A.; Mendell, J.T. A small piece in the cancer puzzle: MicroRNAs as tumor suppressors and oncogenes. *Oncogene* **2006**, *25*, 6188–6196. [CrossRef]
11. Schwarzenbach, H.; Hoon, D.S.B.; Pantel, K. Cell-free nucleic acids as biomarkers in cancer patients. *Nat. Rev. Cancer* **2011**, *11*, 426–437. [CrossRef] [PubMed]
12. Hanke, M.; Hoefig, K.; Merz, H.; Feller, A.C.; Kausch, I.; Jocham, D.; Warnecke, J.M.; Sczakiel, G. A robust methodology to study urine microRNA as tumor marker: MicroRNA-126 and microRNA-182 are related to urinary bladder cancer. *Urol. Oncol. Semin. Orig. Investig.* **2010**, *28*, 655–661. [CrossRef] [PubMed]
13. Xie, Y.; Todd, N.W.; Liu, Z.Q.; Zhan, M.; Fang, H.B.; Peng, H.; Alattar, M.; Deepak, J.; Stass, S.A.; Jiang, F. Altered miRNA expression in sputum for diagnosis of non-small cell lung cancer. *Lung Cancer* **2010**, *67*, 170–176. [CrossRef] [PubMed]
14. Michael, A.; Bajracharya, S.D.; Yuen, P.S.T.; Zhou, H.; Star, R.A.; Illei, G.G.; Alevizos, I. Exosomes from human saliva as a source of microRNA biomarkers. *Oral Dis.* **2010**, *16*, 34–38. [CrossRef] [PubMed]
15. Amorim, M.; Salta, S.; Henrique, R.; Jeronimo, C. Decoding the usefulness of non-coding RNAs as breast cancer markers. *J. Transl. Med.* **2016**, *14*. [CrossRef] [PubMed]
16. Madhavan, D.; Cuk, K.; Burwinkel, B.; Yang, R. Cancer diagnosis and prognosis decoded by blood-based circulating microRNA signatures. *Front. Genet.* **2013**, *4*, 116. [CrossRef] [PubMed]
17. Leidner, R.S.; Li, L.; Thompson, C.L. Dampening Enthusiasm for Circulating MicroRNA in Breast Cancer. *PLoS ONE* **2013**, *8*. [CrossRef] [PubMed]

18. Sala, E.; Mema, E.; Himoto, Y.; Veeraraghavan, H.; Brenton, J.D.; Snyder, A.; Weigelt, B.; Vargas, H.A. Unravelling tumour heterogeneity using next-generation imaging: Radiomics, radiogenomics, and habitat imaging. *Clin. Radiol.* **2017**, *72*, 3–10. [CrossRef]
19. Incoronato, M.; Grimaldi, A.M.; Cavaliere, C.; Inglese, M.; Mirabelli, P.; Monti, S.; Ferbo, U.; Nicolai, E.; Soricelli, A.; Catalano, O.A.; et al. Relationship between functional imaging and immunohistochemical markers and prediction of breast cancer subtype: A PET/MRI study. *Eur. J. Nucl. Med. Mol. Imaging* **2018**. [CrossRef]
20. Catalano, O.A.; Daye, D.; Signore, A.; Iannace, C.; Vangel, M.; Luongo, A.; Catalano, M.; Filomena, M.; Mansi, L.; Soricelli, A.; et al. Staging performance of whole-body DWI, PET/CT and PET/MRI in invasive ductal carcinoma of the breast. *Int. J. Oncol.* **2017**, *51*, 281–288. [CrossRef]
21. Catalano, O.A.; Nicolai, E.; Rosen, B.R.; Luongo, A.; Catalano, M.; Iannace, C.; Guimaraes, A.; Vangel, M.G.; Mahmood, U.; Soricelli, A.; et al. Comparison of CE-FDG-PET/CT with CE-FDG-PET/MR in the evaluation of osseous metastases in breast cancer patients. *Br. J. Cancer* **2015**, *112*, 1452–1460. [CrossRef] [PubMed]
22. Botsikas, D.; Bagetakos, I.; Picarra, M.; Barisits, A.C.D.C.A.; Boudabbous, S.; Montet, X.; Giang Thanh, L.; Mainta, I.; Kalovidouri, A.; Becker, M. What is the diagnostic performance of 18-FDG-PET/MR compared to PET/CT for the N- and M- staging of breast cancer? *Eur. Radiol.* **2019**, *29*, 1787–1798. [CrossRef] [PubMed]
23. Ma, Z.S.; Wang, D.W.; Sun, X.B.; Shi, H.; Pang, T.; Dong, G.Q.; Zhang, C.Q. Quantitative analysis of 3-Tesla magnetic resonance imaging in the differential diagnosis of breast lesions. *Exp. Ther. Med.* **2015**, *9*, 913–918. [CrossRef] [PubMed]
24. Li, L.; Wang, K.; Sun, X.L.; Wang, K.Z.; Sun, Y.Y.; Zhang, G.F.; Shen, B.Z. Parameters of Dynamic Contrast-Enhanced MRI as Imaging Markers for Angiogenesis and Proliferation in Human Breast Cancer. *Med. Sci. Monit.* **2015**, *21*, 376–382. [PubMed]
25. Ma, C.X.; Ellis, M.J. The Cancer Genome Atlas: Clinical Applications for Breast Cancer. *Oncology (New York)* **2013**, *27*, 1263–1269.
26. Matamala, N.; Vargas, M.T.; Gonzalez-Campora, R.; Minambres, R.; Arias, J.I.; Menendez, P.; Andres-Leon, E.; Gomez-Lopez, G.; Yanowsky, K.; Calvete-Candenas, J.; et al. Tumor MicroRNA Expression Profiling Identifies Circulating MicroRNAs for Early Breast Cancer Detection. *Clin. Chem.* **2015**, *61*, 1098–1106. [CrossRef] [PubMed]
27. Ng, E.K.O.; Li, R.F.N.; Shin, V.Y.; Jin, H.C.; Leung, C.P.H.; Ma, E.S.K.; Pang, R.; Chua, D.; Chu, K.M.; Law, W.L.; et al. Circulating microRNAs as Specific Biomarkers for Breast Cancer Detection. *PLoS ONE* **2013**, *8*. [CrossRef]
28. Thakur, S.; Grover, R.K.; Gupta, S.; Yadav, A.K.; Das, B.C. Identification of Specific miRNA Signature in Paired Sera and Tissue Samples of Indian Women with Triple Negative Breast Cancer. *PLoS ONE* **2016**, *11*. [CrossRef]
29. Kodahl, A.R.; Lyng, M.B.; Binder, H.; Cold, S.; Gravgaard, K.; Knoop, A.S.; Ditzel, H.J. Novel circulating microRNA signature as a potential non-invasive multi-marker test in ER-positive early-stage breast cancer: A case control study. *Mol. Oncol.* **2014**, *8*, 874–883. [CrossRef]
30. Chan, M.; Liaw, C.S.; Ji, S.M.; Tan, H.H.; Wong, C.Y.; Thike, A.A.; Tan, P.H.; Ho, G.H.; Lee, A.S.G. Identification of Circulating MicroRNA Signatures for Breast Cancer Detection. *Clin. Cancer Res.* **2013**, *19*, 4477–4487. [CrossRef]
31. Wang, K.; Yuan, Y.; Cho, J.H.; McClarty, S.; Baxter, D.; Galas, D.J. Comparing the MicroRNA Spectrum between Serum and Plasma. *PLoS ONE* **2012**, *7*. [CrossRef] [PubMed]
32. Wang, H.J.; Tan, G.; Dong, L.; Cheng, L.; Li, K.J.; Wang, Z.Y.; Luo, H.F. Circulating MiR-125b as a Marker Predicting Chemoresistance in Breast Cancer. *PLoS ONE* **2012**, *7*. [CrossRef] [PubMed]
33. Mar-Aguilar, F.; Mendoza-Ramirez, J.A.; Malagon-Santiago, I.; Espino-Silva, P.K.; Santuario-Facio, S.K.; Ruiz-Flores, P.; Rodriguez-Padilla, C.; Resendez-Perez, D. Serum circulating microRNA profiling for identification of potential breast cancer biomarkers. *Dis. Mark.* **2013**, *34*, 163–169. [CrossRef]
34. Liu, B.Q.; Su, F.; Chen, M.W.; Li, Y.; Qi, X.Y.; Xiao, J.B.; Li, X.M.; Liu, X.C.; Liang, W.T.; Zhang, Y.F.; et al. Serum miR-21 and miR-125b as markers predicting neoadjuvant chemotherapy response and prognosis in stage II/III breast cancer. *Hum. Pathol.* **2017**, *64*, 44–52. [CrossRef] [PubMed]
35. Catalano, O.A.; Horn, G.L.; Signore, A.; Iannace, C.; Lepore, M.; Vangel, M.; Luongo, A.; Catalano, M.; Lehman, C.; Salvatore, M.; et al. PET/MR in invasive ductal breast cancer: Correlation between imaging markers and histological phenotype. *Br. J. Cancer* **2017**, *116*, 893–902. [CrossRef] [PubMed]
36. Almeida, M.I.; Calin, G.A. The miR-143/miR-145 cluster and the tumor microenvironment: Unexpected roles. *Genome Med.* **2016**, *8*. [CrossRef]

37. Berindan-Neagoe, I.; Calin, G.A. Molecular Pathways: MicroRNAs, Cancer Cells, and Microenvironment. *Clin. Cancer Res.* **2014**, *20*, 6247–6253. [CrossRef]
38. Li, Y.; Wang, Y.; Fan, H.; Zhang, Z.; Li, N. miR-125b-5p inhibits breast cancer cell proliferation, migration and invasion by targeting KIAA1522. *Biochem. Biophys. Res. Commun.* **2018**, *504*, 277–282. [CrossRef]
39. Feliciano, A.; Castellvi, J.; Artero-Castro, A.; Leal, J.A.; Romagosa, C.; Hernandez-Losa, J.; Peg, V.; Fabra, A.; Vidal, F.; Kondoh, H.; et al. miR-125b Acts as a Tumor Suppressor in Breast Tumorigenesis via Its Novel Direct Targets ENPEP, CK2-alpha, CCNJ, and MEGF9. *PLoS ONE* **2013**, *8*. [CrossRef]
40. Koboldt, D.C.; Fulton, R.S.; McLellan, M.D.; Schmidt, H.; Kalicki-Veizer, J.; McMichael, J.F.; Fulton, L.L.; Dooling, D.J.; Ding, L.; Mardis, E.R.; et al. Comprehensive molecular portraits of human breast tumours. *Nature* **2012**, *490*, 61–70. [CrossRef]
41. Parker, J.S.; Mullins, M.; Cheang, M.C.U.; Leung, S.; Voduc, D.; Vickery, T.; Davies, S.; Fauron, C.; He, X.; Hu, Z.; et al. Supervised Risk Predictor of Breast Cancer Based on Intrinsic Subtypes. *J. Clin. Oncol.* **2009**, *27*, 1160–1167. [CrossRef] [PubMed]
42. Molina, R.; Barak, V.; van Dalen, A.; Duffy, M.J.; Einarsson, R.; Gion, M.; Goike, H.; Lamerz, R.; Nap, M.; Soletormos, G.; et al. Tumor markers in breast cancer—European Group on Tumor Markers recommendations. *Tumor Biol.* **2005**, *26*, 281–293. [CrossRef] [PubMed]
43. Mirabelli, P.; Incoronato, M. Usefulness of Traditional Serum Biomarkers for Management of Breast Cancer Patients. *Biomed Res. Int.* **2013**. [CrossRef] [PubMed]
44. Liu, C.; Sun, B.; Xu, B.; Meng, X.; Li, L.; Cong, Y.; Liu, J.; Wang, Q.; Xuan, L.; Song, Q.; et al. A panel containing PD-1, IL-2R alpha, IL-10, and CA15-3 as a biomarker to discriminate breast cancer from benign breast disease. *Cancer Manag. Res.* **2018**, *10*, 1749–1761. [CrossRef] [PubMed]
45. Zaleski, M.; Kobilay, M.; Schroeder, L.; Debald, M.; Semaan, A.; Hettwer, K.; Uhlig, S.; Kuhn, W.; Hartmann, G.; Holdenrieder, S. Improved sensitivity for detection of breast cancer by combination of miR-34a and tumor markers CA 15-3 or CEA. *Oncotarget* **2018**, *9*, 22523–22536. [CrossRef] [PubMed]
46. Zajkowska, M.; Glazewska, E.K.; Bedkowska, G.E.; Chorazy, P.; Szmitkowski, M.; Lawicki, S. Diagnostic Power of Vascular Endothelial Growth Factor and Macrophage Colony-Stimulating Factor in Breast Cancer Patients Based on ROC Analysis. *Mediat. Inflamm.* **2016**. [CrossRef]
47. Kirschner, M.B.; Edelman, J.J.B.; Kao, S.C.H.; Vallely, M.P.; van Zandwijk, N.; Reid, G. The Impact of Hemolysis on Cell-Free microRNA Biomarkers. *Front. Genet.* **2013**, *4*, 94. [CrossRef] [PubMed]
48. Catalano, O.A.; Rosen, B.R.; Sahani, D.V.; Hahn, P.F.; Guimaraes, A.R.; Vangel, M.G.; Nicolai, E.; Soricelli, A.; Salvatore, M. Clinical Impact of PET/MR Imaging in Patients with Cancer Undergoing Same-Day PET/CT: Initial Experience in 134 Patients-A Hypothesis-generating Exploratory Study. *Radiology* **2013**, *269*, 857–869. [CrossRef]
49. Pace, L.; Nicolai, E.; Luongo, A.; Aiello, M.; Catalano, O.A.; Soricelli, A.; Salvatore, M. Comparison of whole-body PET/CT and PET/MRI in breast cancer patients: Lesion detection and quantitation of 18F-deoxyglucose uptake in lesions and in normal organ tissues. *Eur. J. Radiol.* **2014**, *83*, 289–296. [CrossRef]
50. Veronesi, U.; Zurrida, S.; Viale, G.; Galimberti, V.; Arnone, P.; Nole, F. Rethinking TNM: A Breast Cancer Classification to Guide to Treatment and Facilitate Research. *Breast J.* **2009**, *15*, 291–295. [CrossRef]
51. Inglese, M.; Cavaliere, C.; Monti, S.; Forte, E.; Incoronato, M.; Nicolai, E.; Salvatore, M.; Aiello, M. A multi-parametric PET/MRI study of breast cancer: Evaluation of DCE-MRI pharmacokinetic models and correlation with diffusion and functional parameters. *NMR Biomed.* **2018**, e4026. [CrossRef] [PubMed]
52. Monti, S.; Aiello, M.; Incoronato, M.; Grimaldi, A.M.; Moscarino, M.; Mirabelli, P.; Ferbo, U.; Cavaliere, C.; Salvatore, M. DCE-MRI Pharmacokinetic-Based Phenotyping of Invasive Ductal Carcinoma: A Radiomic Study for Prediction of Histological Outcomes. *Contrast Media Mol. Imaging* **2018**. [CrossRef] [PubMed]
53. Mirabelli, P.; Incoronato, M.; Coppola, L.; Infante, T.; Parente, C.A.; Nicolai, E.; Soricelli, A.; Salvatore, M. SDN biobank: Bioresource of human samples associated with functional and/or morphological bioimaging results for the study of oncological, cardiological, neurological, and metabolic diseases. *Open J. Bioresour.* **2017**, *4*. [CrossRef]
54. Bellingham, S.A.; Coleman, B.M.; Hill, A.F. Small RNA deep sequencing reveals a distinct miRNA signature released in exosomes from prion-infected neuronal cells. *Nucleic Acids Res.* **2012**, *40*, 10937–10949. [CrossRef] [PubMed]

55. Pfaffl, M.W.; Tichopad, A.; Prgomet, C.; Neuvians, T.P. Determination of stable housekeeping genes, differentially regulated target genes and sample integrity: BestKeeper—Excel-based tool using pair-wise correlations. *Biotechnol. Lett.* **2004**, *26*, 509–515. [CrossRef] [PubMed]
56. Colaprico, A.; Silva, T.C.; Olsen, C.; Garofano, L.; Cava, C.; Garolini, D.; Sabedot, T.S.; Malta, T.M.; Pagnotta, S.M.; Castiglioni, I.; et al. TCGAbiolinks: An R/Bioconductor package for integrative analysis of TCGA data. *Nucleic Acids Res.* **2016**, *44*. [CrossRef] [PubMed]

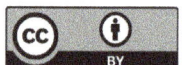 © 2019 by the authors. Licensee MDPI, Basel, Switzerland. This article is an open access article distributed under the terms and conditions of the Creative Commons Attribution (CC BY) license (http://creativecommons.org/licenses/by/4.0/).

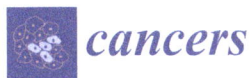

Article

Automated Definition of Skeletal Disease Burden in Metastatic Prostate Carcinoma: A 3D Analysis of SPECT/CT Images

Francesco Fiz [1,*], Helmut Dittmann [1], Cristina Campi [2], Matthias Weissinger [1], Samine Sahbai [3], Matthias Reimold [1], Arnulf Stenzl [4], Michele Piana [5], Gianmario Sambuceti [6] and Christian la Fougère [1,7]

1. Department of Nuclear Medicine and Clinical Molecular Imaging, University Hospital Tübingen, 72076 Tübingen, Germany; helmut.dittmann@med.uni-tuebingen.de (H.D.); matthias.weissinger@med.uni-tuebingen.de (M.W.); Matthias.Reimold@med.uni-tuebingen.de (M.R.); christian.lafougere@med.uni-tuebingen.de (C.l.F.)
2. Department of Medicine-DIMED, Nuclear Medicine Unit, University Hospital of Padua, 35128 Padua, Italy; cristina.campi@gmail.com
3. Nuclear Medicine Unit, Hospital Universitaire Henri Mondor, 94010 Créteil, France; sam.sahbai@gmail.com
4. Department of Urology, University Hospital Tübingen, 72076 Tübingen, Germany; urologie@med.uni-tuebingen.de
5. Department of Mathematics, University of Genoa, 16146 Genoa, Italy; piana@dima.unige.it
6. Department of Health Sciences, Nuclear Medicine Unit, University of Genoa, 16146 Genoa, Italy; sambuceti@unige.it
7. iFIT Cluster of Excellence, University of Tübingen, 72076 Tübingen, Germany
* Correspondence: Francesco.Fiz@med.uni-tuebingen.de; Tel.: +49-07071-29-86410

Received: 22 May 2019; Accepted: 19 June 2019; Published: 21 June 2019

Abstract: To meet the current need for skeletal tumor-load estimation in castration-resistant prostate cancer (CRPC), we developed a novel approach based on adaptive bone segmentation. In this study, we compared the program output with existing estimates and with the radiological outcome. Seventy-six whole-body single-photon emission computed tomographies/x-ray computed tomography with 3,3-diphosphono-1,2-propanedicarboxylic acid from mCRPC patients were analyzed. The software identified the whole skeletal volume (S_{Vol}) and classified the voxels metastases (M_{Vol}) or normal bone (B_{Vol}). S_{Vol} was compared with the estimation of a commercial software. M_{Vol} was compared with manual assessment and with prostate specific antigen (PSA) levels. Counts/voxel were extracted from M_{Vol} and B_{Vol}. After six cycles of ^{223}RaCl2-therapy every patient was re-evaluated as having progressive disease (PD), stable disease (SD), or a partial response (PR). S_{Vol} correlated with that of the commercial software (R = 0.99, $p < 0.001$). M_{Vol} correlated with the manually-counted lesions (R = 0.61, $p < 0.001$) and PSA (R = 0.46, $p < 0.01$). PD had a lower counts/voxel in M_{Vol} than PR/SD (715 ± 190 vs. 975 ± 215 and 1058 ± 255, $p < 0.05$ and $p < 0.01$) and B_{Vol} (PD 275 ± 60, PR 515 ± 188 and SD 528 ± 162 counts/voxel, $p < 0.001$). Segmentation-based tumor load correlated with radiological/laboratory indices. Uptake was linked with the clinical outcome, suggesting that metastases in PD patients have a lower affinity for bone-seeking radionuclides and might benefit less from bone-targeted radioisotope therapies.

Keywords: mCRPC; SPECT/CT; Computer-assisted diagnosis; XOFIGO; Therapy response assessment

1. Introduction

Castration-resistant prostate cancer (CRPC) is defined by rising prostate specific antigen (PSA) levels under androgen blockade and by the eventual diffuse metastatic spread [1–3]. In these patients, skeletal metastases can represent the most relevant prognostic factor, by impairing the static function of the skeleton and by reducing the available space for hematopoiesis [4–6].

Diffuse skeletal CRPC metastatization, once considered a terminal diagnosis, can today be managed by many different approaches, including new-generations of taxanes, second-line hormonal therapy, and radioisotope treatments [7–12]. As these medications might have varying effectiveness and cause different side effects, the choice of therapy sequence usually requires multidisciplinary disease-management. Nevertheless, the most effective sequence of systemic treatments is still a matter of discussion and patient-specific components are likely to play a relevant role [13–15].

Being able to assess treatment response reliably is a pre-requisite for therapy selection and sequencing. Response evaluation may be performed either by analyzing tumor marker blood levels or by serial imaging. Serum PSA level is the most used marker, but alkaline phosphatase might also be helpful in assessing metastasis-dependent bone turnover [16,17].

Circulating markers are, however, dependent on the degree of tumor differentiation and can be altered by concomitant therapies [18–20]. On the other hand, evaluating medical imaging, whether morphological or radioisotope-based, can be challenging in the presence of a high number of metastases or in case of therapy-related changes, such as the "flare" phenomenon [21].

Obtaining an automated evaluation of the skeletal tumor burden is one of the greatest current unmet clinical needs; in recent years, an increasing number of software applications have been developed for this purpose [22]. Existing applications are mostly based on automated thresholding, using standardized uptake value on positron emission tomography (PET) or count values on bone scans; in this setting, telling apart metastases-related uptake from other non-malignant sources of increased bone turnover can be challenging.

To improve the reliability of metastases detection and to obtain a reliable estimation of tumor load, we developed a specific computational tool based on segmentation analysis. This algorithm uses the computed tomography (CT) information to identify and segment all hyperdense localizations within the skeletal system automatically to define the overall metastatic bone compartment. In a second step, information from the co-registered single-photon emission computed tomography (SPECT) or PET images can be extracted for this volume. In this study, we tested this approach on a series of CRPC patients and validated the analysis against different clinical parameters.

2. Results

2.1. Volumetric Assessment and Comparison between Systems

The estimate of total osseous tissue (skeletal volume S_{Vol}, sum of metastases volume M_{Vol}, trabecular volume B_{Vol}, and cortical volume C_{Vol}) showed a tight concordance between our software (EXCALIBUR, University of Genoa, Genoa, Italy) and the commercial application. Mean global skeletal volume was in fact 3875 ± 1513 mL and 3881 ± 1499 mL as measured by the commercial software application and by our computational program, respectively (R = 0.99, $p < 0.001$). Mean counts/voxel were 439 ± 71 and 435 ± 61, respectively, with an R correlation index of 0.92 ($p < 0.001$, data not shown). Mean M_{Vol} was 362 ± 249 mL (range 85–1194 mL), corresponding to 27 ± 20% of the total trabecular bone.

The majority of tumor burden was located within the axial skeleton and in the hipbones (M_{Vol} 335 ± 140 mL); 61 patients (81%) had skeletal localizations within the appendicular long bones (M_{Vol} 32 ± 19 mL).

2.2. Volume Characteristics

Mean Hounsfield density was comparable for M_{Vol} (590 ± 136) and C_{Vol} (531 ± 92) but was significantly lower for B_{Vol} (251 ± 78, $p < 0.001$). Higher tracer activity was measured within M_{Vol} (939 ± 279 mean counts/voxel), as compared to B_{Vol} (462 ± 196 mean counts/voxel, $p < 0.001$). Activity concentration within C_{Vol} was even lower (271 ± 106 mean counts/voxel), see Table 1. Mean counts/voxel were directly correlated to mean Hounsfielf Units (HU) for both M_{Vol} (R = 0.52, p < 0.01) and B_{Vol} (R = 0.74, p < 0.001, Figure 1).

Table 1. Radiological and laboratory parameters in patients with or without superscan.

Parameter	All Patients	Superscan	Non-Superscan	p-Value
Mean M_{Vol} (mL)	357 ± 257	527 ± 304	245 ± 187	<0.001
Number of counted lesions	74 ± 30	106 ± 22	61 ± 23	<0.001
INV%	27 ± 20%	40 ± 23%	21 ± 16%	<0.01
PSA (ng/mL)	539 ± 754	1235 ± 959	257 ± 407	<0.001
B_{Vol} mean counts/voxel	466 ± 198	565 ± 243	428 ± 164	NS
M_{Vol} mean counts/voxel	947 ± 277	1104 ± 291	886 ± 251	<0.05
B_{Vol} mean HU	251 ± 78	319 ± 78	223 ± 59	<0.01
M_{Vol} mean HU	590 ± 136	693 ± 132	549 ± 115	<0.001

M_{Vol}: Metastases Volume; INV%: Invasion% or M_{Vol}/B_{Vol} ratio PSA: Prostate-specific antigen; B_{Vol}: Trabecular bone volume; HU: Hounsfield Unit.

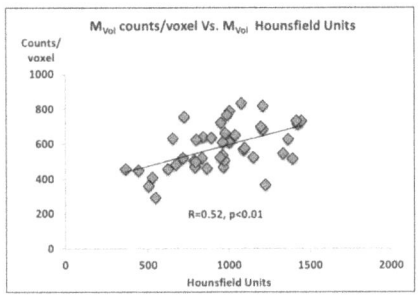
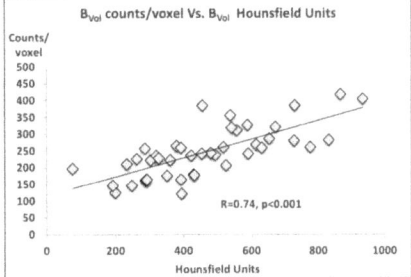
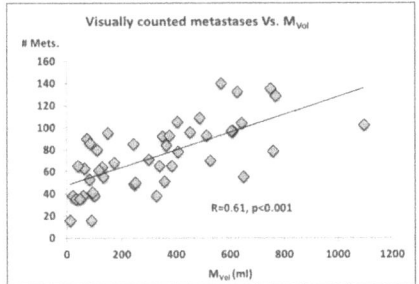
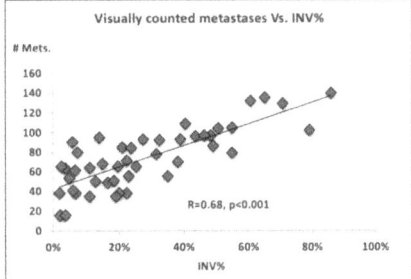

Figure 1. Correlation between counts/voxel and Hounsfield density as well as between volumes and number of metastases. A higher density corresponded to higher mean counts/voxel (top panels). Furthermore, a close correlation was observed between the volumetric estimates and the manual count of metastatic lesions (bottom panels). M_{Vol} = voxels metastases; B_{Vol} = normal bone; INV% = percent of bone invaded by metastases (M_{Vol}/B_{Vol}).

2.3. Tumor Volume, Number of Lesions, and PSA Level

The software based semi-automatic lesion identification (M_{Vol}) and the manual lesion count showed a tight correlation, for the whole skeletal system (R = 0.61, p < 0.001, Figure 1) and the axial segments (R = 0.64, p < 0.001), but not for the appendicular ones (R = 0.07, p = 0.52). Likewise, the number of manually counted lesions correlated with the percent of invasion of the trabecular bone by metastases (INV%) within the whole (R = 0.68) as well as axial (R = 0.69) skeleton, p < 0.001, Figure 1.

Remarkably, PSA level as a marker of tumor load correlated with our measures of bone involvement (M_{Vol} R = 0.46, p < 0.01; number of manually counted lesions R = 0.67, p < 0.001; mean HU of M_{Vol} R = 0.42, p < 0.01; mean HU B_{Vol} R = 0.52, p < 0.001; and M_{Vol}/B_{Vol} ratio R = 0.75, p < 0.001).

2.4. Impact of Superscan Status

Twelve patients (16%) were classified as superscan. CRPC patients with a superscan had a higher mean HU than non-superscan patients in B_{Vol} ($p < 0.001$ Figure 2) as well as in M_{Vol} ($p < 0.01$, Figure 2).

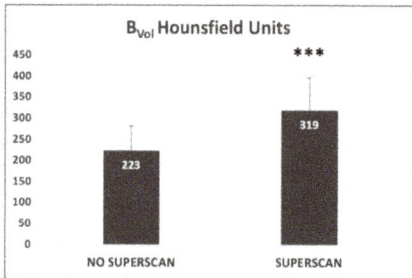
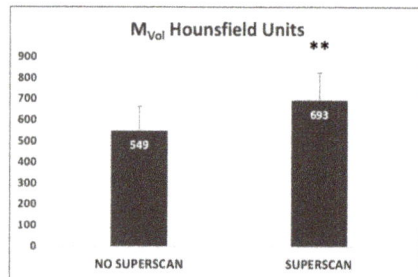
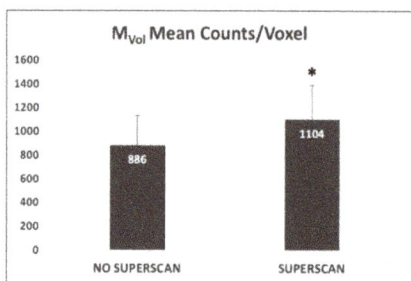
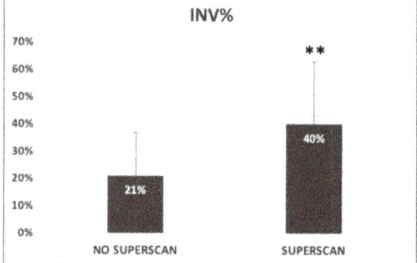

Figure 2. Comparison between superscan and non-superscan patients. Superscan subjects showed a higher density in trabecular bone volume (B_{Vol}) as well as in metastases volume (M_{Vol}) (upper panels). A higher counting rate was observed in the M_{Vol} of superscan patients (bottom left). Finally, percent of trabecular bone space invaded by metastatic lesions was higher in the superscan subjects (bottom right). * $p < 0.05$, ** $p < 0.01$, *** $p < 0.001$. INV% Percent of bone invaded by metastases (M_{Vol}/B_{Vol}).

Mean counts/voxel in M_{Vol} were higher in superscan subjects than in non-superscan (1104 ± 291 vs. 886 ± 251, $p < 0.05$, Figure 2); conversely, mean counts/voxel in B_{Vol} were not significantly different between the two subpopulations.

Finally, superscan was associated with a higher INV% of trabecular bone by osteoblastic lesions (M_{Vol}/B_{Vol} ratio: 40 ± 23% vs. 21 ± 16%, $p < 0.01$, Figure 5), which was reflected, at qualitative analysis, by a higher number of visually observable metastases (Number of metastases = 106 ± 22 vs. 61 ± 23, $p < 0.001$). See Table 1 for a detailed analysis.

2.5. Therapy Response Assessment

According to the response assessment criteria, which are further detailed in the Material and Methods, 21 patients (28%) were classified with progressive disease (PD), while 35 subjects (46%) were classified with stable disease (SD), and 20 patients (26%) with a partial response (PR).

Patients who presented a PD status after the therapy completion exhibited a markedly lower activity in the M_{Vol} (715 ± 190 counts) in the pre-therapy scan, when compared to those with PR (N = 20, 975 ± 215 counts, $p < 0.05$) or SD (N = 35, 1058 ± 255 counts, $p < 0.01$). Of note, similar findings were found within B_{Vol}, where patients with PD displayed the lowest activity (PD 275 ± 60, PR 515 ± 188 and SD 528 ± 162 counts, $p < 0.001$). See Figure 3.

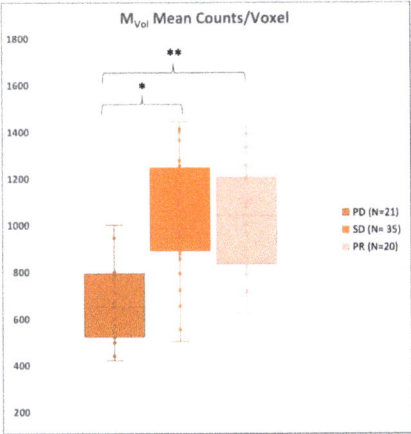
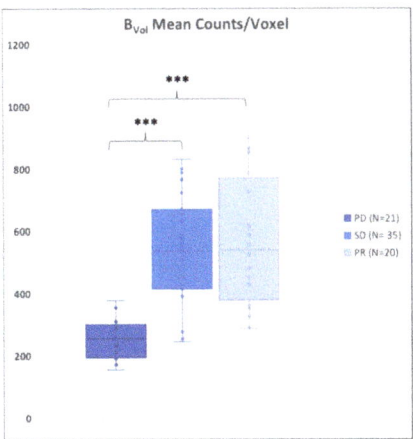

Figure 3. Radioactivity concentration according to response. Patients with progressive disease (PD) after the radioisotope therapy displayed a significantly lower radioactivity concentration at the baseline imaging in metastases volume (M_{Vol}) as well as in trabecular bone volume (B_{Vol}). * $p < 0.05$, ** $p < 0.01$, *** $p < 0.001$. SD = stable disease; PR = partial response.

At receiver operating characteristics (ROC) analysis, both M_{Vol} and B_{Vol} mean counts/voxel were predictive of therapy effectiveness (M_{Vol} 0.895 and B_{Vol} 0.943 for, $p < 0.001$). The best threshold value of mean counts/voxel for discriminating patients with progressive disease was in fact 805 in the M_{Vol} (sensitivity 84%, specificity 81%) and 385 in the B_{Vol} (sensitivity 84%, specificity 100%). No differences were observed in absolute volume of metastases (M_{Vol}) across the therapy outcome groups. See Figure 4.

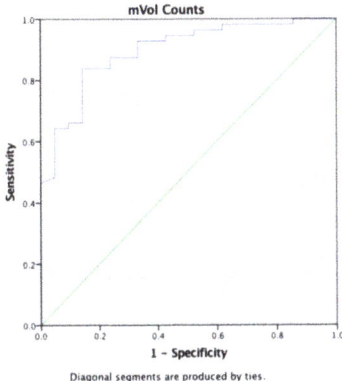
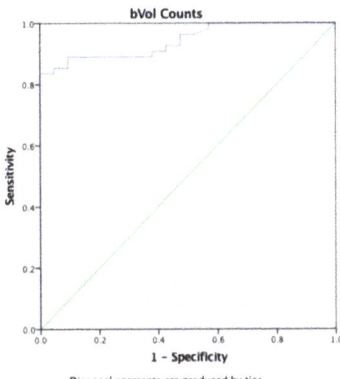

Figure 4. Receiver operating characteristics (ROC) curve of metastases volume (M_{Vol}) and trabecular bone volume (B_{Vol}) counts/voxel values according to progression. Radioactivity concentration was able to discriminate patients with a progressive disease in M_{Vol} as well as in B_{Vol}.

Patients presenting a superscan pattern of radioactivity distribution were evenly distributed among the three groups (PD: 3/21 or 14%, SD 6/35 or 17%, and PR 3/20 15%, p = non significant.

PSA levels showed considerable variations during the therapy. On average, starting from staging to the end of the therapy, it increased by 135 ± 99% in PD patients and by 27 ± 81% in PR subjects. Conversely, PSA decreased by 40 ± 16% in SD patients. However, due to the marked spread of the

PSA-level course among patients, no statistically significant difference could be demonstrated among these groups.

See Table 2 for a detailed analysis.

Table 2. Radiological and laboratory parameters according to response.

Parameter	PD	SD	PR	PD vs. PR	PD vs. SD	PR vs. SD
Mean M_{Vol} (mL)	245 ± 312	342 ± 203	373 ± 254	NS	NS	NS
Number of counted lesions	56 ± 25	80 ± 33	79 ± 26	NS	NS	NS
M_{Vol}/B_{Vol}	19 ± 8%	29 ± 17%	31 ± 23	NS	NS	NS
PSA (ng/mL)	353 ± 540	446 ± 539	746 ± 1004	NS	NS	NS
B_{Vol} mean counts/voxel	275 ± 60	528 ± 162	515 ± 188	<0.001	<0.001	NS
M_{Vol} mean counts/voxel	715 ± 190	1058 ± 255	975 ± 219	<0.05	<0.01	NS
B_{Vol} mean HU	232 ± 81	253 ± 68	264 ± 82	NS	NS	NS
M_{Vol} mean HU	545 ± 157	605 ± 120	610 ± 127	NS	NS	NS

PD: Progressive disease; SD: Stable disease; PR: Partial response; M_{Vol}: Metastases volume; INV%: Invasion% or M_{Vol}/B_{Vol}; PSA: Prostate-specific antigen; B_{Vol}: trabecular bone volume; HU: Hounsfield Units.

3. Discussion

The present paper describes a computational approach to the problem of skeletal tumor burden quantification by means of SPECT/CT data. The robustness of the bone recognition was testified by the tight correlation between the total bone volume as detected by our approach and by a commercial application. The automated identification of bone tumor volume could not be compared with a reference standard, as, to the best of our knowledge, a commercially available CT-based tumor burden estimator does not yet exist. However, the estimates provided by this software tool show a tight concordance with the traditional measures of tumor burden performed with imaging and blood tests.

In our analysis, we considered both the raw figure of tumor volume as well as the percent of invasion, in other words, the ratio between tumor and trabecular volume. Both estimators strongly correlated with the number of manually counted lesions as well as with the PSA values.

As expected, patients with a superscan status at planar bone scans presented a higher tumor volume as well as a higher percent of trabecular bone invaded by bone metastases. These patients presented also a higher bone metastases density and counting rate; however, mean counts in trabecular bone did not significantly differ from those in the trabecular bone of non-superscan patients.

However, the distribution of radioactivity into the metastases, as well as into the trabecular bone, appears to play an important role in the therapeutic effectiveness of ^{223}RaCl$_2$. Previous studies have in fact shown that the distribution of the bone scan tracers mirrors that of ^{223}RaCl$_2$ [23,24]. In our population, patients who were found to have a disease progression at the end of the therapy presented a lower counting rate at the baseline SPECT/CT not only within the known tumor lesions, but also in the trabecular bone. It might be hypothesized that a lower counting rate at SPECT/CT could correspond to a lesser ^{223}RaCl$_2$ avidity and thus to a reduced absorbed dose. Thus, one might hypothesize that micrometastases (if present) in trabecular bone exhibiting only a low counting rate will receive an insufficient therapeutic dose. It is worth noting that tumor volume was conversely and not significantly different across patients with partial response, stable, or progressive disease. As a consequence, semi-quantitative evaluation of bone tracer uptake at baseline might be useful for ^{223}RaCl$_2$ therapy stratification.

Patients presenting with a superscan finding were equally distributed in the three response groups, in other words, the presence of a superscan was not per se associated with imaging-based therapy response in our population. Actually, the role of this imaging feature in predicting therapy response in patients treated with ^{223}RaCl$_2$ has not been extensively studied. A previous report demonstrated a trend for shorter survival in those patients when compared to those with less than six metastases [25]; however, the relatively low frequency of this condition does not allow us to reach definite conclusions, unless large-scale studies are planned. Nonetheless, our data might suggest that some superscan patients might indeed benefit from a ^{223}RaCl$_2$ treatment.

The robustness of the generated volumetric data and the clinical relevance of the information that has been derived from this analysis suggest a relevant potential for the computer-enhanced evaluation of tumor burden. The relevance of such approaches is testified to by the growing number of computer-assisted techniques, which have been developed in the last few decades to estimate the tumor burden [22]. Different approaches have been presented, for example, the bone-scan index, which is designed to be applied to planar bone scintigraphy [26], but was subject to false-positive findings in the event of a flare phenomenon [27]. Moreover, new 3D-segmentation algorithms have been introduced for PET/CT, one based on a ^{18}F-NaF PET-threshold and requiring specific threshold determination for each individual scanner [28], the other using the tracer uptake of ^{68}Ga-PSMA (prostate-specific membrane antigen) [29], that might be of special interest for upcoming, but currently not approved, PSMA radio-ligand therapies. The main difference of our approach lies on the use of CT-density contrast instead of the PET information for defining tumor volume as well as the applicability to any CT-based hybrid imaging, PET/CT and SPECT/CT, the latter being more widely available and less cost intensive, which is a major advantage of our current approach with SPECT/CT. Finally, the use of bone seeking tracers might better reflect the uptake of ^{223}RaCl$_2$ and thus predict the radiation to the metastases. One algorithm included a segmentation.

Some limitations have to be mentioned. A possible source of error could be a misclassification of non-tumor-related bone thickening [30]. The application automatically excludes non-bone hyperdensity (e.g., vascular calcification) from the edge detection. Likewise, voxel belonging to the spinal canal and hypodense areas (such as bone cysts) are also sorted out. Our approach was shown to be congruent with the estimation of bone volume as provided by a standard commercial software. However, a comparison to an independent imaging-based reference standard provided by means of magnetic resonance or PSMA-PET/CT was not available. Moreover, comparison with other approved methods of tumor load determination, based on planar data, such as the bone scan index [31], was not possible because of their intrinsic difference.

Another significant limitation is that in the SPECT/CT analysis, the limited resolution of the single-photon technique could underestimate the counts in smaller volumes. Finally, we evaluated the therapy response only in subjects who completed the entire ^{223}RaCl$_2$ therapy. This decision was made in order to have a homogenous population and to be able to perform a therapy effectiveness evaluation at the same time point after baseline staging. However, this choice excluded patients who interrupted the therapy due to tumor-progress or because of toxicity; therefore, the information presented in this manuscript applies only to the patient population with a relatively better prognosis [32]. Further studies could shed light on the correlation among tumor load, tracer distribution, and overall survival in patients with in-therapy progression.

4. Materials and Methods

4.1. Patient Population

Seventy-six consecutive patients suffering from CRPC, who underwent whole-body ^{99m}Tc-bisphosphonate-SPECT/CT (mean age 69.5 ± 7, age range 55.5–80.8), were retrospectively analyzed. All examinations were performed for staging in patients with multiple bone lesions, before radionuclide therapy using ^{223}RaCl2. Inclusion criteria comprised histologically confirmed prostate cancer, evidence of prostate specific antigen (PSA) increase under maximal androgen blockade, and presence of clinically symptomatic as well as radiologically confirmed osteoblastic skeletal metastases. Exclusion criteria were the presence of metal implants impeding the analysis of either the axial or the appendicular skeleton (e.g., bilateral total hip replacement, extensive spondylosyndesis, etc.), absence of a signed informed consent, and inability to complete the planned six cycles of ^{223}RaCl$_2$-therapy.

Any previous therapy or combination of treatments was admitted. The PSA level at the time of the scan was recorded.

All patients gave written informed consent for the retrospective analysis of the pseudonymized clinical SPECT/CT data. The investigations were conducted in accordance with the Helsinki Declaration and with national regulations, after approval by the ethics committee of the University of Tübingen. All patients signed a specific consent form, detailing the use of imaging as well as of laboratory data for research purposes.

4.2. Patients' Follow Up

Patients were followed up with throughout the execution of the radionuclide therapy, which included six ^{223}RaCl$_2$ administrations (one per month). A whole-body SPECT/CT scan was carried out at the end of therapy. This scan was re-evaluated by an experienced viewer who was blinded to the results of the computational analysis and who stratified the patients according to therapy response as follows: if new lesions were detected (whether on CT or in the SPECT images), the case was classified as progressive disease (PD). On the contrary, if no new lesions were observed, the patient was considered having a stable disease (SD). Finally, if no new lesions were observed and the uptake intensity was visibly diminished, the case was judged as partial response (PR). This study was approved by the Local Ethics Committee of the University of Tübinngen (No. 747/2017BO1) on 9 March 2015.

4.3. Scan Protocol

Patients were scanned on a hybrid SPECT/CT device (Discovery 670 Pro, GE Healthcare, Chicago, IL, USA), three hours after injection of 8–10 MBq/Kg of ^{99m}Tc-3,3-diphosphono-1,2-propanedicarboxylic acid (CIS bio, Berlin, Germany). To minimize artifacts caused by the presence of radioactive urine in the excretory system, patients were asked to drink at least 1000 mL of water during the uptake time and to void immediately before the scan. No urinary bladder catheterization was used.

The acquisition protocol comprised a whole-body planar scan. This part was followed by a whole-body SPECT/CT scan, from vertex up to mid-distal femur, which was obtained by reconstructing and fusing three sequential fields-of-view on a dedicated workstation (Xeleris 3®, GE Healthcare, Chicago, IL, USA). SPECT acquisition was carried out with the two camera heads in H-Mode; parameters for each field-of-view were as follows: energy window 140.5 ± 1 0%, angular step 6°, time per step 15″. The transaxial field-of-view and pixel size of the reconstructed SPECT images were 54 cm and 5 × 5 mm, respectively, with a matrix size of 128 × 128. SPECT raw data were reconstructed using ordered-subset expectation maximization iterative protocol (2 iterations, 10 subsets).

The technical parameters of the 16-detector row, helical CT scanner included a gantry rotation speed of 0.8 s and a table speed of 20 mm per gantry rotation. The scan was performed at 120 kV voltage and 10–80 mA current. A dose modulation system (OptiDose®, GE Healthcare, Chicago, IL, USA) was applied to optimize total exposure according to the patient's body size. No contrast medium was injected.

4.4. Image Analysis

Segmentation of bone volumes was performed on the CT data according to the previously validated method [33–35]. Briefly, the algorithm identified the skeleton on CT images by assuming that compact bone is the structure with the highest X-ray attenuation coefficient in the human body. This assumption implies a stark HU value difference between soft tissue and cortical bone. The program functions by reading the HU values of every voxel in any given slice horizontally; when it encounters a sharp variation of HU density, it assumes that it had reached the bone outer border. From that point, it samples a 2-pixel ring, which corresponds to the cortical bone. It then samples the average density of this cortical bone volume. Thereafter, it categorizes every voxel on the inside of this volume as trabecular bone (bone volume, B_{Vol}) or as osteoblastic metastases volume (M_{Vol}). This is done by using the mean density of the cortical volume as the cutoff value, assuming the osteoblastic metastases will have an average density at least equal to that of cortical bone. Therefore, the final output of this process consists of the following volumes:

- Cortical Volume (C_{Vol}): the bone surface
- Trabecular Volume (B_{Vol}): the normal trabecular bone
- Metastases Volume (M_{Vol}): osteoblastic metastases (tumor burden)
- Skeletal Volume (S_{Vol}): entire skeletal volume (sum of C_{Vol}, B_{Vol}, and M_{Vol})
- %INV: percent of invasion (M_{Vol}/B_{Vol} ratio)

A graphical overview of the segmentation process and an example of the program's work on the original slices are shown in Figures 5 and 6.

For details on the mathematical rationale underlying the bone recognition algorithm, please see the original work from Sambuceti et al. [33]. For an overview on the principle of tumor burden estimation, we refer to our previous work [6].

After an initial automatic segmentation, the program displayed the resulting images to the operator, who could manually exclude all benign hyperdensities (e.g., osteochondrosis, osteophytes, metal implants). Purely lytic areas, having a HU inferior to 30, were automatically removed.

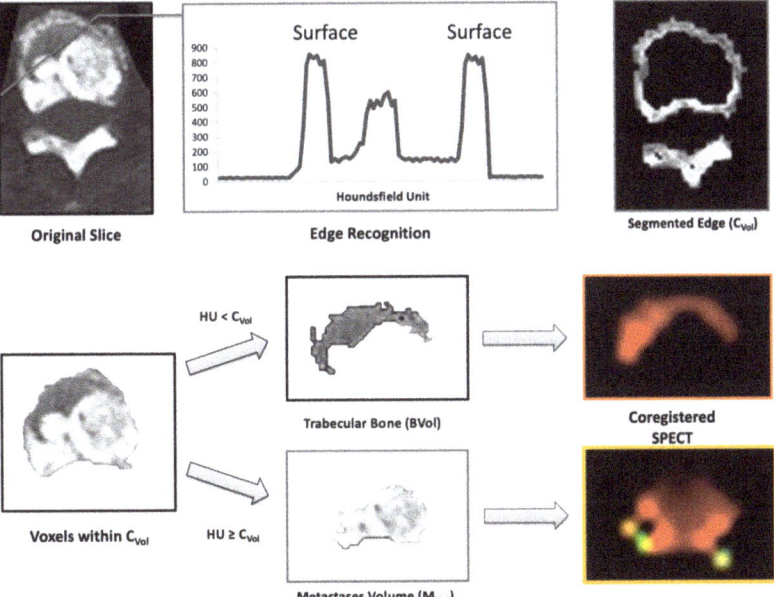

Figure 5. Functioning of the segmentation process. The software analyzes sequentially the Hounsfield Unit (HU) density of voxel within a single slice (top left). The bone border is identified as an increase of HU values (top center). After definition of the cortical volume (C_{Vol}, top right), its mean HU density is calculated. This value is used to classify all voxels located on the inside of C_{Vol} as pertinent to bone metastases (M_{Vol}) or to normal trabecular bone (B_{Vol}, middle and left bottom panels). Afterwards, mean counts/voxel are extracted from the co-registered images (bottom right).

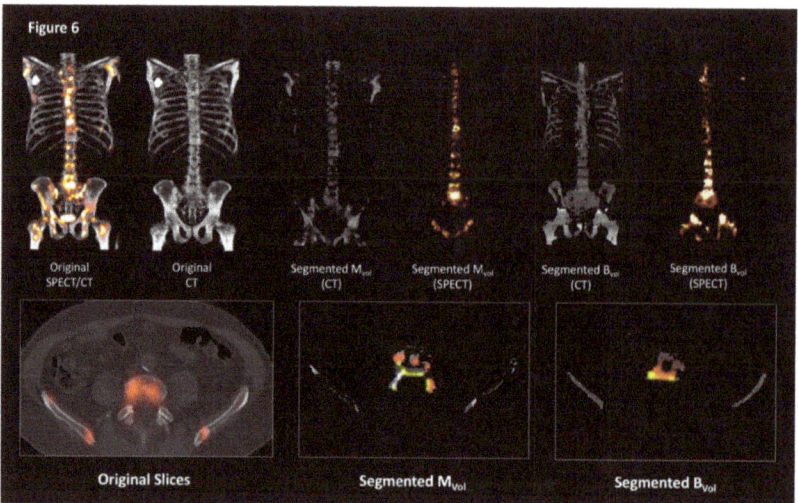

Figure 6. Examples of the segmentation output. Three-dimensional maximum intensity projections representations (top panels) and transaxial views (bottom panels) of the original images (left) and of the processed imaging outputs (center and right).

In the next step, masks corresponding to the M_{Vol} and the B_{Vol} were generated and exported onto the co-registered SPECT images; here, mean radioactivity concentration (counts/voxel) was calculated. The program's output included the volume (in mL), the mean HU density, and the mean counts of both volumes M_{Vol} and B_{Vol}. For the purpose of the present study, the skull was excluded from the analysis. Separate computations were then conducted for the whole-body skeleton (the whole skeleton from atlas until the distal femurs), the axial skeleton (vertebrae and sternum), and the appendicular bones (humeral and femoral shafts).

4.5. Validation of the Computational Technique and Comparison with Controls

In order to correlate the information obtained by the new program with known indices, we compared the magnitude of volumes, density values, and tracer distribution with approved radiological, clinical, and laboratory standards of reference. In the first step, we aimed to verify the correctness of the bone identification by our program. To do so, we compared the total S_{Vol} with a volumetric estimate of the whole skeleton obtained by a licensed commercial application (QMetrix®, General Electric, Boston, MA, USA). This comparison was done to ensure that our method could correctly recognize the bone volume on the CT images.

In the second step, we compared the M_{Vol} (as an estimate of the tumor burden) with the absolute number of metastatic lesions, which were manually counted on the SPECT/CT images by an expert reader. Finally, M_{Vol}, mean M_{Vol} HU, average M_{Vol} counts, and ratio between M_{Vol} and B_{Vol} were correlated to PSA levels.

To further stratify disease aggressiveness, both HU values and counts of M_{Vol} were compared between patients with or without a superscan finding at planar imaging. Superscan was defined as the presence of uniformly increased activity within the skeleton, with very faint or absent visualization of the renal system [36].

4.6. Statistical Analysis

Data are presented as mean ±standard deviation. The t-test for unpaired data was used to compare values between patients' subgroups. To verify the probability of therapy response as a function of the measured counts within the segmented volumes, ROC analyses were performed, and areas-under-curve (AUC) calculated. Correlations between indices were assessed with bivariate analyses, using Pearson's R index. Prevalence of superscan patients among groups was tested using the Chi-squared test.

A p-value of <0.05 was considered significant. The SPSS statistical program (SPSS®, v. 21.0, IBM, Armonk NY, USA) was employed.

5. Conclusions

This study aimed to contribute to the transition to tailored treatments in the field of metastasized castration-resistant prostate cancer. The availability of reliable indices of disease burden and the capability to measure therapy response accurately, as well to predict its clinical course, are key in ensuring the best possible treatment to every single patient. The present paper presents a method by which disease-specific indices, mirroring the corresponding parameters of disease status, can be obtained. The capability to extract this data can potentially be used, pending further studies, to ameliorate the imaging-based disease stratification and to improve the therapeutic schedule, therefore improving treatment effectiveness in these patients.

Author Contributions: Individual contribution are as follows: Conceptualization: F.F., C.l.F and G.S.; methodology: M.R., H.D., C.C. and A.S.; Software: C.C. and M.P.; Formal analysis: M.W. ans S.S.; Visualization: M.W. and S.S.; Writing (draft preparation): F.F., M.W. and H.D.; Writing (review and editing): F.F., C.l.F., H.D., A.S., M.P. and G.S.; Supervision: C.l.F.

Funding: This research received no external funding.

Conflicts of Interest: The authors declare no conflict of interest.

References

1. Seruga, B.; Ocana, A.; Tannock, I.F. Drug resistance in metastatic castration-resistant prostate cancer. *Nat. Rev. Clin. Oncol.* **2011**, *8*, 12–23. [CrossRef] [PubMed]
2. Cookson, M.S.; Roth, B.J.; Dahm, P.; Engstrom, C.; Freedland, S.J.; Hussain, M.; Lin, D.W.; Lowrance, W.T.; Murad, M.H.; Oh, W.K.; et al. Castration-resistant prostate cancer: AUA Guideline. *J. Urol.* **2013**, *190*, 429–438. [CrossRef] [PubMed]
3. Bubendorf, L.; Schopfer, A.; Wagner, U.; Sauter, G.; Moch, H.; Willi, N.; Gasser, T.C.; Mihatsch, M.J. Metastatic patterns of prostate cancer: An autopsy study of 1589 patients. *Hum. Pathol.* **2000**, *31*, 578–583. [CrossRef] [PubMed]
4. Huang, X.; Chau, C.H.; Figg, W.D. Challenges to improved therapeutics for metastatic castrate resistant prostate cancer: From recent successes and failures. *J. Hematol. Oncol.* **2012**, *5*, 35. [CrossRef] [PubMed]
5. Benjamin, R. Neurologic complications of prostate cancer. *Am. Fam. Physician* **2002**, *65*, 1834–1840. [PubMed]
6. Fiz, F.; Sahbai, S.; Campi, C.; Weissinger, M.; Dittmann, H.; Marini, C.; Piana, M.; Sambuceti, G.; la Fougere, C. Tumor Burden and Intraosseous Metabolic Activity as Predictors of Bone Marrow Failure during Radioisotope Therapy in Metastasized Prostate Cancer Patients. *Biomed. Res. Int.* **2017**, *2017*, 3905216. [CrossRef] [PubMed]
7. Kantoff, P.W.; Higano, C.S.; Shore, N.D.; Berger, E.R.; Small, E.J.; Penson, D.F.; Redfern, C.H.; Ferrari, A.C.; Dreicer, R.; Sims, R.B.; et al. Sipuleucel-T immunotherapy for castration-resistant prostate cancer. *N. Engl. J. Med.* **2010**, *363*, 411–422. [CrossRef] [PubMed]
8. Kwon, E.D.; Drake, C.G.; Scher, H.I.; Fizazi, K.; Bossi, A.; van den Eertwegh, A.J.; Krainer, M.; Houede, N.; Santos, R.; Mahammedi, H.; et al. Ipilimumab versus placebo after radiotherapy in patients with metastatic castration-resistant prostate cancer that had progressed after docetaxel chemotherapy (CA184-043): A multicentre, randomised, double-blind, phase 3 trial. *Lancet Oncol.* **2014**, *15*, 700–712. [CrossRef]
9. Pezaro, C.J.; Omlin, A.G.; Altavilla, A.; Lorente, D.; Ferraldeschi, R.; Bianchini, D.; Dearnaley, D.; Parker, C.; de Bono, J.S.; Attard, G. Activity of cabazitaxel in castration-resistant prostate cancer progressing after docetaxel and next-generation endocrine agents. *Eur. Urol.* **2014**, *66*, 459–465. [CrossRef] [PubMed]

10. Hoskin, P.; Sartor, O.; O'Sullivan, J.M.; Johannessen, D.C.; Helle, S.I.; Logue, J.; Bottomley, D.; Nilsson, S.; Vogelzang, N.J.; Fang, F.; et al. Efficacy and safety of radium-223 dichloride in patients with castration-resistant prostate cancer and symptomatic bone metastases, with or without previous docetaxel use: A prespecified subgroup analysis from the randomised, double-blind, phase 3 ALSYMPCA trial. *Lancet Oncol.* **2014**, *15*, 1397–1406. [CrossRef]
11. Kratochwil, C.; Giesel, F.L.; Stefanova, M.; Benesova, M.; Bronzel, M.; Afshar-Oromieh, A.; Mier, W.; Eder, M.; Kopka, K.; Haberkorn, U. PSMA-Targeted Radionuclide Therapy of Metastatic Castration-Resistant Prostate Cancer with 177Lu-Labeled PSMA-617. *J. Nucl. Med.* **2016**, *57*, 1170–1176. [CrossRef] [PubMed]
12. Kratochwil, C.; Bruchertseifer, F.; Giesel, F.L.; Weis, M.; Verburg, F.A.; Mottaghy, F.; Kopka, K.; Apostolidis, C.; Haberkorn, U.; Morgenstern, A. 225Ac-PSMA-617 for PSMA-Targeted alpha-Radiation Therapy of Metastatic Castration-Resistant Prostate Cancer. *J. Nucl. Med.* **2016**, *57*, 1941–1944. [CrossRef] [PubMed]
13. Sartor, A.O.; Fitzpatrick, J.M. Urologists and oncologists: Adapting to a new treatment paradigm in castration-resistant prostate cancer (CRPC). *BJU Int.* **2012**, *110*, 328–335. [CrossRef] [PubMed]
14. Sartor, O. State-of-the-Art Management for the Patient with Castration-Resistant Prostate Cancer in 2012. *Am. Soc. Clin. Oncol. Educ. Book* **2012**, 289–291. [CrossRef]
15. Chung, P.H.; Gayed, B.A.; Thoreson, G.R.; Raj, G.V. Emerging drugs for prostate cancer. *Expert Opin. Emerg. Drugs* **2013**, *18*, 533–550. [CrossRef]
16. Yu, E.Y.; Gulati, R.; Telesca, D.; Jiang, P.; Tam, S.; Russell, K.J.; Nelson, P.S.; Etzioni, R.D.; Higano, C.S. Duration of first off-treatment interval is prognostic for time to castration resistance and death in men with biochemical relapse of prostate cancer treated on a prospective trial of intermittent androgen deprivation. *J. Clin. Oncol.* **2010**, *28*, 2668–2673. [CrossRef]
17. Bahl, A.K.; Bertelli, G.; Lewis, P.D.; Jenkins, P.; Aziz, A.; Davies, P.J.; Persad, R.; Smith, C.G.; Hurley, K.; Mason, M.D. Correlation of elevated alkaline phosphatase (ALP) and survival in metastatic castration-resistant prostate cancer (CRPC) treated with docetaxel chemotherapy: Results of SWSW Uro-oncology Group study from three U.K. centers. *J. Clin. Oncol.* **2011**, *29*, 206. [CrossRef]
18. Piper, C.; van Erps, T.; Pfister, D.J.; Epplen, R.; Porres, D.; Heidenreich, A. Frequency and prognostic significance of the PSA flare-up phenomenon in men with castration-resistant prostate cancer (CRPC) who undergo docetaxel-based chemotherapy. *J. Clin. Oncol.* **2012**, *30*, 92. [CrossRef]
19. Schroder, F.H.; Tombal, B.; Miller, K.; Boccon-Gibod, L.; Shore, N.D.; Crawford, E.D.; Moul, J.; Olesen, T.K.; Persson, B.E. Changes in alkaline phosphatase levels in patients with prostate cancer receiving degarelix or leuprolide: Results from a 12-month, comparative, phase III study. *BJU Int.* **2010**, *106*, 182–187. [CrossRef]
20. Qin, J.; Liu, X.; Laffin, B.; Chen, X.; Choy, G.; Jeter, C.R.; Calhoun-Davis, T.; Li, H.; Palapattu, G.S.; Pang, S.; et al. The PSA(-/lo) prostate cancer cell population harbors self-renewing long-term tumor-propagating cells that resist castration. *Cell Stem Cell* **2012**, *10*, 556–569. [CrossRef]
21. Pollen, J.J.; Witztum, K.F.; Ashburn, W.L. The flare phenomenon on radionuclide bone scan in metastatic prostate cancer. *AJR Am. J. Roentgenol.* **1984**, *142*, 773–776. [CrossRef] [PubMed]
22. Fiz, F.; Dittman, H.; Campi, C.; Morbelli, S.; Marini, C.; Brignone, M.; Bauckneht, M.; Piva, R.; Massone, A.M.; Piana, M.; et al. Assessment of Skeletal Tumor Load in Metastasized Castration-Resistant Prostate Cancer Patients: A Review of Available Methods and an Overview on Future Perspectives. *Bioengineering* **2018**, *5*, 58. [CrossRef] [PubMed]
23. Carrasquillo, J.A.; O'Donoghue, J.A.; Pandit-Taskar, N.; Humm, J.L.; Rathkopf, D.E.; Slovin, S.F.; Williamson, M.J.; Lacuna, K.; Aksnes, A.K.; Larson, S.M.; et al. Phase I pharmacokinetic and biodistribution study with escalating doses of (2)(2)(3)Ra-dichloride in men with castration-resistant metastatic prostate cancer. *Eur. J. Nucl. Med. Mol. Imaging* **2013**, *40*, 1384–1393. [CrossRef] [PubMed]
24. Pacilio, M.; Ventroni, G.; De Vincentis, G.; Cassano, B.; Pellegrini, R.; Di Castro, E.; Frantellizzi, V.; Follacchio, G.A.; Garkavaya, T.; Lorenzon, L.; et al. Dosimetry of bone metastases in targeted radionuclide therapy with alpha-emitting (223)Ra-dichloride. *Eur. J. Nucl. Med. Mol. Imaging* **2016**, *43*, 21–33. [CrossRef] [PubMed]
25. Fosbol, M.O.; Petersen, P.M.; Kjaer, A.; Mortensen, J. (223)Ra Therapy of Advanced Metastatic Castration-Resistant Prostate Cancer: Quantitative Assessment of Skeletal Tumor Burden for Prognostication of Clinical Outcome and Hematologic Toxicity. *J. Nucl. Med.* **2018**, *59*, 596–602. [CrossRef] [PubMed]

26. Petersen, L.J.; Mortensen, J.C.; Bertelsen, H.; Zacho, H.D. Computer-assisted interpretation of planar whole-body bone scintigraphy in patients with newly diagnosed prostate cancer. *Nucl. Med. Commun.* **2015**, *36*, 679–685. [CrossRef]
27. Ryan, C.J.; Shah, S.; Efstathiou, E.; Smith, M.R.; Taplin, M.E.; Bubley, G.J.; Logothetis, C.J.; Kheoh, T.; Kilian, C.; Haqq, C.M.; et al. Phase II study of abiraterone acetate in chemotherapy-naive metastatic castration-resistant prostate cancer displaying bone flare discordant with serologic response. *Clin. Cancer Res.* **2011**, *17*, 4854–4861. [CrossRef] [PubMed]
28. Rohren, E.M.; Etchebehere, E.C.; Araujo, J.C.; Hobbs, B.P.; Swanston, N.M.; Everding, M.; Moody, T.; Macapinlac, H.A. Determination of Skeletal Tumor Burden on 18F-Fluoride PET/CT. *J. Nucl. Med.* **2015**, *56*, 1507–1512. [CrossRef]
29. Bieth, M.; Kronke, M.; Tauber, R.; Dahlbender, M.; Retz, M.; Nekolla, S.G.; Menze, B.; Maurer, T.; Eiber, M.; Schwaiger, M. Exploring New Multimodal Quantitative Imaging Indices for the Assessment of Osseous Tumor Burden in Prostate Cancer Using 68Ga-PSMA PET/CT. *J. Nucl. Med.* **2017**, *58*, 1632–1637. [CrossRef]
30. Horger, M.; Bares, R. The role of single-photon emission computed tomography/computed tomography in benign and malignant bone disease. *Semin. Nucl. Med.* **2006**, *36*, 286–294. [CrossRef]
31. Nakajima, K.; Edenbrandt, L.; Mizokami, A. Bone scan index: A new biomarker of bone metastasis in patients with prostate cancer. *Int. J. Urol.* **2017**, *24*, 668–673. [CrossRef] [PubMed]
32. Dadhania, S.; Alonzi, R.; Douglas, S.; Gogbashian, A.; Hughes, R.; Dalili, D.; Vasdev, N.; Adshead, J.; Lane, T.; Westbury, C.; et al. Single-centre Experience of Use of Radium 223 with Clinical Outcomes Based on Number of Cycles and Bone Marrow Toxicity. *Anticancer Res.* **2018**, *38*, 5423–5427. [CrossRef] [PubMed]
33. Sambuceti, G.; Brignone, M.; Marini, C.; Massollo, M.; Fiz, F.; Morbelli, S.; Buschiazzo, A.; Campi, C.; Piva, R.; Massone, A.M.; et al. Estimating the whole bone-marrow asset in humans by a computational approach to integrated PET/CT imaging. *Eur. J. Nucl. Med. Mol. Imaging* **2012**, *39*, 1326–1338. [CrossRef] [PubMed]
34. Fiz, F.; Marini, C.; Piva, R.; Miglino, M.; Massollo, M.; Bongioanni, F.; Morbelli, S.; Bottoni, G.; Campi, C.; Bacigalupo, A.; et al. Adult advanced chronic lymphocytic leukemia: Computational analysis of whole-body CT documents a bone structure alteration. *Radiology* **2014**, *271*, 805–813. [CrossRef] [PubMed]
35. Fiz, F.; Marini, C.; Campi, C.; Massone, A.M.; Podesta, M.; Bottoni, G.; Piva, R.; Bongioanni, F.; Bacigalupo, A.; Piana, M.; et al. Allogeneic cell transplant expands bone marrow distribution by colonizing previously abandoned areas: An FDG PET/CT analysis. *Blood* **2015**, *125*, 4095–4102. [CrossRef] [PubMed]
36. Constable, A.R.; Cranage, R.W. Recognition of the superscan in prostatic bone scintigraphy. *Br. J. Radiol.* **1981**, *54*, 122–125. [CrossRef] [PubMed]

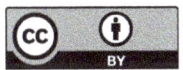 © 2019 by the authors. Licensee MDPI, Basel, Switzerland. This article is an open access article distributed under the terms and conditions of the Creative Commons Attribution (CC BY) license (http://creativecommons.org/licenses/by/4.0/).

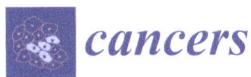

Article

Diffusion-Weighted Imaging Can Differentiate between Malignant and Benign Pleural Diseases

Katsuo Usuda [1,*], Shun Iwai [1], Aika Funasaki [1], Atsushi Sekimura [1], Nozomu Motono [1], Munetaka Matoba [2], Mariko Doai [2], Sohsuke Yamada [3], Yoshimichi Ueda [4] and Hidetaka Uramoto [1]

1. Department of Thoracic Surgery, Kanazawa Medical University, Ishikawa 920-0293, Japan; mhg1214@kanazawa-med.ac.jp (S.I.); aicarby@kanazawa-med.ac.jp (A.F.); a24seki@kanazawa-med.ac.jp (A.S.); motono@kanazawa-med.ac.jp (N.M.); hidetaka@kanazawa-med.ac.jp (H.U.)
2. Department of Radiology, Kanazawa Medical University, Ishikawa 920-0293, Japan; m-matoba@kanazawa-med.ac.jp (M.M.); doaimari@kanazawa-med.ac.jp (M.D.)
3. Department of Pathology and Laboratory Medicine, Kanazawa Medical University, Ishikawa 920-0293, Japan; sohsuke@kanazawa-med.ac.jp
4. Department of Pathophysiological and Experimental Pathology, Kanazawa Medical University, Ishikawa 920-0293, Japan; z-ueda@kanazawa-med.ac.jp
* Correspondence: usuda@kanazawa-med.ac.jp; Tel.: +81-76-286-2211; Fax: +81-76-286-1207

Received: 1 May 2019; Accepted: 3 June 2019; Published: 12 June 2019

Abstract: It is not clear whether magnetic resonance imaging (MRI) is useful for the assessment of pleural diseases. The aim of this study is to determine whether diffusion-weighted magnetic resonance imaging (DWI) can differentiate malignant pleural mesothelioma (MPM) from pleural dissemination of lung cancer, empyema or pleural effusion. The DWI was calibrated with the b value of 0 and 800 s/mm^2. There were 11 MPMs (8 epithelioid and 3 biphasic), 10 pleural disseminations of lung cancer, 10 empyemas, and 12 pleural effusions. The apparent diffusion coefficient (ADC) of the pleural diseases was $1.22 \pm 0.25 \times 10^{-3}$ mm^2/s in the MPMs, $1.31 \pm 0.49 \times 10^{-3}$ mm^2/s in the pleural disseminations, $2.01 \pm 0.45 \times 10^{-3}$ mm^2/s in the empyemas and $3.76 \pm 0.62 \times 10^{-3}$ mm^2/s in the pleural effusions. The ADC of the MPMs and the pleural disseminations were significantly lower than the ADC of the empyemas and the pleural effusions. Concerning the diffusion pattern of DWI, all 11 MPMs showed strong continuous diffusion, 9 of 10 pleural disseminations showed strong scattered diffusion and 1 pleural dissemination showed strong continuous diffusion, all 10 empyemas showed weak continuous diffusion, and all 12 pleural effusions showed no decreased diffusion. DWI can evaluate pleural diseases morphologically and qualitatively, and thus differentiate between malignant and benign pleural diseases.

Keywords: magnetic resonance imaging; diffusion-weighted imaging; malignant pleural mesothelioma; pleural dissemination; empyema; pleural effusion

1. Introduction

Malignant pleural mesothelioma (MPM) is a highly lethal disease with limited therapeutic options that are difficult for patients to endure. Computed tomography (CT) is the primary imaging modality used to evaluate MPM and accurately track the spread of the primary tumor, the intrathoracic lymphadenopathy, as well as the extrathoracic spread. Early diagnosis of MPM is usually difficult in the modality of a chest CT, because pleural thickness or pleural effusion due to MPM can resemble a benign disease on a CT scan image. Additional imaging modalities, such as magnetic resonance imaging (MRI) and fluoro-2-deoxy-glucose positron emission tomography/computed tomography

(FDG-PET/CT), have emerged in recent years and are complementary to CT for disease staging and evaluation of patients with MPM [1]. There have been several recent research papers that have shown that MRI is the best modality for the assessment of the pleural interface, characterization of complex pleural effusion, and identification of exudate and hemorrhages, and staging accuracy [2]. MRI is more accurate than CT in staging evaluation of local invasions in the endothoracic fascia or single chest wall focus (68% vs. 46%) and the diaphragm (82% vs. 55%) [3]. Diffusion-weighted magnetic resonance imaging (DWI) has reportedly been useful in differentiating malignant pleural diseases from benign alterations [4]. DWI utilizes the random, translational motion, or so-called Brownian movement, of water molecules in biologic tissue [5]. DWI has been used for brain imaging, mainly for the assessment of acute ischemic strokes, intracranial tumors and demyelinating diseases [6].

The purpose of this study was to determine whether DWI can differentiate MPM from pleural dissemination of lung cancer, empyema, or pleural effusion.

2. Results

Below is shown typical radiological imaging of an MPM (Figure 1), a pleural dissemination of lung cancer (Figure 2), an empyema (Figure 3) and a pleural effusion (Figure 4).

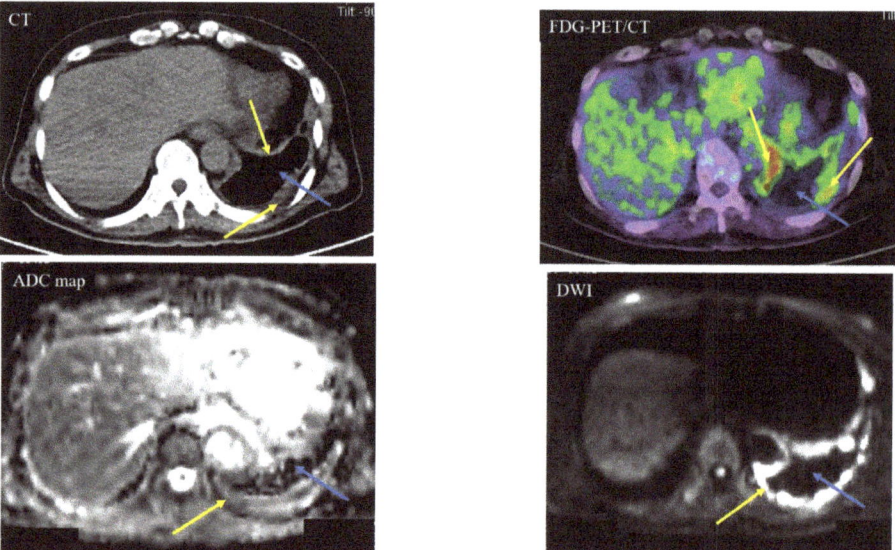

Figure 1. Case 1—Malignant Pleural Mesothelioma (MPM). A 64-year-old male with MPM (cT4N2M0). The yellow arrows indicate the MPM. The blue arrows indicate pleural effusion. Computed tomography (CT) showed left pleural thickness of the MPM. The apparent diffusion coefficient (ADC) of the MPM was 0.84×10^{-3} mm^2/s (positive) and the ADC of the pleural fluid was 3.95×10^{-3} mm^2/s (negative). Fluorodeoxyglucose (FDG)-position emission tomography (PET)/CT showed partial accumulation (standardized uptake value (SUV)max: 12.39) of FDG on the MPM.

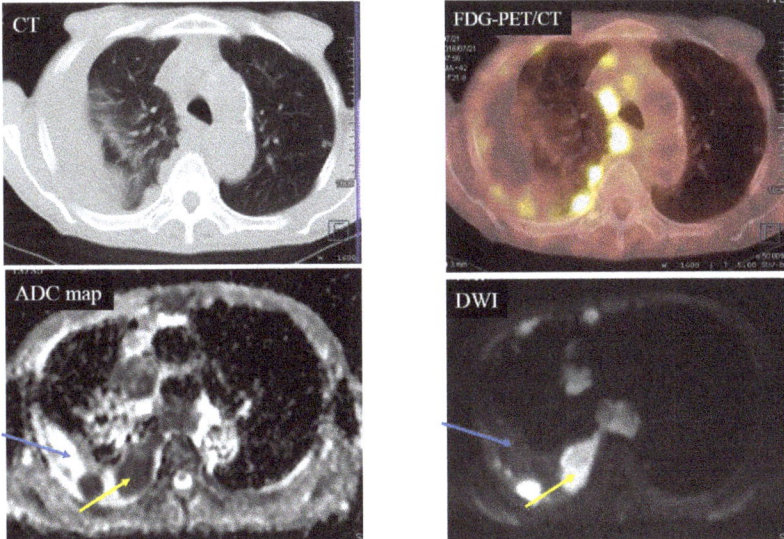

Figure 2. Case 2—Pleural dissemination of lung cancer. An 81-year-old male with pleural dissemination of a large cell neuroendocrine carcinoma. The yellow arrows indicate pleural dissemination. The blue arrows indicate pleural fluid. The apparent diffusion coefficient (ADC) of the pleural dissemination was 0.67×10^{-3} mm^2/s (positive) and the ADC of the pleural fluid was 3.03×10^{-3} mm^2/s (negative). Fluorodeoxyglucose-position emission tomography/computed tomography (FDG-PET/CT) showed scattered accumulation (standardized uptake value (SUVmax): 14.7) of the FDG on the pleural dissemination.

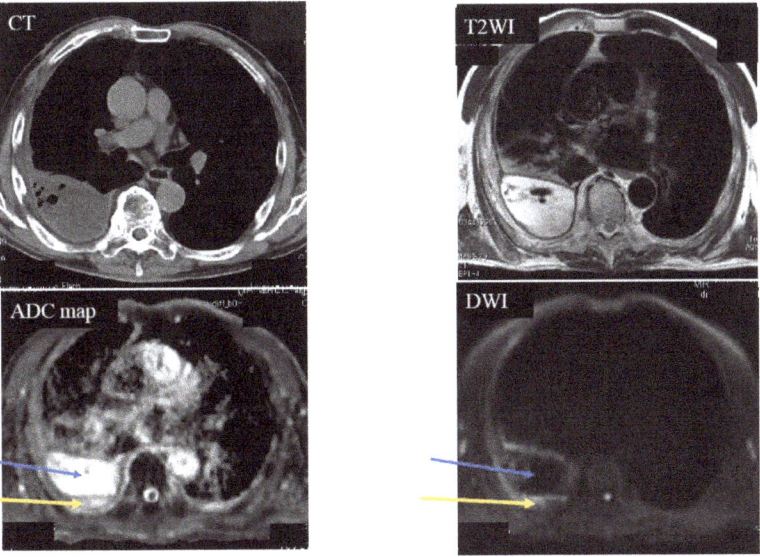

Figure 3. Case 3—Empyema. A 70-year-old male with right empyema. The yellow arrows indicate pleural thickness. The blue arrows indicate pleural fluid. The apparent diffusion coefficient (ADC) of the pleural thickness was 1.82×10^{-3} mm^2/s (negative) and the ADC of the pleural fluid was 3.95×10^{-3} mm^2/s (negative).

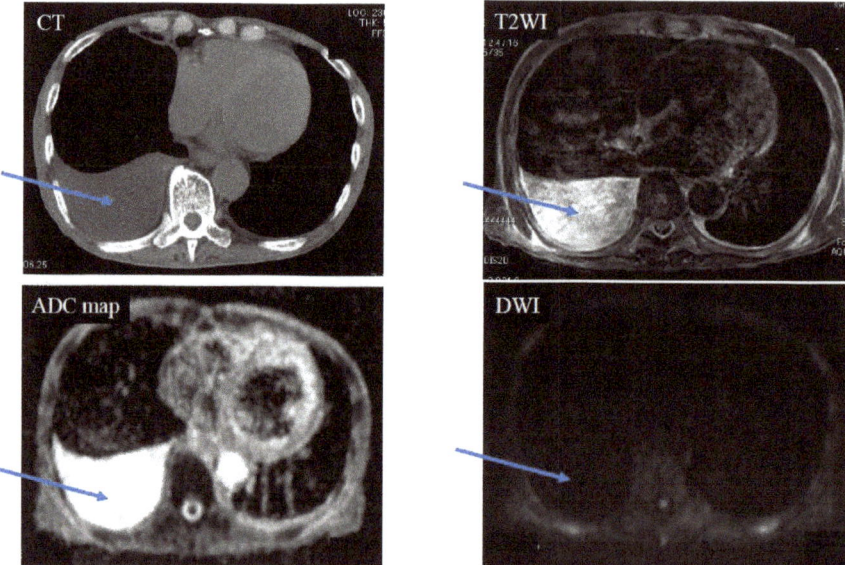

Figure 4. Case 4—Pleural effusion due to exudative pleurisy in a 79-year-old male, who suffered from right pneumonia. The blue arrows indicate pleural fluid. Pleural effusion was not seen in diffusion weighted magnetic resonance imaging (DWI). The apparent diffusion coefficient (ADC) of pleural fluid was 4.02×10^{-3} mm^2/s (negative).

Diffusion patterns based on pleural lesions are shown in Table 1. All 11 cases of MPM showed strong continuous diffusion. Nine of the 10 pleural disseminations showed strong scattered diffusion, and one pleural dissemination showed strong continuous diffusion. All 10 empyemas showed weak continuous diffusion. All 12 pleural effusions showed no decreased diffusion.

The ADC values of the pleural diseases were $1.22 \pm 0.25 \times 10^{-3}$ mm^2/s in the MPMs, $1.31 \pm 0.49 \times 10^{-3}$ mm^2/s in the pleural disseminations, $2.01 \pm 0.45 \times 10^{-3}$ mm^2/s in the empyemas and $3.76 \pm 0.62 \times 10^{-3}$ mm^2/s in the pleural effusions (Figure 5). The ADC of the MPMs was significantly lower than that of the empyemas ($P = 0.0007$) and the pleural effusions ($P < 0.0001$). The ADC values of the pleural disseminations were significantly lower than that of the empyemas ($P = 0.0086$) and the pleural effusions ($P < 0.0001$). The ADC of the MPM was not significantly different from that of pleural dissemination.

There were eight epithelioid and three biphasic MPMs. The ADC ($1.23 \pm 0.26 \times 10^{-3}$ mm^2/s) of the epithelioid MPMs was not significantly higher than the ADC ($1.17 \pm 0.21 \times 10^{-3}$ mm^2/s) of the biphasic MPMs ($P = 0.73$).

Of the 10 pleural disseminations of lung cancer, seven were adenocarcinomas, two were small cell carcinomas, and one was large cell neuroendocrine carcinoma (LCNEC). The ADC of the pleural dissemination was $1.63 \pm 0.13 \times 10^{-3}$ mm^2/s in adenocarcinomas, $0.68 \pm 0.18 \times 10^{-3}$ mm^2/s in small cell carcinomas, and 0.67×10^{-3} mm^2/s in a LCNEC. The ADC of adenocarcinomas was significantly higher than that of small cell carcinomas ($P = 0.0002$).

Six of the pleural effusions were exudative, two were caused by atelectasis, two were caused by malignant uterus tumors, one was caused by trauma, and one was caused by asbestosis. Because the two patients with malignant uterus tumors had negative results of pleural cytology and did not have pleural dissemination, the causes of pleural effusion in the malignant uterus tumors were not clear.

Table 1. Diffusion patterns of DWI for pleural lesions.

	Diffusion Pattern	Strong Continuous	Strong Scattered	Weak Continuous	No Decreased	No. of Cases
Diagnosis	MPM	11	0	0	0	11
	Pleural dissemination	1	9	0	0	10
	Empyema	0	0	10	0	10
	Pleural effusion	0	0	0	12	12
No. of cases		12	9	10	12	43

MPM: Malignant Pleural Mesothelioma.

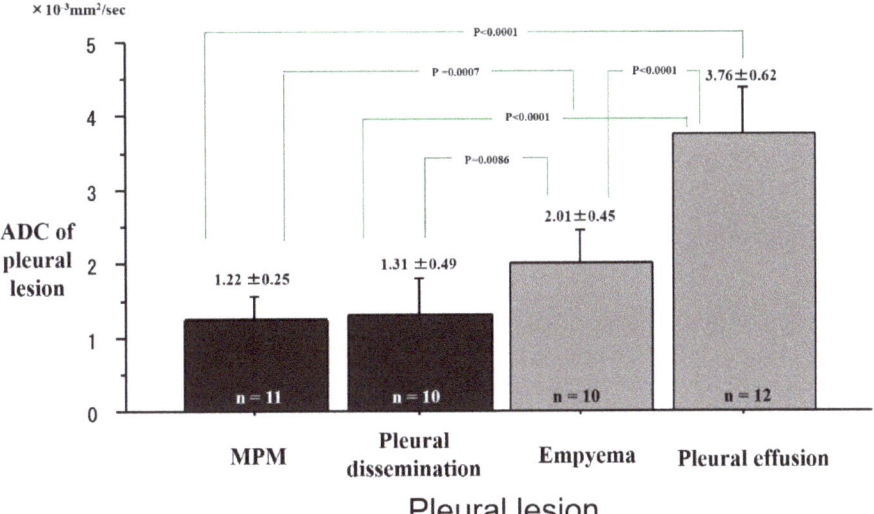

Figure 5. Differences of apparent diffusion coefficient (ADC) of pleural lesions. Mean ADCs were $1.22 \pm 0.25 \times 10^{-3}$ mm^2/s in Malignant Pleural Mesothelioma (MPM), $1.31 \pm 0.49 \times 10^{-3}$ mm^2/s in pleural dissemination, $2.01 \pm 0.45 \times 10^{-3}$ mm^2/s in empyema, and $3.76 \pm 0.62 \times 10^{-3}$ mm^2/s on pleural effusion. The ADC of the MPM was significantly lower than that of empyema ($P = 0.0007$) or pleural effusion ($P < 0.0001$). The ADC of pleural dissemination was significantly lower than that of empyema ($P = 0.0086$) or pleural effusion ($P < 0.0001$).

The ADC values of the pleural fluid were $3.87 \pm 0.29 \times 10^{-3}$ mm^2/s in MPMs, $3.59 \pm 0.57 \times 10^{-3}$ mm^2/s in the pleural disseminations, $2.40 \pm 1.26 \times 10^{-3}$ mm^2/s in the empyemas, and $3.94 \pm 0.27 \times 10^{-3}$ mm^2/s in the pleural effusions (Figure 6). The ADC of pleural fluid was significantly lower in the empyemas than in the MPMs ($P = 0.0023$), the pleural disseminations ($P = 0.0286$) and the pleural effusions ($P = 0.0009$). No significant differences in pleural fluid were found in MPMs, pleural disseminations, and pleural effusions.

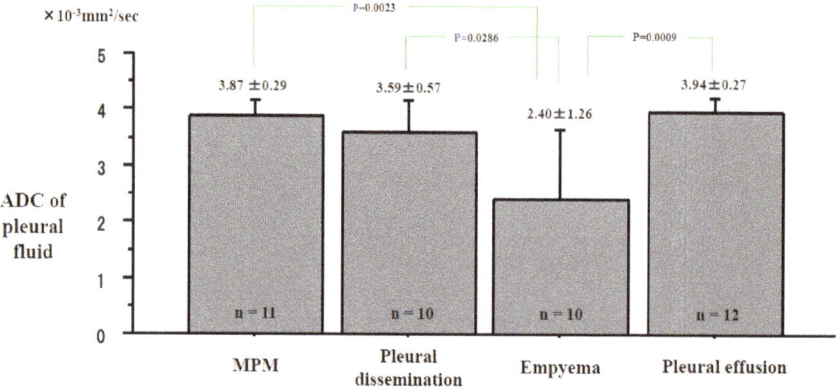

Pleural lesion

Figure 6. Differences in the apparent diffusion coefficient (ADC) of the pleural effusion inside the pleural lesions. The ADCs of pleural fluid were $3.87 \pm 0.29 \times 10^{-3}$ mm^2/s in Malignant Pleural Mesothelioma (MPM), $3.59 \pm 0.57 \times 10^{-3}$ mm^2/s in the pleural dissemination, $2.40 \pm 1.26 \times 10^{-3}$ mm^2/s in the empyema, and $3.94 \pm 0.27 \times 10^{-3}$ mm^2/s in the pleural effusion.

3. Discussion

DWI can be used to detect the restricted diffusion of water molecules in the body. Evidence has shown the advantage of DWI for functional information of neoplasm [7]. It has been reported that DWI has the potential for differential diagnosis of pulmonary nodules and masses, and evaluation of N factor/M factor/stage of lung cancer [8–11]. Two reports of meta-analysis concluded that DWI was an accurate modality to evaluate N factor of lung cancer [12,13].

Diagnosing MPM correctly in its early phases is very difficult with CT because of fewer symptoms, less pleural thickness or pleural effusion. At this stage, a chest CT would be performed to assess the pleural disease, but the MPM might not be detected. MRI is an important adjunctive imaging examination in thoracic oncologic imaging that is applied as a problem-solving tool to evaluate chest wall invasion, intraspinal extension, and cardiac/vascular invasion [14]. Moreover, functional MR imaging modality, such as DWI and dynamic contrast material–enhanced MR imaging modality, have already proven effective in differentiating malignant from benign pleural diseases and assessing chest wall and diaphragmatic involvement [15–19]. As this research has shown, DWI can diagnose an MPM as a malignant tumor with strong continuous diffusion over the entire circumference of the pleural with an ADC of less than 1.70×10^{-3} mm^2/s. The MPMs present marked restricted diffusion of the pleural tumor in DWI [20].

Coolen et al. [4] reported that visual evaluation of pleural pointillism was denoted by the presence of multiple, hyperintense pleural spots on high-b-value DWI. It is useful to differentiate MPM from benign alterations, which perform substantially better than mediastinal pleural thickness and shrinking lung. Pleural pointillism could be used to provide guidance for biopsies and thoracoscopic evaluations. In our article, one MPM also had hyperintense pleural diffusion on DWI, which we expressed as "strong continuous diffusion". Strong continuous diffusion and pleural pointillism can be seen in DWI of MPMs. Although pleural pointillism on high-b-value DWI had better sensitivity and accuracy than pleural thickness and lung shrinkage, the specificity was not significantly better, which suggests that the three parameters should complement, rather than substitute, one another. Gill et al. [19] also reported that the ADC value ($1.31 \pm 0.15 \times 10^{-3}$ mm^2/s) of the epithelioid MPMs was statistically higher than that ($1.01 \pm 0.11 \times 10^{-3}$ mm^2/s) of the biphasic MPMs (P = 0.00024). In our study, we could not repeat the results from Gill's article due to small sample size.

MRI has advantages over FDG-PET/CT due to its excellent soft tissue contrast and absence of ionizing radiation [7]. Uptake of FDG in FDG-PET/CT is not always tumor specific, as seen in benign inflammatory lesions, which can make accurate staging of MPMs difficult [21]. Although FDG-PET/CT is more effective than CT for differentiating malignant from benign pleural diseases [22], its utility is limited to assessing the primary tumor extension and the nodal status of MPM [23]. In general, FDG-PET/CT can detect thicker parts of MPMs, but not thinner parts of MPMs.

DWI could diagnose pleural dissemination from lung cancer as a malignant tumor with strong scattered diffusion along the pleura when the ADC was less than 1.70×10^{-3} mm^2/s. Pleural metastasis from breast cancer can be detected with DWI [24]. Moreover, DWI can evaluate pleural lesions morphologically and qualitatively, while also differentiating between malignant pleural diseases and benign pleural diseases. We have also shown that DWI can differentiate MPM from pleural dissemination.

In our cases of empyema, The ADC of the pleural effusion decreased due to pus. The ADC of pleural fluid in empyemas was significantly lower than the ADC of the MPMs, the pleural disseminations, and the pleural effusions. Abscesses and thrombi impede the diffusivity of water molecules due to their hyperviscous nature [7,25]. Therefore, the ADC value of empyema was significantly lower without a significant decreased diffusion of the pleura. To diagnose empyema, the ADC value of pleura and pleural cavity must be carefully evaluated.

MRI has proven superior to CT in the characterization of pleural fluid [26]. Pleural fluid is typically hypointense on T1-weighted imaging and hyperintense on T2-weighted imaging [2]. As shown in this article, when a patient with pleural fluid shows no decreased diffusion in DWI, and when the ADC of the pleural fluid is higher, the pleural disease can be identified as benign.

MRIs have several advantages. They do not involve contrast agents and examinations take less time. Furthermore, MRIs do not have the downside of radiation exposure and are suitable for children with negative reactions to radiation [27]. On the other hand, an MRI is not a viable option for people with devices, such as pacemakers, or tattoos. In addition, MRI examinations are loud, and can cause some patients anxiety.

Limitations

There are two important limitations in this study. First, this study was performed at a single institution and dealt with a small number of patients, which unavoidably introduced selection bias. Second, we could not acquire consent forms from all the patients who developed pleural lesions in the period from March 2015 to February 2019. Due to these limitations, our sample size was small. Our ADC measurements were repeated three times and the minimum ADC value was recorded. Thus, this ADC may not fully represent the whole tumor. There is no overwhelming agreement in the literature concerning optimal DWI techniques and image analysis procedures, including region of interest (ROI) size and placement.

Nevertheless, DWI has two limitations. First, some of the more common benign diseases which present decreased diffusion and lower ADC values in DWI are pulmonary abscesses and empyemas with histopathological necrosis. Second, mucinous adenocarcinomas were usually hypointense in DWI and showed higher ADC values, which could be misjudged as benign lesions in DWI [28]. Since mucinous adenocarcinomas had lower cellularity than tubular adenocarcinomas, it had lower DWI signal intensity and higher ADC values than tubular adenocarcinoma in the ano-rectal region [29].

4. Patients and Methods

4.1. Eligibility

The study protocol for evaluating pleural lesions with CT and MRI with DWI was approved by the ethical committee of Kanazawa Medical University (the approval number: No.189, the approval date:

25th January 2012). After discussing the risks and benefits of the examinations with their surgeons, we obtained written informed consents for CT and MRI from each patient.

4.2. Patients

A total of 43 patients with pleural diseases or pleural effusions underwent CT scans and MRI examinations and were enrolled in this study in the period from March 2015 to February 2019. Exclusion criteria were unwillingness to undergo an MRI examination, and the general issues that exclude most patients from getting an MRI (e.g., incompatible implanted medical devices, claustrophobia, and tattoos).

The diagnosis of MPM and pleural dissemination of lung cancers were confirmed histopathologically by biopsy or surgical procedure. The diagnosis of empyema was confirmed by positive culture of pleural effusion or by purulent pleural effusion. The diagnosis of pleural effusion was confirmed by negative cytology and negative culture of pleural effusion.

There were 11 MPMs, 10 pleural disseminations of lung cancers, 10 empyemas and 12 pleural effusions.

4.3. Magnetic Resonance Imaging (MRI)

The 1.5 T superconducting magnetic scanner (Magnetom Avanto; Siemens, Erlangen, Germany) with two anterior six-channel body phased-array coils and two posterior spinal clusters (six-channels each) was used for MRI examinations. The conventional MRI consisted of a coronal T1-weighted spin-echo sequence and coronal and axial T2-weighted fast spin-echo sequences. DWI using a single-shot echo-planar technique were performed under SPAIR (spectral attenuated inversion recovery) with respiratory triggered scan with the following parameter: b value = 0 and 800 s/mm^2; TR/TE/flip angle, 3000–4500/65/90; diffusion gradient encoding in three orthogonal directions; receiver bandwidth, 2442 Hz/Px; voxel size, 2.7 × 2.7 × 6.0 mm; field of view, 350 mm; matrix size, 128 × 128; number of excitations, 5; section thickness, 6 mm and section gap, 0 mm. After image reconstruction, a 2-dimensional (2D) round or elliptical ROI was marked on the lesion which was detected visually on the ADC map with reference to T1-weighted or CT image by a radiologist (M.D.) with 26 years of MRI experience who was unaware of the patients' clinical data. The procedure was done three times and we recorded the minimum apparent diffusion coefficient (ADC) value. A consensus was reached if there were any differences of opinion. The optical cutoff value (OCV) of ADC for diagnosing malignancy in DWI was determined to be 1.70×10^{-3} mm^2/s using the receiver operating characteristics (ROC) curve, as previously described [8]. Pleural lesions with an ADC value of the same or less than the OCV were classified as positive. Pleural lesions with ADC value of more than the OCV or those that could not be detected on DWI were classified as negative. Diffusion pattern of DWI were divided into 4 categories: ① strong continuous diffusion, ② strong scattered diffusion, ③ weak continuous diffusion and ④ no decreased diffusion.

FDG-PET/CTs were also used for the evaluation. FDG-PET/CTs were done with a dedicated PET camera (SIEMENS Biograph Sensation 16, Erlangen Germany). All patients fasted for 6 hours before the scans. The OCV of maximum standardized uptake value (SUVmax) for diagnosing malignancy in FDG-PET/CT was determined to be 4.45 using the ROC curve, as previously described [8].

4.4. Statistical Analysis

Using StatView for Windows (Version 5.0; SAS Institute Inc. Cary, NC, USA), statistical analysis was performed. The data is presented as the mean ± standard deviation. A two-tailed Student t test was used for comparison of ADC values of various pleural lesions. A p-value of <0.05 was deemed statistically significant.

5. Conclusions

DWI can evaluate pleural diseases morphologically and qualitatively, while also differentiating between malignant pleural diseases and benign pleural diseases. DWI has the ability to differentiate MPM from pleural dissemination.

Author Contributions: Conceptualization, K.U.; methodology, M.M. and M.D.; formal analysis, S.Y.; investigation, Y.U.; resources, S.I. and A.F.; data curation, A.S. and N.M.; writing—original draft preparation, K.U.; writing—review and editing, K.U.; supervision, H.U.

Funding: This study was supported partly by a Grant-in-Aid for Scientific Research from the Ministry of Education, Culture, Sports, Science and Technology, Japan (Grant number: 16K10694) and by 2017 Grant-in-Aid of the Magnetic Health Science Foundation, Japan.

Acknowledgments: We are grateful to Keiya Hirata of the MRI Center, Kanazawa Medical University, for technical assistance. We are grateful to Dustin Keeling for proofreading this paper.

Conflicts of Interest: All authors have no conflict of interest to declare.

References

1. Nickell, L.T., Jr.; Lichtenberger, J.P., 3rd; Khorashadi, L.; Abbott, G.F.; Carter, B.W. Multimodality imaging for characterization, classification, and staging of malignant pleural mesothelioma. *Radiographics* **2014**, *34*, 1692–1706. [CrossRef] [PubMed]
2. Pessôa, F.M.; de Melo, A.S.; Souza, A.S.; de Souza, L.S.; Hochhegger, B.; Zanetti, G.; Marchiori, E. Applications of magnetic resonance imaging of the thorax in pleural diseases: A state-of-the-art review. *Lung* **2016**, *194*, 501–509. [CrossRef] [PubMed]
3. Heelan, R.T. Staging of malignant pleural mesothelioma: Comparison of CT and MR imaging. *Am. J. Roentgenol* **1999**, *172*, 1039–1047. [CrossRef] [PubMed]
4. Coolen, J.; De Keyzer, F.; Nafteux, P.; De Wever, W.; Dooms, C.; Vansteenkiste, J.; Derweduwen, A.; Roebben, I.; Verbeken, E.; De Leyn, P.; et al. Malignant pleural mesothelioma: Visual assessment by using pleural pointillism at diffusion-weighted MR imaging. *Radiology* **2015**, *274*, 576–584. [CrossRef] [PubMed]
5. Le Bihan, D.; Breton, E.; Lallemand, D.; Aubin, M.L.; Vignaud, J.; Laval-Jeantet, M. Separation of diffusion and perfusion in intravoxel incoherent motion MR imaging. *Radiology* **1988**, *168*, 497–505. [CrossRef] [PubMed]
6. Tien, R.D.; Felsberg, G.J.; Friedman, H.; Brown, M.; MacFall, J. MR imaging of high-grade cerebral gliomas: Value of diffusion-weighted echoplanar plus sequences. *Am. J. Roentgenol.* **1994**, *162*, 671–676. [CrossRef] [PubMed]
7. Kwee, T.C.; Takahara, T.; Ochiai, R.; Koh, D.M.; Ohno, Y.; Nakanishi, K.; Niwa, T.; Chenevert, T.L.; Luijten, P.R.; Alavi, A. Complementary roles of whole-body diffusion-weighted MRI and 18F-FDG PET: The state of the art and potential applications. *J. Nucl. Med.* **2010**, *51*, 1549–1558. [CrossRef] [PubMed]
8. Usuda, K.; Sagawa, M.; Motono, N.; Ueno, M.; Tanaka, M.; Machida, Y.; Matoba, M.; Kuginuki, Y.; Taniguchi, M.; Ueda, Y.; et al. Advantages of diffusion-weighted imaging over positron emission tomography-computed tomography in assessment of hilar and mediastinal lymph node in lung cancer. *Ann. Surg. Oncol.* **2013**, *20*, 1676–1683. [CrossRef]
9. Li, B.; Li, Q.; Chen, C.; Guan, Y.; Liu, S. A systematic review and meta-analysis of the accuracy of diffusion-weighted MRI in the detection of malignant pulmonary nodules and masses. *Acad. Radiol.* **2014**, *21*, 21–29. [CrossRef] [PubMed]
10. Shen, G.; Jia, Z.; Deng, H. Apparent diffusion coefficient values of diffusion-weighted imaging for distinguishing focal pulmonary lesions and characterizing the subtype of lung cancer: A meta-analysis. *Eur. Radiol.* **2016**, *26*, 556–566. [CrossRef]
11. Usuda, K.; Zhao, X.T.; Sagawa, M.; Matoba, M.; Kuginuki, Y.; Ueda, Y.; Sakuma, T. Diffusion-weighted imaging is superior to positron emission tomography in the detection and nodal assessment of lung cancers. *Ann. Thorac. Surg.* **2011**, *91*, 1689–1695. [CrossRef] [PubMed]
12. Peerlings, J.; Troost, E.G.; Nelemans, P.J.; Cobben, D.C.; de Boer, J.C.; Hoffmann, A.L.; Beets-Tan, R.G. The diagnostic value of MR Imaging in determining the lymph node status of patients with non-small cell lung cancer: A meta-analysis. *Radiology* **2016**, *281*, 86–98. [CrossRef] [PubMed]

13. Shen, G.; Hu, S.; Deng, H.; Kuang, A. Performance of DWI in the nodal characterization and assessment of lung cancer: A meta-analysis. *Am. J. Roentgenol.* **2016**, *206*, 283–290. [CrossRef] [PubMed]
14. Hayes, S.A.; Plodkowski, A.J.; Ginsberg, M.S. Imaging of Thoracic Cavity Tumors. *Surgical Oncology Clinics* **2014**, *23*, 709–733. [CrossRef] [PubMed]
15. Hierholzer, J.; Luo, L.; Bittner, R.C.; Stroszczynski, C.; Schröder, R.J.; Schoenfeld, N.; Dorow, P.; Loddenkemper, R.; Grassot, A. MRI and CT in the differential diagnosis of disease. *Chest* **2000**, *118*, 604–609. [CrossRef] [PubMed]
16. Luo, L.; Hierholzer, J.; Bittner, R.C.; Chen, J.; Huang, L. Magnetic resonance i pleural maging in distinguishing malignant from benign pleural disease. *Chin. Med. J.* **2001**, *114*, 645–649.
17. Luna, A.; Sanchez-Gonzalez, J.; Caro, P. Diffusion weighted imaging of the chest. *Magn. Reason. Imaging Clin. N. Am.* **2011**, *19*, 69–94. [CrossRef] [PubMed]
18. Coolen, J.; De Keyzer, F.; Nafteux, P.; De Wever, W.; Dooms, C.; Vansteenkiste, J.; Roebben, I.; Verbeken, E.; De Leyn, P.; Van Raemdonck, D.; et al. Malignant pleural disease: Diagnosis by using diffusion-weighted and dynamic contrast-enhanced MR imaging-initial experience. *Radiology* **2012**, *263*, 884–892. [CrossRef] [PubMed]
19. Gill, R.R.; Umeoka, S.; Mamata, H.; Tilleman, T.R.; Stanwell, P.; Woodhams, R.; Padera, R.F.; Sugarbaker, D.J.; Hatabu, H. Diffusion-weighted MRI of malignant pleural mesothelioma: Preliminary assessment of apparent diffusion coefficient in histologic subtypes. *Am. J. Roentgenol.* **2010**, *195*, W125–W130. [CrossRef] [PubMed]
20. Bonomi, M.; De Filippis, C.; Lopci, E.; Gianoncelli, L.; Rizzardi, G.; Cerchiaro, E.; Bortolotti, L.; Zanello, A.; Ceresoli, G.L. Clinical staging of malignant pleural mesothelioma: Current perspectives. *Lung Cancer Target Ther.* **2017**, *8*, 127–139. [CrossRef]
21. Jaruskova, M.; Belohlavek, O. Role of FDG-PET and PET/CT in the diagnosis of prolonged febrile states. *Eur. J. Nucl. Med. Mol. Imaging* **2006**, *33*, 913–918. [CrossRef] [PubMed]
22. Flores, R.M.; Akhurst, T.; Gonen, M.; Larson, S.M.; Rusch, V.W. Positron emission tomography defines metastatic disease but not locoregional disease in patients with malignant pleural mesothelioma. *J. Thorac. Cardiovasc. Surg.* **2003**, *126*, 11–16. [CrossRef]
23. Otsuka, H.; Terazawa, K.; Morita, N.; Otomi, Y.; Yamashita, K.; Nishitani, H. Is FDG-PET/CT useful for managing malignant pleural mesothelioma? *J. Med. Investig.* **2009**, *56*, 16–20. [CrossRef] [PubMed]
24. Yang, S.M.; Kim, S.H.; Kang, B.J.; Song, B.J. Extramammary findings on breast MRI: Prevalence and imaging characteristics favoring malignancy detection: A retrospective analysis. *World J. Surg. Oncol.* **2016**, *14*, 119. [CrossRef] [PubMed]
25. Desprechins, B.; Stadnik, T.; Koerts, G.; Shabana, W.; Breucq, C.; Osteaux, M. Use of diffusion-weighted MR imaging in differential diagnosis between intracerebral necrotic tumors and cerebral abscesses. *Am. J. Neuroradiol.* **1999**, *20*, 1252–1257. [PubMed]
26. Qureshi, N.R.; Gleeson, F.V. Imaging of pleural disease. *Clin. Chest Med.* **2006**, *27*, 193–213. [CrossRef] [PubMed]
27. Darge, K.; Jaramillo, D.; Siegel, M.J. Whole-body MRI in children: Current status and future applications. *Eur. J. Radiol.* **2008**, *68*, 289–298. [CrossRef] [PubMed]
28. Usuda, K.; Sagawa, M.; Motono, N.; Ueno, M.; Tanaka, M.; Machida, Y.; Tonami, H. Diagnostic performance of diffusion weighted imaging of malignant and benign pulmonary nodules and masses: Comparison with positron emission tomography. *Asian Pac. J. Cancer Prev.* **2014**, *15*, 4629–4635. [CrossRef] [PubMed]
29. Nasu, K.; Kuroki, Y.; Minami, M. Diffusion-weighted imaging findings of mucinous carcinoma arising in the ano-rectal region. Comparison of apparent diffusion coefficient with that of tubular adenocarcinoma. *Jpn. J. Radiol.* **2012**, *30*, 120–127. [CrossRef] [PubMed]

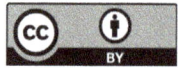

© 2019 by the authors. Licensee MDPI, Basel, Switzerland. This article is an open access article distributed under the terms and conditions of the Creative Commons Attribution (CC BY) license (http://creativecommons.org/licenses/by/4.0/).

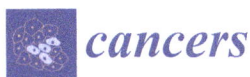

Article

Machine-Learning-Based Prediction of Treatment Outcomes Using MR Imaging-Derived Quantitative Tumor Information in Patients with Sinonasal Squamous Cell Carcinomas: A Preliminary Study

Noriyuki Fujima [1,*], Yukie Shimizu [1], Daisuke Yoshida [1], Satoshi Kano [2], Takatsugu Mizumachi [2], Akihiro Homma [2], Koichi Yasuda [3], Rikiya Onimaru [3], Osamu Sakai [4], Kohsuke Kudo [1] and Hiroki Shirato [3,5]

1. Department of Diagnostic and Interventional Radiology, Hokkaido University Hospital, Sapporo 060-8638, Hokkaido, Japan; yshimizu1222@yahoo.co.jp (Y.S.); panacea-hok@umin.net (D.Y.); kkudo@huhp.hokudai.ac.jp (K.K.)
2. Department of Otolaryngology-Head and Neck Surgery, Hokkaido University Graduate School of Medicine, Sapporo 060-8638, Hokkaido, Japan; skano@med.hokudai.ac.jp (S.K.); mizumati@med.hokudai.ac.jp (T.M.); ak-homma@med.hokudai.ac.jp (A.H.)
3. Department of Radiation Medicine, Hokkaido University Graduate School of Medicine, Sapporo 060-8638, Hokkaido, Japan; kyasuda@med.hokudai.ac.jp (K.Y.); ronimaru@med.hokudai.ac.jp (R.O.); shirato@med.hokudai.ac.jp (H.S.)
4. Departments of Radiology, Otolaryngology-Head and Neck Surgery, and Radiation Oncology, Boston Medical Center, Boston University School of Medicine, Boston, MA 02118, USA; Osamu.Sakai@bmc.org
5. The Global Station for Quantum Medical Science and Engineering, Global Institution for Collaborative Research and Education, Sapporo 060-0808, Hokkaido, Japan
* Correspondence: Noriyuki.Fujima@mb9.seikyou.ne.jp; Tel.: +81-117-065-977; Fax: +81-117-067-876

Received: 18 April 2019; Accepted: 6 June 2019; Published: 10 June 2019

Abstract: The purpose of this study was to determine the predictive power for treatment outcome of a machine-learning algorithm combining magnetic resonance imaging (MRI)-derived data in patients with sinonasal squamous cell carcinomas (SCCs). Thirty-six primary lesions in 36 patients were evaluated. Quantitative morphological parameters and intratumoral characteristics from T2-weighted images, tumor perfusion parameters from arterial spin labeling (ASL) and tumor diffusion parameters of five diffusion models from multi-b-value diffusion-weighted imaging (DWI) were obtained. Machine learning by a non-linear support vector machine (SVM) was used to construct the best diagnostic algorithm for the prediction of local control and failure. The diagnostic accuracy was evaluated using a 9-fold cross-validation scheme, dividing patients into training and validation sets. Classification criteria for the division of local control and failure in nine training sets could be constructed with a mean sensitivity of 0.98, specificity of 0.91, positive predictive value (PPV) of 0.94, negative predictive value (NPV) of 0.97, and accuracy of 0.96. The nine validation data sets showed a mean sensitivity of 1.0, specificity of 0.82, PPV of 0.86, NPV of 1.0, and accuracy of 0.92. In conclusion, a machine-learning algorithm using various MR imaging-derived data can be helpful for the prediction of treatment outcomes in patients with sinonasal SCCs.

Keywords: magnetic resonance imaging; machine learning; diffusion; perfusion; texture analysis; squamous cell carcinoma of the head and neck

1. Introduction

Multimodal treatment such as a combination of surgery, chemotherapy and radiotherapy is the standard treatment methods for head and neck squamous cell carcinomas (SCCs), including nasal cavity or paranasal sinus SCCs [1]. Superselective arterial infusion of cisplatin with concomitant radiotherapy has been widely recognized as a preferred treatment method for maxillary SCCs because of its high local control rate and good prognosis, especially in patients with advanced diseases [2]. In performing such nonsurgical therapy, the ability to predict treatment outcome, for instance whether local control will be achieved, is very important. High-accuracy data-based predictions based on individualized risk categories could help optimize management such as the selection of chemotherapy (e.g., decisions about whether to perform induction chemotherapy) and the best post-treatment follow-up strategy. In this way, truly personalized precision medicine may result from image-based data.

To assess and predict treatment outcomes, information about tumor, node, metastasis (TNM) staging and tumor size have been conventionally used. However, several studies have reported that such tumor conventional morphological information is not necessarily promising for predicting treatment outcomes [3,4]. In contrast, a wide variety of information can be obtained for any tumor from imaging such as quantitative tumor shape data [5], intratumoral textural parameters [6] and tumor functional information such as tumor tissue perfusion information from perfusion-weighted imaging [4,7] and tumor microstructural characteristics from diffusion-weighted imaging (DWI) [8–10]. Especially, several studies identified associations between diffusion parameters derived from DWI and various histopathological features, e.g. expression of Ki-67, p53, degree of tumor cellularity, etc. [11,12]. Tumor perfusion parameters derived from dynamic contrast enhanced (DCE) technique were also reported its correlation to tumor histopathological features such as p16 status and vascular endothelial growth factor (VEGF) expression [13]. Another report demonstrated even conventional magnetic resonance (MR) T1 weighted image (T1WI) and T2 weighted image (T2WI) showed the correlation to several histopathological features with the use of histogram image analysis [14]. In contrast, as another approach by different imaging modality, positron-emission tomography (PET) with ^{18}F-fluorodeoxyglucose (FDG) depicts a tumor's rate of glucose metabolism. Several reports indicated FDG-PET imaging parameters provided significant correlations to many histopathological features [15–19]. However, FDG-PET scanning was a little invasive because of its radiation exposure. In using MR imaging, most abovementioned tumor characteristics can be obtained completely non-invasively without the use of contrast agent and radiation exposure. Several of these MR derived parameters have been reported as independent predictors for treatment outcomes [4,8,20–23]. If we can efficiently integrate these data, prediction of the treatment outcome with high diagnostic accuracy may be obtained.

Conventional multiparametric analysis is an important diagnostic method and will continue to provide clinically useful cut-off values for parameters. However, a more advanced analysis technique is needed to handle the variety of tumor characteristics that are now available. Recently, machine-learning algorithms have been reported to select various parameters effectively in medical imaging analysis including the assessment of head and neck SCC as a kind of artificial intelligence-based diagnostic technique [24,25], however, the number of reports is very limited and they have focused exclusively on intratumoral texture analysis parameters only; the utility of tumor functional information such as tumor perfusion and diffusion is still uncertain. The utilization of advanced parameters by machine learning may achieve ever-better predictive results by integrating data on numerous tumor characteristics.

The aim of this study was to determine the power of a machine-learning algorithm integrating multiple quantitative MR imaging data including shape parameters, intratumoral texture, perfusion and diffusion to predict treatment outcomes in patients with sinonasal SCCs.

2. Results

Fourteen patients were revealed to have local failure. Of these 14 patients, local failure was proven in 11 by surgical biopsy with histological demonstration of residual SCC. In three patients, a large new mass lesion was observed during the follow-up period. The remaining 22 patients were determined to have local control by clinical observation throughout follow-up (mean 57 mos; range 34–86 mos). Imaging analyses of the primary sites were successfully performed in all patients. Details of obtained tumor morphological and intratumoral characteristics, perfusion and diffusion parameters are summarized in Table 1.

Table 1. Data of patients with local control and failure.

			Treatment Outcome	
			Local Control	Local Failure
Patients' Characteristics (no. of patients)	T-stage	T1	0	0
		T2	1	0
		T3	10	3
		T4	11	11
	N-stage	N0	18	12
		N1	2	0
		N2	2	2
		N3	0	0
Morphological Parameters		Tumor volume (mL)	25.3 ± 16.5	34.3 ± 28.6
		Surface area (cm^2)	50.4 ± 18.7	69.6 ± 29.7
		Sphericity	0.71 ± 0.08	0.61 ± 0.11
Intratumoral Characteristics Parameters		Relative mean signal	3.8 ± 0.6	3.4 ± 0.6
		Coefficient of variance	0.12 ± 0.02	0.14 ± 0.04
		Contrast	35.1 ± 6	41.3 ± 8.6
		Correlation	0.84 ± 0.02	0.86 ± 0.03
		Energy ($\times 10^{-3}$)	1.5 ± 0.3	1.2 ± 0.4
		Homogeneity	0.28 ± 0.03	0.26 ± 0.03
Perfusion Parameters		Absolute TBF (mL/100g/min)	156.7 ± 32.9	133.7 ± 29.3
		Relative TBF	7.47 ± 0.83	6.25 ± 1.22
Diffusion Parameters		ADC ($\times 10^{-3}$ mm^2/s)	0.91 ± 0.1	0.87 ± 0.13
		f ($\times 10^2$ %)	0.16 ± 0.05	0.16 ± 0.07
		D* ($\times 10^{-3}$ mm^2/s)	19.5 ± 7.5	16.7 ± 5.7
		D ($\times 10^{-3}$ mm^2/s)	0.75 ± 0.06	0.73 ± 0.09
		K	0.73 ± 0.07	0.76 ± 0.08
		D_k ($\times 10^{-3}$ mm^2/s)	1.24 ± 0.14	1.22 ± 0.19
		alpha (α)	0.69 ± 0.07	0.67 ± 0.08
		DDC ($\times 10^{-3}$ mm^2/s)	1.14 ± 0.12	1.12 ± 0.17
		f_1 ($\times 10^2$ %)	0.14 ± 0.04	0.13 ± 0.04
		f_2 ($\times 10^2$ %)	0.23 ± 0.04	0.25 ± 0.05
		f_3 ($\times 10^2$ %)	0.62 ± 0.06	0.61 ± 0.08
		D_1 ($\times 10^{-3}$ mm^2/s)	32.9 ± 7.8	28.1 ± 6.5
		D_2 ($\times 10^{-3}$ mm^2/s)	1.03 ± 0.16	0.92 ± 0.15
		D_3 ($\times 10^{-3}$ mm^2/s)	0.64 ± 0.07	0.62 ± 0.1

Data are means ± standard deviations. TBF, tumor blood flow; ADC, apparent diffusion coefficient; f, perfusion fraction; D*, fast diffusion coefficient; D, true diffusion coefficient; K, kurtosis value; D_k, kurtosis corrected diffusion coefficient; α, diffusion heterogeneity; DDC, distributed diffusion coefficient; f_1, perfusion-related diffusion fraction; f_2, intermediate diffusion fraction; f_3, slow diffusion fraction; D_1, perfusion-related diffusion coefficient; D_2, intermediate diffusion coefficient; D_3, slow diffusion coefficient.

In the support vector machine (SVM) analysis, classification criteria for the discernment of local control versus failure in the training set data could be constructed with a sensitivity of 0.98, specificity of 0.91, positive predictive value of 0.94, negative predictive value of 0.97 and accuracy of 0.96, as a mean value obtained from the nine test set data. In the parameter selection process, the five top-ranked features in all nine training data sets included the perfusion parameter of relative tumor blood flow (TBF), morphological parameter of tumor sphericity, and texture parameter of contrast. In addition, the morphological parameter of tumor volume was selected six times, the diffusion parameter of intermediate diffusion coefficient (D_2) in tri-exponential model DWI five times, the diffusion parameter of perfusion fraction f in the intravoxel incoherent motion (IVIM) DWI model three times, the texture parameter of energy twice, and both diffusion parameters of apparent diffusion coefficient (ADC) and patient characteristics of T-stage once. Details of results for training group data are presented in Table 2.

Table 2. Results of the Training Set Data (n=32 in each set).

Set No.	Sensitivity	Specificity	PPV	NPV	Accuracy
1	1	0.92	0.95	1	0.97
Top 5 ranked variables: Sphericity, Relative TBF, Contrast, D2, f					
2	1	1	1	1	1
Top 5 ranked variables: Relative TBF, Sphericity, Contrast, T-stage, Tumor volume					
3	1	0.85	0.9	1	0.94
Top 5 ranked variables: Relative TBF, Contrast, Sphericity, Tumor volume, f					
4	0.95	0.78	0.91	0.9	0.91
Top 5 ranked variables: Relative TBF, Sphericity, D2, Energy, Contrast					
5	1	1	1	1	1
Top 5 ranked variables: Sphericity, Relative TBF, D2, Contrast, Tumor volume					
6	1	0.85	0.9	1	0.94
Top 5 ranked variables: Relative TBF, Sphericity, f, Contrast, Energy					
7	1	0.92	0.95	1	0.97
Top 5 ranked variables: Sphericity, Relative TBF, Contrast, Tumor volume, ADC					
8	0.94	0.93	0.94	0.93	0.94
Top 5 ranked variables: Relative TBF, Sphericity, Contrast, D2, Tumor volume					
9	0.95	0.9	0.95	0.9	0.94
Top 5 ranked variables: Relative TBF, Sphericity, D2, Contrast, Tumor volume					
Average	0.98	0.91	0.94	0.97	0.96

PPV, positive predictive value; NPV, negative predictive value; TBF, tumor blood flow; D_2, intermediate diffusion coefficient; f, perfusion fraction; ADC, apparent diffusion coefficient.

The classification algorithm for the discernment of local control versus failure obtained by training set data was further used for the classification in the validation set data. Group assignment in the validation data set was achieved with a sensitivity of 1.0, specificity of 0.82, positive predictive value of 0.86, negative predictive value of 1.0 and accuracy of 0.92; these values were the means of total 36 validation data (4 × 9 validation sets).

3. Discussion

Our findings revealed that a machine-learning-derived diagnostic algorithm by pre-treatment MR imaging-derived tumor data can highly predict the treatment outcome of local control versus failure in patients with sinonasal SCCs. To the best of our knowledge, the current study is the first report to indicate the utility of a machine learning-based diagnosis derived from quantitative morphological, intratumoral, perfusion and diffusion data. This diagnostic ability can be useful as a kind of artificial intelligence-based technique. Being able to predict the local outcome of the primary tumor would have a significant impact on treatment decision. If a poor outcome after chemoradiation therapy is strongly indicated, additional or alternate treatment plan such as induction chemotherapy, earlier salvage surgery after the chemoradiotherapy, or surgical resection prior to chemoradiation therapy may be offered. Follow-up strategy after the treatment such as the frequency and duration of the imaging follow-up may be also optimized individually, depending on the pre-treatment risks.

Quantitative morphological shape characteristics of tumors (i.e., sphericity) were recently reported to be useful for the prediction of treatment outcomes in head and neck SCC as an advanced morphological parameter compared to TNM stage and tumor size [5,23]. Intratumoral heterogeneity was also indicated as a prognostic factor in head and neck SCC patients [26,27]; in these reports, tumors with high degree of intratumoral heterogeneity demonstrated a tendency for poor prognoses. In contrast, tumor perfusion and diffusion are considered to be major tumor functional parameters that indirectly reflect biological processes; thus, these may be related to individual treatment sensitivity. In previous reports, tumor perfusion was described as an important predictor of the treatment outcome [4]. Lower tumor perfusion was related to poor treatment outcome in these reports, probably because of the relation between tumor hypoxia and lower tumor perfusion [28,29]. Tumor diffusion was also significantly related to treatment outcome in head and neck SCC patients; in numerous ADC studies [30], low ADC was related to a good treatment outcome. Additionally, non-Gaussian diffusion parameters beyond ADC values have been recently shown to be useful for treatment outcome prediction [8].

The various characteristics of tumor shape, intratumoral characteristics, and tumor perfusion and diffusion are expected to reflect different types of biological conditions. Multiparametric use of these data were suggested to allow each parameter's diagnostic power to be expressed. A previous study used multiparametric analysis employing both ADC values and tumor perfusion information, and concluded that the combination of diffusion and perfusion data was helpful for diagnosis [31]. However, diagnostic performance was not still complete, probably because simple cut-offs are insufficient to fully reflect tumor biology. In the current study, the machine-learning algorithm seemed to emphasize all effective parameters sufficiently. The high diagnostic accuracy of treatment outcome prediction obtained by the present study is probably due to the effective use of numerous tumor characteristics with an ideal determination strategy. The various characteristics differ from patient to patient; non-invasive acquisition of numerous tumor characteristics using advanced MR imaging sequence and post-processing techniques and determination of the diagnostic strategy using this machine-learning algorithm should contribute greatly to individualized precision medicine for sinonasal SCC patients.

The current study has several limitations. First, the number of patients was quite small. However, sinonasal SCC are not very common, and it would be a challenge to investigate a larger number of sinonasal SCC patients who received advanced MR imaging protocol and long-term follow-up. The results of the present study should be regarded as preliminary. Second, analysis of intratumoral characteristics was performed only in T2WI. Arterial spin labeling (ASL) and DWI were acquired with the use of large pixel size to obtain sufficient signal-to-noise ratios; therefore, especially complex intratumoral analysis such as second-order texture was somewhat difficult. Additionally, post-contrast-enhanced T1WI is somewhat invasive, and differences in readout schemes such as 2D or 3D acquisition affect intratumoral texture data. Third, although a few studies which performed radiomics approach to predict treatment outcome in patients with head and neck cancer were recently reported [32–35], whether diagnostic power obtained in the current study will be superior or not compared to previous reports is still unclear. It was because patient characteristics, treatment method, follow-up strategy, imaging technique and diagnostic model construction algorism were quite different among these studies. Further analysis to address these limitations will be needed.

4. Materials and Methods

4.1. Subjects

This retrospective study was approved by the institutional review board of Hokkaido University Hospital (ID: 017-0322, date of approval: 28th February 2018), and the requirement to obtain written informed consent was waived. From September 2010 to October 2015, 36 consecutive patients with histopathologically proven sinonasal SCCs who were referred to our hospital to undergo superselective arterial infusion of cisplatin with concomitant radiotherapy were enrolled in this study. Patient characteristics are summarized in Table 3.

The treatment regimen was a superselective arterial infusion of cisplatin with concomitant radiotherapy for all patients. Superselective transarterial infusion therapy with cisplatin (100–120 mg/m^2 per week for 4 weeks) via the dominant feeding arteries to the primary tumor was performed using a microcatheter, with concurrent radiotherapy of a total of 70 Gy in 35 fractions with curative intent.

Table 3. Patient characteristics (n = 36).

	Number of Patients
Age	
Range	43–73
Median	59
Average	58.7
Gender	
Male	28
Female	8
Primary tumor site	
Nasal cavity	6
Paranasal sinus	30
T-stage	
T1	0
T2	1
T3	13
T4a	17
T4b	5
N-stage	
N0	30
N1	2
N2	4
N3	0
Smoking status	
Tabacco smokers	31
Packs-years	
Range	2–161
Median	34
Average	40.4
Alcohol use	
Occasional or non-drinker	10
Moderate use	6
Heavy use	20

4.2. MR Imaging Protocol

All MR imaging was performed using a 3.0-Tesla unit (Achieva TX; Philips Healthcare, Best, The Netherlands) with a 16-channel neurovascular coil. MR imaging including conventional anatomical imaging of spin-echo (SE) T1WIs, turbo spin-echo (TSE) fat-suppressed (Fs) T2WIs, ASL and multiple b-value DWI was performed before treatment in all patients. The patients were instructed not to swallow, move their tongues, open their mouths, or make any other voluntary motion during the MR scan. All axial slices were placed in parallel with the anterior commissure-posterior commissure line.

4.2.1. Conventional MR Imaging Acquisition

Conventional MR imaging sequences were obtained to evaluate the primary tumor including axial SE T1WIs (TR, 450 ms; TE, 10 ms; field of view (FOV), 240 × 240 mm; 512 × 512 matrix; slice thickness, 5 mm; inter-slice gap, 30%; scanning time, 2 min 12 s), and axial TSE Fs-T2WIs (TR, 4500 ms; TE, 70 ms; TSE factor, 9; FOV, 240 × 240 mm; 512 × 512 matrix; slice thickness, 5 mm; inter-slice gap, 30%; scanning time, 2 min 06 s). Coronal TSE T2WIs (TR, 4,500 ms; TE, 70 ms; TSE factor, 9; FOV, 240 × 240 mm; matrix, 512 × 512; slice thickness, 4 mm; inter-slice gap, 30%; scanning time, 2 min 06 s) were also obtained as a supporting tool for ASL acquisition (*see below*).

4.2.2. ASL Acquisition

For the ASL imaging, a pseudo-continuous ASL (pCASL) technique was used. The acquisition of pCASL was performed using multi-shot spin-echo echo-planar imaging to obtain control and labeled images. The labeling slab was placed just under the bifurcation of the internal and external carotid arteries using coronal T2WIs as a reference for the placement of the labeling plane by carefully detecting the vessel flow void. Control images were obtained without the labeling of arterial water, using the same imaging scheme as the labeled images. The acquisition parameters of the pCASL were as follows: labeling duration, 1650 ms; post-label delay, 1280 ms; TR, 3619 ms; TE, 18 ms; flip angle, 90°; number of shots, two; FOV, 230 × 230 mm; matrix, 80 × 80; slice thickness, 5 mm; number of slices, 15; acceleration factor for parallel imaging, two; scanning time, 5 min 11 s. ASL-based perfusion-weighted images were obtained by subtracting values of the control from the labeled images.

4.2.3. DWI Acquisition

The DWI acquisition used single-shot spin-echo echo-planar imaging (EPI) with three orthogonal motion-probing gradients. Twelve b-values (0, 10, 20, 30, 50, 80, 100, 200, 400, 800, 1,000, and 2000 s/mm^2) were used. Other imaging parameters were: TR, 4500 ms; TE, 64 ms; DELTA (large delta; gradient time interval), 30.1 ms; delta (small delta; gradient duration), 24.3 ms; flip angle, 90°; FOV, 230 × 230 mm; 64 × 64 matrix; slice thickness, 5 mm × 20 slices; voxel size 3.59 × 3.59 × 5.00 mm; parallel imaging acceleration factor, 2; numbers of signal averages, b-value of 0–100 s/mm^2 (one average), 200–800 s/mm^2 (two averages) and 1000–2000 s/mm^2 (three averages); scanning time, 4 min 37 s.

4.3. Data Analysis

4.3.1. ROI Delineation

A board-certified neuroradiologist with ten years' experience in head and neck imaging delineated each tumor with a polygonal region-of-interest (ROI) on Fs-T2WIs, ASL subtraction images and DWI b0 images. The ROI of the axial Fs-T2WI was placed first; then almost the same ROI was delineated with reference to the Fs-T2WI ROI so that the same region was delineated for all sequences. For the DWI analysis, the tumor ROI on the b0 image was copied on the echo planar imaging (EPI) of the respective b-values. Any area suspected of being a necrotic or a cystic lesion was excluded from the ROI. If the tumor extended into two or more slices, all slices were delineated respectively. In addition, the medial pterygoid muscle of the healthy side was also delineated with a polygonal ROI on Fs-T2WI and ASL images for the relative T2WI signal intensity and perfusion parameter calculation with reference to the axial Fs-T2WI.

4.3.2. Analysis of Fs-T2WI for Morphological and Intratumoral Data

For the analysis of morphological characteristics, we calculated the tumor volume and tumor surface area from the morphological shape of all selected tumor voxels with the delineated tumor ROI on Fs-T2WI. The sphericity of each tumor was calculated by a previously reported method [23]. For the intra-tumoral characteristics analysis, we calculated the relative Fs-T2WI mean signal intensity (=mean signal on tumor ROI/ the medial pterygoid muscle ROI), the coefficient of variance (CV) in the tumor ROI and the textural parameters within the ROI. Textural features included the contrast, correlation, energy, and homogeneity, based on gray-level co-occurrence matrix (GLCM) features, namely, spatially detailed signal intensity data within the tumor ROI; GLCM were previously described the most common and sensitive texture descriptor to calculate lesion heterogeneity in greater detail from the texture data [36]. Texture parameters were calculated based on a previously reported method [37].

4.3.3. ASL and DWI Analysis

We calculated the TBF of the pCASL from the signal data in ASL subtraction images using the previously described equation [7]. Both absolute and relative TBF values were calculated, with absolute TBF being the mean TBF value in the delineated tumor ROI, and relative TBF being that value divided by the medial pterygoid muscle blood flow, i.e., the mean value in the muscle ROI [7]. From the diffusion signal data, we calculated each parameter of mono-exponential function (i.e., ADC), bi-exponential function so-called IVIM (the perfusion fraction f, the pseudo-diffusion coefficient D*, and the true diffusion coefficient D), the tri-exponential function (the perfusion-related diffusion fraction f_1 and coefficient D_1, the intermediate diffusion fraction f_2 and coefficient D_2, and the slow diffusion fraction f_3 and coefficient D_3), the stretched exponential model (SEM) (diffusion heterogeneity α and distributed diffusion coefficient DDC) and the diffusion kurtosis imaging (DKI) (kurtosis value K and kurtosis-corrected diffusion coefficient D_k). Using the signal intensities of all 12 b-values, we calculated the bi-exponential and tri-exponential function parameters. Assessments of the ADC, SEM and DKI usually target tissue diffusion (except for the perfusion-related signal), and we therefore used the signal intensity of six b-values (0, 200, 400, 800, 1000 and 2000 s/mm^2) for the parameter calculations of ADC, DKI and SEM. To perform these parameter calculations, we used the previously reported calculation method [38]. In-house developed program by MATLAB ver. 2015a (MathWorks, Natick, MA, USA) was used for the above-described calculations.

4.4. Determination of the Clinical Outcome

In all patients, clinical and radiological follow-up was performed for ≥ 2 years after treatment to determine the final diagnosis of local control/failure at the primary site. During follow-up period, if residual/recurrent tumor was suspected by visual inspection or radiological assessment (e.g., development of mass like lesion in post-treatment granulation tissue), surgical resection was performed to confirm the presence of histological residual/recurrent tumor. If patient's consent for the surgical resection was not obtained, careful observation was continued. Local failure was defined by the histopathological confirmation of SCC in biopsied or surgically resected tissue, or the observation of clearly development/enlargement of a mass lesion arisen from post-treatment granulation. Local control was defined by histopathological confirmation of the absence of SCC by surgical resection and no enlargement of soft tissue in post-treatment granulation throughout the follow-up period.

4.5. Statistical Analysis Based on Machine Learning Algorithm

A machine-learning algorithm by non-linear SVM with radial basis function was used to obtain the best diagnostic algorithm for the differentiation of local control versus failure groups. The kernel size (γ) and regularization parameter (C) with the best performance to predict the local control versus failure group was determined by the grid-search technique within ranges of 2^{-20} to 2^{10} for γ and from 2^{-10} to 2^{10} for C. In the feature-selection process, we performed backward sequential selection to determine the ranking in all features as well as the best diagnostic algorithm. This method is based on an iterative technique in which the starting condition includes all features. With each iteration, the feature with the least impact on improving the diagnostic performance for the differentiation of local control versus failure is eliminated. Features are removed one by one, and the rank of each feature is determined by the number of the iteration in which it was eliminated. Higher ranked features are explained that remained through the longest number of iterations. Ultimately, several highly ranked features that showed the highest diagnostic accuracy for predicting local control versus failure groups were included in the final established diagnostic model [39]. To avoid the possibility of overfitting with the use of leave-one-out cross-validation technique, the accuracy of the prediction was evaluated through a 9-fold cross-validation scheme. The data were randomly divided into 9 equal-size subsets (i.e. four patients each), of which eight subsets of the 32 (4 × 8) patients were used for training and the remaining one of four (4 × 1) patients for validating. The mean diagnostic accuracy over 9 repetitions was calculated for all possible combinations of features to find the combination of features with the highest predictive power. The overall analytic process is summarized in Figure 1. All of the analysis was performed using MATLAB ver. 2015a.

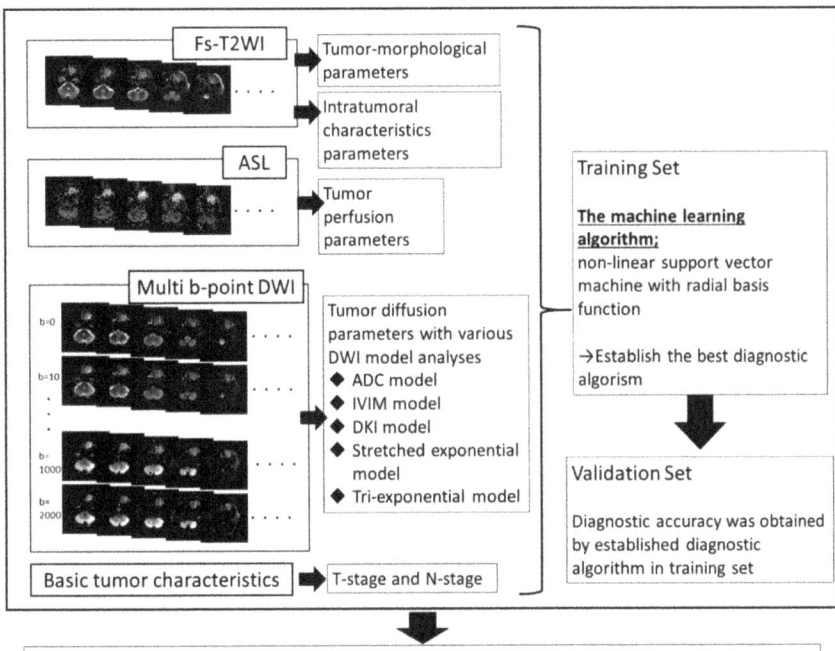

Figure 1. The overall process for parameter acquisition and machine-learning analysis.

Morphological and intratumoral data from Fs-T2WI, perfusion data from ASL and diffusion data from DWI were respectively obtained by post-processing image analysis. The diagnostic algorithm was constructed by the machine-learning technique from all the obtained parameters in the training set patient group; then, the diagnostic accuracy of the constructed algorithm was calculated from the data in the validation set. This process was repetitively performed 9 times in each set of training and validation groups in a total cross-validation analysis.

5. Conclusions

The integration of quantitative tumor morphological, intratumoral textural, perfusion and diffusion data with the machine-learning-based analysis might be highly accurate at predicting treatment outcomes in patients with sinonasal SCC. This information could help in making decisions regarding treatment options such as details of treatment planning, additional treatment, and follow-up strategies, and thus to improved patient prognoses.

Author Contributions: Conceptualization, N.F.; Methodology, N.F.; Software, Y.S.; Validation, Y.S. and D.Y.; Formal Analysis, N.F., Y.S., D.Y. and K.K.; Investigation, S.K., T.M. and A.H.; Resources, K.Y. and R.O.; Data Curation, N.F., Y.S. and K.K.; Writing—Original Draft Preparation, N.F. and O.S.; Writing—Review & Editing, Y.S., S.K., T.M., A.H., K.Y., R.O., K.K. and H.S.; Visualization, Y.S., D.Y. and O.S.; Supervision, H.S.; Project Administration, N.F. and K.K.; Funding Acquisition, N.F.

Funding: This study has received funding by grant support from Ministry of Education, Culture, Sports, Science and Technology-Japan (ID; 18K07661).

Conflicts of Interest: The authors declare no conflict of interest.

References

1. Wong, S.J.; Harari, P.M.; Garden, A.S.; Schwartz, M.; Bellm, L.; Chen, A.; Curran, W.J.; Murphy, B.A.; Ang, K.K. Longitudinal Oncology Registry of Head and Neck Carcinoma (LORHAN): Analysis of chemoradiation treatment approaches in the United States. *Cancer* **2011**, *117*, 1679–1686. [CrossRef] [PubMed]
2. Homma, A.; Sakashita, T.; Yoshida, D.; Onimaru, R.; Tsuchiya, K.; Suzuki, F.; Yasuda, K.; Hatakeyama, H.; Furusawa, J.; Mizumachi, T.; et al. Superselective intra-arterial cisplatin infusion and concomitant radiotherapy for maxillary sinus cancer. *Br. J. Cancer* **2013**, *109*, 2980–2986. [CrossRef] [PubMed]
3. Cao, Y.; Popovtzer, A.; Li, D.; Chepeha, D.B.; Moyer, J.S.; Prince, M.E.; Worden, F.; Teknos, T.; Bradford, C.; Mukherji, S.K.; et al. Early prediction of outcome in advanced head-and-neck cancer based on tumor blood volume alterations during therapy: A prospective study. *Int. J. Radiat. Oncol. Biol. Phys.* **2008**, *72*, 1287–1290. [CrossRef] [PubMed]
4. Fujima, N.; Yoshida, D.; Sakashita, T.; Homma, A.; Tsukahara, A.; Tha, K.K.; Kudo, K.; Shirato, H. Usefulness of Pseudocontinuous Arterial Spin-Labeling for the Assessment of Patients with Head and Neck Squamous Cell Carcinoma by Measuring Tumor Blood Flow in the Pretreatment and Early Treatment Period. *Am. J. Neuroradiol.* **2016**, *37*, 342–348. [CrossRef] [PubMed]
5. Apostolova, I.; Steffen, I.G.; Wedel, F.; Lougovski, A.; Marnitz, S.; Derlin, T.; Amthauer, H.; Buchert, R.; Hofheinz, F.; Brenner, W. Asphericity of pretherapeutic tumour FDG uptake provides independent prognostic value in head-and-neck cancer. *Eur. Radiol.* **2014**, *24*, 2077–2087. [CrossRef] [PubMed]
6. Buch, K.; Fujita, A.; Li, B.; Kawashima, Y.; Qureshi, M.M.; Sakai, O. Using Texture Analysis to Determine Human Papillomavirus Status of Oropharyngeal Squamous Cell Carcinomas on CT. *Am. J. Neuroradiol.* **2015**, *36*, 1343–1348. [CrossRef] [PubMed]
7. Fujima, N.; Kudo, K.; Tsukahara, A.; Yoshida, D.; Sakashita, T.; Homma, A.; Tha, K.K.; Shirato, H. Measurement of tumor blood flow in head and neck squamous cell carcinoma by pseudo-continuous arterial spin labeling: Comparison with dynamic contrast-enhanced MRI. *J. Magn. Reson. Imaging* **2015**, *41*, 983–991. [CrossRef] [PubMed]
8. Fujima, N.; Yoshida, D.; Sakashita, T.; Homma, A.; Tsukahara, A.; Shimizu, Y.; Tha, K.K.; Kudo, K.; Shirato, H. Prediction of the treatment outcome using intravoxel incoherent motion and diffusional kurtosis imaging in nasal or sinonasal squamous cell carcinoma patients. *Eur. Radiol.* **2017**, *27*, 956–965. [CrossRef]
9. Surov, A.; Stumpp, P.; Meyer, H.J.; Gawlitza, M.; Hohn, A.K.; Boehm, A.; Sabri, O.; Kahn, T.; Purz, S. Simultaneous (18)F-FDG-PET/MRI: Associations between diffusion, glucose metabolism and histopathological parameters in patients with head and neck squamous cell carcinoma. *Oral Oncol.* **2016**, *58*, 14–20. [CrossRef]
10. Swartz, J.E.; Driessen, J.P.; van Kempen, P.M.W.; de Bree, R.; Janssen, L.M.; Pameijer, F.A.; Terhaard, C.H.J.; Philippens, M.E.P.; Willems, S. Influence of tumor and microenvironment characteristics on diffusion-weighted imaging in oropharyngeal carcinoma: A pilot study. *Oral Oncol.* **2018**, *77*, 9–15. [CrossRef]
11. Meyer, H.J.; Leifels, L.; Hamerla, G.; Höhn, A.K.; Surov, A. ADC-histogram analysis in head and neck squamous cell carcinoma. Associations with different histopathological features including expression of EGFR, VEGF, HIF-1α, Her 2 and p53. A preliminary study. *Magn. Reson. Imaging* **2018**, *54*, 214–217. [CrossRef] [PubMed]
12. Surov, A.; Meyer, H.J.; Winter, K.; Richter, C.; Hoehn, A.K. Histogram analysis parameters of apparent diffusion coefficient reflect tumor cellularity and proliferation activity in head and neck squamous cell carcinoma. *Oncotarget* **2018**, *9*, 23599–23607. [CrossRef] [PubMed]
13. Meyer, H.J.; Leifels, L.; Hamerla, G.; Höhn, A.K.; Surov, A. Associations between Histogram Analysis Parameters Derived from DCE-MRI and Histopathological Features including Expression of EGFR, p16, VEGF, Hif1-alpha, and p53 in HNSCC. *Contrast Media Mol. Imaging* **2019**, *2019*, 5081909. [CrossRef] [PubMed]
14. Meyer, H.J.; Leifels, L.; Hamerla, G.; Höhn, A.K.; Surov, A. Histogram Analysis Parameters Derived from Conventional T1- and T2-Weighted Images Can Predict Different Histopathological Features Including Expression of Ki67, EGFR, VEGF, HIF-1α, and p53 and Cell Count in Head and Neck Squamous Cell Carcinoma. *Mol. Imaging Biol.* **2019**. [CrossRef] [PubMed]

15. Grönroos, T.J.; Lehtiö, K.; Söderström, K.O.; Kronqvist, P.; Laine, J.; Eskola, O.; Viljanen, T.; Grénman, R.; Solin, O.; Minn, H. Hypoxia, blood flow and metabolism in squamous-cell carcinoma of the head and neck: Correlations between multiple immunohistochemical parameters and PET. *BMC Cancer* **2014**, *14*, 876. [CrossRef] [PubMed]
16. Rasmussen, G.B.; Vogelius, I.R.; Rasmussen, J.H.; Schumaker, L.; Ioffe, O.; Cullen, K.; Fischer, B.M.; Therkildsen, M.H.; Specht, L.; Bentzen, S.M. Immunohistochemical biomarkers and FDG uptake on PET/CT in head and neck squamous cell carcinoma. *Acta Oncol.* **2015**, *54*, 1408–1415. [CrossRef]
17. Surov, A.; Meyer, H.J.; Wienke, A. Can Imaging Parameters Provide Information Regarding Histopathology in Head and Neck Squamous Cell Carcinoma? A Meta-Analysis. *Transl. Oncol.* **2018**, *11*, 498–503. [CrossRef]
18. Surov, A.; Meyer, H.J.; Höhn, A.K.; Winter, K.; Sabri, O.; Purz, S. Associations between 18F-FDG-PET and complex histopathological parameters including tumor cell count and expression of KI 67, EGFR, VEGF, HIF-1α and p53 in head and neck squamous cell carcinoma. *Mol. Imaging Biol.* **2019**, *21*, 368–374. [CrossRef]
19. Zhao, K.; Yang, S.Y.; Zhou, S.H.; Dong, M.J.; Bao, Y.Y.; Yao, H.T. Fluorodeoxyglucose uptake in laryngeal carcinoma is associated with the expression of glucose transporter-1 and hypoxia-inducible-factor-1α and the phosphoinositide 3-kinase/protein kinase B pathway. *Oncol. Lett.* **2014**, *7*, 984–990. [CrossRef]
20. Chen, Y.; Ren, W.; Zheng, D.; Zhong, J.; Liu, X.; Yue, Q.; Liu, M.; Xiao, Y.; Chen, W.; Chan, Q.; et al. Diffusion kurtosis imaging predicts neoadjuvant chemotherapy responses within 4 days in advanced nasopharyngeal carcinoma patients. *J. Magn. Reson. Imaging* **2015**, *42*, 1354–1361. [CrossRef]
21. Paudyal, R.; Oh, J.H.; Riaz, N.; Venigalla, P.; Li, J.; Hatzoglou, V.; Leeman, J.; Nunez, D.A.; Lu, Y.; Deasy, J.O.; et al. Intravoxel incoherent motion diffusion-weighted MRI during chemoradiation therapy to characterize and monitor treatment response in human papillomavirus head and neck squamous cell carcinoma. *J. Magn. Reson. Imaging* **2017**, *45*, 1013–1023. [CrossRef] [PubMed]
22. Noij, D.P.; Martens, R.M.; Marcus, J.T.; de Bree, R.; Leemans, C.R.; Castelijns, J.A.; de Jong, M.C.; de Graaf, P. Intravoxel incoherent motion magnetic resonance imaging in head and neck cancer: A systematic review of the diagnostic and prognostic value. *Oral Oncol.* **2017**, *68*, 81–91. [CrossRef] [PubMed]
23. Fujima, N.; Hirata, K.; Shiga, T.; Yasuda, K.; Onimaru, R.; Tsuchiya, K.; Kano, S.; Mizumachi, T.; Homma, A.; Kudo, K.; et al. Semi-quantitative analysis of pre-treatment morphological and intratumoral characteristics using (18)F-fluorodeoxyglucose positron-emission tomography as predictors of treatment outcome in nasal and paranasal squamous cell carcinoma. *Quant. Imaging Med. Surg.* **2018**, *8*, 788–795. [CrossRef] [PubMed]
24. Parmar, C.; Grossmann, P.; Rietveld, D.; Rietbergen, M.M.; Lambin, P.; Aerts, H.J. Radiomic Machine-Learning Classifiers for Prognostic Biomarkers of Head and Neck Cancer. *Front. Oncol.* **2015**, *5*, 272. [CrossRef] [PubMed]
25. Leger, S.; Zwanenburg, A.; Pilz, K.; Lohaus, F.; Linge, A.; Zophel, K.; Kotzerke, J.; Schreiber, A.; Tinhofer, I.; Budach, V.; et al. A comparative study of machine learning methods for time-to-event survival data for radiomics risk modelling. *Sci. Rep.* **2017**, *7*, 13206. [CrossRef]
26. Kuno, H.; Qureshi, M.M.; Chapman, M.N.; Li, B.; Andreu-Arasa, V.C.; Onoue, K.; Truong, M.T.; Sakai, O. CT Texture Analysis Potentially Predicts Local Failure in Head and Neck Squamous Cell Carcinoma Treated with Chemoradiotherapy. *Am. J. Neuroradiol.* **2017**, *38*, 2334–2340. [CrossRef]
27. Cheng, N.M.; Fang, Y.H.; Chang, J.T.; Huang, C.G.; Tsan, D.L.; Ng, S.H.; Wang, H.M.; Lin, C.Y.; Liao, C.T.; Yen, T.C. Textural features of pretreatment 18F-FDG PET/CT images: Prognostic significance in patients with advanced T-stage oropharyngeal squamous cell carcinoma. *Eur. J. Nucl. Med. Mol. Imaging* **2013**, *54*, 1703–1709. [CrossRef]
28. Newbold, K.; Castellano, I.; Charles-Edwards, E.; Mears, D.; Sohaib, A.; Leach, M.; Rhys-Evans, P.; Clarke, P.; Fisher, C.; Harrington, K.; et al. An exploratory study into the role of dynamic contrast-enhanced magnetic resonance imaging or perfusion computed tomography for detection of intratumoral hypoxia in head-and-neck cancer. *Int. J. Radiat. Oncol. Biol. Phys.* **2009**, *74*, 29–37. [CrossRef]
29. Donaldson, S.B.; Betts, G.; Bonington, S.C.; Homer, J.J.; Slevin, N.J.; Kershaw, L.E.; Valentine, H.; West, C.M.; Buckley, D.L. Perfusion estimated with rapid dynamic contrast-enhanced magnetic resonance imaging correlates inversely with vascular endothelial growth factor expression and pimonidazole staining in head-and-neck cancer: A pilot study. *Int. J. Radiat. Oncol. Biol. Phys.* **2011**, *81*, 1176–1183. [CrossRef]
30. King, A.D.; Thoeny, H.C. Functional MRI for the prediction of treatment response in head and neck squamous cell carcinoma: Potential and limitations. *Cancer Imaging* **2016**, *16*, 23. [CrossRef]

31. Chawla, S.; Kim, S.; Dougherty, L.; Wang, S.; Loevner, L.A.; Quon, H.; Poptani, H. Pretreatment diffusion-weighted and dynamic contrast-enhanced MRI for prediction of local treatment response in squamous cell carcinomas of the head and neck. *Am. J. Roentgenol.* **2013**, *200*, 35–43. [CrossRef] [PubMed]
32. Jethanandani, A.; Lin, T.A.; Volpe, S.; Elhalawani, H.; Mohamed, A.S.R.; Yang, P.; Fuller, C.D. Exploring Applications of Radiomics in Magnetic Resonance Imaging of Head and Neck Cancer: A Systematic Review. *Front. Oncol.* **2018**, *8*, 131. [CrossRef] [PubMed]
33. Wang, G.; He, L.; Yuan, C.; Huang, Y.; Liu, Z.; Liang, C. Pretreatment MR imaging radiomics signatures for response prediction to induction chemotherapy in patients with nasopharyngeal carcinoma. *Eur. J. Radiol.* **2018**, *98*, 100–106. [CrossRef]
34. Zhang, B.; He, X.; Ouyang, F.; Gu, D.; Dong, Y.; Zhang, L.; Mo, X.; Huang, W.; Tian, J.; Zhang, S. Radiomic machine-learning classifiers for prognostic biomarkers of advanced nasopharyngeal carcinoma. *Cancer Lett.* **2017**, *403*, 21–27. [CrossRef] [PubMed]
35. Zhang, B.; Tian, J.; Dong, D.; Gu, D.; Dong, Y.; Zhang, L.; Lian, Z.; Liu, J.; Luo, X.; Pei, S.; et al. Radiomics Features of Multiparametric MRI as Novel Prognostic Factors in Advanced Nasopharyngeal Carcinoma. *Clin. Cancer Res.* **2017**, *23*, 4259–4269. [CrossRef] [PubMed]
36. Vujasinovic, T.; Pribic, J.; Kanjer, K.; Milosevic, N.T.; Tomasevic, Z.; Milovanovic, Z.; Nikolic-Vukosavljevic, D.; Radulovic, M. Gray-Level Co-Occurrence Matrix Texture Analysis of Breast Tumor Images in Prognosis of Distant Metastasis Risk. *Microsc. Microanal.* **2015**, *21*, 646–654. [CrossRef] [PubMed]
37. Fujima, N.; Homma, A.; Harada, T.; Shimizu, Y.; Tha, K.K.; Kano, S.; Mizumachi, T.; Li, R.; Kudo, K.; Shirato, H. The utility of MRI histogram and texture analysis for the prediction of histological diagnosis in head and neck malignancies. *Cancer Imaging* **2019**, *19*, 5. [CrossRef] [PubMed]
38. Fujima, N.; Sakashita, T.; Homma, A.; Shimizu, Y.; Yoshida, A.; Harada, T.; Tha, K.K.; Kudo, K.; Shirato, H. Advanced diffusion models in head and neck squamous cell carcinoma patients: Goodness of fit, relationships among diffusion parameters and comparison with dynamic contrast-enhanced perfusion. *Magn. Reson. Imaging* **2017**, *36*, 16–23. [CrossRef] [PubMed]
39. Xu, X.; Zhang, X.; Tian, Q.; Wang, H.; Cui, L.B.; Li, S.; Tang, X.; Li, B.; Dolz, J.; Ayed, I.B.; et al. Quantitative Identification of Nonmuscle-Invasive and Muscle-Invasive Bladder Carcinomas: A Multiparametric MRI Radiomics Analysis. *J. Magn. Reson. Imaging* **2018**. [CrossRef]

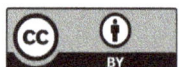

© 2019 by the authors. Licensee MDPI, Basel, Switzerland. This article is an open access article distributed under the terms and conditions of the Creative Commons Attribution (CC BY) license (http://creativecommons.org/licenses/by/4.0/).

MDPI
St. Alban-Anlage 66
4052 Basel
Switzerland
Tel. +41 61 683 77 34
Fax +41 61 302 89 18
www.mdpi.com

Cancers Editorial Office
E-mail: cancers@mdpi.com
www.mdpi.com/journal/cancers